# Handbook of
# Head Trauma

Acute Care to Recovery

# CRITICAL ISSUES IN NEUROPSYCHOLOGY

*Series Editors*

Antonio E. Puente
*University of North Carolina, Wilmington*

Cecil R. Reynolds
*Texas A&M University*

*Current Volumes in this Series*

A Continuation Order Plan is available for this series. A continuation order will bring
delivery of each new volume immediately upon publication. Volumes are billed only
upon actual shipment. For further information please contact the publisher.

# Handbook of Head Trauma

## Acute Care to Recovery

Edited by
## Charles J. Long
and
## Leslie K. Ross

*Memphis State University and*
*University of Tennessee Center for the Health Sciences*
*Memphis, Tennessee*

PLENUM PRESS • NEW YORK AND LONDON

Library of Congress Cataloging-in-Publication Data

Handbook of head trauma : acute care to recovery / edited by Charles
J. Long and Leslie K. Ross.
        p.    cm. -- (Critical issues in neuropsychology)
     Includes bibliographical references and index.
     ISBN 0-306-43947-6
     1. Brain damage.  2. Brain damage--Patients--Rehabilitation.
I. Long, Charles J., 1935-    .  II. Ross, Leslie K.  III. Series.
     [DNLM: 1. Brain Injuries--psychology.  2. Brain Injuries-
-rehabilitation.    WL 354 H236]
     RC387.5.H27  1992
     617.4'81044--dc20
     DNLM/DLC
     for Library of Congress                                    92-21764
                                                                     CIP

ISBN 0-306-43947-6

© 1992 Plenum Press, New York
A Division of Plenum Publishing Corporation
233 Spring Street, New York, N.Y. 10013

Printed in the United States of America

# Contributors

Thomas F. Bergquist • Spain Rehabilitation Center, Department of Rehab Medicine, University of Alabama at Birmingham School of Medicine, Birmingham, Alabama

Gerald Bennett • Spain Rehabilitation Center, Department of Rehab Medicine, University of Alabama at Birmingham School of Medicine, Birmingham, Alabama

Sandra G. Caldwell • Spain Rehabilitation Center, Department of Rehab Medicine, University of Alabama at Birmingham School of Medicine, Birmingham, Alabama

Linda Warren Duke • Spain Rehabilitation Center, Department of Rehab Medicine, University of Alabama at Birmingham School of Medicine, Birmingham, Alabama

Claudio A. Feler • Semmes Murphy Clinic, Memphis, Tennessee

Janice Gambach • Department of Psychiatry, Southern Illinois University School of Medicine, Springfield, Illinois

David A. Gansler • Boston Veterans Medical Center, Boston, Massachusetts

Gerald Goldstein • VA Medical Center, Pittsburgh, Pennsylvania

William Drew Gouvier • Department of Psychology, Louisiana State University, Baton Rouge, Louisiana

Bobby G. Greer • College of Education, Memphis State University, Memphis, Tennessee

Bruce P. Hermann • Regional EpiCare Center, Memphis, Tennessee

W. L. Hutcherson • The Rehab Hospital in Mechanicsburg, Mechanicsburg, Pennsylvania

Warren T. Jackson • Department of Psychology, Louisiana State University, Baton Rouge, Louisiana

Christy L. Jones • Department of Psychology, Memphis State University, Memphis, Tennessee

Mary Anne Knack • Department of Counseling and Personnel Services, Memphis State University, Memphis, Tennessee

Charles J. Long • Department of Psychology, Memphis State University, and University of Tennessee Center for the Health Sciences, Memphis, Tennessee

Robert L. Mapou • HIV Behavioral Medicine Research Program, Henry M. Jackson Foundation for the Advancement of Military Medicine, Rockville, Maryland

Robert J. McCaffrey • Department of Psychology, State University of New York at Albany, Albany, New York

Michael McCue • Behavioral Neuropsychology Associates, Pittsburgh, Pennsylvania

Joseph H. Miller • Memphis Neurosciences Center, Methodist Hospitals of Memphis, University of Tennessee School of Medicine, Memphis, Tennessee

Thomas A. Novack • Spain Rehabilitation Center, Department of Rehab Medicine, University of Alabama at Birmingham School of Medicine, Birmingham, Alabama

Randolph W. Parks • Department of Psychiatry, Southern Illinois University School of Medicine, Springfield, Illinois

Andrew J. Phay • Alvin C. York VA Medical Center, Murfreesboro, Tennessee

Marvin H. Podd • Department of Psychology, National Navy Medical Center, Bethesda, Maryland

Antonio E. Puente • Department of Psychology, University of North Carolina at Wilmington, Wilmington, North Carolina

Robert L. Pusakulich • Department of Psychology, VA Medical Center, Memphis, Tennessee

Rob Roberts • College of Education, Memphis State University, Memphis, Tennessee

Leslie K. Ross • Department of Psychology, Memphis State University, and University of Tennessee Center for the Health Sciences, Memphis, Tennessee

Maureen E. Schmitter • Department of Psychology, Memphis State University, Memphis, Tennessee

Donald P. Seelig • Psychological Consultation and Treatment Center, Fort Washington, Maryland

Daniel E. Stanczak • Neuropsychology Department, Baylor University Institute for Rehabilitation, Dallas, Texas

Donald A. Taylor • Cumberland Hospital, New Kent, Virginia

Sandra Vicari • Department of Psychiatry, Southern Illinois University School of Medicine, Springfield, Illinois

Clarence B. Watridge • Department of Neurosurgery, University Physicians Foundation, University of Tennessee Center for the Health Sciences, Memphis, Tennessee

Sherry L. Weathers • Spain Rehabilitation Center, Department of Rehab Medicine, University of Alabama at Birmingham School of Medicine, Birmingham, Alabama

Danny Wedding • Institute of Medicine, National Academy of Sciences, Washington, DC

J. Michael Williams • Neuropsychology Laboratory, Hahnemann University, Philadelphia, Pennsylvania

Ronald F. Zec • Departments of Psychiatry and Internal Medicine (Division of Neurology), and the Center for Alzheimer Disease and Related Disorders, Southern Illinois University School of Medicine, Springfield, Illinois

# Preface

Health-care professionals in the United States have made tremendous strides in the assessment and treatment of head injury over the past 20 years. Much of the effort of the 1970s related to the development of an understanding of the problems and the needs of head-injured survivors. During the 1980s, rehabilitation programs were developed to meet these needs. We have now progressed from near ignorance concerning the pervasive consequences of head injury to a reasonably sound understanding of both its direct and indirect effects. The nature and extent of our knowledge remain severely limited, however. Perhaps the 1990s (the Decade of the Brain) will be the period during which we specialize and refine our procedures and outline new directions for the rehabilitation of head-injured individuals.

With the advances in medical technology, the number of patients surviving severe head injuries is increasing. Survival often does not presume the functionality that characterizes the most desirable quality of life, however. Challenged with lives that are medically stable but radically altered with regard to cognition, personality, and emotion, head trauma survivors and their families are confronted with both the task of recovery and adaptation to a new, and often more limited, life-style.

Individuals experiencing a head injury are, without warning, involved in an accident that will not only permanently change their own life but will also have a significant impact on their family and larger support network. Families of head-injury victims have complained about both the lack and inconsistency of information that is provided during this time. They feel caught up in an endless flow of specialists, each dealing with a small facet of the problem. At the other end of the continuum, some families have limited contact with medical/rehabilitation specialists due to a lack of financial resources.

It is surely apparent to the medical/health professionals who work with head-injured individuals that no one specialty can solve all the problems or answer all the questions that will arise following head injury. While each profession focuses on a specific aspect of the recovery problem, what is done in one specialty can have significant consequences in other aspects of treatment. For this reason, although we cannot be specialists in all the aspects of rehabilitation, it is advantageous to be knowledgeable of the terminology and procedures employed in other specialty areas (e.g., neurosurgery and vocational planning) and the problems that each specialty faces in working with head-injured individuals.

Much remains to be done to enhance our understanding of head injury and to better assist both head-injured individuals and their families. We need to improve our methods for acute-care management and for determining the severity and nature of injury. We also need to gain a better understanding of neurological, cognitive, emotional, social, and vocational variables and how these variables interact to influence the rehabilitation process and eventual outcome. Finally, we should develop a more effective means of matching rehabilitation resources with patient needs.

Given the complex nature of traumatic brain injury, a comprehensive approach is vital to the conceptualization and treatment of its survivors. This book attempts to offer a fairly comprehensive compendium of information regarding clinical aspects of head injury by focusing on head injury from acute care to recovery. While, due to space limitations, this book does not provide sections from a number of disciplines such as physical, occupational, and speech therapy, it does attempt to bring together a diverse group of professionals who deal with head injury.

In general, the book is arranged to follow relevant issues (for both the patient and the family) in a temporal fashion, consistent with the progress of treatment and recovery. The chapters present diverse approaches and address theoretical issues that emphasize practical clinical applications. In addition to discussing traditional concepts of brain–behavior relationships, the topics covered in this book are reflective of the growth that has occurred in the field through the years.

Appropriately, the first section of this book begins with the neurosurgeon's perspective on head trauma. These chapters discuss issues involved in the initial management of the different types of head trauma and the various treatment decision strategies employed by the neurosurgeon. At this stage of treatment, the focus is on preserving and minimizing neurological damage due to secondary complications. These chapters will provide the reader with an appreciation of how, at this stage of acute care, diagnosis and treatment considerations occur in a compressed time frame of minutes or hours.

As the patient recovers physically, the concern shifts to assessing the functional consequences of head injury; these issues are addressed in Part II. In order to develop realistic rehabilitation goals, it is important to understand the neuropsychological strengths and weaknesses of the patient. The role and contribution of the clinical interview in neuropsychological assessment is presented in Chapter 3. For example, the interview can be a major means of establishing the patient's premorbid level of functioning. Other chapters in this section outline various difficulties, such as seizure disorders, that may influence a patient's outcome. Chapter 4 presents information on how to assess and understand head injury's potential effects on cognition and on social and emotional adjustment. Chapter 5 discusses the cognitive basis of behavioral disorders that often follow head injury, as well as the relationship between cognitive deficits and neuropathology. The last two chapters in this section deal with integrating the information that is obtained from the neuropsychological assessment. A theoretical model of brain–behavior relationships is presented in Chapter 6. The use of a "cortical functions model" should assist clinical neuropsychologists in describing a patient's cognitive functional status and in constructing relevant rehabilitation programs for the patient. The last chapter of this section is a more "applied" approach to the integration of neuropsychological data. That is, it addresses the referral questions often made by neurologists, neurosurgeons, attorneys, insurance companies, and government agencies (e.g., "What will the patient's cognitive functioning be at some point in the future and/or what was his or her premorbid level of cognitive functioning?"). As the authors point out, it is necessary to evaluate and integrate demographic variables, personality characteristics, and social variables with a patient's performance on neuropsychological tests.

Rehabilitation goals and treatment programs become important as the patient continues his or her recovery, and this broad area is discussed in Part III. The diversity of rehabilitation issues can be seen by simply glancing at the chapter titles in the table of contents. For example, there is a discussion of theoretical concerns related to the delivery of rehabilitative services (Chapter 8). Another chapter presents a theoretical perspective to rehabilitation (drawn from cognitive psychology) that offers a potential basis for the development of a cognitive theory of intervention (Chapter 10). Other chapters discuss specific treatment modalities (e.g., pharmacologic intervention, Chapter 9) and specific areas in which cognitive rehabilitation has been employed (e.g., memory deficits, Chapter 11; attention/concentration impairments, Chapters 12 and 14; disorders of executive functioning, Chapter 13).

Part IV addresses the difficult area of outcome prediction following head injury. As Jones (Chapter 15) points out, being able to predict a patient's outcome following head injury is important since head injury is the most expensive and time-consuming form of medical emergency for the American public. There has been slow progress in the area of outcome prediction and rehabilitation, partly because of the lack of a well-defined conceptualization of the course of recovery. Being able to present a model of recovery would facilitate the design of effective and cost-productive programs by (a) aiding the family's understanding of the recovery process, (b) setting realistic rehabilitation goals, and (c) being better able to evaluate the head-injured person's progress. Jones presents an empirical study that investigates the course of recovery and the factors that make this process unique to each individual. Chapter 16 addresses the issue of outcome by using an assessment battery that is tailored for the acute-care brain injury environment, the Hahnemann Orientation and Memory Examination. This battery represents a comprehensive and efficient clinical tracking system—assessing cognitive abilities at the earliest stages of recovery that can potentially enhance the management of trauma patients, in addition to being useful in predicting outcome and placing patients in the best possible discharge setting. The last chapter of this section, Chapter 17, is more traditional in its discussion of outcome predictors. That is, topics such as the pathophysiology of head injury, the use of brain-imaging techniques, the use of clinical neurophysiological monitors, age, the neurological examination (e.g., Glasgow Coma Score), intracranial pressure, etc., are addressed.

Part V consists of several chapters examining the use of psychotherapy with cognitively impaired individuals and the family's role in the rehabilitation process. The authors of Chapter 18 present a framework for the application of group psychotherapy principles to cognitively impaired adults and their families. Chapter 19 acknowledges the extreme burden placed on family members by head-injured individuals and the importance of defining a role for families in the rehabilitation program that allows them to impact the recovery process. In order to clearly establish the family's role, the authors of this chapter state, ". . . professionals must overcome some of their well-established prejudices against having family members participating in a rehabilitation program." Chapter 20 focuses on intervention with head-injured families through the family systems approach. This chapter not only acknowledges the stressors that stem from the trauma itself, but it also considers findings that many of the families were "dysfunctional" prior to the occurrence of the head injury. Therefore, such "dysfunctions" will compound any therapeutic interventions involving the family.

The last section of this book deals with the final stages of recovery: vocational evaluation and job-oriented rehabilitation. Chapter 21 focuses on the vocational evaluation process, the testing instruments that are particularly useful in assessing persons with head injury, and program planning as it relates to reentry into the community. Chapter 22 offers programmatic recommendations for comprehensive job-oriented rehabilitation for persons who have sustained a head injury. The next chapter, Chapter 23, discusses pragmatic issues about whether patients with cognitive limitations should return to driving. Finally, the last chapter presents a general approach to forensic issues (Social Security and workmen's compensation) in head trauma. This chapter provides information about how to decrease ambiguity and provide the courts with the best possible neuropsychological data so that a proper administrative and/or legal decision may be reached.

The authors hope that this book proves to be beneficial by providing useful information and clinically related material to a diverse group of professionals who have an interest in head injury. We believe that pertinent information is offered by individuals in the forefront of the work in traumatic brain injury. These professionals give insight into the neurological, psychological, and vocational methods of their respective specialties. In addition, they explain the role each aspect of treatment plays in the sequential process of recovery. We feel that learning and sharing more knowledge in this area, specifically in a multidisciplinary fashion, is essential given the multitude of issues that emerge in this population. We hope this book may help to challenge others to continue this investigation.

Charles J. Long
Leslie K. Ross

*Memphis, Tennessee*

# Contents

## Part II. NEUROPSYCHOLOGICAL ASSESSMENT OF HEAD-INJURED INDIVIDUALS

Chapter 3
USE OF HISTORY IN NEUROPSYCHOLOGICAL ASSESSMENTS ......... 35

*Andrew J. Phay*

Chapter 4
NEUROPSYCHOLOGICAL ASSESSMENT OF PATIENTS WITH EPILEPSY    57

*Bruce P. Hermann*

Chapter 5
NEUROPATHOLOGY AND NEUROPSYCHOLOGY OF BEHAVIORAL
    DISTURBANCES FOLLOWING TRAUMATIC BRAIN INJURY ........ 75

*Robert L. Mapou*

Chapter 6
USING A MODEL OF COGNITIVE FUNCTION TO PLAN COGNITIVE

*Robert L. Pusakulich*

Chapter 7

*Charles J. Long and Maureen E. Schmitter*

**Part III. INPATIENT AND OUTPATIENT REHABILITATION**

Chapter 8
ACUTE REHABILITATION OF THE HEAD-INJURED INDIVIDUAL:

*Daniel E. Stanczak and W. L. Hutcherson*

Chapter 9
## THE USE OF PHARMACOLOGY IN THE TREATMENT OF HEAD-INJURED PATIENTS

*Leslie K. Ross*

Chapter 10
## COGNITIVE REHABILITATION AFTER HEAD TRAUMA: TOWARD AN INTEGRATED COGNITIVE/BEHAVIORAL PERSPECTIVE ON INTERVENTION

*Linda Warren Duke, Sherry L. Weathers, Sandra G. Caldwell,
and Thomas A. Novack*

Chapter 11
MEMORY REHABILITATION ...................................... 191

*Gerald Goldstein*

Chapter 12
THE EFFICACY OF ATTENTION-REMEDIATION PROGRAMS FOR
    TRAUMATICALLY BRAIN-INJURED SURVIVORS ................. 203

*Robert J. McCaffrey and David A. Gansler*

Chapter 13
THE EXECUTIVE BOARD SYSTEM: AN INNOVATIVE APPROACH TO
    COGNITIVE–BEHAVIORAL REHABILITATION IN PATIENTS WITH
    TRAUMATIC BRAIN INJURY ................................... 219

*Ronald F. Zec, Randolph W. Parks, Janice Gambach, and Sandra Vicari*

Chapter 14
COMPUTER-ASSISTED COGNITIVE REMEDIATION OF ATTENTION
      DISORDERS FOLLOWING MILD CLOSED HEAD INJURIES ......... 231

*Marvin H. Podd and Donald P. Seelig*

## Part IV. OUTCOME PREDICTION FOLLOWING HEAD INJURY

Chapter 15
RECOVERY FROM HEAD TRAUMA: A CURVILINEAR PROCESS? ....... 247

*Christy L. Jones*

Chapter 16

*J. Michael Williams*

Chapter 17

*Donald A. Taylor*

## Part V. INDIVIDUAL THERAPY AND FAMILY ISSUES IN REHABILITATION

### Chapter 18
### GROUP PSYCHOTHERAPY WITH BRAIN-DAMAGED ADULTS AND THEIR FAMILIES

*Warren T. Jackson and William Drew Gouvier*

### Chapter 19
### FAMILY INVOLVEMENT IN COGNITIVE RECOVERY FOLLOWING TRAUMATIC BRAIN INJURY

*Thomas A. Novack, Thomas F. Bergquist, and Gerald Bennett*

## Chapter 23
## NEUROLOGICAL IMPAIRMENT AND DRIVING ABILITY .............. 417

*Danny Wedding*

## Chapter 24
## FORENSIC ISSUES IN HEAD TRAUMA: NEUROPSYCHOLOGICAL
## PERSPECTIVES OF SOCIAL SECURITY DISABILITY AND WORKER'S
## COMPENSATION ............................................. 425

*Antonio E. Puente*

# I

# Background Issues of Head Injury

NOTE. In view of the rapid developments in neurosurgical treatment of traumatic brain injury, certain procedures outlined in Chapter 1 have been modified. Since the intent of the early chapters of the book is to provide the readers with a general overview of neurosurgical intervention rather than specific information regarding how to do it, it was decided not to make such changes in the text.

# Management and Evaluation of Head Trauma

## JOSEPH H. MILLER

### INTRODUCTION

Various specialists who deal with the prevention, treatment, care, and rehabilitation of head injuries have recognized for years the magnitude of the problem. However, it was under the leadership of Dr. Murray Goldstein, Director of the National Institute of Neurological Disorders and Stroke of the National Institutes of Health, that an organized effort on a national basis was begun to give widespread attention to the head injury "epidemic" problem. Dr. Goldstein's efforts resulted in the formation of the Intra-agency Head Injury Task Force, with its first formal report published in June of 1989 (Goldstein, 1990). This report gives startling figures: "someone receives a head injury every fifteen seconds in the United States. A conservative estimate puts the total of head injuries at over two million per year, with 500,000 severe enough to require hospital admission. Seventy-five thousand to 100,000 persons die each year as a result of brain injury. It is the leading cause of disability in children and young adults and is also the principal cause of brain damage in young adults. Five thousand new cases of epilepsy caused by head trauma are reported each year. Related medical and legal bills often leave families with near or total financial ruin. The economic cost alone approaches 25 billion dollars per year."

JOSEPH H. MILLER • Memphis Neurosciences Center, Methodist Hospitals of Memphis, University of Tennessee School of Medicine, Memphis, Tennessee 38104.

*HANDBOOK OF HEAD TRAUMA: Acute Care to Recovery*, edited by Charles J. Long and Leslie K. Ross. Plenum Press, New York, 1992.

## MANAGEMENT

The management of head trauma is divided into three categories (Table 1.1). The first category is the immediate support of the unconscious patient (which includes patients who have sustained head trauma). Not infrequently head trauma is associated with other metabolic or chemical problems, and the general principles of managing the unconscious patient apply equally to the patient with known head trauma.

The second category of evaluating the patient with an altered level of consciousness includes the evaluation of six physiological functions that provide an indication of the patient's current neurological level. A standardized baseline for the neurological evaluation can be established by the physician through the evaluation of a patient's neurological level, history, and neurological trend. The sine qua non of neurological evaluation is to determine whether the patient is getting better or worse.

The third category of evaluation of the head injury patient is classification of the type of injury. The Memphis Neurosciences Center has a method of classifying head injuries based on clinical and anatomical observations made in the initial evaluation of a patient. The severity of the injury is classified as either minor or major, with consideration of possible complications that could arise. The type of head injury is frequently clarified or expanded by the various head-imaging techniques subsequent to the immediate support, examination, and clinical and anatomical classification.

## IMMEDIATE SUPPORT OF THE UNCONSCIOUS PATIENT

The immediate support of the unconscious patient involves evaluating a dozen parameters to determine if various vital systems are being supported and making any alterations needed for support. These parameters are divided into four groups and are called "The Dirty Dozen of Unconsciousness" (Table 1.2).

The first group involves the recognition and determination of three things that the brain requires: (1) oxygen, (2) blood, and (3) glucose. One must be certain that these three requirements are being provided in the initial support. The second group includes three things that are fatal if not corrected: (1) increased intracranial pressure, (2) changes in pH, and (3) results of suicide or overdose. The third set of parameters are the "Symptomatic Three": (1) temperature abnormalities, (2) seizures, and (3) extreme agitation. The fourth three are called the "Three Don't Forgets" and include (1) cornea, skin, and catheter care, (2) the avoidance of superficial nerve compression, and (3) lab tests. The patient is most vulnerable for increased brain damage and complications from the time that unconsciousness develops until definitive tests such as a CAT scan are done and the appropriate

TABLE 1.1.   Three Categories of Evaluating
the Head-Injured or Unconscious Patient

---

1. Immediate support of the unconscious patient
2. Six functions to be evaluated
3. Classification of type of head injury

---

TABLE 1.2.  Immediate Support of the Unconscious
Patient (Dirty Dozen of Unconsciousness)

| | |
|---|---|
| Required three | "Three don't forgets" |
| $O_2$ | Cornea, skin, catheter care |
| Cerebral blood flow | Avoid nerve compression |
| Glucose | Lab tests |
| Fatal three | —Neuro EKG |
| Increased intracranial pressure | —Coma I profile |
| pH | —Coma II profile |
| Suicide–overdose | |
| Symptomatic three | |
| Temperature | |
| Seizures | |
| Agitation | |

treatment accomplished. The physician is also vulnerable medico-legally in this emergent environment; however, if these parameters are properly recognized, addressed, and corrected, all possible emergency care has been provided.

## Required Three

### *Oxygen Requirement*

The brain requires 3.3 cm³ of oxygen per 100 g of brain per min (Kety & Schmidt, 1948). If this is reduced to 2.5 cm³, mental changes develop; and at 2 cm³ the patient becomes comatose (Plum & Posner, 1972). In order to assure that the brain of a comatose patient receives the required amount of oxygen, the patient is suctioned and oxygenated with a mask. During this time 1 mg of atropine is given intravenously to reduce the effect of the sympathetic discharge and tracheal vagal stimulation produced by intubation. During hypoxemia this discharge can cause cardiac arrhythmias or arrest. The patient is then intubated and ventilated. It is desirable to keep the arterial oxygen partial pressure close to 100 mm Hg and the arterial carbon dioxide partial pressure at 30 to 35 mm Hg.

### *Cerebral Blood Flow Requirement*

The cerebral blood flow requirement is about 55 cm³ per 100 g of brain per min. At 27 cm³ the patient becomes comatose. Many times the physician is left with the decision whether or not to give blood to an acutely ill patient. With the advent of the tremendous spread of AIDS, this decision reaches monumental proportions. In the acutely ill patient who is still undergoing evaluation, the mean arterial pressure should be kept at about 100 mm Hg and the hematocrit (HCT) between 25 and 30.

If the patient is chronically ill and has been under observation, with these parameters observation may be continued during the study period. However, in the case of an undiagnosed, acutely ill patient who has deteriorated to the point where survival is in question, it is our policy to administer blood when the hematocrit is below 25 and the arterial pressure cannot be maintained in a reasonable range. If the patient is hypotensive, the cause is most likely extracerebral. The administration of 800 mg of dopamine in 500 cm$^3$ of 5% dextrose in water (D5W) and titrated, beginning at 5 cm$^3$ per h, may correct the hypotension quickly if the hypotensive episode is not due to blood loss. If extreme hypertension is present in the absence of an intracranial mass, the secondary vasoconstriction of the cerebral arterioles may produce cerebral ischemia. This is initially treated by administering 5 to 10 mg of Apresoline intravenously with titration every 4 to 6 h as needed. If this does not work and the hypertension remains extreme, 50 mg of Nipride is given in 250 cm$^3$ of 5% dextrose in water (D5W) and starting titration at 5 cm$^3$ every hour. This is a last resort since loss of autoregulation may occur and last for several hours and, in some instances, intracranial pressure may increase.

## Cerebral Glucose Requirement

The brain requires 5.5 cm$^3$ of glucose per 100 g of brain per min (Plum & Posner, 1972). The brain normally contains 2 g of stored glucose, which prorates to about a 90-min reserve. If the brain is without glucose after this time limit, processes begin that cause additional brain tissue destruction; thus, it is imperative that virtually every unconscious patient in which the etiology is unknown receive glucose immediately. This should be administered intravenously in a 50 cm$^3$ solution of 50% glucose containing 100 mg of thiamine. If the glucose is not low, this is essentially harmless; but it provides dramatic results when needed.

## Fatal Three

The next group of parameters has come to be known as the "Fatal Three" since, if they are not corrected, the patient may not survive. These include (1) increased intracranial pressure, (2) changes in the pH, and (3) attempts at suicide or overdose.

## Increased Intracranial Pressure

Consideration of a patient with increased intracranial pressure includes (1) immediate action, (2) surgical treatment, and (3) nonsurgical treatment.

The immediate actions required with increased intracranial pressure as the cause of unconsciousness include hyperventilation and elevation of the head. The tidal volume should be 15 cm$^3$ per kg of body weight, with a respiratory rate of 12 breaths per min. Laboratory parameters need to be maintained at an arterial carbon dioxide partial pressure of 25 to 30 mm Hg (Plum & Posner, 1980). In addition, mannitol is given at 0.5 to 1.0 g/kg body weight in 3 to 5 min and is repeated as needed. Twenty to forty milligrams of Lasix is pushed intravenously over 5 minutes. Steroids are considered, particularly if there is a history of malignancy. If used, 20 mg of Decadron is given intravenously, followed by 6 mg every 4 h until the definite need for steroids can be established.

An immediate CAT scan is the next step in the management of the head-injured patient. Facilities that receive head-injured or acutely unconscious patients should have a CAT scan available on a 24-h basis. The trend now is to have the CAT scanner in the emergency department in order to avoid delays in the ongoing treatment and allow immediate scanning. The results of the CAT scan may provide the treating physician with significant diagnostic information. If a patient has changes in the level of consciousness and is acutely ill from increased intracranial pressure, certain CAT scan results indicate the need for immediate surgery. These include (1) epidural hematoma, (2) subdural hematoma, (3) lobar or opercular intracerebral hematoma, (4) cerebellar hematoma, or (5) cerebellar infarct.

If these lesions are neither revealed nor suspected, one considers continued use of steroids, antibiotics, and mannitol. During treatment with mannitol, urinary output should be measured every hour and electrolytes measured every 6 h. If the basal cisterns are absent on the CAT scan, but a surgical lesion is not present and the patient remains acutely ill from increased intracranial pressure, then the intracranial pressure is monitored.

## pH Changes

The next parameter to be evaluated in the unconscious patient is the change in blood pH (hydrogen ion concentration). It is not rare for a patient to be admitted with a head injury who actually became unconscious before the accident occurred. Often the unconsciousness is out of proportion to the injury, and it may be difficult to designate the etiology of the unconsciousness. If the patient is hyperventilating, metabolic acidosis or respiratory alkalosis should be suspected; and the appropriate lab tests should be ordered so that the cause can be identified. However, if the patient is hypoventilating, metabolic alkalosis or respiratory acidosis should be suspected; and as before, the appropriate lab tests should be ordered.

If an acidosis is present, it may be lethal if left untreated. Differential diagnosis includes diabetes and uremia, which the laboratory results may rule in or out. If diabetes or uremia is not present, one must suspect the possibility of poisoning.

The treatment of possible poisoning requires the immediate intravenous administration of sodium bicarbonate to combat acidosis in a dose of 1 mEq/kg of body weight. If a respiratory acidosis has developed and the patient is hypoventilating, mechanical ventilation is necessary to decrease the arterial carbon dioxide partial pressure. If a metabolic alkalosis is present, differential diagnosis should be considered in older patients who have been on diuretics or in patients with liver failure or sepsis. Patients on diuretics who become symptomatic show a characteristic laboratory picture of hyponatremia, hypokalemia, and alkalosis. An acute respiratory alkalosis causes one to suspect salicylate poisoning. This may later become a metabolic acidosis.

## Attempts at Suicide or Overdose

The third potentially fatal cause of unconsciousness is attempted suicide by overdose, gases, or poisons. The three immediate cardinal actions include (1) the maintenance of vital signs, (2) intubation and ventilation, and (3) support of blood volume and blood pressure. If the patient is suspected of taking an overdose, the second step is to get rid of the material that has not yet been absorbed. If the patient is conscious, vomiting may be induced by the use of 30 cm$^3$ of syrup of ipecac followed by 6 ounces of water. This should be repeated in 30 min if vomiting has not occurred. Apomorphine, 0.01 mg/kg body weight, may also be given intravenously. If respiratory depression is produced, this must be countered with 0.1 mg of naloxone. If the patient is unconscious, gastric lavage with a 34 French catheter is indicated. The patient is placed head down on the left side, and a measured 300 cm$^3$ of water or ½ normal saline is used for the lavage. There must be an exchange of a measured amount of fluid so that, if the fluid is being leaked out of the stomach into the abdomen, it can be noted and lavage discontinued. After all possible material has been removed from the stomach and the exchange of fluid from the abdomen remains clear, 2 tablespoons or 30 to 50 g of activated charcoal in water is given to deactivate the material left in the crevices of the stomach.

If the identity of the material ingested is in question, a poison center should be contacted to assist in this determination. The treating physician should always remember that many suicide attempts involve the ingestion of different drugs including alcohol, sedatives, narcotics, and whatever other medications were available to the patient at the time of the attempt. Treatment varies according to the type of poison involved.

## Symptomatic Three

The third group of problems that one must deal with in the acutely injured or ill patient includes the "Symptomatic Three." These are (1) temperature abnormalities, (2) seizures, and (3) agitation.

### Temperature Abnormalities

Hyperthermia and hypothermia should not be forgotten as possible factors when evaluating an unconscious patient. In the average person coma results if body temperature increases to 42°C (107.6°F) (Plum & Posner, 1972) or if it falls to 26°C (78.8°F) (Duguid, Simpson, & Stavers, 1961). It would not be unlikely for a person to be transported from a football field with a suspected head injury, when the actual loss of consciousness resulted from hyperthermia. Neither would it be unlikely to discover that a patient found unconscious at home, presumably from a head injury, was a victim of hypothermia. This is not an uncommon finding with older people following disconnection of their utilities. When a patient has a fever of undetermined cause and CAT scan results indicate that no intracranial mass is present, blood cultures should be ordered and a lumbar puncture performed.

### Seizures

If the patient presents in status epilepticus, it may not be evident whether the seizures began before or after the head trauma. If the etiology is not known, two intravenous lines are started, an immediate (STAT) coma profile is obtained, and anticonvulsant blood levels are determined. One intravenous line is used to administer 100 mg of thiamine and a 50 cm³ solution of 50% glucose. Fifty milligrams of Dilantin is given intravenously every minute until 1000 mg has been accomplished in 20 min. In the other intravenous line, Valium, 2 to 10 mg, is titrated as a quick-acting drug to have a more immediate effect on the seizures. Ativan, 1 to 2 mg, can be given intravenously as an alternate to the Valium. When this is accomplished, one waits 30 min. If the patient is still seizuring, 100 mg of phenobarbital is given intravenously; then 50 mg is administered every 15 min to a total dose of 500 mg. During this maneuver, it is necessary to be prepared to treat respiratory depression should it develop. After 30 min, if the seizuring is still occurring, the patient is given a neuromuscular blockade of Pavulon, 4 to 5 mg, intravenously and placed under halothane or barbiturate anesthesia for 2 to 3 h.

## Agitation

Unconscious patients may be agitated and can be very difficult to manage. Often the imaging techniques are not satisfactory because of movement. Since it is imperative that any type of structural or mass lesion be identified, the best imaging possible must be accomplished with good technique before one rules out a mass lesion. It is therefore imperative that the patient's movement be controlled. This is achieved by the use of 1 mg of Stadol intravenously. If this does not readily work, then 1/2 to 1 mg of Versed is used. Valium, 5 to 10 mg, or Ativan, 1 to 2 mg, is also occasionally used, as it was commonly used in the past. If the patient is an elderly individual, respiratory depression may be noted, but this is extremely rare. Significant depression in which support ventilation was required occurred in only one of 100 consecutive cases.

## Three Don't Forgets

In keeping with the evaluation of the unconscious patient, some problems have been listed as the "Three Don't Forgets." Attention must be given to (1) cornea, skin, and catheter care, (2) superficial nerve compression, and (3) laboratory profile.

## Cornea, Skin, and Catheter Care

Ophthalmic ointment is used every 8 h as needed to prevent the drying out of the eyes. It may be necessary to close the eyelids with tape. This is usually changed frequently for pupillary evaluation, but it should be changed at least every 12 h.

## Superficial Nerve Compression

In addition, superficial nerve compression must be avoided. It is not rare to see a secondary ulnar nerve neuropathy from compression of a superficial nerve at the elbow that had not been recognized and guarded against during the patient's unconsciousness.

## Laboratory Support

Lastly, appropriate laboratory support is needed. This includes an EKG and the ability to recognize EKG changes that might be produced by neurological abnormalities. Coma I and Coma II Lab Profiles have been developed (Table 1.3). This makes ordering the laboratory studies in an acute environment easier, more accurate, and, by arrangement with the laboratory, cheaper. The Coma I Profile includes, from arterial blood, the pH, $pCO_2$, $HCO_3$, HCT, and $O_2$ saturation. From the venous blood, the Na, K, Cl, $CO_2$, Ca, glucose, BUN, and osmolarity are determined. The Coma II Profile includes all of the above plus alcohol, ammonia, porphyrin screen, magnesium, and urine drug screen of 56 different drugs.

TABLE 1.3. Coma Profiles

Coma I profile
  Arterial blood: pH, $pCO_2$, $pO_2$, $HCO_3$, HCT, $O_2$ saturation
  Venous blood: Na, K, Cl, $CO_2$, Ca, glucose, BUN, osmolarity
Coma II profile
  All of I plus: Alcohol, ammonia, porphyrin screen, magnesium, urine drug screen (56 drugs)

Equipment needed to accomplish immediate support of the unconscious patient includes equipment for monitoring intracranial pressure. Twenty-two drugs are needed in the ER and ICU for the support as described (Table 1.4).

## EVALUATION OF NEUROLOGICAL LEVELS

The importance of developing experience and understanding of the neurological evaluation of the acutely ill patient with an altered level of consciousness from structural or metabolic lesions cannot be overemphasized. It is through this understanding that one determines whether or not the patient's unconsciousness is most likely due to a structural lesion or to a metabolic lesion. The monograph by Plum and Posner details the evaluation

TABLE 1.4. Twenty-two Drugs Needed in the ER or
ICU for the Emergency Treatment of Head Trauma

| Drug | Amount |
| --- | --- |
| Atropine | 1 mg IV |
| Dopamine | 800 mg in 500 cm³ D5W |
| Apresoline | 10 mg |
| Nipride | 50 mg in 250 cm³ D5W |
| Thiamine | 100 mg IV |
| Glucose | 50 mg of 50% solution IV |
| Mannitol | 1g/kg |
| Lasix | 40 mg in D5W |
| Decadron | 20 mg IV, then mg q4h |
| Sodium bicarbonate | 1 mEq/kg IV |
| Syrup of ipecac | 30 cm³ |
| Apomorphine | 6 mg IV |
| Activated charcoal | 2 tbs (30 to 50 g) |
| Naloxone | 0.4 mg diluted in 10 cm³ saline |
| Physostigmine | 1 mg |
| Valium | 10 mg (or Ativan) |
| Dilantin | 1 g |
| Phenobarbital | 500 mg |
| Pavulon | 4 to 5 mg IV |
| Stadol | 1 mg IV |
| Versed | ½ to 1 mg IV |
| Ophthalmic ointment | |

and support of their monumental work. We have learned from them and, for many years, have heavily relied on their approach to the problem and have confirmed that their approach is accurate and beneficial. More detailed descriptions may be obtained from their monograph. The following technique of evaluating the unconscious patient has been developed primarily from their work. Below is a summary of how we use it. When evaluating the acutely ill patient or the patient with acute head trauma, it is necessary to consider three coma conditions (Table 1.5), three coma questions (Table 1.6), and six physiological functions (Table 1.7).

## Three Coma Conditions

When a patient exhibits a changing level of consciousness, the cause of the unconsciousness may be due to a supratentorial mass, a subtentorial mass or destructive lesion, or metabolic alterations.

## Three Coma Questions

The three coma questions must be answered pertaining to the level of the brain involved, the nature of the involvement, and the direction that the disease process is taking (i.e., whether the patient is getting better or worse).

## Six Functions to Be Examined

The following outline is a method of evaluating the patient. Upon the completion of the evaluation, the physician will usually know whether or not the patient has a structural or metabolic lesion and, thus, have some direction for this initial evaluation. If the cause of unconsciousness is not definitely determined, an immediate CT scan is required.

The six functions to be examined include the state of consciousness, pattern of respiration, pupillary reflexes, ocular movements, motor function, and specific lab tests to be used in the unconscious patient.

The state of consciousness may be evaluated by the use of many coma scales. The coma scale adopted by the Memphis Neurosciences Center includes the Ransohoff coma scale (Ransohoff & Fleischer, 1975) which is simple, easily understood, and standardizes communication among the staff.

The evaluation of the pattern of breathing will often help determine the level of the brain that is involved. Changes in the pattern of breathing may reveal a change in one direction or the other.

The pupillary reflexes are the sine qua non of determining the difference between metabolic causes of unconsciousness and structural causes. It is extremely unusual for

TABLE 1.5.   Three Coma Conditions

1. Supratentorial mass lesions
2. Subtentorial mass or destructive lesions
3. Metabolic disorders

TABLE 1.6.    Three Coma Questions

1. Where is the lesion in the brain?
2. What is the lesion in the brain?
3. Is the patient getting better or worse?

a patient to regress neurologically due to a structural lesion and not show some pupillary change.

The evaluation of ocular movements will frequently reveal additional evidence pointing to the location of the brain lesion.

The motor function also is important in determining location and regression of the neurological patient.

The lab tests may make the diagnosis and confirm evidence of adequate support to the brain. The lab tests are used as previously listed and include the neurological exam, EKG, Coma I, and Coma II Profile.

There are several coma scales used around the world. The Glasgow Coma Scale is commonly used and is necessary if one is reporting work or doing research that might be compared with other publications.

However, in the Memphis Neurosciences Center, the six physiological functions to be studied first include the evaluation of the level of consciousness by the Ransohoff Coma Scale. This Coma Scale, in conjunction with the other functions, gives a clearer understanding of the individual patient and has been easily learned by the nurses in the recovery room, intensive care units, emergency room, and on the neurological and neurosurgical floors. The significance of the other physiological functions is frequently recognized by them.

The states of consciousness as determined by Ransohoff (Ransohoff & Fleischer, 1975) may be graded by I to VI. Grade I represents an alert patient who responds immediately to questions; he may be disoriented and confused, but follows complex commands. He may be Grade I only because he was rendered unconscious. Grade II includes the drowsy patient who is confused, uninterested, does not lapse into sleep when undisturbed, and follows only simple commands. Grade III indicates the stuporous patient who sleeps when not disturbed, but responds briskly and appropriately to mildly noxious stimuli. Grade IV is deep stupor; the patient responds defensively to prolonged noxious stimuli. The first level of coma is Grade V in which there is no appropriate response to any stimuli but reflex movement of decorticate and decerebrate responses are present. Grade VI, or deep coma, is flaccidity with no response to any stimulation. As one develops

TABLE 1.7.    Six Functions to Be Examined

1. State of consciousness
2. Pattern of respiration
3. Pupillary reflexes
4. Ocular movements
5. Motor function
6. Lab tests in coma

experience with this coma scale, it becomes much more meaningful and functional in evaluating the individual patient. For instance, a patient who goes to sleep in the emergency room with two IVs, a catheter, frequent blood pressure determinations, and other neurological examinations obviously has suffered serious injury. The significant injury can be sensed at Grade III. I have yet to discover anyone without a significant injury who could sleep in that environment.

The patterns of breathing as outlined by Plum and Posner, in our experience, are not common; but, when present, they become very meaningful. Forebrain injury is quite common and often seen in a conscious patient who is cooperative enough to take in five deep breaths. A normal individual will continue to breathe, but it is considered abnormal if there is a period of apnea beyond 10 seconds. This is termed posthyperventilation apnea and is a sign of a forebrain injury.

The most well-known and characteristic of all breathing patterns is that of Cheyne–Stokes respiration. This is a sign of a deep cerebral hemisphere or diencephalon lesion, and it includes an ascending and descending crescendo with a period of apnea of about 20% of the entire respiratory cycle. The interesting thing here is that, if this respiratory pattern is noted in trauma at this stage, the patient is still probably in a reversible situation; but, if the respiratory pattern changes to one level below, reversibility is not as likely. Therefore, if the patient has an essentially normal respiratory pattern which changes to that of Cheyne–Stokes, an immediate evaluation must exclude cranial mass or a metabolic lesion as the cause. Central neurogenic hyperventilation may be caused by a midbrain or a midpontine lesion. Apneusis or breath holding may be caused by mid or caudal pontine lesions; cluster breathing may result from low pons or high medulla lesions; and ataxic breathing may be triggered by a lesion in the dorsomedial medulla or respiratory center itself. When ataxic breathing is identified, virtually all these patients need mechanical support and immediate determination as to the etiology.

A clear understanding as to the evaluation of the pupils and pupillary reflexes is helpful and frequently meaningful. In our experience it is very unusual for a patient to die of an intracranial structural lesion without some type of pupillary change, even though it may not be one of dilated and fixed pupils. Metabolic and diencephalic lesions cause small and reactive pupils, tectal lesions elicit very large fixed pupils with hippus, midbrain lesions produce pupils that are fixed in the midposition, and pontine lesions result in pinpoint pupils that are reactive under magnification. Uncal herniation causes third nerve compression and a unilateral, dilated, and fixed pupil. If this develops in a patient who has been conscious and with a decreasing level of consciousness, it is virtually always an immediate surgical emergency. Any delay is likely to result in death or permanent brain injury.

A general understanding of the ocular movements in the unconscious patient is important. The following are rare findings but quite meaningful when recognized. Spontaneous movements include roving eye movements, nystagmus, and the nystagmoid jerking of one eye. Roving eye movements are usually associated with metabolic problems but are being increasingly recognized in certain types of brain injuries. Retraction and convergence nystagmus are seen in midbrain lesions and ocular bobbing in pontine lesions. Nystagmoid jerking of one eye is most often due to a lesion in the pons and on that side.

Gaze abnormalities include the categories of lateral conjugate, lateral dysconjugate, and vertical. Lateral dysconjugate and vertical are assumed to be brain stem lesions. Lateral conjugate can be either a cerebral or a brain stem lesion. If the eyes are conjugately deviated to the right, ice water is placed in the left ear under proper conditions. If the eyes move across the midline to the left, this is a sign of proper functioning of the brain stem. If the eyes do not move or move to the midline only, this is assumed to represent a brain stem lesion.

Tests that one uses in evaluating eye movements include the eyelid and corneal reflexes, oculocephalic reflexes, and oculovestibular reflexes. They are well described in the literature.

The fifth function is that of evaluating the motor system. There are a large number of motor abnormalities that may be noted. These can be divided into specific or nonspecific abnormalities. Specific abnormalities include those that are seen only in metabolic lesions. Specific motor abnormalities are considered to be signs of metabolic etiology only. Nonspecific motor abnormalities include paratonia, snouting, grasp reflexes, decorticate, decerebrate, flaccidity, focal weaknesses, and seizures. Specific abnormalities include tremor, asterixis, and multifocal myoclonus.

The lab tests are used as previously listed and include the neuro EKG, Coma I and Coma II Profile.

## CLASSIFICATION AND COMPLICATIONS OF HEAD INJURIES

The third category of evaluating the head injury patient includes a classification to identify the specific type of injury. The Memphis Neurosciences Center has developed a classification of head injuries that is to be used in the initial evaluation of the patient in the emergency room and is based on anatomical and clinical perimeters (Table 1.8). From the classification point of view, there are three categories that must be determined. One must consider whether the patient has sustained a minor or major injury and what the possible complications might be. This classification, when used initially in the emergency room, defines a minor injury as one that involves the scalp only. Any injury that involves the skull, brain, or blood vessels of the brain initially should be considered a major injury. A patient brought to the emergency room alive with a head injury usually survives; but if he does not, it is almost always because of complications. Therefore, complications of head injuries are to be considered at the time of the initial evaluation of the head injury patient.

### Minor Head Injuries

In this classification one may have a major scalp injury; but, if the scalp only is involved, it is considered a minor head injury. These include scalp contusions, scalp lacerations and/or avulsions, and subgaleal hematomas. Subgaleal hematomas are usually resolved spontaneously and rarely require aspiration except in blood dyscrasia. Surgical drainage virtually never is needed.

### Major Head Injuries

If in the initial evaluation the skull, brain, or blood vessels of the brain are potentially involved, it is considered a major injury. Injuries to the skull include linear fracture, depressed fracture, and basilar fracture. Lesions of the brain include cerebral concussion,

TABLE 1.8.   Clinical and Anatomical Classification of Head
Injuries and Complications to Be Used in the Initial Evaluation

| | |
|---|---|
| Minor head injury | Complications |
|   Scalp contusion |   Hematomas |
|   Scalp laceration and/or avulsion |     Epidural |
|   Subgaleal hematoma |     Subdural |
| |     Intracerebral |
| Major head injury |   All Others |
|   Skull |     CSF |
|     Linear fracture |       Rhinorrhea |
|     Depressed fracture |       Otorrhea |
|     Basilar fracture |       Pneumocephalus |
|   Cerebral |     Vascular |
|     Cerebral concussion |       Subarachnoid hemorrhage |
|     Cerebral contusion |       Occlusions |
|     Cerebral laceration |         Thrombosis |
|   Shearing forces |         Spasm |
|   Penetrating wounds |         Embolization |
|   Laceration by depressed fragment |       A–V fistula or aneurysm |
|   Vessels |     Infections |
|     Arteries |       Osteomyelitis |
|     Veins |       Meningitis |
|     Large sinuses |       Abscess |
| |     Miscellaneous |
| |       Cerebral edema |
| |       Hydrocephalus |
| |       Seizures |

cerebral contusion, and cerebral laceration. The mechanism of laceration is usually determined by the injury (shearing forces, penetrating wounds, or laceration by depressed fragments or objects). If the arteries, veins, or large sinuses of the brain are potentially involved, it is initially considered a major injury.

## Complications

Even with severe wounds, most patients who arrive in the emergency room alive will survive. There are many changes that occur in the brain secondary to injury, and one is referred to the extensive literature concerning this. However, in the initial acute phase there are several complications that can develop which may cause death or permanent impairment that otherwise would not occur if recognized early. The following classification of complications is utilized. Complications include hematomas and all others. Hematomas are so important in the acute head injury, particularly in one that is getting worse, that these stand out alone since they may be readily corrected by surgery if done soon enough. The hematomas include epidural, subdural, and intracerebral hematoma. These have differences in clinical presentations, and the massive literature on head injuries may be consulted for their clinical descriptions.

Other complications are listed under the heading "all others" and are to be considered in the initial evaluation of the acutely head injured patient. These include the cerebrospinal fluid complications of rhinorrhea, otorrhea, and pneumocephalus which are listed under this category. Also included are the vascular complications of subarachnoid hemorrhage, occlusion by thrombus, spasm, or embolization, and traumatic arteriovenous fistula or aneurysms. Infections of osteomyelitis, meningitis, abscess, and/or empyema are also considered. Miscellaneous complications include cerebral edema, hydrocephalus, and seizures.

It is important to determine whether or not a skull fracture is present. Because a skull fracture may be missed on a CAT scan, it continues to be routine to obtain an adequate skull x-ray. A recent report showed, under multivariate analysis, that skull fractures are the only independent significant risk factor in predicting intracranial hemorrhage in adolescents. The routine skull x-ray was felt mandatory in all head injuries in adolescents (Chan, Mann, Yue, & Fan, 1990). If a skull fracture is found, immediate CT is suggested. Other evaluations by Jane (Dacy, Alves, Rimel, Winn, & Jane, 1986) and associates found that in 610 patients with a Glasgow Coma Scale of 13 to 15, 10.8% had a skull fracture; 7.6% of those had a hematoma that required a craniotomy. Of the total group 3% had surgery, and there was 1% without skull fracture who required surgery. Twenty percent of those with skull fracture required surgery. Two patients with Glasgow Coma Scale of 15 and negative skull x-ray required surgery; therefore, an awake patient with a head injury does not necessarily mean that a trivial injury was sustained. Clinically, cerebral concussion represents a loss of consciousness without a permanent impairment. The pathology of concussion has not been clearly worked out. As more attention has been directed to this and more information obtained, more residual problems have been noted. In the initial evaluation, cerebral concussion and cerebral contusion differ only in quantity. Contusion assumes changes in cells and axons which may or may not recover, and the complications of hemorrhage, edema, and infarction are seen. Traumatic cerebral contusion is usually wedge-shaped, with the widest areas at the surface and tapering to the white matter. The distribution is more likely to be frontal and temporal. The lesion is mainly subcortical; and, as a result, the incidence of seizures is low. Traumatic cerebral lacerations are frequently superficial, and therefore seizures are more common.

A very high percentage of patients unconscious from a head injury have hematomas. Syndromes of the epidural, subdural, or intracerebral hematomas are well delineated in the literature. Traumatic intracerebral hematomas, however, are becoming more recognized and are associated with swelling from necrotic tissue, edema, and mass effect of the hematoma. Acute and chronic hematomas are commonly seen in the elderly, alcoholics, and also in infant shaking. Acute intracerebral hematoma is almost always associated with contusions and/or lacerations and is primarily a secondary result.

It is helpful to determine whether or not the head was fixed at the time of the blow. If the head was fixed, the lesion is usually on the surface under the blow. If the head was not fixed, the largest lesion may be of the contra coup type. If there has been a shearing component, contusions may be related to the bony surfaces of the skull in the frontal or temporal lobes.

This classification utilizes the history and the clinical information derived from the examination. It proceeds to the imaging studies of skull x-rays, CAT scan, and/or MRI. Frequently this more clearly delineates the initial evaluation and clarifies any discrepancy noted. The CAT scan and/or MRI are mandatory in major head injuries since it is not uncommon to see totally unsuspected lesions based on the initial evaluation.

## REFERENCES

Chan, K., Mann, K. S., Yue, C. P., & Fan, Y. W. (1990). The significance of skull fracture in acute traumatic intracranial hematomas in adolescence: A prospective study. *Journal of Neurosurgery*, *72*, 189–194.

Dacy, R. D., Alves, W. M., Rimel, R. W., Winn, H. R., & Jane, J. A. (1986). Neurosurgical complications after apparently minor head injury. *Journal of Neurosurgery*, *65*, 203–210.

Duguid, H., Simpson, R. D., & Stavers, J. M. (1961). Accidental hypothermia. *Lancet*, *2*, 1213–1219.

Goldstein, M. (1990). Traumatic brain injury: A silent epidemic. Editorial. *Annals of Neurology*, *27*, 327.

Kety, S. S., & Schmidt, C. F. (1948). The nitrous oxide method for the quantitative determination of cerebral blood flow in man; theory, procedure and normal values. *Journal of Clinical Investigation*, *27*, 476–483.

Plum, F., & Posner, J. B. (1972). *The diagnosis of stupor and coma* (2nd ed.) (p. 197). Philadelphia: Davis.

Plum, F., & Posner, J. B. (1980). *The diagnosis of stupor and coma* (3rd ed.) (p. 34). Philadelphia: Davis.

Ransohoff, J., & Fleischer, A. (1975). Head injuries. *Journal of the American Medical Association*, *8*, 861–864.

# 2

# Initial Management of Head Trauma

## CLAUDIO A. FELER and CLARENCE B. WATRIDGE

### INTRODUCTION

In the United States, trauma is the leading cause of death in people 18 to 40 years of age. Of those who die, the majority have significant central nervous system injury. In those patients who remain disabled, central nervous system injuries are predominant.

The objectives of early management in the head-injured patient are early diagnosis, provision of appropriate therapy for that diagnosis, prevention of secondary injury to the brain, and normalization of the brain's physiologic milieu.

### GENERAL APPROACH TO TRAUMA

Historical information is important, both regarding the past medical history (including drug abuse) and the mode of injury. For example, chronic alcohol abusers may have preexisting brain atrophy, providing greater tolerance to intracranial mass lesions. However, they are also subject to coagulopathy on the basis of underlying liver dysfunction. Patients with known epilepsy should be maintained on their anticonvulsants because cerebral blood flow is markedly increased during a seizure, with a resultant increase in intracranial pressure.

Knowledge of the mechanism of injury will help in differentiation of central nervous system lesions. Patients who have blunt trauma will differ from patients who have deceleration types of injuries, and the latter will differ from those who have penetrating injuries to the skull and brain. In addition, the mechanism of injury (whether it be deceleration or acceleration injury) will benefit the examiner in the index of suspicion for

CLAUDIO A. FELER • Semmes Murphy Clinic, Memphis, Tennessee 38103.     CLARENCE B. WATRIDGE • Department of Neurosurgery, University Physicians Foundation, University of Tennessee Center for the Health Sciences, Memphis, Tennessee 38103.

*HANDBOOK OF HEAD TRAUMA: Acute Care to Recovery*, edited by Charles J. Long and Leslie K. Ross. Plenum Press, New York, 1992.

spine injury. The mechanism of injury may be more important in appropriately analyzing spine injuries than analyzing brain injuries, as the CAT scan has become the mainstay of evaluation of the head trauma patient. Computerized tomography, as well as conventional roentgenography, has maintained a stable role in evaluations of spine injuries. Victims who have significant head trauma are not always able to give a good history, nor are they able to relate their symptoms. It is very common for patients with significant head trauma and spine trauma to be unable to relate symptoms that would lead to the diagnosis of other system injuries. To this end, a multidisciplinary approach is utilized to evaluate the entire patient for evidence of other system injuries. Even with this approach, it is very common for patients experiencing significant head trauma and loss of consciousness to have complaints arise as they awaken from their coma, and these complaints may lead to the later diagnosis of other unsuspected injuries. Management of patients with significant trauma has been facilitated by the trauma center multidisciplinary approach method of care.

The first priority in examination of the head-injured patient is evaluation of the vital signs. The usual ABCs of cardiopulmonary resuscitation remain paramount when treating the head-injured patient. An adequate airway, breathing, and circulatory parameters are obtained and stabilized prior to proceeding with evaluation and treatment of neurologic and spine injuries.

## NEUROLOGIC TRAUMA

Repeated, careful neurologic assessments are essential to caring for patients with closed head injuries. These provide the physician with an idea of the course of the patient's progress. A victim of trauma with a steadily improving neurologic examination allows for continued observation and continuation of the current treatment plan. However, the patient who is progressively worsening in his neurologic functions demands a change in the diagnostic protocol and institution of an appropriate treatment plan to stop the neurologic worsening. Ideally, this assessment is reproducible and quickly obtainable. To this end, the Glasgow Coma Scale has been developed (Teasdale & Jennett, 1974). While it is not a complete neurologic examination, it does provide an assessment of the level of consciousness and satisfies the above criteria.

In the Glasgow Coma Scale, an evaluation is made for eye opening, verbal response, and motor capacity (Table 2.1). It is important to recognize that this scale has some

TABLE 2.1.  Glasgow Coma Scale

| Modality assessed | Score | Modality assessed | Score | Modality assessed | Score |
|---|---|---|---|---|---|
| Verbal response | | Eye opening | | Motor response | |
| None | 1 | None | 1 | None | 1 |
| Incomprehensible sounds | 2 | To pain | 2 | Abnormal extension | 2 |
| Inappropriate words | 3 | To speech | 3 | Abnormal flexion | 3 |
| Confused | 4 | Spontaneously | 4 | Withdraws | 5 |
| Oriented | 5 | | | Localizes | 5 |
| | | | | Obeys | 6 |

shortcomings. The score may vary from side to side in a given patient. If this occurs, both sides should be scored independently to avoid later confusion. Additionally, the scale is not valid in preverbal children or in those patients with preexisting deafness or mutism. Using the Glasgow scale, all patients with a score of 7 or less are in coma, as are most of the patients with a score of 8.

In addition to the above evaluation, the mini-neurologic examination includes observation of the vital signs, respiratory pattern, and an examination of the pupils and eye movements. Examination of the head will reveal scalp lacerations and underlying skull fractures suggestive of contaminated brain. The presence of bilateral periorbital hematomas (raccoon eyes), blood and cerebrospinal fluid (CSF) emanating from the ear (CSF otorrhea), or blood and CSF draining from the nose (CSF rhinorrhea) are indicative of basilar skull fractures. Lateralizing or focal findings are important and must be investigated and their etiology identified. If the CAT scan of the head does not demonstrate a lesion capable of causing a focal deficit, it must be explained by some other mechanism. Cerebral arteriography is necessary in such a patient to rule out a dissection of the carotid artery, which can cause distal embolization or arterial occlusion resulting in brain ischemia, thus mimicking the same signs as intracranial mass lesions such as intracranial subdural epidural hemorrhage. In the comatose patient, cortical dysfunction may be masked by the patient's poor level of function and other signs of a carotid artery lesion; such signs include a Horner's syndrome, which may be the only sign suggestive of a carotid artery dissection in the comatose patient (Watridge, Muhlbauer, & Lowery, 1989).

At a minimum, the comatose patient should have roentgenograms of the chest, pelvis, and entire spinal axis. Adequate cervical spine films may be difficult to obtain. However, the patient should be managed as having a spine fracture until it has been clearly disproven. After the patient's vital signs are stabilized, an emergency CAT scan of the head is obtained for a specific diagnosis of the head injury.

In the comatose patient (i.e., Glasgow coma score of less than 9) initial intervention consists of intubation, oxygenation, hyperventilation, and elevation of the head. The patient's systemic blood pressure is supported if necessary. Intracranial pressure monitoring is instituted in all of these patients with a Glasgow coma score of 7 or less.

## MANAGEMENT OF INTRACRANIAL PRESSURE

Hyperventilation has the effect of decreasing intracranial pressure (Lundberg, Kjallquist, & Bien, 1959). The mechanism of this effect is mediated by a decrease in bicarbonate in the central nervous system, which causes vasoconstriction and a resultant decrease in cerebral blood flow, thus lowering intracranial pressure. This paradox of reduction of cerebral blood flow to decrease intracranial pressure allows for a presumed improvement in cerebral perfusion pressure. Intubation should be accomplished carefully so that an occult cervical spine injury is not aggravated. In addition, patients with obvious basilar skull fracture or midface fractures should not be nasally intubated for fear of violating the skull base and brain.

Subsequent to establishment of an adequate airway, the next priority is blood pressure control. Patients may be in shock for various reasons, such as hypovolemia from hemorrhage. Any obvious external bleeding is tamponed with a pressure dressing. Large-bore intravenous lines are placed. Fluids are administered liberally until a blood pressure greater than 100 systolic is established. The composition of these intravenous fluids is critical and should be isoosmolar if crystalloid. Hypoosmolar fluids may be expected to contribute to or cause cerebral edema as a result of their free water content. Plasma expanders, such as 5% albumin, may be used. In the trauma setting with shock, replacement of blood volume with whole blood is preferred. Hyperglycemia should be avoided, as in animal models of stroke this condition has been shown to be deleterious (Myers & Yamaguchi, 1977; Plum, 1983). To obtain adequate blood pressure, vasoactive compounds may be necessary and, in this case, these compounds should be mixed in normal saline if compatible.

Intracranial pressure monitoring will allow for diagnosis and specific treatment of raised intracranial pressure. Once a systemic blood pressure greater than 100 systolic is obtained, treatment modalities for lowering raised intracranial pressure exist. Furosemide (a loop diuretic) and mannitol (a hyperosmolar diuretic) produce profound diuresis. The net effect is dehydration of the extracellular space and decreased intracranial pressure.

In the early evaluation of the trauma victim with coincident head trauma, hypertension may be present. This hypertension should not be vigorously controlled, because the presence of hypertension may indicate a high intracranial pressure. The presence of Cushing's triad (hypertension, bradycardia, and respiratory irregularity) is ominous and should be recognized as indicative of significantly increased intracranial pressure (Cushing, 1901).

Any patient with a Glasgow coma score of less than 7 is presumed to have increased intracranial pressure. While the definitive management of increased intracranial pressure is diagnosis specific, prior to obtaining a diagnostic study, management of the patient with presumed increased intracranial pressure may be done empirically. Although intracranial pressure monitoring has not been shown to be more effective than empiric therapy for increased intracranial pressure in decreasing morbidity and mortality, it has become widely accepted. Monitoring of the intracranial pressure allows specific therapy for increased intracranial pressure and is utilized in most trauma centers. Patients with Glasgow coma scores of 8 or greater are observed closely for any signs of deterioration, as has been mentioned in previous sections.

The Monroe–Kellie doctrine dictates that the skull is essentially a closed space with a fixed volume; thus, pressure within the skull is governed by changes in volume (Monroe, 1783; Kellie, 1824). The contents of the skull include brain parenchyma, CSF, and blood. Acute changes in any of these constituents will cause a fluctuation in the intracranial pressure. Maneuvers to decrease intracranial pressure include elevation of the head (thus promoting venous return), hyperventilation, and dehydration. Barbiturates such as pentobarbital have also been used in the management of increased intracranial pressure (Marshall, Smith, & Shapiro, 1976).

In the setting of the multiple-trauma patient, many causes for increased intracranial pressure may exist. These include parenchymal edema, decreased venous drainage, and intracranial hematomas. Management of increased intracranial pressure and blood pressure are critical to prevention of secondary injury. Injured brain commonly has deficits of normal autoregulatory capacity, and cerebral blood flow is passively dependent on systemic blood pressure (Overgaard & Tweed, 1974). Cerebral perfusion is a function of blood pressure and intracranial pressure. It may be calculated as cerebral perfusion pressure equals mean arterial blood pressure less intracranial pressure. Adequate perfusion is maintained with a cerebral perfusion pressure greater than 40 Torr.

## TRAUMATIC NEUROLOGIC DIAGNOSES

The basis for rational management of the head-injured patient is predicated on accurate identification of the specific pathologic processes involved. While the various pathologic processes seen in severe closed head injuries are distinct, they often coexist in a given patient. For example, contrecoup contusions may be present in someone who has an epidural hematoma. For the purpose of this discussion each pathologic process will be discussed independently. In any given patient, however, each must be correctly identified and appropriately managed.

## CONCUSSION

Patients often present with a history of transient loss of consciousness following a blow to the head. These victims complain of varying degrees of anterograde and retrograde amnesia. Those who have a normal neurologic examination at the time of presentation and remain so for 24 hours have had a concussion. The diagnosis of concussion is a discharge diagnosis. The term "concussion" is a clinical diagnosis and not based on pathologic findings. At the time of presentation, the patient must be treated as if he or she has a severe head injury. Patients who have had head trauma with transient loss of consciousness can have the development of a delayed intracranial hemorrhage, which may cause their neurologic condition to deteriorate. The time between the trauma and the deterioration of neurologic status is termed the "lucid interval." For these reasons, patients who have suffered significant head trauma, with resultant concussion, are generally admitted to the hospital for observation and/or computerized axial tomography of the head.

## SCALP INJURIES

Trauma victims commonly have scalp injuries. The presence of a scalp laceration raises the index of suspicion for brain injury. Absence of a scalp injury does not, however, rule out a head injury. Such scalp injuries include contusions, lacerations, and degloving injuries. Scalp contusions require no direct management. Scalp lacerations are repaired primarily when not associated with an underlying depressed skull fracture. In the presence of a compound depressed skull fracture, operative management is recommended. This operative procedure requires debridement, irrigation, and layered closure of the compound head injury. Degloving or scalping injuries may be extensive and require copious irrigation, debridement, and reconstruction of the scalp.

## SKULL FRACTURES

The presence of a linear skull fracture on plain skull roentgenogram suggests a potential for secondary brain injury. These fractures may cause tearing of arterial or venous structures, giving rise to epidural bleeding and the formation of an epidural hematoma. Computerized axial tomography of the head is obtained to make this diagnosis. No intervention is required for an adult linear skull fracture, unless a complication such as epidural hemorrhage is present. Certain linear skull fractures are more commonly associated with epidural hemorrhage than others; these fractures are those that cross meningeal arterial grooves. Children with linear skull fractures, however, should be observed for the presence of a "growing" skull fracture. This is one which occurs when there is injury to the leptomeninges with resultant CSF in meninges sequestered in the skull fracture. The presence of a growing skull fracture requires craniotomy for closure of the dura and repair of the fracture.

Depressed skull fractures may be open or closed injuries (Figure 2.1). Goals of management are dependent upon the type of injury. Those patients with open depressed skull fractures are taken to surgery emergently for debridement and elevation of the fracture. The primary goals are decontamination of the brain and dural closure. This is essential to decreasing the risk of infectious complications such as brain abscesses. Closed depressed skull fractures may be electively elevated for cosmetic purposes. Elevation is not felt to change neurologic outcome in these latter cases. Depressed skull fractures that are closed and over large venous sinuses are generally left unoperated.

Basilar skull fractures with CSF fistula are treated with elevation of the head. This reduces the intracranial pressure and thus diminishes leaking of the spinal fluid. Patients are not placed on prophylactic antibiotics but are observed for possible meningitis. Prophylactic antimicrobial therapy is felt to promote infection by resistant bacteria. Usually these injuries do not require operative intervention. Occasionally craniotomy is needed for dural

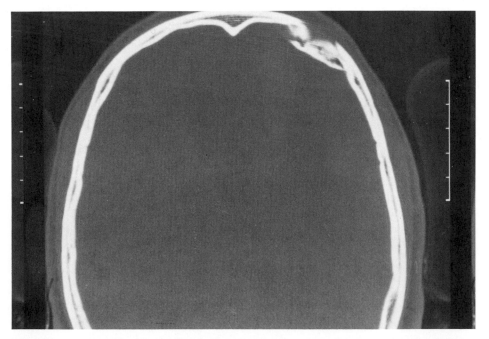

FIGURE 2.1.  CT scan demonstrating a closed depressed skull fracture involving both the inner and outer tables of the skull.

closure. An exception to this rule is the severe cranial facial trauma with cranial base and sinus fractures, causing the same situation as an open depressed skull fracture. When extensive skull fractures and cranial base fractures exist simultaneously, extensive facial fracture repair, sinus exoneration, and dural closure are recommended.

## INTRACRANIAL HEMATOMAS

Epidural hematomas are typically a complication of linear skull fracture (Figure 2.2). These hematomas result from a laceration of meningeal arteries, venous structures, or bleeding from the diploe of the skull. Not infrequently a lucid interval is seen, during which the patient is neurologically normal prior to deterioration from the mass lesion in the head. During this lucid interval, the patient may develop a progressive deterioration of the level of consciousness as the clot expands. Sudden deterioration can occur, resulting from brain herniation caused by shift of the brain from the mass lesion of the clot. These patients must be managed expeditiously by removal of the mass lesion to avoid permanent neurologic

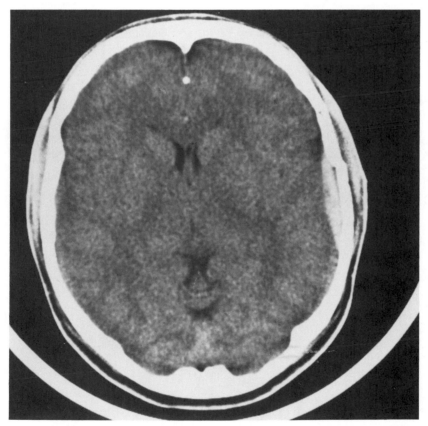

FIGURE 2.2. Epidural hematoma demonstrated in the left parietal area.

sequelae or death. The goals of surgery are removal of the mass lesion and hemostasis. Commonly, the brain is spared significant primary damage as the skull absorbs much of the force of the injury. With expedient diagnosis and surgery, excellent outcomes are seen in patients presenting in an alert state. Primary brain injury may also be coexistent with an epidural hematoma, with subsequent poor results (even with appropriate removal of the epidural hemorrhage).

Subdural hematomas are frequently associated with significant primary brain injury (Figure 2.3). Classically, these hematomas are thought to result from bleeding of bridging veins from dura to brain surface. However, they often result from superficial brain contusions and lacerations of the cortex and pia arachnoid. Arterial bleeding may well be the origin of some subdural clots. This group of patients is more difficult to manage than those with epidural hematomas because of a higher incidence of primary brain injury and subsequent severe cerebral edema and swelling. In those patients with severe injuries, intracranial pressure monitoring is utilized and plays a significant role in patient management.

Those patients sustaining superficial contusions without laceration of the pia arachnoid often have pronounced subarachnoid hemorrhage. Trauma is the most common cause of this disorder. While subarachnoid hemorrhage is often seen in patients with severe head injury, unlike aneurysmal subarachnoid hemorrhage, symptomatic cerebral vasospasm is rarely seen. These patients must, however, be followed carefully for progressive hydrocephalus as this is a common complication of severe traumatic subarachnoid hemorrhage.

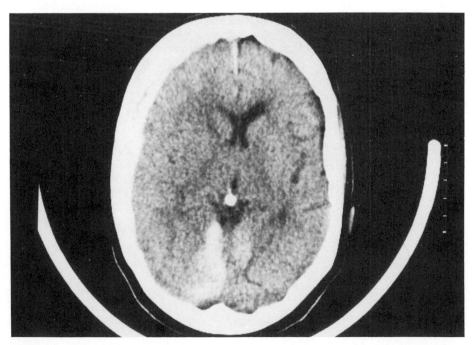

FIGURE 2.3. CT scan demonstrating a right frontoparietal acute subdural hematoma with shift of the midline.

## CEREBRAL CONTUSIONS

Contusions of the brain are managed conservatively when possible. These are most often located at the tips of the temporal lobes or on the inferior surfaces of the frontal lobes, but they may also be located on the frontal and occipital poles (Figure 2.4). These gliding contusions are seen in contrecoup injuries and result from the brain striking the calvarium at the brain–bone interface. Deeper contusions may also be seen. Medical management of these injuries is indicated in most cases. This management includes hyperventilation, head elevation, and diuresis to a hyperosmolar state, as outlined previously. Steroids are used by some in treating the surrounding edema, but this has not been shown scientifically to be of benefit. The indication for surgical management is neurologic decompensation in the face of optimal medical therapy, or persistent elevation of intracranial pressure in the face of a mass lesion without neurologic decompensation. Surgical management involves resection of the involved hemorrhagic clot and contused brain.

## INTRACEREBRAL HEMATOMA

Intracerebral hematomas are managed in much the same way as extensive contusions. An attempt to manage these with medical therapy is always carried out. Intracranial

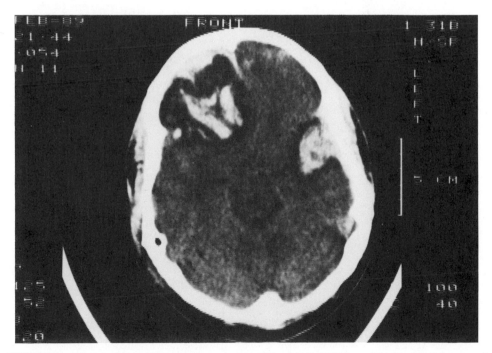

FIGURE 2.4. CT scans demonstrate extensive contusions of the right frontal lobe and the tip of the left temporal lobe.

pressure monitoring is used in those patients with Glasgow coma scores of 7 or less. Surgical intervention is reserved for those patients exhibiting intolerance to the clot in the face of maximal medical therapy, or persistently elevated intracranial pressure in the face of optimal medical therapy. Often these hematomas are deep in the brain or within eloquent brain locations. The choice of a surgical approach must take this into account to minimize further damage to the brain secondary to the surgery.

## PENETRATING BRAIN INJURY

Penetrating injuries include missile and stab wounds, as well as compound depressed skull fractures (Figure 2.5A,B). The primary goal of management in penetrating injuries is decontamination of the brain. In the case of missile injury, treatment includes local wound

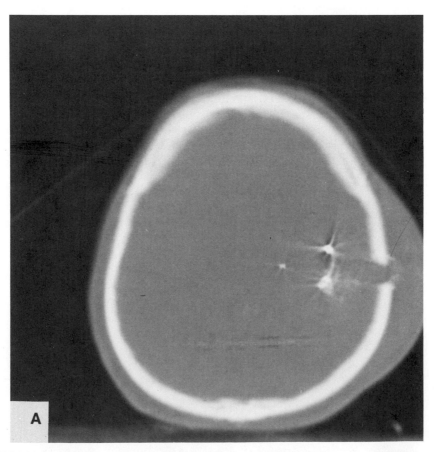

FIGURE 2.5. (A) CT scan bone windows clearly show the bony defect caused by the entering bullet as well as metallic fragments in brain parenchyma. (B) CT scan demonstrates intraparenchymal bullet fragments with associated hematoma.

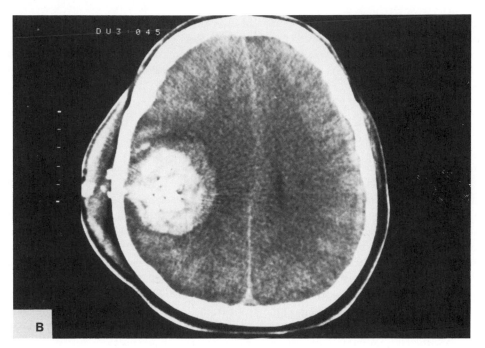

FIGURE 2.5. (*Continued*)

debridement as well as removal of bony and missile fragments within the brain paren-chyma. Additional pathology is often present, such as contusion and intracerebral and extracerebral hematomas. These lesions are removed at the time of local wound debride-ment and decontamination. Closure of the dura is important to avoid CSF fistula and further contamination. Patient selection for surgical intervention is important. Those patients presenting with a Glasgow coma score of 3 have been demonstrated to have lethal injuries and should be managed without surgical intervention (Clark, Muhlbauer, Watridge, & Ray, 1986). Patients suffering missile wounds typically have complicated courses, especially if a high-velocity injury is present, as secondary edema is a prominent feature of the injury. Intracranial pressure monitoring is helpful in these patients. Perioperative antibiotics are administered to assist in wound sterilization.

## DIFFUSE AXONAL INJURY

Diffuse axonal shear injuries are the result of rapid deceleration. Typically these patients will present deeply comatose, with an absence of focal supratentorial findings on neurologic examination. They may also demonstrate variable brain stem findings. The pathologic process is axonal disruption, and lesions are prevalent in the deep white matter, such as the corpus callosum. The CAT scan of the brain may be normal or show evidence of increased pressure secondary to diffuse edema. These patients are managed with an intracranial pressure monitor and subsequent intracranial pressure control. The prognosis for this group of patients is guarded and highly variable. Those patients who demonstrate diffuse axonal shear and normal-to-low intracranial pressures seem to have a worse outcome than those patients who have closed head trauma and controllable increased intracranial pressure.

## TRAUMATIC CAROTID DISSECTION

Trauma patients may exhibit a subtle injury causing neurologic manifestations that may mimic intracranial mass lesions. These symptoms may be due to local cerebral ischemia secondary to an arterial occlusion. In trauma patients, the most common cause of the arterial occlusion results from traumatic carotid dissection. In this situation, distal embolization may occur, which causes a local cerebral infarction resulting in focal neurologic deficits in the distribution of that arterial supply. Patients may also experience progressive occlusion of the carotid dissection, resulting in massive cerebral infarctions and death. A high index of suspicion is needed for the diagnosis of this entity. Any trauma patient who exhibits focal neurologic deficits which are unexplained by computerized axial tomography of the head, spinal cord injury, or peripheral nerve injury should be evaluated for traumatic carotid artery dissection. Management of this disorder is primarily conservative, with anticoagulation, since surgical treatment of traumatic carotid artery dissections is hazardous.

## GENERAL NEURO-TRAUMA CONSIDERATIONS

In addition to the above-discussed care for the head-injured patient, special attention must be given to the general care of these patients. Skin care is of paramount importance in order to avoid skin necrosis from decubitus ulcers and subsequent infection. The patient may require a special mattress or bed to decrease sacral pressure if frequent turning and rolling of the patient is insufficient. Comatose patients have an inordinately high basal metabolic rate and thus have significant nutritional needs (Clifton, Robertson, & Choi, 1986). Pulmonary care is of paramount importance as well. Appropriate attention to pulmonary care will prevent hypoxemia (which, of course, is an additional insult to the injured brain). Commonly, patients with severe head trauma require extended periods of ventilator support, either for therapeutic reasons, or due to inadequate ventilatory drive.

## CONCLUSION

The emergency management of the head-injured patient must be expedient and appropriate for the specific pathologic process. To this end, the necessary evaluation (both at the bedside and through diagnostic tests) must be performed efficiently and without flaw. Only through these measures can a significant impact be made for these critically injured patients.

## REFERENCES

Clark, W. C., Muhlbauer, M. S., Watridge, C. B., & Ray, M. W. (1986). Analysis of 76 civilian craniocerebral gunshot wounds. *Journal of Neurosurgery, 65*, 9–14.

Clifton, G. L., Robertson, C. S., & Choi, S. C. (1986). Assessment of nutritional requirements of head-injured patients. *Journal of Neurosurgery, 64*, 895.

Cushing, H. (1901). Concerning a definite regulatory mechanism of the vaso-motor center which controls blood pressure during cerebral compression. *Johns Hopkins Bulletin, 12*, 290–292.

Kellie, G. (1824). An account of the appearances observed in the dissection of two of the three individuals presumed to have perished in the storm of the 3rd, and whose bodies were discovered in the vicinity of Leith on the morning of the 4th November, 1821, with some reflections on the pathology of the brain. *Transactions of the Medicochirurgical Society of Edinburgh, 1*, 84–169.

Lundberg, N., Kjallquist, A., & Bien, C. (1959). Reduction of increased intracranial pressure by hyperventilation. *Acta Psychiatrica Scandinavica, 34*, 4–64.

Marshall, L. F., Smith, R. W., & Shapiro, H. M. (1976). The outcome with aggressive treatment in head injuries. Part II: Acute and chronic barbiturate administration in the management of head injury. *Journal of Neurosurgery, 50*, 26–30.

Monroe, A. (1783). *Observations on the structure and function of the nervous system.* Edinburgh: Creech and Johnson.

Myers, R. E., & Yamaguchi, S. (1977). Nervous system effects of cardiac arrest in monkeys. *Archives of Neurology, 34*, 65.

Overgaard, S., & Tweed, W. A. (1974). Cerebral circulation after head injury. I: Cerebral blood flow and its regulation after closed head injury and emphasis on clinical correlation. *Journal of Neurosurgery, 41*, 531–541.

Plum, F. (1983). What causes infarction in ischemic brain? The Robert Wartenberg lecture. *Neurology, 33*, 272.

Teasdale, G., & Jennett, B. (1974). Assessment of coma and impaired consciousness. A practical scale. *Lancet, 2*, 81–83.

Watridge, C. B., Muhlbauer, M. S., & Lowery, R. D. (1989). Traumatic carotid artery dissection: Diagnosis and treatment. *Journal of Neurosurgery, 71*, 854–857.

II

# Neuropsychological Assessment of Head-Injured Individuals

# 3

# Use of History in Neuropsychological Assessments

## ANDREW J. PHAY

The only value of neuropsychological testing in the hands of an experienced neuropsychologist is to support the conclusions already reached through interview and history taking. While this opening salvo is hyperbole, it is probably correct for the majority of cases. The purpose of this chapter is to offer suggestions to the clinician as to how he/she can conduct a richer (i.e., more informative about brain–behavior relationships) interview and history in the course of the neuropsychological assessment. An inference to be taken from the following discussion is that neuropsychological assessments which omit or skimp on the clinical interview and history can be misleading or invalid, often grossly so. The value of this chapter to the reader will vary with the reader's experience and extent to which he/she shares this author's assumption on the value and role of interviewing and history taking in neuropsychological assessments.

One purpose of the clinical interview is to evaluate the patient's current status. Current status is meant to include the traditional mental status and a description of current behavior, environmental stresses, and social supports for the patient. A clinical history typically should include a psychiatric history, medical history, childhood history (including a full educational history), family history, sex and marital history, military history, and a work history. In addition, contact with at least one person who knows the patient is often essential in order to determine patient reliability and obtain information which may be unavailable to the patient. For instance, behavior during a seizure or information concealed by the patient may be revealed. Neuropsychological assessments involving testing, a current status, history, and contact with a family member are often quite time-consuming. Unfortunately there is no quick and easy way to do adequate assessments of individuals.

Several ways in which a thorough current status and history can be valuable in

ANDREW J. PHAY • Alvin C. York VA Medical Center, Murfreesboro, Tennessee 37130.

*HANDBOOK OF HEAD TRAUMA: Acute Care to Recovery*, edited by Charles J. Long and Leslie K. Ross. Plenum Press, New York, 1992.

neuropsychological assessments and interventions will be discussed. An outline of these comments is presented in Table 3.1.

## DESCRIBE THE PATIENT'S FUNCTIONING

### Premorbid Functioning

*Problems of Measurement of Current Intellectual Ability*

The diagnostic importance of the current status and patient history information is enormous because this allows current functioning to be compared with the patient's

TABLE 3.1.  Neuropsychological Assessment:
Current Status and History

I. Describe the patient's functioning
  A. Premorbid functioning
    1. Problems of measurement of current intellectural ability
    2. Methods of measuring premorbid intelligence
      a. Hold–don't hold
      b. Regression equation
      c. Current status and history
    3. False-positive errors in measuring premorbid levels
      a. Learning disablity
      b. Low premorbid I.Q.
      c. Previous deficits
      d. Transient disorder
    4. False-negative errors in measuring premorbid levels
      a. Superior premorbid I.Q.
      b. Islands of superior ability
      c. Current overachievers
  B. Current functioning
    1. Differential diagnosis
      a. Unreported behavior or denied behavior
      b. Familial disorders/behavioral
      c. Premorbid functioning
      d. Multiple diagnoses
      e. Baseline determination for future diagnoses
      f. Etiology of symptoms
      g. Localization of lesions
    2. Severity
II. Facilitate test usage and interpretation
  A. Focus the assessment
  B. Minimize the bias of the testing milieu
  C. Limit unjustified inferences
  D. Describe an individual, not just a syndrome
  E. Develop rapport with the patient
  F. Give face validity to the evaluation results
III. Discover points of intervention
  A. Patient interventions
  B. Family interventions
  C. Environmental interventions

premorbid functioning. There are at least two major problems in our attempts to assess a decline in the patient's level of intellectual functioning. First, I.Q. or the psychometric measurement of intelligence does not always reflect an individual's level of intellectual functioning. Second, we rarely have a premorbid I.Q. assessment and therefore have to rely on less valid measures than a standardized test of intelligence.

The lack of a perfect correlation between I.Q. and intelligence or intellectual functioning is partly due to the ambiguity of what intelligence means. Intelligence is a concept which has different meanings to different investigators and is continually undergoing revision (Matarazzo, 1972). The failure of formal tests of intelligence to always reflect intelligence is recognized by virtually every major researcher on intelligence (Matarazzo, 1972). Every clinical/counseling psychologist has probably encountered unimpaired patients whose daily activities suggest they are functioning at a level different from their formally assessed level of intelligence. Examples of this discrepancy are graduate students who are not exceptionally bright but nevertheless are able to function adequately academically because they work extremely hard. As Wechsler (1949) stated: "general intelligence cannot be equated with intellectual ability however broadly defined, but must be regarded as a manifestation of the personality as a whole" (p. 78). In summary, the best test of intelligence is no more than a good estimate of current intellectual functioning.

*Methods of Measuring Premorbid Intelligence*

Despite the lack of agreement of what the term "intelligence" means, when no premorbid tests are available, three major approaches are used to assess this factor. They are: the use of hold–don't hold test comparisons; a regression equation based on patient demographic characteristics; and the patient's history. Wechsler attempted to contrast scores from the Wechsler intelligence scales (Wechsler–Bellevue, WAIS, WAIS-R) subtests which were not affected by a decline in intellectual functioning (hold tests) and those subtests which were affected (Matarazzo, 1972). Variations of hold–don't hold comparisons have been refined by: (1) specifying subtests for particular diagnostic categories (e.g., depression) (Kraus, 1966); (2) the use of a series of subtest combinations (Hewson, 1949); and (3) the development of a test of intelligence which has as its primary purpose the measurement of this hold–don't hold difference (Shipley, 1940). While these comparisons are sometimes helpful in determining a decline in intellectual functioning due to numerous factors, they are very inadequate when used alone (Ahuja, 1975; Aita, Armitage, Reitan, & Rabinowitz, 1947; Fisher & Parsons, 1962; Matarazzo, 1972; McKeever, 1961; McKeever & Gerstein, 1958; Parker, 1957; Phay, 1990a,b; Prado & Taub, 1966; Reitan, 1962; Russell, 1972; Savage, 1970; Wheeler & Wilkins, 1951; Yates, 1956). For example, demented patients evidence a decline on all Wechsler subtest scores (Storris & Doerr, 1980). The heavy loading of time subtests on don't hold tests excessively penalizes those patients who are slow for other than pathological reasons (e.g., cautious approach to testing or lack of motivation). The free response format of many of the hold tests sometimes unduly penalizes unimpaired persons who tend to give brief answers or refuse to give an answer unless they are certain of its accuracy (i.e., they won't respond based on partial or uncertain knowledge). The hold tests also unduly penalize dyslexic persons. Difference scores between hold and don't hold tests also commonly arise among "normals" due to varying interests, practices, experiences, and aptitudes. For a fuller discussion of these problems, see Matarazzo (1972).

The failure of the hold–don't hold difference scores to always reflect a decline in intellectual functioning has led to the development of a regression equation based on the patient's age, sex, race, education, and occupation (Klesges, Sanches, & Stanton, 1981: Klesges, Wildening, & Golden, 1981; Wilson, Rosenbaum, & Brown, 1979). While this regression equation is helpful, it is obviously not always correct (Bolter, Gouvier, Veneklasen, & Long, 1982; Gouvier, Bolter, Veneklasen, & Long, 1982). This equation assumes that age, sex, race, education, and occupation collectively have the same meaning across individuals.

*Example A: Overestimation of premorbid I.Q.* Mr. A. was a 39-year-old, white male who had completed the eleventh grade and worked as a guard and driver for a local business. His premorbid I.Q., according to the regression equation, was 96. His WAIS F.S.I.Q. was 60. Five years later he was retested on the WAIS, obtaining a F.S.I.Q. of 76. Mr. A.'s history revealed that he had been promoted through school automatically, regardless of academic achievement. In fact, he stated that he was never failed. He also reported dropping out of a remedial reading class after the first session because the other children made fun of him. He said he learned to speak with his fists. He claimed that during his high school years he was often bullied, scapegoated, poor in reading, writing, and spelling, clumsy, a daydreamer, often in fights, often tardy for school or skipped school, was lonely, frequently punished, and good in sports. At age 44, his reading skills were at a 3.1 grade level (Gates–McKillop–Horowitz Reading Diagnostic Tests). He reported that his math skills were his forte; they were assessed to be at a 7.5 grade level (Stanford Diagnostic Mathematics Test, Blue Level). He evidenced reversal of figures at both testing times. While Mr. A.'s clinical picture was not a simple one, given his long history of fighting and significant head trauma prior to our first assessment, the regression equation appears to have overestimated his premorbid level of intelligence.

*Example B: Underestimation of premorbid I.Q.* Mr. B. was a white, 63-year-old male who dropped out of school after the eleventh grade and has spent his life as a factory worker. His full-scale estimated I.Q. based on the regression equation was 107.60. However, Mr. B.'s history revealed that all four of his children went to college. Two of the four children were Merit Scholars. The I.Q. of one of the non-Merit Scholar children was assessed by the military to be about 170. Mr. B. built his own house and did all the electrical work. He did woodworking, welding, plumbing, and roofing. He enjoyed reading Bertrand Russell, Carlos Castenada, and lay books on Einstein's theories. Some of his favorite T.V. programs included Nova, Nature, and National Geographic. He subscribed to, read, and understood *Science*, *High Technology*, *Natural Science*, *Scientific American*, and other science magazines. He tuned his car, has repaired his T.V., and was often consulted by friends when a motor needed repair. Obviously, the regression equation significantly underestimated Mr. B.'s intelligence. If Mr. B. were afflicted with a dementing disorder, the dementia would have to be quite progressed before his current I.Q. level dropped below his underestimated premorbid I.Q. level.

In essence, the estimated premorbid I.Q. of patients who are atypical for any of the demographic characteristics are likely to be in error when using this regression equation. Thus, both hold–don't hold tests and a regression equation are sometimes inadequate in the assessment of premorbid level of intellectual functioning.

What is recommended for the determination of both the premorbid and current levels of intellectual functioning is the use of a completed current status and history (which includes the demographic features in the regression equation) in conjunction with a standardized test of intelligence capable of reflecting hold–don't hold differences. This combination of history and intelligence test data improves one's accuracy over both hold–don't hold difference scores and the regression equation.

## False-Positive Errors in Measuring Premorbid Levels

One of the most common errors likely to be made in the assessment of the premorbid level of intellectual functioning when a current status and history are not taken are false-positive errors—saying there is a loss of functioning when there isn't. Three common false-positive errors involve overlooking: (1) the existence of a low premorbid I.Q. which is attributed to a recent decline in I.Q., (2) the effects of a transient disorder which impairs cognitive functioning (e.g., depression) for indications of recent, permanent cognitive loss, and (3) previous deficits unrelated to the most recent loss. All of these errors are less likely when a full current status and history are obtained.

> *Example C: Recent head trauma or low premorbid I.Q.* Mr. C. was referred for evaluation due to possible cognitive loss from a recent head trauma. His WAIS F.S.I.Q. was in the Borderline Retarded Range. Upon taking the history, it was discovered that Mr. C. had only a 7th grade education, always had enormous difficulty with reading, writing, and math, disliked all subjects, and failed often. He reversed letters as a child. It appeared likely that he never functioned at a 7th grade level and had passed due to the school's "generosity." Neither of his parents had completed high school. His father was a longshoreman and his mother a housewife. Two of three brothers had not finished high school. His one sister was still in school. While Mr. C.'s mother denied any problems during her pregnancy or his birth, Mr. C. had fallen down the stairs and hit his head when six years old. He was hospitalized, but there were no observed sequelae. Throughout his life he was involved in numerous fights and car accidents. While this is not a simple case, it is clear that Mr. C.'s level of intellectual functioning had been quite low prior to the recent head trauma. Indeed, he and his mother denied any symptoms of cognitive loss after the recent head trauma.

> *Example D (from L. Hartlage, 1983, personal communication): Dementia or low premorbid I.Q.* Mr. D. was a 62-year-old male who ran his family farm. He was referred for assessment for possible dementia. Significant cognitive loss had been reported over the last several months. Neuropsychological assessment suggested that Mr. D. had significant multiple cognitive deficits. Upon eliciting Mr. D.'s history, it was discovered that he had not completed high school and that his mother had been the real manager of the farm, regularly giving explicit instructions to Mr. D. about his duties. Since his mother had died a year previously, Mr. D. no longer had someone to tell him what to do and therefore was unable to function at his previous level.

Transient loss of cognitive functioning is sometimes observed in depressed patients whether they are young or old (Henry, Weingarten, & Murphy, 1973; Miller, 1975; Weingarten, Cohen, Murphy, Martello, & Gerdt, 1981). The misdiagnosis of depressed patients as demented is particularly common among the elderly (Marsden & Harrison, 1972; Ron, Toone, Gorralda, & Lishman, 1979; Beck, Benson, Scheibel, Spar, & Rubenstein, 1982; Maletta, Pirozzola, Thompson, & Mortimer, 1982; Post, 1975). Taking a careful current status and history can often rule out or confirm depression. Of course, neurological impairment and depression can occur concomitantly as Lishman (1978) stated:

> It is perhaps worth emphasizing that the normal psychiatric history remains important even when the presenting complaints have a markedly organic flavor. Where the questions arise of a differential diagnosis between functional and organic mental illness, all parts of the standard psychiatric inquiry will need to be completed. Previous reactions to stress and symptoms observed during previous episodes of ill-health, may help to clarify the significance of the present clinical features . . . there is still a need to know about premorbid patterns of functioning, special vulnerabilities, and details of the patient's social and family setting. Such information may throw light upon the content of the illness and on special factors which will need to be borne in mind in management. Knowledge of the level achieved in education and at work can similarly be valuable in assessing present evidence of intellectual decline. [p. 111]

We have seen many patients who have a history of numerous incidents of possible CNS damage (Example C). Determining the effects of the most recent trauma or disease is often not possible. While we ask about changes due to each incident, we have to remind ourselves that the recent changes may not have occurred had the patient's brain been previously undamaged. Failure to get a history will lead the examiner to attribute all observed loss to the recent incident. Even head trauma as a child may permanently alter a person's brain functioning without evidencing either permanent structural or clinical changes.

*False-Negative Errors in Measuring Premorbid Levels*

The failure to discover cognitive loss when it has occurred sometimes arises with (1) patients who demonstrated premorbid underachievement (Example B); (2) patients whose unique experience enables them to perform well on some tasks of cognitive functioning; and (3) patients with mild deficits who work hard to compensate for these deficits. It is of importance to remember that there is a normal variability among cognitive functions in persons of the same general intellectual level and that the onset of insidiously progressive disorders (e.g., SDAT) is never known.

> *Example E (from W. G. Rosen, 1983, personal communication): Premorbid islands of superior ability*. Mrs. E. was evaluated for dementia at the age of 76. She had complaints of memory loss: forgetting conversations, missing appointments, and having difficulty keeping to her typically busy schedule. Testing revealed a mild memory impairment. Her drawings on the Rosen Drawing Test were excellent, which certainly is not a typical picture of a demented patient. Seven months later Mrs. E. was again tested. Her memory was much worse, and she complained of greater difficulties. It appeared that she was suffering from a dementing process; however, contrary to typical demented patients, her drawings on the Rosen Drawing Test were remarkably good. Mrs. E.'s history revealed the source of her atypicality. Mrs. E. had been a painter in her mid-20s and had stopped her artistic career to raise a family. At the age of 52 she got her B.A., a Masters of Fine Arts Degree, and became involved in numerous art organizations. Mrs. E. had exceptional premorbid skills in drawing.

Much of the discussion on the importance of the patient's current status and history can be summed up in a quote of Swiercinsky (1978):

> For many differential diagnostic questions, it is essential that the neuropsychologist know the detailed background leading to the present neurological condition of the patient. Current symptoms need to be diagnosed as recently acquired or long-standing. Dyslexia may be due to a lesion affecting Wernicke's area of the dominant hemisphere and be part of a current process. Or, the patient may have exhibited dyslexia or dyslexialike characteristics all of his life. One way to help determine this is to obtain details about the schooling history, reading habits, etc. of the patient. Also, knowledge of whether or not the patient grew up in an intellectually stimulating environment or a relatively deprived environment offers valuable clues for determining the etiology of presenting symptoms. If the necessary history is unavailable, the information must be obtained either from the patient, if possible, or through separate interviews with family members. [pp. 99–100]

## Current Functioning

*Differential Diagnosis*

The current level and characteristics of a patient's intellectual functioning can also be elucidated by the patient's current status and history. This information assists us in determining both the diagnosis and the severity of the dysfunction.

Differential diagnosis is facilitated by the current status and history in the following eight circumstances: (1) when symptoms are unreported; (2) when patients are of questionable reliability or veracity; (3) when there is a familial incidence of common disorders or behaviors; (4) when determination of premorbid functioning is crucial to diagnosis; (5) when there may be more than one disorder; (6) when follow-up assessments are necessary to determine diagnosis; (7) when the etiology of the symptom is important; and (8) when the localization of the lesion site is of significance.

Unreported and unreliable reports of symptoms or denial of behavior are common problems. Patients omit clinically significant behavior or provide unreliable reports for many different reasons. They may respond only to questions posed by the examiner, who might fail to ask all the pertinent questions. The patient may be unaware of or unable to communicate his behavior, or he may avoid or deny behavior he doesn't want the examiner to know about.

*Example F: A patient may interpret symptoms differently from others.* Mr. F.'s evaluation of his own behavior was different from his wife's and our evaluation; this led Mr. F. to overlook abnormal behavior which he considered normal. Mr. F. had reported, in his current status and history, recurrent episodes of depression as characterized by dysphoria, brooding, excessive guilt, insomnia, significant recent weight loss, psychomotor retardation (worse in the day and better at night), early morning awakening, decreased ability to concentrate, less enjoyment from all activities, and fatigue. He denied any symptoms of mania or hypomania. It was not until his wife was contacted that a different diagnostic picture emerged. She reported recurrent manic episodes characterized by unusual energy, pressured speech, sleep less than three hours a night, increased irritability, hyperactivity, provocativeness, impulsiveness, small financial indiscretions, and recurrent depressive and manic episodes for 13 years. He was given a DSM-III diagnosis of Bipolar Disorder, depressed without psychotic features (296.52). Mr. F. thought of his manic episodes as times when he was feeling normal. Until his wife was contacted, he was diagnosed and treated as a unipolar depressive.

Similarly, depressives may deny or minimize depressive symptoms because they don't want to be considered complainers or "crazy," are not currently experiencing dysphoria, or cannot think of a suitable reason for their depression. Misreporting of symptoms and their severity is sufficiently common among patients to warrant attempts to contact a family member of every patient.

*Example G: A patient may not report symptoms unless explicitly questioned.* One patient referred to the neuropsychology lab for assessment of possible cognitive deficits due to alcoholism was a 59-year-old veteran with a B.S. in engineering who had worked all his life, was highly verbal, was married, and had several children. While there were some indications of mild cognitive loss, perhaps reversible with abstinence, his current level of intellectual functioning was above that of most veterans. He was easy to test, always appropriate, and tried hard to give his best performance. Usually a current status is one of the first assessment procedures with patients, but for some reason he had spent several hours in testing prior to a current status being obtained. To the surprise of the examiner, in the current status interview the patient reported severe depression and visual and auditory hallucinations over the last 30–40 years. He hallucinated several people talking and making comments on his behavior, plans, and thoughts. These hallucinations occurred in many different places, did not always involve the same individuals, were not related to drinking (in fact, the voices tended to subside when he drank), and sometimes told the patient to hurt himself or someone else or that someone was talking about him. Initially, the hallucinations troubled and frightened the patient, but he came to accept them and no longer believed they were strange experiences. He assumed many other people have similar experiences which they also do not discuss with others. The patient's old medical records verified a lifelong history of hallucinations and a diagnosis of schizophrenia. Interviewing had picked up what our testing had missed.

Similarly, patients frequently do not report relevant childhood events unless specifically questioned about them. For example, patients may fail to report information about head trauma as a child, premature birth, dyslexia, or forced changes in hand preference as a child.

> *Example H: Explicit questioning on handedness.* Mr. H. wrote with his right hand. However, he was left-footed and left-eyed. During questioning, he revealed he had been forced to write with his right hand as a child, did everything else (such as throwing a ball) with his left hand, considered himself left-handed, and had a nickname of "Lefty" throughout high school. He was still called "Lefty" by his close friends. His history of a forced change in his writing hand greatly altered our assessment of his motor functioning which revealed superior speed and dexterity in his left leg, arm, and hand.

Patients may fail to report behavior because they are unaware of it, such as when suffering from dementia or memory loss for events associated with head trauma or a seizure. Or the patient may be aware of his behavior but be unable to report it accurately because of aphasia. Clearly we have to rely on family members for information in such cases.

> *Example I: Avoids reporting or denies behavior.* One 34-year-old male patient sent for neuropsychological evaluation had stabbed and seriously injured someone prior to admission. Mr. I. denied any memory of the event and reported a 14-year history of seizures. The attending psychiatrist thought Mr. I.'s violent behavior might be the result of a seizure. While the history could not prove whether or not this violent episode was related to a seizure, it clearly indicated that antisocial behavior was a lifelong characteristic. Mr. I. had a history of running away from home as an adolescent, stealing as a child, numerous arrests as an adult, expulsion from high school, a very sporadic employment history with many different kinds of jobs, frequent absences from work, divorce, failure to pay child support, lack of a permanent address, and a history of drug abuse (including cocaine, Quaaludes, marijuana, heroin, and prescribed pain killers). The clinical impression of Mr. I. was that, despite his revelations, he was minimizing or denying much of his previous antisocial behavior.

> *Example J: Exaggeration of a symptom cluster.* Mr. J. was seen after having been charged with killing a man during an explosive episode. Mr. J. had been evaluated by us several years previously. Consequently, there were two evaluations on him. In his first evaluation he appeared to have an intellectual level well within the Retarded Range while in the second evaluation he appeared to be functioning well within Borderline Retarded Range. This increase in I.Q. may have been due to a recovery of function from a significant head trauma he had suffered about a year prior to the first assessment. On both occasions he evidenced a severe learning disability, marital discord, alcoholism, a long history of antisocial behavior, including sudden violent outbursts and anxiety and depression. However, on the second evaluation he admitted to schizophrenic symptoms which he had explicitly denied on his first evaluation. Furthermore, both his wife and mother (at the time of his first evaluation) had explicitly denied schizophrenic symptoms. While corroborating Mr. J.'s reports of his other symptoms, he did not appear schizophrenic to his examiners at either time. His discharge papers from the military many years ago had mentioned anxiety but not schizophrenia. Based on the interviews with the patient, his wife, and his mother, his military discharge papers, clinical impressions, and test results, it was suggested that (though Mr. J. had many serious problems) his reported schizophrenic symptoms were of questionable validity.

The current status and history from family members is often helpful in confirming or disconfirming a diagnostic suspicion (i.e., when the examiner is uncertain of the reliability or validity of the patient's report).

> *Examples K and L: Questionable validity.* Mr. K. and Mr. L. were both suspected of being alcoholics by all the ward staff, despite the fact that they reported drinking only occasionally.

Mr. K. also had a history of head trauma which could at least partially explain his impaired test results. When we spoke with Mr. K.'s mother, she reported that her son had abused alcohol for 20–25 years and had been in numerous detox centers and rehabilitation programs. On the other hand, when we spoke with Mr. L.'s daughter, wife, and private physician about Mr. L.'s possible alcoholism, all denied it and reported very mild drinking habits. Based on the consistency of these reports, the clinical impression that the patient, his daughter, and his wife were not consciously attempting to distort or hide facts, and Mr. L.'s test results, it was concluded that the staff had probably mislabeled Mr. L. as an alcoholic.

Discovering disorders and symptoms in the family members of patients can often point in certain diagnostic directions or help to confirm diagnostic suspicions. The number of medical and psychiatric disorders which can present with cognitive, emotional, or "hysterical" symptoms which have a familial incidence significantly greater than chance is large and includes Huntington's disease, narcolepsy, progressive muscular dystrophies, epilepsy, Pick's disease, diabetes mellitus, depression, schizophrenia, dyslexia, manic depression, alcoholism, hyperactivity, and many others. Furthermore, some disorders are highly associated with other disorders in families. For instance, depression and alcoholism often occur in the same family (Winokur, Codoret, Baker, & Dorzab, 1975; Winokur, 1977).

In addition to the high familial occurrence of medical/psychiatric disorders, the occurrence of physical and psychological characteristics among the patient's family members is too important to be ignored. For example, the average correlation between parents and their children or between siblings on measures of intelligence is about +0.50 (Erlenmeyer-Kimling & Jarvik, 1963; Jensen, 1969). Similarly, academic skills which reflect intellectual ability (such as reading, spelling, and arithmetic) also are highly positively correlated between parents and their offspring (Matarazzo, 1972).

A second example of the importance of familial characteristics is that of the presence or absence of left-handedness in family members. This has been related to hemisphere lateralization of verbal functions; equal frequency of left or right hemisphere damage resulting in language disturbances in left-handed persons (Hecaen & Sauquet, 1972); clinical impressions that learning-disabled children have a high incidence of family members who are left-handed, -footed, and -eyed (Denckla, 1978); the relationship of the outcome for speech, language, and intellectual handicap in infantile hemiplegics (Annett, 1973); and the relationship of laterality differences for auditory and visual perception in both right- and left-handers (Zurif & Bryden, 1969; Hines & Satz, 1971).

Premorbid functioning in the determination of the differential diagnosis is almost always important. The current status and history in the assessment of premorbid level of intelligence is the sine qua non of a diagnosis of dementia (Wells, 1977; Joynt & Shoulson, 1979). The differential diagnosis of multi-infarct from other dementias relies heavily on a history of the evolving symptoms picture. Similarly, a personal and family history can suggest the possible etiology of the dementia due to alcoholism, Huntington's disease, heavy metal intoxication, etc. An accurate diagnosis of the type of dementia greatly affects patient treatment, prognosis, and family counseling.

It is common to have patients with multiple problems which are only partly covered in the presenting symptoms. There are two difficulties which often arise in the assessment of these patients. The first difficulty is that secondary or tertiary problems which are not directly related to the primary or presenting symptoms are often overlooked. For example, depression is often overlooked (or labeled as understandable and not treated) in neurological patients. Learning disabilities are also frequently overlooked. The second difficulty is that there are few norms for patients with multiple disorders. Typically the patients referred for neuropsychological assessments present difficult diagnostic questions. These patients usually have multiple disorders and atypical symptom pictures. While there are normative data on alcoholics, there are no norms for alcoholics who also suffer from head trauma, seizure disorders, diabetes, or are self-medicating an underlying biological depression with alcohol. It is rare that we see an alcoholic, a depressive, or a learning-disabled person whose significant problems are limited to the presenting complaint(s). Brain-damaged patients are often depressed. Schizophrenics often have a poor educational background, grow up in an unstable familial environment, treat their symptoms with alcohol, and/or receive significant dosages of major tranquilizers. Stroke patients often have hypertension, severe familial and financial stress, and the significance of their academic training and intellectual environment vary enormously. "Pure" alcoholics or "pure" right hemisphere stroke patients are seldom seen. A good current status and history minimizes the possibility of overlooking biological or environmental factors which may influence a patient's cognitive and intellectual functioning.

> *Example M: Multiple problems.* Mr. M. had pneumonia as a 6-month-old infant, rheumatic fever and "chorea" at age 8, and later developed a head twitch and bilateral tremor in his upper extremities. He has been emotionally labile all of his life. As a child and adolescent he was in many fights but denied ever having been knocked unconscious. It was discovered in the 8th grade that he could neither read nor cite the alphabet. He worked hard to overcome his reading disability and now, at age 40, reads at a 7th or 8th grade level (Gates–MacGinitie Reading Tests, level F). Mr. M. has experienced significant maternal neglect throughout his life. Fortunately, his father was very affectionate and Mr. M.'s lifelong emotional support. About a year prior to our assessment of Mr. M., his father had died. Mr. M. was experiencing increasing depression. Alcoholism and probably an underlying biological depression were evident throughout Mr. M.'s family. Mr. M.'s brother, mother, one of two maternal uncles, two of three maternal aunts, and his maternal grandmother were probably alcoholics. As an adult, Mr. M. suffered numerous head traumas in which he lost consciousness (two driving accidents and at least one of his numerous fights). He had a seizure disorder for which he takes Dilantin which has lessened his seizure frequency to about one per week. He was divorced from a drug addict, but denied having abused drugs or alcohol himself. Mr. M. was very depressed, unable to return to his former employment, and was trying to give emotional support to his sister who recently experienced considerable stress.

The question is: where does one find appropriate norms for this patient? There are none. Patients are often more complex than our normative data. The point is not that normative data are valueless but that their value is limited.

> *Example N: Head trauma and lifelong depression.* Mr. N. was seen a month after suffering a head trauma. Mr. N. evidenced significant cognitive impairments, particularly of right hemisphere dysfunction, which had not existed the day before his trauma. His affective and cognitive disturbances were all attributed to his recent trauma. Upon interviewing the patient's wife, it was discovered that for the last two years the patient had been quite withdrawn, afraid to leave his home, go to work, or ride the trains. He drank heavily, was happy only when drinking, and talked of moving to California and starting over. He was fatigued; had initial, middle, and terminal insomnia; and had a decreased appetite. He quit reading (which he used to enjoy immensely), quit watching T.V., and lost interest in all his usual activities. He also felt guilty about not going to work, had mentioned suicidal ideation (no plan or stated intent), had withdrawn from religious activities, and had said he no longer loved his daughter. In essence, his behavior sounded like a Major Depressive Episode. It was recommended that the patient be evaluated for somatic and psychological treatment for his depression.

Obtaining baseline data can be helpful in plotting the course of a known disorder or in the diagnosis of a suspected, but unproven, deficit. It is common to see patients about whom one is uncertain if they have seizures, are in early stages of a dementing process, or are evidencing deficits due to their depression rather than their head trauma. It is good to keep in mind that cognitive symptoms usually predate a diagnosis of dementia. Indeed, we have no way to diagnose the onset of insidious dementing processes or psychopathological processes. Documenting and charting change in the functioning level of patients can be extremely valuable in making the diagnosis or in determining the course of a dementia in its early stages, the focus of a seizure, the effects of mild head trauma, or neurosurgery. The use of a repeated current status, as well as repeated tests, can help document that change.

The etiology of the symptoms can sometimes be suggested or determined through the use of the current status and history. (See discussions of dementia and familial disorders/behavior discussed above.) Localization of lesions can be suggested in the current status and history. Moderate to severe language, motor, visual-spatial, or cognitive deficits are easy to spot in the initial interview by observing, listening to, and questioning the patient. Even mild deficits are often suggested. Questions which inquire about any changes in the patient's vision, hearing, sense of balance, ability to feel objects, taste, smell, gait, upper and lower limbs (strength and dexterity), speech production/articulation/comprehension, reading, ability to find one's way, telling time, dressing, eating, hobbies, using tools, recognizing friends, etc., often elicit localizing information. This current status, when used with a patient and a family member, augments formal neuropsychological testing results. General questions such as "How has your husband's memory been?" typically elicit little information. Indeed, the term "memory" is often used as a euphemism for any kind of cognitive deficit. It is usually more informative if the examiner is explicit. For example, "Can your husband do crossword puzzles as well as he used to?" is a better question than "Has there been any change in your husband's hobbies?"

> *Example O (from H. Kohn, 1984, personal communication): Localization.* Mr. O. was admitted to the hospital for trauma to his left hemisphere. He was right-handed. He was unable to read a map, get around in large-scale space, and couldn't organize space. The students investigating Mr. O. were quite excited because he seemed to be a patient who had an anomalous organization of brain function. Dr. Kohn asked his students to get a history before coming to any conclusions. Mr. O.'s history revealed that he could never read a map, had always had a hard time driving around, and was always very poor in art. That was the end of the anomalous brain. This patient had apparently compensated for his visual-spatial difficulties by use of his language skills. When his language skills became impaired due to the trauma to the left hemisphere, he could no longer compensate.

## Severity

The current status and history may reflect the severity of the patient's deficits or extent of his recovery better than tests. Two examples come to mind. The first example is a patient who one knows is impaired but does not realize how impaired until we discover from the history that the patient had an unusually high premorbid I.Q. The second example is a patient who reports functioning at a higher or lower level at home than in the hospital.

> *Example P: Underestimation of premorbid I.Q.* A 22-year-old male with a recent history of paranoid behavior (dx. schizophreniform disorder) and a head trauma a month after initial mental health hospitalization appeared to be demented on our tests. Given the relative lack of variability across various intellectual tasks, a low morbid I.Q. was suspected. The patient claimed that he had

some college education, but his veracity was questionable. During an interview with the patient's mother, she brought a copy of a certification of excellence her son had received upon completing high school, a copy of a list of books her son had bought while serving in the military (which included books on business management, technical writing, computers, biology, geometry, trigonometry, and geology), and also reported that her son had had some college, though his grades had not been good. Based on the history from the patient's mother, the most reasonable explanation for much of the patient's poor performance was his high dosage of Haldol (20 mg T.I.D.). Repeat testing was recommended after the patient was taken off this medication.

*Example Q: Underestimation of current functioning.* Mr. Q. was seen in cognitive remediation sessions. He had suffered severe brain damage due to encephalitis. He had progressed to the point of being able to say two-word responses and remember this author's name. When comments were made on this progress, his mother (who came to all the sessions and was the principal therapist for her son) said he did much better at home. She proceeded to relate examples of her son initiating language and nonverbal behavior with family members. She also recalled instances in which her son remembered where various articles of food were kept in the house; the names, health status, and cities in which his grandparents lived; and occasions when he was able to form compound questions and responses.

The importance of the current status and history in diagnostic assessment is well summarized by DeJong (1979):

> A good clinical history often holds the key to diagnosis. This is true in the medical history, surgical history, and psychiatric history. It is especially true in the neurologic history, where a carefully obtained, properly analyzed, detailed account of the patient's symptoms, past and present, may lead to an accurate discernment of the nature and location of the disease process. A skillfully taken history, with a careful analysis and interpretation of the chief complaints and of the course of the illness, will very frequently indicate the probable diagnosis, even before physical, neurologic, and laboratory examinations are carried out. In many instances the physician learns more from what the patient says and how he says it than from any other avenue of inquiry. Every neurologic examination must be preceded by an accurate history if it is possible to obtain one. Many errors in diagnosis are due to incomplete or inaccurate histories. [p. 7]

## FACILITATE TEST USAGE AND INTERPRETATION

When they are given first, the current status and history help to screen for deficits, suggesting what areas of behavior may be impaired and what tests are most likely to give valuable information. Luria (1966) discusses the importance of the preliminary conversation, generally a portion of the current status and history, in screening for possible deficits:

> An investigation for the purpose of establishing the topical diagnosis of brain lesions must begin with a preliminary conversation with the patient. The more care and attention to detail paid during this conversation, the more precise and purposeful the subsequent clinical psychological investigation of the patient will be. This preliminary conversation has a twofold purpose. First, it enables the investigator to form a general idea of the state of the patient's consciousness, of the level and peculiarities of his personality, of his attitude toward himself and his situation. Second, it brings to light the patient's principal complaints and exposes the group of pathological phenomena that may be of localizing significance and that must be studied with special care. As a rule, the basic hypotheses concerning the nature and sometimes, the location of the pathological process are formed during this preliminary conversation with the patient, and the rest of the investigation serves to confirm, modify, or refute these hypotheses. Knowledge of the patient's premorbid state frequently has a very important bearing on the evaluation of such behavioral manifestations as slowness or quickness of response and emotionality or restraint, for such manifestations may either be a sign of disease or indicate individual traits in the patient's makeup. [pp. 309–310]

Similarly, Filskov and Leli (1981) have stated:

> Although frequently neglected, the following answers should be obtained to questions about past events. The early history should be traced: any birth injury, including forceps delivery, anoxia, or a necessity to use the intensive care nursery should be reported. Uncontrolled high fevers, disease involving the CNS (e.g., meningitis, encephalitis), head injuries with loss of consciousness, and seizures for whatever cause should be recorded, along with the age, a description of the course of recovery, any after effects, and type of treatment. A careful school history, including adjustment problems, learning disabilities, as well as academic strengths, should be noted for adults. A prior psychiatric record, along with careful questioning regarding the reasons for any hospitalizations is essential to understand past and present environmental stresses and patterns of coping for the person. Understanding a person's premorbid coping abilities is important, yet frequently neglected. Such factors as stress tolerance and degree of psychopathology in a person's life before the onset of a brain disorder can alter the extent of adaptation or compensation that is seen. The person who has strong internal resources can obviously cope better than someone who has never had those capabilities. [pp. 548–549]

For instance, a patient who appears moderately demented upon interview would usually be more appropriately assessed with an instrument like the Mattis Dementia Rating Scale than the WAIS-R which discriminates poorly at low levels of intellectual functioning. With an aphasic patient, you may wish to begin with a Boston Diagnostic Aphasia Examination–Revised, the Aphasia Screening Test of the Halstead–Reitan, or the language subtests of the Luria–Nebraska Neuropsychological Battery to document the extent and characteristics of his deficits before trying any other assessment techniques involving language. An initial conversation will often give the first clues of aphasia, depression, malingering, or dementia. The more knowledgeable and experienced the interviewer, the more that can be gained from the interview. Furthermore, one can form accurate impressions without being aware of which cues lead to their formation. A skilled professional notices unusual voice quality, gait and limb disturbances, subtle language aberrations, etc. Many of the observations, which must be pointed out to the student, have become second nature to the experienced clinician. There is no substitute for experience. In addition to an initial interview, it is often helpful to have a patient attempt to fill out a history questionnaire at the beginning of the assessment. The patient's ability to fill out the form can tell one a great deal about his reading and writing skills and knowledge of grammar and spelling as well as his history. When asked to evaluate patients whose primary language is not English, one often gets a much fuller and more accurate current status and history when they are given in the patient's primary language.

## Minimize the Bias of the Testing Milieu

The assessment milieu is an artificial situation which distorts testing results in at least three ways. First, the assessment milieu typically maximizes motivation and minimizes organizational ability. A patient may put forth his best possible effort so that the test results overestimate his daily functioning. Outside of the testing situation, where he has no authority figure instructing him on appropriate behavior, and is not explicitly told to try his best or what to do, he may not put forth as much effort. The patient with moderate to severe deficits is unable to compensate sufficiently to give an adequate performance. However, when the patient has mild deficits or the testing situation compensates for the patient's deficits (e.g., supplying structure and direction to frontal lobe patients), the patient's deficits may go unobserved on neuropsychological tests.

Often patients with memory complaints do well on memory tests. One's first impulse is to reduce cognitive dissonance by discounting the patient's report. However, it may be that the fault lies with the tests, one's ignorance of the patient's premorbid level of memory ability, or the explicitness of the test may compensate for the patient's losses. Life doesn't often tell you what is important for you to remember. If you can't decide what to remember and you can't or don't attend or concentrate, then your recall of daily events will be poor though you may do well on tests of memory. The current status and history gives information about the patient's functioning in environments which are much less structured and less directed, and they sample a much greater range of behavior.

Second, testing results may miss the impaired patient whose deficits are too slight for our tests to pick up. Patients who are characterized by themselves or their family as having impaired memory (while performing within normal limits on all neurological, radiological, and neuropsychological tests) may be experiencing changes due to a dementing process too subtle for neuropsychological tests to elicit.

Third, some patients refuse to try to minimally comply with testing requirements, resulting in an assessment which underestimates their daily functioning. While this situation occurs more often with psychiatric patients, it may also occur with neurological patients. The importance of relating the results of our formal assessment procedures to the patient's current status and history is well stated by Goldstein (1959):

> Today it is hardly understandable that the solution to the problem was not discovered earlier, namely; to consider the symptoms not only in relation to the dysfunction of limited parts of the brain but in relation to the individual in whom they appear; in other words, to consider them as performances of the sick individual. The concentration of study not on the single symptom but on the behavior of the total personality of the patient, during examination and in everyday life, made it more and more evident that the symptoms could only be correctly evaluated if one considered them in relation to the condition of the total psychophysical personality. This instigated an intensive study of each single symptom in relation to the behavior of the total patient at a given moment, which in turn, became the point of departure for the concept of the so-called organismic approach to psychopathology in general. [p. 183]

## Limit Unjustified Inference

It is the experience of this author that the more information available on a patient, the less likely incorrect speculations about the patient's functioning are made. Information confines and limits our theorizing about the patient. A thorough assessment lessens the unwanted intrusions of the examiner's bias. In essence, ignorance begets bias.

## Describe an Individual, not Just a Syndrome

The current status and history reveal information about the patient which portray the patient more as an individual and less as a syndrome. We have all observed our and other staff members' attitudes change toward a patient after discovering similarities with the patient. Learning that a brain damaged patient plays chess, enjoyed gardening, wrote songs, played ball with his or her son, rode horses, or was a good cook often humanizes that individual for us. One of the functions a psychologist serves is to present the patient as a person to the staff who read his/her report. It can facilitate the growth of understanding and empathy in students to require the reading of biographies or autobiographies authored by an impaired individual or someone close to them which discusses the relationship between the disorder or impairment and the person. Head injury occurs inside a person who lives among other persons.

Park and Claiborne (1976) and Landes (1964) are excellent sources for firsthand accounts of *adult psychiatric disorders*. Other accounts are: Barnes (1971), Beers (1908), Benziger (1969), Bruch (1978), Burton (1974), Davis (1979), Donaldson (1976), Edwards (1981), Endler (1982), Evans (1954), Farmer (1972), Frank (1958), Freeman (1951, 1969, 1980), Freeman and Roy (1976), Gotkin (1975), Hayward (1977), Howland (1974), Keyes (1981), Knauth (1975), Knight (1950), Liu (1979), Logan (1976), Moore (1955), Murphy (1968), Naylor (1977), Neary (1975), Olsen (1974), Parker (1972), Peters (1978), Reed (1976), Rhodes and Freeman (1964), Schreber (1955), Sizemore and Pidttillo (1977), Sturgeon (1979), Ward and Farrelli (1982), and Wechsler, Wechsler, and Karpf (1972).

Accounts of *childhood psychiatric problems* include: Anonymous (1951), Anonymous (1967), Craig (1972, 1978), D'Ambrosio (1970, 1978), Foy (1970), Green (1964), Hayden (1980), Kaufman (1981), Lane (1976), Lane and Pillard (1978), Lorenz (1963), MacCracken (1976), Maclean (1977), and Phillips (1975).

Accounts of *adult neurological patients* include: Adam (1974), Armstrong (1979), Brownstein (1980), Dorros (1981), Gardner (1974), Greenblatt (1972), Griffith (1970), Gunther (1949), Heymanns (1977), Luria (1972), Mee (1978), Sachs (1983, 1985), and Wint (1967).

A good reference for accounts of childhood neurological disorders can be found in Featherstone (1980). Other accounts not mentioned in Featherstone (1980) include Brown (1976), Collins (1980), Friedman (1974), Greenfield (1970, 1978), Kaufman (1976), Kupfer (1982), Landvater (1976), Lynch (1979), Napear (1970), Nason (1974), Natchez (1975), Ottenberg (1978), Schaefer (1978), and White (1972). None of these lists are even close to being comprehensive.

The accounts of psychiatric patients (including schizophrenics, depressives, multiple personalities, etc.) were lumped together for two reasons. First, in several of these accounts, there is a disagreement about diagnosis both among professionals and between those treated and those treating. Second, while there have been enormous advances in the treatment and diagnosis of psychiatric patients, not the least of which is DSM-III-R, it is not clear that the boundaries drawn among various psychiatric disorders and among subtypes of each of these disorders have been accurately delineated. Nor is it certain that the right questions are being asked to enable significant advances in our future understanding of these disorders. To go further, too often the categorization of patients as psychiatric or neurological reflects both current methods of assessment and our ignorance of the disorders. A diagnostic label can minimize the likelihood that the patient will receive all of the interventions which might be of assistance to him. In essence, the diagnosis is too often treated rather than the individual. This polemic is not to be construed as an attack upon psychiatric diagnosis or DSM-III-R. The former appears to be necessary for appropriate treatment and the latter a significant improvement in our efforts at classification of mental disorders. Rather, the limitations of a label in describing an individual's functioning are underlined.

## Develop Rapport with the Patient

The use of the current status and history can facilitate establishing a good rapport with the patient. The examiner seems concerned about the patient as a person. A partnership can be formed with patients. Partially as a result of a focus on the individual rather than the syndrome, patients are often willing to do an enormous amount of work in the assessment process. It is common for the patient to spend ten or more hours in testing, interviewing, and filling out forms without complaint.

## Give Face Validity to the Evaluation Results

A current status and history makes neuropsychological assessments more convincing both to other professionals and to the patients and their families. This "face validity" can be particularly important if you are trying to convince the neurologist, patient, or family members of the need for a particular intervention. Even when other professionals disagree with well-documented findings, they usually respect a thorough job. Similarly, patients and their family members are often more receptive to feedback about their impairments when there is a thorough assessment, even though they may have previously discounted similar conclusions from others. If a neuropsychologist wishes to influence other professionals, patients, and their family members, he must both be good and appear to others to be good at his job.

## DISCOVER POINTS OF INTERVENTION

The current status and history can facilitate the beginning of psychotherapy or counseling with the patient. Problem areas can often be pinpointed, and the therapist can be given an immediate and good grasp of the patient's background and problems. A thorough history is particularly important since many therapists focus their energies on therapy exchanges and current behavior/problems and are neglectful of getting a full history. Excellent assessments and descriptions of the individual patient are often prerequisites to a successful intervention.

> *Example R: History in psychotherapy.* Mr. R.'s physical and cognitive functioning were deteriorating due to multiple sclerosis. Within the past two years while his illness was progressing, he had separated from his wife (reportedly because she was having affairs) and his mother had died. He was unsure if he could still function sexually, was anxious about becoming dependent on others, and had significant financial problems. Despite all of these reverses, he had a girlfriend, was only mildly dysphoric, had only a few mild somatic symptoms of depression, and was actively making plans for the future. Clearly the diagnosis of multiple sclerosis and a description which was limited to Mr. R.'s physical and cognitive deficits were very inadequate in giving direction to his psychotherapist.

> *Example S: Marital counseling resulting from changes due to deficits.* Mr. S. had a ruptured left hemisphere aneurysm at the age of 40, three years before we initially saw him. He had residual expressive aphasia and some comprehensive language deficits in addition to a right-sided weakness. He was able to walk with a cane and was willing to put forth an enormous effort in all of his remediation therapies. It was discovered (on taking a history from the patient and his wife) that, premorbidly, the patient had had a very responsible job, gotten his younger brother and father a job with the same firm, and made virtually all the household decisions. Not surprisingly, his cognitive impairments and his inability to return to work had resulted in considerable changes in his marital relationship. Based on the patient's history, the possibility of marital therapy was explored with this couple. They finally agreed and appeared to profit from this intervention.

There are many examples of potentially significant areas of exploration found in patient histories. For instance, there are probably very different family dynamics involved when a patient with an average I.Q. has siblings who all appear to have a lower I.Q. or, conversely, all have a higher I.Q. The obvious question that arises is whether this patient was treated differently in his family. Another example is the patient who, from the family history, appears to be at risk for hypertension. Obviously, the patient's diet may need to be discussed. Other facts which suggest a need for further discussion in psychotherapy are being single throughout adult life, being the only one of several children who is living with the parents, having a marital relationship which is described in very different terms by the patient and his spouse, possessing such an intense resentment of authority that the patient is likely to be more receptive to a nonauthoritarian therapist, etc. If this kind of information is not gathered during the assessment portion of intervention with the patient, it is often overlooked.

Incidentally, relatively little work has been done on the special characteristics, techniques, and approaches of psychotherapy with brain-damaged individuals. There are many potential dissertations in this area.

## Family Intervention

The need for interventions with the family members of the patient often first surfaces in the patient's current status and history. We tell our interns that, if you can offer substantial benefits to family members, you often help the patient as well, albeit indirectly. The family may need counseling on the genetics of Huntington's disease, likelihood of developing high blood pressure, psychotherapy, knowledge about the expected course of SDAT, referral sources for a dyslexic child, information about the patient's diet, assistance in applying for disability benefits, etc. There are situations (such as with demented or schizophrenic patients) when the only useful intervention one can make on behalf of the patient is to help that patient's family cope with the patient.

## Environmental Interventions

The preliminary assessment of existing and needed environmental, social, and financial supports of the patient is in the current status and history. For instance, are there family members in the immediate vicinity with whom the patient might be able to live upon discharge? Does the social worker need to apply for military, VA, or Social Security payments on behalf of the patient? Is the patient's family likely to be willing to assist in rehabilitative efforts with the patient? The involvement and support of the patient's family is often critical to the speed and extent of recovery (Golden, 1978; Lezak, 1976). Is there a family member who can oversee the patient's medication? Does an environmental engineer need to inspect the patient's house and make recommendations concerning the installation of environmental aids such as clocks with large numbers, handrails, a passageway for a wheelchair? Is the patient's family aware of the immense need for routine and structure in the life of a brain-damaged patient? Does the family need counseling in order not to overly infantilize the patient out of sympathy for his suffering, or because its easier for an intact person to perform the patient's chores than assist or wait on the patient to do it (e.g., dressing or hygiene)? All of us frequently perform the role of consultants to our patients and their families.

As Sax *et al.* (1983) have pointed out in discussing patients with Huntington's disease:

We have also observed that individuals with a similar degree of neurologic impairment have different abilities to cope with the disease, depending on affective state and the family and occupational support available to the patient. Effective counseling can enhance a patient's functional level. [p. 33]

In summary, there are many important reasons to take a thorough current status and history, some of which have been discussed here. It is an assessment procedure which relies heavily upon the knowledge, thoroughness, and curiosity of the examiner as well as a commitment to evaluate the person, not just the symptoms.

Before concluding this chapter, it should be mentioned that it is not always possible or appropriate to take a thorough current status and history. It is very time-consuming, easily taking 3 hours. A neuropsychologist's workload may be too extensive to allow him to spend 3+ hours on history taking. The patient may not be able to endure lengthy assessment procedures, so that a brief history and selected neuropsychological tests may be a more efficient assessment approach. An evaluation may be needed quickly, for instance if the patient is scheduled for surgery in two days. The patient's rehabilitation program may be so intensive that he is seldom available for assessment procedures. Everyone encounters situations in which it is not possible to conduct a thorough assessment. Furthermore, a current status and history is sometimes of little or no value in the evaluation of the patient. An obvious example is the comatose patient. It is clear that one does not need a history to determine the cognitive functioning of the patient. It takes very little information to diagnose a lateralized lesion in a hemiparetic or hemianoptic patient. It is not appropriate to take a full current status and history when conducting research with a specific focus not involving the patient's past behavior. Indeed one can argue that the appearance of a Major Depressive Episode subsequent to a stroke is sufficient to warrant a trial of antidepressant medication, regardless of whether a premorbid positive or negative history for depression exists. It is not intended to suggest that current status and history is a panacea or should be used alone. Rather, the current status and history greatly adds to, reinforces, and complements a thorough testing protocol.

## REFERENCES

Adam, R. C. (1974). *Living with mysterious epilepsy: My 48 year victory over fear*. New York: Exposition Press.
Ahuja, V. (1975). Comparison between deterioration in depressives as obtained from WAIS index (Wechsler) and revised WAIS index (J Kraus). *Journal of Psychological Researches, 21*, 98–101.
Aita, J. A., Armitage, S. G., Reitan, R. M., & Rabinowitz, A. (1947). The use of certain psychological tests in the evaluation of brain injury. *Journal of General Psychology, 37*, 25–44.
Annett, M. (1973). Laterality of childhood hemiplegia and the growth of speech and intelligence. *Cortex, 9*, 4–33.
Anonymous. (1951). *Autobiography of a schizophrenic girl*. New York: Grune & Stratton.
Anonymous. (1967). *Go ask Alice*. Englewood Cliffs, NJ: Prentice–Hall.
Armstrong, A. O. (1979). *Cry Babel: The nightmare of aphasia and a courageous woman's struggle to rebuild her life*. New York: Doubleday.
Barnes, M. (1971). *Two accounts of a journey through madness*. New York: Ballantine.
Beck, J. C., Benson, D. F., Scheibel, A. B., Spar, J. E., & Rubenstein, L. Z. (1982). Dementia in the elderly: The silent epidemic. *Annals of Internal Medicine, 97*, 231–241.
Beers, C. (1921). *A mind that found itself: An autobiography*. New York: Longmans, Green.
Benziger, B. F. (1969). *The prison of my mind*. New York: Walker.

Bolter, J., Gouvier, W., Veneklasen, J., & Long, C. J. (1982). Using demographic information to predict premorbid I.Q.: A test of clinical validity with head trauma patients. *Clinical Neuropsychology, 2*, 171–174.

Brown, H. (1976). *Yesterday's child*. New York: Signet.

Brownstein, K. O. (1980). *Brainstorm: A personal story*. New York: Avon.

Bruch, H. (1978). *The golden cage: The enigma of anorexia nervosa*. New York: Vintage.

Burton M. (1974). *An alcoholic in the family*. Philadelphia: Lippincott.

Collins, P. (1980). *Your daughter is brain damaged: A mother's story*. New York: Dutton.

Craig, E. (1978). *One, two, three—The story of Matt, a feral child*. New York: McGraw–Hill.

Craig, E. (1972). *P. S. Your not listening*. New York: Richard W. Baron.

D'Ambrosio, R. (1970). *No language but a cry*. New York: Doubleday.

D'Ambrosio, R. (1978) *Leonora*. New York: McGraw–Hill .

Davis, B. K. (1979). *Letters to my husband's analyst*. New York: Hawthorn Books.

DeJong, R. N. (1979). *The neurological examination: Incorporating the fundamentals of neuroanatomy and neurophysiology* (4th ed.). New York: Harper & Row.

Denckla, M. B. (1978). Minimal brain dysfunction. In J. S. Chall & A. F. Marisky (Eds.), *Education and the brain*. Chicago: University of Chicago Press.

Donaldson, K. (1976). *Insanity inside out*. New York: Crown Publishers.

Dorros, S. (1981). *Parkinson's: A patient's view*. Washington, DC: Seven Locks Press.

Edwards, H. (1981). *What happened to my mother*. New York: Harper & Row.

Endler, N. S. (1982). *Holiday of darkness: A psychologist's personal journey out of his depression*. New York: Wiley.

Erlenmeyer-Kimling, L., & Jarvik, L. F. (1963). Genetics and intelligence: A review. *Science, 142*, 1477–1479.

Evans, J. (1954). *Three men: An experiment in the biography of emotion*. New York: Knopf.

Farmer, F. (1972). *Will there really be a morning?* New York: Putnam.

Featherstone, H. (1980). *A difference in the family life with a disabled child*. New York: Basic Books.

Filskov, S. B., & Leli, D. A. (1981). Assessment of the individual in neuropsychological practice. In S. B. Filskov & T. J. Boll (Eds.), *Handbook of clinical neuropsychology*. New York: Wiley.

Fisher, G. M., & Parsons, P. A. (1962). The effect of intellectual level on the rate of false positive organic diagnoses from the Hewson and Adolescent Ratios. *Journal of Clinical Psychology, 18*, 125–126.

Foy, J. G. (1970). *Gone is shadow's child*. Plainfield, NJ: Logos.

Frank, G. (1958). *Judy*. New York: Harper & Row.

Freeman, L. (1951). *Fight against fears*. New York: Warner Books.

Freeman, L. (1969). *Farewell to fear*. New York: Putnam.

Freeman, L. (1980). *Too deep for tears*. New York: Hawthorn/ Dutton.

Freeman, L., & Roy, J. (1976). *Betrayal*. New York: Stein & Day.

Friedman, M. (1974). *The story of Josh*. New York: Praeger.

Gardner, H. (1974). *The shattered mind*. New York: Vintage Books.

Golden, C. J. (1978). *Diagnosis and rehabilitation in clinical neuropsychology*. Springfield, IL: Thomas.

Goldstein, K. (1959).

Gotkin, J. P. (1975). Too much anger, too many tears. *A personal triumph over psychiatry*. New York: Quadrangle/ The New York Times Book Co.

Gouvier, W., Bolter, J., Veneklasen, J., & Long, C. J. (1982). Predicting verbal and performance I.Q. from demographic data: Further findings with head trauma patients. *Clinical Neuropsychology, 5*, 119–121.

Green, H. (1964). *I never promised you a rose garden*. New York: Signet.

Greenblatt, M. H. (1972). *Multiple sclerosis and me*. Springfield, IL: Thomas.

Greenfield, J. (1970). *A child called Noah. A family journal*. New York: Holt, Rinehart & Winston.

Greenfield, J. (1978). *A place for Noah*. New York: Holt, Rinehart & Winston.

Griffith, V. E. (1970). *A stroke in the family. A manual of home therapy*. New York: Delacorte Press.

Gunther, J. (1949). *Death be not proud: A memoir*. New York: Harper & Row.

Hayden, T. L. (1980). *One child*. New York: Putnam.

Hayward, B. (1977). *Haywire*. New York: A. A. Knopf.

Hecaen, H., & Sauguet, J. (1972). Cerebral dominance in left handed subjects. *Cortex, 8*, 19–48.

Henry, G. M., Weingarten, H., & Murphy, D. L. (1973). Influence of affective states and psychoactive drugs on verbal learning and memory. *American Journal of Psychiatry*, *130*, 966–971.

Hewson, L. (1949). The Wechsler–Bellevue Scale and the Substitution Test as aids in neuropsychiatric diagnosis. *Journal of Nervous & Mental Disorders*, *109*, 158–266.

Heymanns, B. (1977). *Bittersweet triumph*. New York: Doubleday.

Hines, D., & Satz, P. (1971). Superiority of right visual halffields in right handers for recall of digits presented at varying rates. *Neuropsychologia*, *9*, 21–25.

Howland, B. (1974). *W-3*. New York: Viking.

Jensen, A. R. (1969). How much can we boost I.Q. and scholastic achievement? *Harvard Educational Review*, *39*, 1–123.

Joynt, R. J., & Shoulson, I. (1979). Dementia. In K. M. Heilman & E. Valenstein (Eds.), *Clinical neuropsychology*. New York: Oxford University Press.

Kaufman, B. N. (1976). *Son rise*. New York: Warner.

Kaufman, B. N. (1981). *A miracle to believe in*. New York: Doubleday.

Keyes, D. (1981). *The minds of Billy Milligan*. New York: Bantam Books.

Klesges, R. C., Sanches, V. C., & Stanton, A. L. (1981). Cross validation of an adult premorbid functioning index. *Clinical Neuropsychology*, *3*, 13–15.

Klesges, R. C., Wildening, G. N., & Golden, C. J. (1981). Premorbid indices of intelligence: A review. *Clinical Neuropsychology*, *3*, 32–39.

Knauth, P. (1975). *A season in hell*. New York: Harper & Row.

Knight, J. (1950). *The story of my psychoanalysis*. New York: McGraw–Hill.

Kraus, J. (1966). On the method of indirect assessment of intellectual impairment: A modified WAIS index. *Journal of Clinical Psychology*, *22*, 66–69.

Kupfer, F. (1982). *Before and after Zachariah. A family story about a different kind of courage*. New York: Delacorte Press.

Landis, C. (1964). *Varieties of psychopathological experience*. New York: Holt, Rinehart & Winston.

Landvater, D. (1976). *David*. Englewood Cliffs, NJ: Prentice–Hall.

Lane, H. (1976). *The wild boy of Averyron*. Cambridge, MA: Harvard University Press.

Lane, H., & Pillard, R. (1978). *The wild boy of Burundi. A study of an outcast child*. New York: Random House.

Lezak, M. D. (1976). *Neuropsychological assessment*. New York: Oxford University Press.

Lishman, A. I. (1978). *Organic psychiatry: The psychological consequences of cerebral disorder*. Oxford, England: Blackwell Scientific Publications.

Liu, A. (1979). *Solitaire*. New York: Harper & Row.

Logan J. (1976). *Josh: My up & down in & out life*. New York: Delacorte Press.

Lorenz, S. E. (1963). *There is always tomorrow*. New York: Holt, Rinehart & Winston.

Luria, A. R. (1966). *Higher cortical functions*. New York: Basic Books.

Luria, A. R. (1972). *The man with a shattered world*. Chicago: Henry Regnery.

Lynch, M. (1979). *Mary, Fran and Mo*. New York: St. Martin's Press.

MacCracken, M. (1976). *Lovey, a very special child*. Philadelphia: Lippincott.

McKeever, W. F. (1961). The validity of the Hewson ratios: A critique of Wolff's study. *Journal of Nervous & Mental Disease*, *132*, 417–419.

McKeever, W. F., & Gerstein, A. I. (1958). Validity of the Hewson ratios: Investigation of a fundamental methodological consideration. *Journal of Consulting Psychology*, *22*, 150.

Maclean, C. (1977). *The wolf children*. New York: Penguin Books.

Maletta, G. J., Pirozzola, F. J., Thompson, G., & Mortimer, J. A. (1982). Organic mental disorders in a geriatric outpatient population. *American Journal of Psychiatry*, *139*, 521–523.

Marsden, C. D., & Harrison, M. J. G. (1972). Outcome of investigation of patients with senile dementia. *British Medical Journal*, *2*, 249–252.

Matarazzo, J. (1972). *Wechsler's measurement and appraisal of adult intelligence* (5th ed.). Baltimore: Williams & Wilkins.

Mee, C. L., Jr. (1978). *Seizure*. New York: M. Evans.

Miller, W. R. (1975). Psychological deficit in depression. *Psychological Bulletin*, *82*, 238–260.

Moore, W. L. (1955). *The mind of chains. The autobiography of a schizophrenic*. New York: Exposition Press.

Murphy, F. (1968). *The Frank Murphy story*. New York: Dodd, Mead.

Napear, P. (1970). *Brain child, a mother's diary*. New York: Harper & Row.

Nason, M. D. (1974). *Tara*. New York: Hawthorn Books.

Natchez, G. (1975). *Gideon a boy who hates learning in school*. New York: Basic Books.

Naylor, P. (1977). *Crazy love: An autobiographical account of marriage and madness*. New York: William Morrow.

Neary, J. (1975). *Whom the gods destroy*. New York: Atheneum.

Olsen J. (1974). *The man with the candy. The story of the Houston mass murders*. New York: Simon & Schuster.

Ottenberg, M. (1978). *The pursuit of hope*. New York: Rawson, Wade.

Park, C. C., & Claiborne, (1976). *You are not alone: Understanding and dealing with mental illness. A guide for patients, families, doctors and other professionals*. Boston: Little, Brown.

Parker, B. (1972). *A mingled yarn chronicle of a troubled family*. New Haven, CT: Yale University Press.

Parker, J. W. (1957). The validity of some current tests for organicity. *Journal of Consulting & Clinical Psychology*, *21*, 425–428.

Peters, C. (1978). *Tell me who I am before I die*. New York: Rawson.

Phay, A. (1990a). Shipley Institute of Living Scale: Part I Moderator variables. *Medical Psychotherapy—An International Journal*, *3*, 1–15.

Phay, A. (1990b). Shipley Institute of Living Scale: Part II Assessment of intelligence and cognitive deterioration. *Medical Psychotherapy—An International Journal*, *3*, 17–35.

Phillips, L. (1975). *I love you, I hate you*. New York: Harper & Row.

Post, F. (1975). Dementia, depression and pseudo-dementia. In D. F. Benson & D. Blumer (Eds.), *Psychiatric aspects of neurological disease*. New York: Grune & Stratton.

Prado, W. M., & Taub, D. V. (1966). Accurate prediction of individual intellectual functioning by the Shipley–Hartford. *Journal of Clinical Psychology*, *22*, 294–296.

Reed, D. (1976). *Anna*. New York: Basic Books.

Reitan, R. M. (1962). Psychological deficit. *Annual Review of Psychology*, *13*, 415–444.

Rhodes, L., & Freeman, L. (1964). *Chastise me with scorpions*. New York: Putnam.

Ron, M. A., Toone, B. K., Gorralda, M. E., & Lishman, W. A. (1979). Diagnostic accuracy in presenile dementia. *British Journal of Psychiatry*, *134*, 161–168

Russell, E. (1972). WAIS factor analysis with brain-damaged subjects using criterion measures. *Journal of Consulting and Clinical Psychology*, *39*, 133–139.

Sachs, O. (1983). *Awakenings*. New York: Dutton.

Sachs, O. (1985). *The man who mistook his wife for a hat*. New York: Summit Books.

Savage, R. D. (1970). Intellectual assessment. In P. Mittler (Ed.), *The psychological assessment of mental and physical handicaps*. London: Methuen.

Sax, D. S., O'Donnell, B., Butters, N., Menzer, L., Montgomery, K., & Kayne, H. L. (1983). Computer tomographic, neurologic and neuropsychological correlates of Huntington's disease. *International Journal of Neuroscience*, *18*, 21–36.

Schaefer, N. (1978). *Does she know she's there?* New York: Doubleday.

Schreber, D. (1955). *Memoirs of my nervous illness*. London: William Dawson.

Shipley, W. C. (1940). A self-administering scale for measuring intellectual impairment and deterioration. *Journal of Psychology*, *9*, 371–377.

Sizemore, C. C., & Pidttillo, E. S. (1977). *I'm Eve*. New York: BJ Publishing Group.

Sturgeon, W. (1979). *Depression: How to recognize it, how to treat it and how to grow from it*. Englewood Cliffs, NJ: Prentice–Hall.

Swiercinsky, D. (1978). *Adult neuropsychological evaluation*. Springfield, IL: Thomas.

Ward, W., & Farrelli, L. (1982). *The healing of Lia, a true account of multiple personalities*. New York: Macmillan Co.

Wechsler, D. (1949). Cognitive, conative, and non-intellective intelligence. *The American Psychologist*, *3*, 78–83.

Wechsler, J. A., Wechsler, N. F., & Karpf, H. W. (1972). *In a darkness*. New York: Norton.

Weingarten, H., Cohen, R. M., Murphy, D. L., Martello, J., & Gerdt, C. (1981). Cognitive processes in depression. *Archives of General Psychiatry*, *38*, 42–47.

Wells, C. (1977). Diagnostic evaluation and treatment in dementia. In C. Wells (Ed.), *Dementia*. Philadelphia: Davis.

Wheeler, J. I., & Wilkins, W. L. (1951). The validity of the Hewson ratios. *Journal of Consulting Psychology*, *15*, 163–166.

White, R. (1972). *Be not afraid. The story of a tragically afflicted child and his stubbornly courageous family*. New York: Dial Press.

Wilson, R. S., Rosenbaum, G., & Brown, G. (1979). The problem of premorbid intelligence in neuropsychological assessment. *Journal of Clinical Neuropsychology, 1*, 49–53.

Winokur, G. (1977). Genetic patterns as they affect psychiatric diagnosis. In V. M. Rakoff, H. C. Stancer, & H. B.
Kedward (Eds.), *Psychiatric diagnosis*. New York: Brunner/Mazel.

Winokur, G., Codoret, R., Baker, M., & Dorzab, J. (1975). Depression spectrum disease vs. pure depressive
disease: Some further data. *British Journal of Psychiatry, 127*, 75–77.

Wint, G. (1967). *The third killer. Meditation on a stroke*. New York: Abelard-Schuman.

Yates, A.J. (1956). The use of vocabulary in the measurement of intellectual deterioration—A review. *Journal of
Mental Science, 102*, 409–440.

Zurif, E. B., & Bryden, M. P. (1969). Familial handedness and left–right difference in auditory and visual
perception. *Neuropsychologia, 7*, 179–187.

# 4

# Neuropsychological Assessment of Patients with Epilepsy

## BRUCE P. HERMANN

Epilepsy is one of the most prevalent neurological disorders, affecting from 1 to 2% of the population or some two to four million Americans (National Commission for the Control of Epilepsy and Its Consequences, 1978). Epilepsy can seriously affect an individual's quality of life because of its potential to impair cognition, personality, and behavior (Dodrill, 1981; Hermann & Whitman, 1984). Because the majority of cases (some 75–80%) begin before the age of 18, epilepsy can be considered to be a disorder of largely childhood and adolescent onset and to, therefore, have the potential to seriously compromise important aspects of cognitive, social, and behavioral development.

In spite of the prevalence of epilepsy and the potential of several specialty areas within psychology to make a contribution to the care of individuals with epilepsy, psychology has, for some reason, never expressed much interest in the disorder (Dodrill, 1981; Mostofsky, 1978). This disinterest is reflected in a lack of training in epilepsy and limited experience in working with clients with epilepsy during formal internship and postdoctoral experiences. As a consequence, practitioners are often less than optimally prepared to deal with the multifaceted problems presented by this population. The purpose of this chapter is to present some suggestions which may prove helpful in the comprehensive assessment of patients with epilepsy. It will concentrate on some suggested areas of inquiry for the clinical interview, provide general and specific recommendations for cognitive assessment, and conclude with suggestions pertaining to the assessment of the patient's psychosocial and behavioral status.

The thrust of this presentation is entirely clinical and is not meant to be a detailed review of the cognitive and behavioral effects of epilepsy. Many such reviews are available elsewhere (Hermann & Whitman, 1984; Rausch, 1985). Further, there will not be an

BRUCE P. HERMANN • Regional EpiCare Center, Memphis, Tennessee 38103.

*HANDBOOK OF HEAD TRAUMA: Acute Care to Recovery*, edited by Charles J. Long and Leslie K. Ross. Plenum Press, New York, 1992.

extended discussion concerning the classification of seizures or the modern management of epilepsy. Several recent texts discuss these topics in depth (e.g., Laidlaw & Richens, 1982). The purpose of this chapter is to provide some background information, suggestions, and experiences which may be helpful in the comprehensive psychological assessment of adults with epilepsy.

First to be discussed will be the clinical interview with the patient with epilepsy. It is important to obtain some information concerning the history and current status of the patient's epilepsy, and the nature of this information will be discussed. Second, several issues related to the neuropsychological assessment of patients with epilepsy will be overviewed. In the course of this discussion, some findings derived from the neuropsychological assessment of patients attending our epilepsy center will be presented. Finally, epilepsy can have a variety of effects on the behavioral, emotional, and social status of the patient. Some of the more pernicious effects will be briefly reviewed, and some suggestions for assessment will be presented.

## THE CLINICAL INTERVIEW

In addition to the usual information that is obtained during a thorough clinical interview prior to the beginning of formal neuropsychological testing, it is important to gather some information concerning the patient's epilepsy. The chronicity of the patient's epilepsy, the severity of the disorder, treatment regimes, and the characteristics of the seizures themselves represent some of the data that should be obtained.

### The Seizures

An easy point of departure for the interview is to have the patient describe his or her seizures. Some patients can give very clear and detailed descriptions of their aura, their behavior during the seizures (although this is generally based on the reports of others), their postictal state, and other relevant details. Other patients may seem to have very little awareness or understanding of their ictal events other than they "pass out" or "black out." However, if the patient is asked the appropriate questions, he or she can often provide the interviewer with fairly detailed information.

Patients can first be questioned as to the nature of the aura or "warning" that they experience in association with their seizures. Most adults with epilepsy suffer from partial seizures and, by definition, have a focal origin to their seizures. This focal origin may be manifested in their aura (i.e., simple partial seizure) and is experienced as an alteration in sensation, cognition, or emotion. It should be emphasized to the patient that the focus of interest here concerns any changes in perception, mood, thoughts, sensations, or feelings immediately (generally) prior to the loss of consciousness. Some patients are very aware of their aura and can provide considerable detail, while other patients cannot spontaneously provide this information. It is not uncommon for a patient to say that he or she does have a warning of some type prior to a seizure, but it is "hard to describe," "difficult to put into words," or "indescribable." In such cases, it is helpful to run through the list of potential simple partial seizures (Table 4.1) and to have the patient simply indicate whether they experience that particular event *immediately prior to losing consciousness*. The reason for

TABLE 4.1. Possible Aura Symptomatology

| | |
|---|---|
| Sensory or somatosensory symptoms | Visual, auditory, olfactory, gustatory, vertiginous, somatosensory |
| Autonomic symptoms | Epigastric sensation, flushing |
| Cognitive symptomatology | Déjà vu, jamais vu, forced thinking, other ideational disturbances |
| Affective symptomatology | Fear, depression, elation, anger |
| Psychosensory symptomatology | Illusions (micropsia, macropsia, metamorphosia) |
| | Auditory or visual hallucinations and illusions |
| Motor symptomatology | |

this emphasis is that some patients will endorse many experiences when they, at first, clearly bear no relation to the ictal event.

It is also worth mentioning to the patient that several of the auras associated with epilepsy can be quite unusual and, at times, frightening. On occasion some patients may be reluctant to admit to some ictal phenomena (i.e., feelings of depersonalization, forced thoughts, visual/auditory illusions, or hallucinations) because of their obvious psychiatric connotations. Therefore, it is important to reassure individuals that a wide array of very unusual sensations and experiences can indeed be part of the seizure disorder.

Once the interviewer has worked through the potential auras, has elicited some positive replies from the patient, and is convinced that these experiences are indeed ictal in nature, then some attempt should be made to arrange these experiences into their usual or typical sequential order. For example, if the patient has indicated that prior to losing consciousness he/she experiences an intense sensation of familiarity (like having lived through this before) or experiences a "rerun" of something that has previously happened in his or her life (déjà vu), a tingling in the left hand, and a very foul smell, then the patient should be asked to identify which of these events is the first identifiable sensation, the second, and so on. This information is occasionally helpful in providing some information as to the localization of the epileptogenic lesion and, at the very least, helps to provide some idea of the phenomenology of the patient's seizures. While these events usually precede a loss of consciousness (complex partial seizure) or generalized tonic–clonic convulsions (secondarily generalized seizure), it is important to determine if the patient also experiences these very same events at other times without losing consciousness. If this is the case, it is some indication that the patient may also suffer from simple partial seizures.

After delineation of the initial ictal events, the patient should be asked to describe what happens during a typical seizure. As a rule, patients are amnesic for the behavior which occurs during complex partial (and, of course, secondarily generalized) seizures; therefore, the patient needs to be asked what others (e.g., spouse, parent) have told them about their behavior during a seizure. Of course, if a family member who has seen the patient's seizures is present, then he or she can provide that information. Some patients may have an aura and then proceed immediately into a generalized tonic–clonic seizure (secondarily generalized seizure), while some may subsequently have an event characterized by clouded consciousness, mumbling, talking and saying words but not making any sense, ambulating, exhibiting a variety of automatisms (lip smacking and chewing movements, fiddling with their clothes or nearby objects), autonomic changes (drooling, flushing of the face), and other seemingly unusual behaviors (complex partial seizure). Again, some patients may be somewhat hesitant to reveal some of their ictal behaviors because of embarrassment, but the patient should be reassured that these behaviors are very typical for complex partial seizures.

At this point the interviewer should have a good sense of the patient's seizure activity. The typical course of ictal events has been obtained, and an attempt to derive some sense of seizure frequency can be derived. For instance, on a weekly or monthly basis, how often do they experience their aura only (simple partial seizure) (with no subsequent loss of consciousness or tonic–clonic activity), how often do they experience the major (tonic–clonic or secondarily generalized) attacks, and how often do they have complex partial seizures? This is always an estimate because some patients may not be aware of all their seizures, may exhibit a form of denial in underestimating their seizure frequency, or may overestimate seizure frequency because they interpret any unusual sensation or experience as an indication of some form of seizure activity.

Lastly, a description of the postictal state should be obtained. Most patients are tired, exhausted, sleepy, and/or suffer from a headache after a complex partial or, especially, tonic–clonic seizure. More interestingly, some patients have emotional or behavioral complications postictally. Occasionally there are patients who experience a postictal psychosis shortly after a flurry of seizures. These patients usually have a clear mentation interictally, but become quite delusional postictally with predominantly religious or paranoid ideation. Other patients may have a period of intense depression which may last for a few days and gradually lift. This is more than a reactive depression caused by unhappiness because a seizure has occurred (although such reactive depressions certainly occur). Rather, it is an organic mood change which may last up to a few days. On the other hand, some patients may report a feeling of great relief, a significant easing of anxiety or tension, and so on. In some patients this appears to be an organic mood change, while in others it seems to be related to the belief that they will not experience a seizure for some time. The postictal mood and behavioral changes which are presumed to be organic in nature are relatively uncommon, but they can be very problematic for the patient.

At some time during the assessment session, after greater rapport has been established with the patient, some inquiry should be made as to how the patient feels about their epilepsy, their perceptions as to how they feel others have treated them because of their epilepsy, and so on. The experiences related by persons with epilepsy are oftentimes surprising in the context of our modern culture. We continue to have patients report that they were excluded from regular classrooms and put in behavior-disordered or MR settings solely because of their epilepsy, or were even barred from the classroom and sent home for homebound tutoring because the seizures were said to be too disruptive for the school setting. From patients who live in small towns we have been told stories of unbelievable social exclusion, sometimes because townspeople thought that epilepsy was contagious. The essential point is that it is very common for people with epilepsy to have experienced differential treatment because of their epilepsy, and it is germane to the assessment process to uncover these experiences and relate them to the patient's current situation and the reason for referral. This point will be returned to later when discussing personality and behavioral assessment.

## Other Background Information

Other information related to the patient's epilepsy should be obtained: for instance, the chronicity of the disorder. At what age did the recurrent seizures begin? Someone with an onset of epilepsy at age 7 is likely to have very different life experiences and opportunities compared to someone with onset at age 20. The latter has proceeded through school without the burden of a chronic neurological disorder; socialization experiences have not been affected by a chronic (and, at times, embarrassing and stigmatizing) disorder. Such an individual would surely have unique stresses which might be very different in nature compared to a patient with a 20-year history of epilepsy.

Antiepileptic medications can be a double-edged sword. They are effective in reducing the frequency of seizures, but some types of antiepileptic medications can have significant side effects in some individuals. Caution is indicated in attempting to assess the effects of the medications on cognition and/or emotional functioning. On occasion the medications clearly have some adverse effects, particularly if the patient has not been treated using modern medical practices. Using the wrong anticonvulsant for the patient's particular seizure type, administering toxic amounts of medication, or prescribing multiple anticonvulsant medications (particularly of the barbiturate type) can have adverse effects on cognition and behavior. However, some patients may clearly erroneously blame all their difficulties on the use of antiepileptic medications. Consultation with the attending physician about the side effects of the patient's medications is often warranted.

## NEUROPSYCHOLOGICAL ASSESSMENT

Patients are referred to our epilepsy center primarily for consideration of epilepsy surgery. As such they have had poorly controlled seizures for a number of years (the average duration of epilepsy is approximately 18 years) and have taken a diversity of anticonvulsant medications in varying combinations; generally, the epilepsy has had significant adverse effects on the quality of their lives. As part of their preoperative work-up, the patients routinely undergo comprehensive neuropsychological evaluation. This testing is conducted in order to provide information which might be of help in identifying the lateralization and localization of the underlying epileptogenic lesion, provide a baseline with which to compare the adequacy of the patient's postoperative cognitive functioning, and provide information which will be of value to other professionals involved in the patient's planning and management (e.g., vocational rehabilitation specialists). To date we have had an extensive experience with this population and have assessed approximately 400 patients.

In the material to follow, I will relate some aspects of our clinical experience which might be of value to those who only occasionally are called on to see a patient with epilepsy. The thrust here is purely descriptive and clinical, and the limitations of such a presentation should be clear. Nevertheless, based on our experience over the years, we have made some alterations in our test battery and in our interpretation of particular tests and findings. Some tests and test batteries have been found to be more helpful than others, and our findings have led to other areas of investigation.

The process of neuropsychological assessment will be discussed in terms of conventional neuropsychological domains (psychometric intelligence; academic achievement; language function; visual–perceptual, visual–spatial, and visual–constructional ability; memory and learning ability; problem solving; attentional abilities; and sensorimotor function. Pertinent data will be presented which may help emphasize some of the points discussed.

## Psychometric Intelligence

As would be expected, the WAIS-R is used to assess overall intellectual ability (Table 4.2). The mean Full Scale IQ for our entire population falls in the low average range, and the lowest subtest scores are Information, Vocabulary, and Digit Symbol. Despite the fact that the mean educational attainment of our population is a high school degree, it seems that relative weaknesses revolve around the patients' fund of general information and vocabulary abilities, both measures of old learning in this group of patients with chronic neurological disorder. The sensitivity of Digit Symbol to organic dysfunction is also seen in this population.

While all patients with complex partial seizures have, by definition, an underlying focal lesion, the WAIS-R IQ discrepancy scores are rarely helpful in suggesting the laterality of the lesion. In a sample of 146 patients who were found (through invasive monitoring of spontaneous seizures) to have a unilateral temporal lobe onset, only 21% (31/146) exhibited a significant (i.e., 15 point) Verbal/Performance IQ split. Most interestingly, of the 31 patients who exhibited a 15-point IQ discrepancy, the discrepancy lateralized to the wrong hemisphere (i.e., contralateral to the hemisphere containing the proven epileptogenic lesion) in 36% of the cases (11/31). These findings emphasize the importance of the rest of the neuropsychological battery if information of lateralizing or localizing significance is desired.

On those occasions where there are no localizing or lateralizing signs on the bulk of the neuropsychological battery, but a significant Verbal/Performance IQ difference exists, we look quite hard for other than neurological reasons to explain the existence of that IQ split. Additionally, I have a fair degree of skepticism about overinterpretation of subtest scatter. We have seen enough patients with right temporal lobe epilepsy with a highly significant strength on Picture Arrangement, and left temporal lobe patients with comparable strength on Similarities, to withhold our enthusiasm regarding such findings. In essence, the findings obtained from the WAIS-R are viewed in the context of the findings derived from the entire neuropsychological battery.

TABLE 4.2.   WAIS-R Scores

| Scale | Mean (S.D.) |
| --- | --- |
| Information | 7.6 (2.9) |
| Digit Span | 8.9 (2.7) |
| Vocabulary | 7.6 (2.5) |
| Arithmetic | 8.8 (2.6) |
| Comprehension | 8.0 (2.9) |
| Similarities | 8.1 (2.6) |
| Picture Completion | 8.7 (2.7) |
| Picture Arrangement | 8.7 (2.8) |
| Block Design | 8.9 (2.6) |
| Object Assembly | 8.8 (2.8) |
| Digit Symbol | 7.6 (2.7) |
| Verbal IQ | 88.8 (11.9) |
| Performance IQ | 89.7 (13.1) |
| Full Scale IQ | 88.4 (11.6) |

## Academic Achievement

We have found the assessment of academic achievement (using the WRAT-R) to be quite helpful for a variety of reasons. First, many patients had the onset of their epilepsy in childhood or adolescence; they therefore were subject to a chronic neurological disorder and (usually) were prescribed many different antiepileptic medications (often barbiturate in nature and, at times, in toxic amounts) during their school years. For this reason they were at a disadvantage during their formal education and, not surprisingly, their achievement suffered. Further, it is not uncommon to encounter patients who were excluded from regular classrooms because the school and/or teachers did not want to deal with their seizures, believing them too disruptive to the classroom situation or simply being afraid of the attacks themselves. Unfortunately, some of these children may have been inappropriately placed in special education classrooms, given homebound tutoring, and so on. The end result is a less than adequate education. Of course the severity of the seizures, the underlying neurological abnormality, absences due to seizures and related hospitalizations and doctor visits, and/or the necessity of multiple anticonvulsants could have had pernicious effects as well. The net result is that academic achievement suffered, and the WRAT-R provides a rough estimate of the adequacy of some of their very basic academic abilities. If serious deficiencies are noted, then further, more detailed assessment of academic achievement can be carried out.

The information derived from the WRAT-R can be extremely helpful in the vocational rehabilitation process, and can also suggest when it would not be appropriate to administer self-report measures such as the MMPI because of compromised word reading ability. The WRAT-R can also occasionally provide some information of potential lateralizing value. In our experience, patients with lesions in a diversity of locations exhibit significantly impaired academic achievement. Therefore, task failure in and of itself is not particularly revealing. However, occasionally a patient with a low average to average IQ will have a significantly higher than expected word reading and word spelling ability, despite the fact that their epilepsy was present throughout the course of their formal education. Such instances raise the hypothesis that the lesion underlying their epilepsy is not located in the dominant hemisphere. Again, this needs to be examined in the context of the entire evaluation.

## Language Function

Patients with epilepsy who do not have an underlying structural lesion rarely have a frank language disorder or present with a classic aphasia. That is not to say, however, that some patients do not have subtle, yet significant, impairments in selected language abilities. We have found it quite helpful to carry out formal assessment of language ability using the Multilingual Aphasia Examination (MAE) (Benton & Hamsher, 1983). The MAE is useful for a variety of reasons. First, it allows a very efficient screening of a diversity of important language functions (visual naming, oral associative fluency, oral spelling, repetition, aural and reading comprehension of individual words and phrases, and a brief Token Test). Second, it provides age and education adjustments, something which is very valuable when dealing with patients who oftentimes have disrupted educational histories. Third, the test provides excellent norms with which to compare the patient to normal controls as well as an aphasic population. Finally, the MAE detects subtle language problems in the epilepsy population (such as comprehension, fluency, or dysnomia) which are relevant in the vocational rehabilitation planning process. In our experience, patients (as a group) do not exhibit ceiling effects on the test. In our epilepsy population, the mean scores fall between the 30th and the 50th percentiles; so, despite the relatively easy nature of the tasks, nonaphasic patients with epilepsy do face some considerable challenges on the MAE (Table 4.3). At the level of the individual patient, the two easiest subtests are Aural Comprehension and Reading Comprehension and, therefore, ceiling effects on these subtests constitute a mild problem.

### Visual–Perceptual, Visual–Spatial, and Visual–Constructional Skill

We have relied on the visual–perceptual and visual–spatial tests of Benton, Hamsher, Varney, and Spreen (1983) (Visual Form Discrimination Test, Judgment of Line Orientation Test, Facial Recognition Test) and, occasionally, the Three Dimensional Block Design Test (most helpful in patients who have structural lesions). Additionally, the Rey Complex Figure and the Hooper Visual Organization Test are administered. The Hooper has proven to be of little value in the assessment of epilepsy patients, while the tests devised by Benton have been quite useful.

The Visual Form Discrimination Test appears sensitive to visual alertness/concentration in patients generally, but it does not appear to be of lateralizing value. We have not examined the lateralizing value of the Line Orientation or Facial Recognition Test. But it is the clinical comparison of the intactness of the patients' performance on the language (MAE) versus visual–perceptual/spatial/constructional tests that has been most helpful in our experience. Relative intactness of language abilities in the context of some impaired performances on the visual–perceptual and spatial measures may (considering the rest of the results) suggest the possibility of right hemisphere dysfunction, and vice versa. It is not unusual, however, for a patient with unilateral temporal lobe onset to their seizures to show scattered impairments in both language and visual–spatial abilities (or to be intact on both dimensions). The individual variability among patients can be striking.

Among those patients with a right temporal lobe epileptogenic lesion, we have not noticed any particular pattern of performance on the visual–perceptual and spatial tests. Patients with identical mesial temporal lobe lesions may show any combination of impairments, or even spared performance, on the measures.

TABLE 4.3.   Multilingual Aphasia
Battery Performance

| Scale | Mean (S.D.)[a] |
| --- | --- |
| Visual Naming | 34.6 (31.3) |
| Sentence Repetition | 35.6 (28.7) |
| Oral Fluency | 32.6 (27.9) |
| Oral Spelling | 38.3 (27.3) |
| Token Test | 49.6 (30.1) |
| Aural Comprehension | 45.9 (26.6) |
| Reading Comprehension | 41.6 (24.5) |

[a]Values presented are percentile scores.

Interestingly, we recently examined the ability of the Rey Complex Figure to discriminate patients with left versus right temporal lobe epilepsy. The protocols were rescored, and interrater reliability was above 0.90. There was no significant difference between the left and right temporal lobe groups on the Rey copy. For our own purposes, we are quite cautious in the interpretation of the results derived from the Rey Complex Figure.

## Memory Function

Most patients presenting to our center suffer from partial seizures and, by definition, therefore have an underlying focal lesion. In the vast majority of the patients, the epileptic focus is in one of the temporal lobes. Therefore, a thorough assessment of memory and learning abilities is one of the most important aspects of the evaluation.

For our own purposes, we have created considerable redundancy in the assessment of memory function. Multiple tests of both verbal and nonverbal memory function (in recognition, immediate, and delayed recall formats) are utilized so as to be able to reliably identify and confirm a consistent material-specific memory impairment or asymmetry. In our experience, a patient may score in the impaired range on one measure of verbal recall but perform adequately on two others. Obviously, the interpretation of such findings would differ from that of findings where a patient consistently exhibited impairment on all measures of verbal learning and recall.

At our center the following memory tests are utilized: Wechsler Memory Scale (Form 1) utilizing Russell's (1975, 1988) procedure; the California Verbal Learning Test (Delis, Kramer, Kaplan, & Ober, 1987); the Recognition Memory Test (Warrington, 1984); and the memory administration of the Rey Complex Figure (15-minute delay). This grouping of tests allows assessment of recognition memory, free recall of both verbal and nonverbal material in both immediate and delayed recall conditions, and uses stimuli of varying complexity. Tables 4.4 and 4.5 present some idea as to the mean performances of our surgical population on the WMS and the CVLT. One interesting aspect concerns the relatively large standard deviations. These findings underscore the variability that is observed in this population in general. This variability is also noted when attempting to

TABLE 4.4. California Verbal Learning Test Performance

| Indices | Mean (S.D.) |
| --- | --- |
| Trial 1 | 4.8 (1.6) |
| Trial 2 | 7.5 (2.2) |
| Trial 3 | 8.8 (2.4) |
| Trial 4 | 9.6 (2.4) |
| Trial 5 | 10.3 (2.6) |
| Interference Trial | 4.9 (2.0) |
| Short Delay Recall | 8.2 (3.5) |
| Long Delay Recall | 8.1 (3.6) |
| Total Words Recalled | 41.2 (9.7) |
| Correct Recognitions | 13.6 (2.4) |
| False Positives | 2.8 (3.0) |

TABLE 4.5.   Wechsler Memory Scale
Performance (Form 1)

| Index | Mean (S.D.) |
|---|---|
| Memory Quotient | 89.4 (19.1) |
| Logical Memory (Immediate)[a] | 8.3 (2.8) |
| Logical Memory (% Recalled) | 63.8 (27.9) |
| Visual Reproduction (Immediate)[a] | 8.9 (2.8) |
| Visual Reproduction (% Recalled) | 65.9 (31.5) |
| Associate Learning (Immediate)[a] | 8.9 (2.9) |

[a]These scales are presented in scaled score format per
method of Osborne and Davis (1978) (mean = 10, standard
deviation = 3).

identify material-specific impairments which are believed to be associated with unilateral temporal lobe dysfunction. At the level of group statistics, one often obtains the expected material-specific memory impairments (verbal versus visual) as a function of the laterality of the underlying temporal lobe epileptogenic lesion (as determined by invasive EEG recording of spontaneous seizures). At the level of the individual patient, however, considerable heterogeneity in findings may be observed, including even the opposite of predicted findings.

Invasive monitoring (subdural strip electrodes or depth electrodes) of spontaneous complex partial seizures of temporal lobe origin most frequently indicate seizure onset from the deeper parts of the temporal lobe, particularly hippocampus. Thus, if one is interested in identifying the site of seizure onset, then memory function in general and delayed memory ability in particular become the findings of most interest.

## Problem Solving

Complex partial seizures most commonly originate from one of the temporal lobes, but occasional patients are encountered who have onset of their complex partial seizures from a frontal lobe. Several investigators have suggested ways to try to distinguish complex partial seizures of temporal versus frontal lobe origin; but, at the level of the individual patient, this is difficult to do with adequate reliability and validity. Neuropsychological evaluation may be helpful in this regard via the use of traditional frontal lobe tests. If, for example, performance was impaired on frontal lobe tests in the context of generally intact memory function, then perhaps a frontal lobe origin of the complex partial seizures would be indicated. The opposite might be true in the context of impaired memory function with regard to intact performance on frontal lobe tasks.

The memory measures have been spelled out previously; to assess the integrity of frontal lobe function, we have relied on the Wisconsin Card Sorting Test (Heaton, 1981), particularly the measure of perseverative responding which is derived from the WCST. One problem which has arisen in regard to the differential identification of complex partial seizures of frontal versus temporal lobe origin is that we have found a sizable proportion of patients with complex partial seizures of verified mesial temporal lobe origin to exhibit significantly elevated perseverative responding (defined as over 19 perseverative responses by Heaton) (Hermann, Wyler, & Richey, 1988). Following an anterior temporal lobectomy, patients do not, as a group, become more perseverative, suggesting that it is not the temporal lobe dysfunction which causes the perseverative responding. There are other possible explanations.

First, there are considerable interconnections between the temporal and frontal regions, and therefore the frontal dysfunction which is noted in temporal lobe epilepsy (i.e., perseverative response tendency) might possibly be caused by propagation of epileptiform activity to the frontal regions. Second, the perseverative responding might be an artifact of more general or widespread compromise of cortical areas. However, in our sample, some 20 to 30% of patients show this perseverative tendency, and all of the patients have a neurological disorder which has been long-standing. Third, the perseverative tendency might be related to some index of the damage caused by repeated seizures or may correlate with the lifetime number of generalized tonic–clonic attacks. Whatever the cause, it does appear that (among patients with chronic temporal lobe epilepsy) indices of "frontal lobe dysfunction" may be obtained when there is no verifiable frontal lobe pathology revealed via either ictal onset of spontaneous seizures, neuroimaging, or clinical neurological exam. Yet it is a clear functional deficit.

We have started to incorporate some of the Luria-like frontal lobe tasks in order to determine whether there is some correspondence between perseverative performance on the WCST and failure on the Luria tasks. Symmetry in findings would lend greater confidence to the interpretation of the results.

## Sensorimotor Function

We utilize the conventional measures of motor function (Grooved Pegboard, Finger Oscillation Test, Grip Strength) and some of Benton's measures of tactile–perceptual function (Tactile Form Perception, Finger Identification Test). The sensory findings are rarely of lateralizing significance in the absence of a structural lesion.

Motor asymmetries are occasionally noted on some of the motor tasks, but rarely do all three measures provide consistent lateralizing information in the absence of a structural lesion. In fact, it is not uncommon for the motor measures to provide contradictory information. In this regard it may be helpful to remember that even when motor asymmetries are obtained in the absence of a structural lesion they may be of some false localizing value. The amygdala is traditionally considered to be among the structures composing the basal ganglia and therefore to play some role in motor function. The amygdala is also among the subcortical structures affected by epilepsy, and it is theoretically possible that motor asymmetries could be so affected. Such an explanation would predict that motor asymmetries should be exacerbated following anterior temporal lobectomy, which most often includes resection of the amygdala; however, this has not been the case in our experience. As suggested previously, it may be possible that motor function could be affected by spread of interictal epileptiform activity from mesial temporal to frontal areas. In such a case, one might predict normalization of motor function in the hand contralateral to the operated hemisphere postoperatively. This, however, has not been the case either. As a result, we place only mild confidence in the motor findings in the absence of an underlying structural lesion.

## EMOTIONAL AND BEHAVIORAL ASSESSMENT

As will become clear in the material to follow, epilepsy is a disorder which has the potential to affect many different facets of a patient's life. Therefore, a comprehensive neuropsychological evaluation should include assessment of possible complications in behavioral, social, and emotional adjustment. In the space available we will not cover traditional assessment procedures such as the MMPI or projective assessment procedures. Rather, the emphasis in this section will concern issues related to psychological and social adjustment in epilepsy and the available procedures and measures with which to assess these special problems.

### Overall Psychosocial Status

In the 1970s Congress established a special commission, the Commission for the Control of Epilepsy and Its Consequences, to survey the current status of epilepsy in the United States. The Commission was instructed to assess many different issues related to epilepsy (including gaps in treatment, education, and research) as well as the problems and needs exhibited by patients with epilepsy and their families. The final report was a landmark document. The Commission reported on the effects of epilepsy on the family unit, relationships between epilepsy and emotional problems, vocational difficulties, academic achievement, financial stress, problems in housing and transportation, the limited training and education that a diversity of professional groups receive about epilepsy, and other important problems faced by people with epilepsy. What becomes very evident is that the assessment of patients with epilepsy requires a broad approach in order to take into consideration the special problems and stresses inherent in the disorder.

The Washington Psychosocial Seizure Inventory (WPSI) can be a helpful measure with which to assess the current psychosocial status of patients with epilepsy (Dodrill, Batzel, Quiesser, & Temkin, 1980). This is a 132-item self-report inventory presented in a yes–no format that assesses a variety of concerns especially pertinent to epilepsy (Family Background, Interpersonal Adjustment, Emotional Adjustment, Vocational Adjustment, Financial Status, Adjustment to Seizures, Medicine and Medical Management, and Overall Psychosocial Functioning). The inventory was devised specifically for the assessment of patients with epilepsy and yields information which is largely complementary to MMPI assessment.

Some of the WPSI scales are particularly helpful. The Vocational and Financial Status scales can help to detect employment difficulties as well as the patient's dissatisfaction with his/her current vocational situation and the financial stresses associated with such a state of affairs. Detection of vocational difficulties is important because referral to the state Department of Rehabilitation Services is often a particularly helpful referral. Surprisingly, it is not uncommon for patients to be unaware of the special services which might be available to them because of their epilepsy.

The Adjustment to Epilepsy scale can also be particularly helpful. Oftentimes patients resent having epilepsy and live in a state of fear regarding the possibility of a seizure, an event which can happen anywhere, anytime, and with little or no warning. Along with the fear of the event itself, the patient may fear embarrassment, disclosure of their epilepsy for all to see, and the potential social consequences of having a seizure in public. Further, some patients resent having to take anticonvulsant medications which can be expensive, have significant side effects, and still not completely control the seizures. The Adjustment to Seizures scale of the WPSI can help assess these problems which can subsequently be a focus of discussion or intervention. The essential point is that the WPSI facilitates an efficient screening of many specific issues related to epilepsy. An adolescent/children's form has just been made available which will help in the screening of special difficulties associated with epilepsy in the developmental years (e.g., academic achievement problems).

An important concept related to the above discussion concerns what has been called "fear of seizures" by Mittan (1986). In a series of detailed interviews with patients with epilepsy, Mittan found that many patients harbored a diversity of misperceptions and fears concerning their epilepsy. For instance, in Mittan's sample, many patients were concerned that they might actually die during a seizure. While there is an increased risk of sudden, unexplained, and unexpected death in epilepsy, the risk is very small. However, patients' perceptions were that the possibility of death was high. In addition to misperceptions regarding the risk to life associated with epilepsy, patients felt that the development of emotional distress, cognitive deterioration, and other adverse events were similarly relatively probable events.

Having these misperceptions regarding the nature and course of epilepsy is troublesome enough, but the patients in Mittan's sample appeared to act on these misperceptions. Sizable proportions of his sample espoused so-called "hazardous first-aid practices," such as wanting objects put in their mouth to keep them from swallowing their tongue, wanting to be restrained or held down during seizures, or wanting an ambulance called with each seizure. These are all unnecessary, unhelpful, and potentially harmful procedures. Further, patients commonly altered their prescribed antiepilepsy drug regimen. For example, some patients would take extra medications if they felt like they might have a seizure that day; they would also take extra medications after a seizure occurred, in hopes of preventing the occurrence of another seizure. They might skip their medications if they felt good and believed that they were unlikely to have a seizure that day. All these alterations are, of course, unhelpful as the pharmacokinetics of the medications (drug half-life, steady state) are what determine seizure control.

Therefore, it should be assumed that oftentimes many patients, even very intelligent patients, will harbor misperceptions of epilepsy and its treatment, will have many seizure-related concerns and fears, and might act on these misperceptions and fears in ways that are not in their best interests. As noted above, the Adjustment to Seizures scale of the WPSI can be helpful in this regard. Additionally, Mittan (1986) has developed a very concise Fear of Seizures scale which can be quite helpful in the assessment of these seizure-related concerns. Recently, Goldstein et al. (1990) developed a revised Fear of Seizures scale, the items of which are on a 5-point Likert scale format. This is very helpful because the degree to which a patient believes that these harmful events might occur can be assessed.

When patients are found who do harbor such fears, we have found that a variety of patient education procedures can be quite helpful. There are now several books written for patients with epilepsy and their families which are well written and address many of these issues. We have also found epilepsy self-help groups to be very helpful. The self-help groups are typically coordinated through the local chapters of the Epilepsy Foundation of America and can be exceptionally helpful in providing patients with education, supportive counseling, and tips as to particularly helpful social service agencies which might meet especially salient needs; they can also serve as a general social outlet.

## Social Support

Epilepsy can be associated with considerable social exclusion. Sometimes this exclusion is exhibited by the family as well as by society at large. At times families exhibit embarrassment regarding a child/sibling with epilepsy, sometimes to the extent that the family member with epilepsy is excluded from a variety of family activities. Similarly, the individual with epilepsy may have a very limited circle of friends, little dating experience, fewer opportunities for marriage, and so on. In such instances the amount of social support that is available to the patient may be limited, and the support which is available may be superficial. Hence, assessment of the quantity and quality of available social support is helpful, and we have utilized the social support questionnaire developed by Sarason, Levine, Basham, & Sarason (1983).

## Life Events

Patients with epilepsy can be vulnerable to a wide variety of stressful life events. Sudden cessation of relationships (even marriage) may occur when epilepsy becomes manifest. Employment, housing, financial security, educational opportunities, transportation alternatives, and other important facets of life can be extremely precarious for patients with epilepsy. We have found it quite helpful to inquire as to significant life events experienced by our patients in the past year. We utilize the Life Experiences Survey of Sarason, Johnson, and Siegel (1978). This allows assessment of a wide range of life events and also allows the respondent to indicate the degree of adversity, or support, caused by the life event in question. This information can also be related to any existent depression or other psychopathology which may be evident.

## Personality

There has been considerable interest in the existence of unusual personality traits in persons with epilepsy. In 1975 Waxman and Geschwind proposed the existence of an interictal syndrome of personality change associated with temporal lobe epilepsy consisting of deepened emotionality, increased religiosity, and hypergraphia. In 1977 the syndrome was expanded by Bear and Fedio to include a larger grouping of 18 traits that were hypothesized to reflect alterations in behavior, affect, and cognition.

The existence of such a syndrome remains of some interest, but it is extremely controversial. In our experience, we occasionally see unusual patients who exhibit a subset of the proposed personality syndrome, but the proportion of patients who show this syndrome is quite small. Nevertheless, the interested neuropsychologist may want to assess the patient for such traits. There are a variety of approaches which are available. First, there is the self-report format which was pioneered by Bear and Fedio. There has been some research into the psychometrics of their inventory and a number of limitations have been noted. A revised and reformatted questionnaire was developed by Stark-Adamec and Adamec (1986). In addition to changing the response format from true–false to a Likert scale, they have investigated the factor structure of the inventory; they also have carried out some investigations inquiring as to the specificity of the traits to temporal lobe epilepsy in particular, epilepsy in general, and, more broadly, chronic illness.

Another assessment methodology consists of semistructured interviews. Dan Mungas and his colleagues (1990) have developed an RDC-like procedure to assess many of the key interictal personality and behavioral traits. The interrater reliability, factor structure, and other important psychometric features of the interview procedure have been investigated by Mungas *et al.* and compared to the self-report format. We used the interview methodology and found it to be an efficient technique which bypasses many of the difficulties inherent in a self-report format.

## Miscellaneous Comments

Finally, a few words should be offered about traditional assessment. We utilize the MMPI in the assessment of the patients who present to our center. As shown in Table 4.6, the two-point code type for our patients is 2–8/8–2.

There is a general elevation of the clinical scales across the MMPI, with emphasis on scales 2 and 8. It should be remembered that the data presented concern patients with relatively intractable seizures; and, therefore, these MMPI results cannot be generalized to the entire population of patients with epilepsy. It has been demonstrated recently that WPSI and MMPI assessment of a community sample of adults with epilepsy produced markedly lower scores (Trostle, 1988). It does appear, however, that patients with intractable seizures who present to tertiary care centers are in considerable emotional distress.

The psychologist who sees patients with epilepsy on a fairly regular basis should be aware of the possible interictal behavioral and emotional complications which include sexual dysfunction, schizophrenia-like psychoses, and other problems (Hermann & Whitman, 1984). Perhaps the problem to be most aware of is depression. Despite the large literature devoted to interesting problems such as personality change, interictal psychosis, and aggressive outbursts, we have found the problem of major depression to be more

TABLE 4.6. MMPI Results

| Scale | Mean (S.D.) |
|-------|-------------|
| L | 54.90 (11.20) |
| F | 58.99 (10.95) |
| K | 51.10 (9.50) |
| Hs | 61.60 (10.99) |
| D | 64.50 (14.20) |
| Hy | 61.70 (12.40) |
| Pd | 60.70 (12.20) |
| Mf | 53.50 (10.70) |
| Pa | 57.90 (10.70) |
| Pt | 60.01 (11.40) |
| Sc | 65.03 (12.50) |
| Ma | 60.20 (11.70) |
| Si | 55.60 (10.70) |

frequent, life-threatening, and injurious to the patients' quality of life. In some cases the anticonvulsant medications, mainly the barbiturates, can contribute to the problem, but the etiology underlying the depression may be biological, social, or both. The important point is that the neuropsychologist should conduct a thorough assessment of emotional/behavioral status, with clear attention to depressive symptomatology.

## CONCLUSION

The neuropsychologist is often in a position to make a significant contribution to improving the quality of life of patients with epilepsy. In order to do so, a comprehensive assessment of current cognitive and emotional/behavioral status is required, along with a knowledge of relevant professionals and community/state/federal agencies which are mandated to provide specialized services to patients with chronic disorders such as epilepsy. An understanding of epilepsy and its potential effects on cognition and social and emotional adjustment will color the psychologist's approach to assessing patients with epilepsy, and it is hoped that this chapter will help in that regard.

## REFERENCES

Bear, D., & Fedio, P. (1977). Quantitative analysis of interictal behavior in temporal lobe epilepsy. *Archives of Neurology, 34*, 454–467.

Benton, A. L., & Hamsher, K. (1983). *Multilingual Aphasia Examination Manual*. Iowa City, IA: AJA Associates, Inc.

Benton, A. L., Hamsher, K., Varney, N. R., & Spreen, O. (1983). *Contributions to neuropsychological assessment: A clinical manual*. New York: Oxford University Press.

Delis, D. C., Kramer, J. H., Kaplan, E., & Ober, B. A. (1987). *California Verbal Learning Test: Research Edition Manual*. New York: The Psychological Corporation.

Dodrill, C. B. (1981). Neuropsychology of epilepsy. In S. B. Filskov & T. J. Boll (Eds.), *Handbook of clinical neuropsychology*. New York: Wiley.

Dodrill, C. B., Batzel, L. W., Quiesser, H. R., & Temkin, N. R. (1980). An objective method for the assessment of psychological and social difficulties among epileptics. *Epilepsia, 21*, 123–135.

Goldstein, J., Seidenberg, M., & Peterson, R. (1990). Fear of seizures and behavioral functioning in adults with epilepsy. *Journal of Epilepsy, 3*, 101–106.

Heaton, R. K. (1981). *Wisconsin Card Sorting Test Manual*. Odessa, FL: Psychological Assessment Resources.

Hermann, B. P., & Whitman, S. (1984). Behavioral and personality correlates of epilepsy: A review, methodological critique, and conceptual model. *Psychological Bulletin, 95*, 451–497.

Hermann, B. P., Wyler, A. R., & Richey, E. T. (1988). Wisconsin Card Sorting Test performance in patients with complex partial seizures of temporal lobe origin. *Journal of Clinical & Experimental Neuropsychology, 10*, 467–476.

Laidlaw, J., & Richens, A. (Eds.). (1982). *A textbook of epilepsy* (2nd ed.). Edinburgh: Churchill Livingstone.

Mittan, R. J. (1986). Fear of seizures. In S. Whitman & B. P. Hermann (Eds.), *Psychopathology in epilepsy: Social dimensions*. New York: Oxford University Press.

Mostofsky, D. I. (1978). Epilepsy: Returning the ghost to psychology. *Professional Psychology, 9*, 87–92.

Mungas, D., Blunden, D., Bennington, K., Stone, A., & Palma, G. (1990). Reliability and validity of scales for assessing behavior in epilepsy. *Psychological Assessment, 2*, 423–431.

National Institutes of Health. (1978). *National Commission for the Control of Epilepsy and Its Consequences. Plan for Nationwide Action on Epilepsy*. (DHEW Publication No. NIH 78-276). Washington, DC: Author.

Osborne, D., & Davis, L. J. (1978). Standard scores for Wechsler Memory Scale subtests. *Journal of Clinical Psychology, 34*, 115–116.

Rausch, R. (1985). Differences in cognitive function with left and right temporal lobe dysfunction. In D. F. Benson & E. Zaidel (Eds.), *The dual brain: Hemispheric specialization in humans*. New York: Guilford Press.

Russell , E. W. (1975). A multiple scoring method for the assessment of complex memory functions. *Journal of Consulting & Clinical Psychology*, *43*, 800–809.

Russell, E. W. (1988). Renorming Russell's version of the Wechsler Memory Scale. *Journal of Clinical & Experimental Neuropsychology*, *10*, 235–249.

Sarason, I. G., Johnson, J. H. , & Siegel, J. M. (1978). Assessing the impact of life changes: Development of the Life Experiences Survey. *Journal of Consulting & Clinical Psychology*, *46*, 932–946.

Sarason, I. G., Levine, H. M., Basham, R. B., & Sarason, B. R. (1983). Assessing social support. The Social Support Questionnaire. *Journal of Personality & Social Psychology*, *44*, 127–139.

Stark-Adamec, C., & Adamec, R. E. (1986). Psychological methodology versus clinical impressions: different perspectives on psychopathology and seizures. In B. K. Doane & K. E. Livingston (Eds.), *The Limbic System: Functional Organization and Clinical Disorders*. New York: Raven Press.

Trostle, J. A. (1988). Social aspects of epilepsy. In W. A. Hauser (Ed.), *Current trends in epilepsy*. Landover, MD: Epilepsy Foundation of America.

Warrington, E. K. (1984). *Recognition Memory Test manual*. Berkshire, England: NFER–Nelson Publishing Co.

Waxman, S. G., & Geschwind, N. (1975). The interictal behavior syndrome of temporal lobe epilepsy. *Archives of General Psychiatry*, *32*, 1580–1588.

# 5

# Neuropathology and Neuropsychology of Behavioral Disturbances following Traumatic Brain Injury

## ROBERT L. MAPOU

The nature of traumatic brain injury (TBI) determines many of the neuropathological features with high predictability. The neuropathological sequelae directly influence the cognitive deficits which occur. These, in turn, impact upon the types of behavioral disturbances associated with TBI. Such disturbances can be distinguished from those seen in other behaviorally disturbed individuals, including those who are developmentally disabled, focally injured, or progressively demented.

This chapter will present hypotheses about the cognitive basis of behavioral disorders which frequently follow TBI. It will also illustrate the application of knowledge about cognitive function to behavioral treatment. First, a brief overview of the neuropathology of TBI will be presented. This will be followed by discussion of the types of cognitive deficits associated with this neuropathology, within the context of a framework of cognition. Illustrations of behavioral disorders associated with specific types of cognitive impairment will be provided next. Included will be examples of behavioral difficulties, treatment options, and case illustrations. The chapter will conclude with some final considerations for behavioral treatment following TBI.

ROBERT L. MAPOU • HIV Behavioral Medicine Research Program, Henry M. Jackson Foundation for the Advancement of Military Medicine, Rockville, Maryland 20850.

*HANDBOOK OF HEAD TRAUMA: Acute Care to Recovery*, edited by Charles J. Long and Leslie K. Ross. Plenum Press, New York, 1992.

## NEUROPATHOLOGY OF TBI

The neuropathology of TBI due to acceleration–deceleration events of the type seen in motor vehicle accidents has been well documented (Auerbach, 1986; Jennett & Teasdale, 1981; Levin, Benton, & Grossman, 1982; Teasdale & Mendelow, 1984). The neuropathological effects are produced by two main events: (1) sudden acceleration and deceleration of the brain within the skull, and (2) focal contact between the brain and the skull. The sequelae of these events are called the *primary* effects of TBI and may include: (1) diffuse cortical white matter (axonal) injury due to stretching and shearing of nerve pathways as the brain rotates on its axis,* (2) similar stretching and shearing of subcortical pathways and the brain stem, and (3) focal damage (contusions, lacerations) to cortical and subcortical brain areas. In particular, the underside of the frontal lobes (orbito-frontal region) and the anterior aspects of the temporal lobes are in close proximity to rough, bony skull and often are abraded when the brain suddenly rotates due to rapid acceleration. Thus, regardless of the location of external impact to the skull, focal damage almost always occurs in orbitofrontal and anterior temporal regions of the cortex.

Blood vessel rupture may result in localized hematomas, which occur most commonly under the dura (e.g., subdural hematoma). Hemorrhaging may occur within the brain (intracerebral hemorrhage) or into the ventricles (intraventricular hemorrhage), and cellular destruction may remain even after the blood has dissipated or has been drained surgically.

There are also several *secondary* effects of TBI. Increased intracranial pressure may be produced by hemorrhaging, edema, or hydrocephalus, often in combination with systemic hypotension, and can lead to focal ischemic damage. Another secondary effect is hypoxia due to systemic hemorrhage or shock, respiratory arrest or chest trauma, vomiting and aspiration, or cardiac arrest. Results of hypoxia may include focal ischemia, especially in watershed regions, or diffuse encephalopathy. Finally, air emboli or small blood clots from primary damage may cause blood vessel blockage and focal ischemic damage.

In sum, the neuropathology of TBI includes diffuse damage to brain pathways, particularly those from the brain stem, and focal damage to frontal and temporal regions. Although these are the most predictable effects of TBI, heterogeneity of neuropathology may be produced by focal damage to other brain regions.

## FRAMEWORK OF COGNITIVE FUNCTIONING

Mapou (1988) presented a framework of cognitive functioning which could be used to guide neuropsychological evaluation. Table 5.1 presents a revised and simplified version of this framework, much of which is derived from the work of Luria (1980).

The framework is hierarchical, and functional integrity at lower levels of complexity (e.g., attention) is usually necessary for full application of functions at higher levels of complexity (e.g., learning). Arousal/attention and executive/motor functions are viewed as basic inputs and outputs, respectively, for the central nervous system. Arousal/attention and

---

*Recent research has suggested that diffuse axonal injury is not simply due to stretching and shearing, but, rather, that axons are "shocked" by accelerational forces and later lose their biochemical and functional integrity. For recent data, see Povlishock (1989).

TABLE 5.1.  Framework of Cognition
for Neuropsychological Evaluation

Arousal and attentional functions
Motor and somatosensory functions
Executive functions
Language functions
Visuospatial functions
Reasoning and problem-solving abilities
Learning and memory functions

executive functions are modality and material nonspecific and tend to be disrupted by any process affecting the brain diffusely. Language and visuospatial functions are material-specific and more focal. Reasoning and problem solving, and learning and memory are more integrated functions, generally requiring intactness of all other cognitive realms (e.g., to learn and remember requires adequate attention and executive functions for encoding, intact ability to consolidate and retain information, and retrieval skills).

## CONSIDERATIONS FOR NEUROPSYCHOLOGICAL ANALYSIS OF BEHAVIORAL DISORDERS

Given the described neuropathological effects of TBI, it is possible to predict certain types of cognitive disturbances. Damage to the brain stem and ascending reticular activating system is associated with the onset of coma and subsequent deficits in arousal and attention (Auerbach, 1986). The frontal lobes and associated pathways also mediate aspects of attention, and damage there is likely to produce impairment. Additionally, deficits in executive function and in reasoning and problem solving are common sequelae of frontal lobe injury (Levin *et al.*, 1982; Levin, Grafman, & Eisenberg, 1987). Finally, damage to the temporal lobes and deeper limbic structures may lead to memory impairment, beyond difficulties produced in new learning by deficits in executive functions (organization) and attention. In sum, the most common deficits observed following TBI are in (1) arousal and attention, (2) executive functioning, (3) reasoning and problem solving, and (4) learning and memory (Ben-Yishay & Diller, 1983; Brooks, 1984; Levin *et al.*, 1982; Prigatano & Fordyce, 1986; Wood, 1987). Deficits in language and/or visuospatial functioning may occur, but tend to be less common and related to focal cortical lesions.

Cognitive deficits must be considered when designing behavioral interventions; otherwise they may fail. Interventions should be developed which "teach to" the TBI patient's spared cognitive functions, while avoiding deficit areas (Crosson, 1987; Malec, 1984; Muir, Haffey, Ott, Karaica, Muir, & Sutko, 1983; Wood, 1984, 1987). Thus, neuropsychological evaluation is an important component of behavioral intervention planning. Pretrauma factors must also be considered, however, as behavioral problems due to cognitive deficits arising from TBI *may* be easier to treat than behavioral problems which existed prior to injury. For example, it is well established that personality disorders are extremely difficult to treat, even in individuals without cognitive deficits. If a person has developed a habitual pattern of behavior prior to injury, it is unlikely that this pattern will change substantially following injury. Thus, rather than attempting to change what the person was like pretrauma, behavioral rehabilitation should focus on approximating the patient's pretrauma behavior.

What follows is a description of behavioral difficulties associated with specific cognitive impairments, along with suggestions for treatment and case illustrations. This description is theoretical, based upon the author's clinical experience, and has been found to be useful when developing behavioral treatments. It remains to collect empirical data which support the descriptions provided. Excluded from discussion are disorders associated with impaired emotional functioning due to damage in deeper brain structures (e.g., limbic system, hypothalamus). Such disorders include secondary affective disorder, intermittent explosive disorder (episodic dyscontrol), and psychosis, which are covered elsewhere (see Silver, Yudofsky, & Hales, 1987).

## DISORDERS OF AROUSAL AND ATTENTION

Impairments in one or more aspects of arousal and attention are ubiquitous following TBI (Auerbach, 1986; Levin *et al.*, 1982, 1987; Van Zomeren, 1981; Van Zomeren & Brouwer, 1987; Van Zomeren, Brouwer, & Deelman, 1984; Wood, 1987) and range from mild to severe. A framework may help to delineate the specific types of impairment. Table 5.2 presents a number of components of attention, based upon empirical work of others, such as Barkley (1989), Mirsky (1987), Parasuraman (1985), Posner (1987), Stuss (1987; Stuss, Stethem, & Pelchat, 1988; Stuss, Stethem, & Poirer, 1987), and Van Zomeren & Brouwer (1987). To some degree, the components are hierarchical, and adequate function at one level requires intact function of those at underlying levels. Although impairments may be observed in all aspects of attention, there may be dissociations (e.g., focused and sustained attention may be intact, in the presence of impairment in span of attention and resistance to interference). The following are examples of commonly observed behavioral difficulties resulting from these impairments.

TABLE 5.2.   Arousal and Attentional Functions

| Function | Definition |
|---|---|
| Lower-order functions (deployment) | |
| Arousal | General level of alertness |
| Orienting response | Automatic, nonpurposeful direction of attention to a stimulus |
| Selective attention | Voluntary direction of attention to a stimulus |
| Shifting attention | Voluntary shifting of attention among stimuli |
| Sustained attention | Maintaining attention on a task without fatigue or performance decrement |
| Higher-order functions (encoding) | |
| Span of attention | Amount of information that can be held consciously in mind at any one moment |
| Resistance to interference | Ability to reaccess old information following performance of a brief task (10 to 20 seconds) |
| Mental manipulation | Ability to hold information in mind, manipulate it, and produce a result |

## Decreased Arousal during Emergence from Coma

At this stage of recovery, arousal is suboptimal, and the patient is usually confused and unable to process information efficiently or completely. Thus, external events are not perceived fully and may be experienced as novel, stressful, and frightening. Reactions which emerge from this confusion are generally undirected and nonspecific, and may include thrashing, yelling, pulling at tubes, or grabbing at moving stimuli. Patients at Levels III and IV of the Rancho Los Amigos Scale of Cognitive Function (Malkmus, Booth, & Kodimer, 1980) present with these types of difficulties.

Behavioral interventions at this stage are relatively simple. Environmental and social stimulation of the patient should be limited. The patient may be given orientation information frequently, since she or he will not retain it. Structured, focused sensory stimulation can also be helpful. By providing attention when the patient is calm rather than agitated, calmness can be positively reinforced. Psychopharmacological interventions may also improve arousal and focused attention, and may include reduction of sedating medications (anticonvulsants, antipsychotics, anxiolytics), use of alternative medications with less sedation (e.g., substituting carbamazepine for phenytoin or phenobarbital), or use of psychostimulants, tricyclic antidepressants, or dopamine agonists (e.g., bromocriptine). Although there have been reports of improvements with such changes, empirical data are limited (Cope, 1987; Evans, Gualtieri, & Patterson, 1987; Glenn, 1986, 1987a,b,c; Gualtieri, 1987; Rose, 1988).

## Persisting Confusional State

This type of patient appears awake and alert, but is persistently disoriented and confused, due to impaired attention. If ambulatory, the patient may wander. Attentional impairments decrease new learning, and the patient is likely to have difficulty benefiting from a behavioral program. Because she or he is verbal and ambulatory, however, staff may assume that the patient is functioning at a higher cognitive level than is actually the case.

Initially, the behavior may have to be controlled through use of one-to-one supervision, and major change is unlikely. An assessment should be made as to whether the patient is able to learn procedurally (i.e., through repetitive actions which do not require conscious recollection). If so, behavioral programs which involve simple response–reinforcer relationships and massed practice can be introduced. Psychopharmacological interventions may be useful to optimize attentional function, although published data demonstrating efficacy are quite limited (Cope, 1987).

> *Case Example.* AA was a 55-year-old male who was 20 months post-TBI, which occurred when he fell backwards off of a porch. AA suffered bilateral frontal and temporal contusions. Although awake, ambulatory, and verbal, he presented with impairments in all aspects of attention, and with receptive and expressive dysphasia. Behaviorally, he wandered, struck out at staff, had difficulty communicating, and was noncompliant in therapy. Initially, he was supervised one-to-one and treated with lithium carbonate, with lorazepam given for extreme agitation. As he exhibited rudimentary learning abilities, a behavioral program was developed in which every 15 minutes of his day was scheduled, with structured activities and one-to-one supervision by staff. Immediate positive reinforcement or limit setting occurred in response to his behavior. Behavioral improvement (decreased frequency of outbursts, increased therapy cooperation) occurred within two weeks.

## Decreased Information Processing Efficiency

At a later stage of recovery, a patient may not appear to have arousal/attentional difficulties, but impairments in higher-order attentional functions are likely to be found on neuropsychological evaluation. Attentional impairments can contribute to decreased language comprehension and/or to decreased new learning. Since the patient may not be fully aware of the problem, compensation for difficulties is unlikely. Impairments in attention can contribute to lowered frustration tolerance and associated agitation.

Psychopharmacological interventions may be used to optimize attentional functioning. Behavioral interventions may become more advanced and may focus on helping the patient to become aware of his/her difficulties and to use compensatory strategies (e.g., requesting repetition, asking speaker to slow down, writing down information). Group and individual psychotherapy may also help to promote awareness and use of strategies. Use of more than one type of stimulus presentation (e.g., verbal instructions, pictures, gestures) may maximize the amount of information which is encoded.

> *Case Example (Mapou, 1987).* BB was a 38-year-old male, 18 months post-TBI after being struck while riding his bicycle. He sustained bitemporal hematomas and a left frontal intracerebral hemorrhage. Neuropsychological testing revealed decreased selective and sustained attention, mildly impaired span of attention, and severely impaired resistance to interference. Behaviorally, BB was noncompliant in therapy and yelled when he did not get his way. He was treated with a low dose of methylphenidate, and dramatic improvement in his behavior was noted. A double-blind, placebo-controlled methylphenidate trial confirmed these improvements, and the medication was maintained. BB subsequently entered a functional skills program and made continued gains in independent living skills.

## Effects of Stress and/or Fatigue on a Fragile System

In higher functioning patients (e.g., those in independent living and/or vocational programs), arousal and attentional problems are less obvious. Impairment may not show on many neuropsychological measures, because these are highly structured. Problems can emerge, however, under conditions of stress, change, or ambiguity, which place demands on complex attentional skills. Behavioral difficulties can also occur when the patient is fatigued, especially later in the day. Problems may be manifested in various ways, including fidgeting, decreased frustration tolerance, or refusal to participate in tasks.

Individual and group psychotherapeutic treatment can be used to help the patient develop insight into his/her difficulties and to anticipate when problems might occur. Behavioral techniques, such as relaxation training, may be helpful to manage stress. Pharmacological interventions such as beta-blockers or carbamazepine for episodic dyscontrol may be used if behavioral problems are severe (Glenn, 1987b).

> *Case Example.* CC was a 33-year-old female who had sustained a TBI in a motor vehicle accident 30 months earlier. She suffered a right temporal hematoma and a right frontal skull fracture. She showed no deficits in lower-order attention, and her span of attention and resistance to interference were within normal limits, although she had slight encoding deficits when information exceeded her span. She was in a vocational rehabilitation program and was generally performing well and learning new tasks (running a computer data base to do payroll management). She easily became frustrated and overloaded, however, when presented with what she perceived as too much new information at once. Her deficits interacted with her high expectations of herself, further increasing her frustration. During these incidents, she became angry and verbally abusive toward her trainers,

and required time away from her work to calm. When reviewing her behavior later, she was able to express awareness of the difficulty and regret for what had occurred. When the problem became so severe that she was at risk for discharge from the program, she was placed on a beta-blocker. Intensive individual and group psychotherapy was used to help her adjust to her disability and to develop cognitive–behavioral strategies to remain calm. She gradually became able to anticipate difficulties, and was able to rest or to remove herself temporarily from her work before losing control. She completed her program successfully, received a job placement, and moved from the rehabilitation center into her own apartment.

## DISORDERS OF EXECUTIVE FUNCTIONING

Executive functions are basic behavioral control functions which allow one to plan, initiate, and execute goal-directed behavior for problem solving, especially in novel, unfamiliar situations (Lezak, 1983; Luria, 1980). In contrast to arousal and attention, which may be conceptualized as basic *input* to the central nervous system, executive functions may be conceptualized as basic *output*. At the simplest level, this includes motor functions. In terms of more complex functioning, this includes the ability to establish, maintain, and shift response set as a function of changing task demands, and associated abilities to monitor one's behavior, to think flexibly and to apply feedback to correct one's errors, and to modulate emotional expression. Additionally, these functions can be conceptualized as central processing mechanisms, which allow an individual to mediate internally his/her responses to external events. These functions are typically associated with the frontal lobes (Luria, 1980; Stuss & Benson, 1986) and are impaired by focal frontal lobe damage, but also by diffuse damage to efferent and afferent frontal pathways.

Executive functions are some of the most advanced and complex cognitive functions, and even mild impairment can substantially disrupt daily functioning (Luria, 1980; Stuss & Benson, 1986). Because of the prevalence of frontal lobe damage in TBI, impairments in executive functioning are common (Brooks, 1984; Levin et al., 1982; Stuss, 1987). Clinically, it is the author's opinion that impairments in attention and executive functioning account for the majority of acquired behavioral difficulties following TBI. A variety of commonly observed impairments in executive functioning are listed in Table 5.3, and this is followed by descriptions of associated behavioral difficulties.

### Disinhibition—Failure of Normal Controls on Behavior

Disinhibited behaviors of a sexual, aggressive, or less threatening nature are frequent after TBI (Wood, 1987). Contributing impairments in executive functioning include impulsivity, inability to control emotional expression, inability to self-monitor and self-correct behavior, and lack of awareness of and concern about the impact of one's behavior on others. Disinhibited behavior should be differentiated from agitation due to attentional disorders on the basis of the patient's level of awareness. This type of difficulty is usually seen in a patient who is fully awake and alert, and is often thought by staff "to know better." Patients who are disinhibited may also evidence "knowing without doing" (Luria, 1980). They may be able to express what the correct behavior should be in a given situation, but are unable to guide their behavior by this knowledge.

Treatment of disinhibited behavior is often difficult and lengthy (Wood, 1987).

TABLE 5.3.    Impairments of Executive Functions

Decreased ability to plan, initiate, and execute behavior
Decreased motivation
Decreased flexibility of thinking
Decreased awareness of behavioral alternatives
Decreased organization and sequencing
Impulsivity
Decreased self-monitoring and self-correcting
"Knowing without doing"
Perseveration
Stimulus-bound behavior
Lack of awareness or concern about impact of behavior
Loss of emotional control
Regression to immature forms of behavior

Environmental modifications, including changes in the actions of others (e.g., repetitive reminders), may work best. Highly structured behavioral programs should include limit setting, teaching alternative behaviors, and frequent positive reinforcement for appropriate behavior. When executive impairments are profound and the patient shows no carryover from repetition and feedback, it may not be possible to discontinue a behavior program, and permanent programming may be necessary.

> *Case Example.* DD was a 29-year-old male, 24 months post-TBI after being struck by a car and suffering a right temporal contusion. He exhibited decreased organizational and sequencing skills, impaired planning, impulsivity, and poor emotional control when stressed. EE was a 33-year-old female, 9 months post-TBI due to a fall while intoxicated, from which she suffered a left subdural hematoma, left hemisphere contusions in the frontal, temporal, and occipital lobes and internal capsule, and a right subdural hematoma. Her cognitive impairments included severe language production deficits, decreased planning and sequencing skills, decreased flexibility of thinking, but some ability to respond to feedback. The two patients formed a friendship, which subsequently led to public masturbation. When their behavior was discussed with them, they expressed embarrassment and the need for control. Despite knowledge, however, they were unable to control their behavior. Initial behavioral interventions allowed them to socialize on a limited basis in public areas, with instructions to "talk but not touch." This did not help them to control their behavior, and so they were then allowed to socialize only with supervision, a plan which remained in effect until one of them was discharged.

### Stimulus-Bound Behavior

The stimulus-bound patient tends to be drawn to what she or he perceives to be salient stimuli, without consideration of other factors. Such patients may wander and enter other patients' rooms, may hoard objects, or may be unable to control eating. In these situations, when a stimulus is present, the patient is pulled to do something with it and acts without thinking (e.g., opens any door which comes into view), although she or he may later be able to express that what she or he did was wrong. Treatment is similar to that used with disinhibited behavior. Although the patient below did not suffer TBI, the example illustrates this type of problem.

*Case Example*. FF was a 35-year-old male with insulin-dependent diabetes mellitus and a history of alcoholism. He was 9 months post-insulin shock coma, and his CT scan was described as normal. His impairments in executive functioning were profound and included decreased flexibility, poor planning and associated impulsivity, and perseveration. On the nursing unit, he took, hoarded, and ate food despite a strict diet. Although able to express the need to follow his diet, he was unable to act upon this knowledge. The behavioral intervention was highly structured and simple: the patient was supervised during all meals, and his room was searched several times daily for food. He was also reminded of his diet and praised when he left the dining room without food. He showed no change in his behavior, and these interventions were maintained until his discharge.

## Decreased Initiation

Wood (1987) has identified disorders of initiation as among the hardest to treat. At the extreme, patients with this problem are unable to initiate any behavior without verbal cuing. They also may be actively resistant when attempts are made to facilitate behavior, and they may lose emotional control. Even when reinforcers can be identified, once they have lost their initial novelty, initiation problems can return. This type of patient is sometimes viewed by staff as deliberately unmotivated or resistant, or as depressed.

Treatment should include an intensive program of positive reinforcement, which begins with frequent reinforcement for any desired behavior. As initiation increases, positive reinforcement can be used to shape behavior gradually. Token programs are very useful, because the patient is able to exchange tokens for a variety for reinforcers, and loss of novelty is less likely. Sometimes, however, reinforcers may have to be primary (e.g., food, sleep) because of the strength of reinforcement required. Consistency in program administration is essential with this type of disorder. Psychopharmacological interventions used to improve arousal and attention may be helpful, although there are no empirical data to support this.

*Case Example*. GG was a 33-year-old male who had suffered a TBI in a fall 12 months earlier. Cognitively, he exhibited decreased arousal and initiation, impulsivity, poor planning, and decreased emotional control. His behavioral difficulties were characterized by a lack of participation and cooperation in therapies, constant complaints of pain, and constant requests to return to bed to alleviate these difficulties. A positive reinforcement program was developed in which he earned telephone and television privileges and visits home for therapy participation and cooperation; desired behaviors were shaped gradually. Additionally, rest periods were scheduled, and his bed was folded and phone disconnected at other times. A series of medication trials to increase arousal was also initiated. Sessions were held with some family members to include them in the behavioral program. Although the program was successful initially, family members eventually interfered with its implementation by insisting that the patient receive phone calls and visits home even when he had failed to earn them.

## CONSIDERATIONS FOR DISORDERS
## OF SPEECH AND LANGUAGE FUNCTIONING

Malec (1984) has reviewed research indicating an association between speech and language impairments and behavioral problems. Difficulties in communication can be extremely frustrating to patients, and when there are associated impairments in attention and/or executive functions, behavioral difficulties are more likely. Several illustrations follow.

## Decreased Communication during Emergence from Coma

At this stage of recovery, language comprehension and production are very limited. Combined with impairments in arousal and attention discussed earlier, language impairments can contribute to frustration and agitation since the ability to communicate needs is limited. Treatment is similar to that described for behavioral difficulties due to impaired arousal/attention at this stage. Multimodal communication, which uses verbal and visual input, may also be helpful. Additionally, attempts should be made to develop an effective communication method for the patient. These types of difficulties are commonly seen in patients at Levels III and IV of the Rancho Scale (Malkmus et al., 1980).

## Nonvocal/Augmentative Communicators

These patients are often unable to get their needs met as rapidly as they would like since they have difficulty getting others to attend and respond to them due to slow communication. When there are impairments in executive functioning, frustration with difficulties may escalate to agitation and aggression. Interventions include helping the patient adjust to his/her communication limitations, teaching her/him to be patient with others, and providing positive reinforcement for waiting and not getting upset with others. It is also helpful to encourage staff to take the time needed for communication. The use of augmentative devices or computers with printers can help the patient prepare his/her communications ahead of time, to ensure a more rapid response from staff.

> *Case Example.* HH was a 23-year-old male, 30 months post-TBI from a motor vehicle accident in which he suffered a cerebral contusion. He was nonvocal, with relatively intact language functions, and communicated using a letter board or laptop computer. He exhibited decreased flexibility of thinking and awareness of alternatives, and decreased emotional control, although when calm, he showed insight into his injury and deficits. Behaviorally, he became angry and struck out at staff when they did not respond rapidly to an immediate need or to his attempts to communicate. The severity of his aggression led to the use of a beta-blocker for behavioral control. Negative consequences occurred in response to his actions (e.g., loss of desired privileges), and he was also provided with counseling to address adjustment to disability issues. The frequency of his outbursts decreased, and speech/language therapy resulted in his becoming vocal. Temporary discontinuation of medication indicated that the medication–behavioral treatment program was the best combination for behavioral control, and so medication was maintained.

## Decreased Language Comprehension

As discussed earlier, language comprehension may be impaired secondary to attentional deficits. Although specific language dysfunction is less common after TBI, it may occur and produce primary impairments in language comprehension. Difficulties are most likely when others speak too rapidly or use lengthy and grammatically complex sentences.

Treatment may include the use of compensatory strategies by staff: talking slowly, in short, simple sentences, with repetition as necessary. Speech/language therapy can be used to help improve comprehension, and to help the patient to recognize impairment and request others to slow down or repeat.

> *Case Example.* AA, discussed earlier, also presented with impairments in language. His inability to communicate increased his frustration with others and contributed to his agitation. Behavioral and pharmacological treatments were described. Additionally, staff simplified their communications with him, and intensive speech/language therapy was provided.

## Decreased Speech and/or Language Production

Patients with impairments in speech/language production, when comprehension is relatively intact, know what they would like to say but are unable to express it. Repeated efforts may lead to failure and associated frustration.

To alleviate these difficulties, it may first be necessary to teach staff the best way to facilitate the patient's effective communication. Patience is essential. Speech/language therapy may be used to address the problem directly.

> *Case Example*. JJ was a 26-year-old male, 12 months post-TBI after being struck while on his bicycle. He sustained bilateral frontal hematomas and a left temporal hematoma. He was severely dysarthric, had moderate word finding difficulties, and impaired executive functions, including decreased emotional control. Additionally, he suffered from pain in his legs; this was often severe, and he had difficulty communicating this to staff. Behaviorally, he lost control rapidly and became physically violent when people did not understand what he was saying. He was tried on several different medications for behavioral control. He was also positively reinforced for being patient and for repeating himself until staff understood him. Treatment was facilitated when his pain was effectively relieved, and outbursts decreased substantially after that.

## CONTRIBUTIONS OF DISORDERS OF VISUOSPATIAL FUNCTIONING

Visuospatial impairments generally do not produce behavioral difficulties but may contribute in a number of ways. Patients with visuospatial perceptual disorders may not recognize staff or other patients and encounter difficulty in interpersonal interactions. They may also tend to enter the wrong room because they cannot differentiate their own room from those of others. This may lead to anger from the patient whose room was entered and could lead to a fight, although the error was unintentional. Patients with disorders of spatial awareness may have difficulty finding their way around the facility, with resulting frustration. When other aspects of cognition are more intact, staff sometimes assume that these patients should be able to find their way around and so do not develop interventions to help them. In all of these instances, use of verbal compensatory strategies and repetition of exposure to the visual stimulus may help to reduce the problem. Cognitive rehabilitation of these skills may be best directed toward functional skills rather than toward discrete cognitive functions (for example, see Tankle, 1988).

> *Case Example*. KK was a 39-year-old male, 4 months post-gunshot wound; the bullet entered the right parieto-occipital region, and bone and bullet fragments were found in the left parieto-occipital region. He had a visual defect in which he saw everything as if looking through a cone, with the smallest end at his eye. Thus, his visual field was narrowest at short distances, but wider at long distances. Although able to see and describe objects when in view and able to complete many functional tasks, he often failed to complete or requested help with simple tasks (e.g., eating) because he could not find needed objects near him. Because he could see, however, staff interpreted this behavior as deliberate noncompliance and were harshly critical. Analysis of the difficulty and discussion with the team eliminated their criticism of his problems.

## CONTRIBUTIONS OF DISORDERS OF REASONING AND PROBLEM-SOLVING

These deficits are often hard to define, but are frequent after TBI (Brooks, 1984; Levin *et al.*, 1982). They overlap deficits in executive functioning and may be difficult to differentiate from them (Goldstein & Levin, 1987). In the cognitive framework described earlier, executive functions have to do with basic behavioral controls, while these abilities are higher-level, require integration of lower-level functions, and may be more influenced by education.

Terms associated with reasoning include judgment, insight, and abstraction skills. Patients with impaired reasoning may lack these skills and may be concrete. Such patients may be unable to understand the reasons for specific treatments despite considerable explanation (at minimum) or may insist that hospitalization or rehabilitation is unnecessary (at worst; but see McGlynn & Schacter, 1989, for a discussion of dissociations between denial of deficit and reasoning impairments). These types of impairments limit the patient's ability to participate in treatment planning. Further, if the patient sees no reason for treatment, she or he is less likely to participate at all.

As with treatment for behavioral problems due to impaired executive functions, treatment for patients with impaired reasoning and problem-solving abilities should use structured, simple stimulus-response types of programs. In some instances when awareness is poor, stereotyped responses may be taught and reinforced (Crosson, Barco, Velozo, Boksta, Cooper, Werts, & Brobeck, 1989). Higher-level behavioral approaches, such as contingency contracting, which require insight into cause–effect relationships, are not likely to be successful. Additionally, extended discussion with the patient, either during program development or in the midst of behavioral interventions, will be ineffective and should be avoided. "Knowing without doing," discussed earlier, may result in staff assuming that a patient can act upon expressed knowledge of consequences, although this is not possible. Yet, well-intentioned staff may attempt to reason with such patients and "talk them down." This frequently leads to circular arguments, escalation of behavior, frustration from staff, and a lack of productive interaction.

## CONTRIBUTION OF DISORDERS OF LEARNING AND MEMORY

Memory deficits are often considered universal in TBI (Levin *et al.*, 1982). As discussed by Wood (1987), the prevalence of impairments in attention, executive functions, learning, and memory after TBI often slows progress in rehabilitation. Deficits in attention and executive functioning will impact on new learning by their effects on encoding and retrieval, and memory consolidation deficits can prevent patients from retaining information which is encoded initially. Any deficits in new learning can have profound effects on progress. For example, slowed learning of what is taught in rehabilitation may increase patient frustration. Learning deficits can interfere with the staff's ability to orient patients because this information is not retained despite repetition. Counseling, which requires retention of material from session to session, may be ineffective. Complex behavioral programs requiring new learning may not have a significant impact.

Patience on the part of staff is essential, and programs should not be changed rapidly if unsuccessful; several weeks may be required before even small improvements occur. Deficits in learning and memory may require the use of immediate and/or very frequent reinforcement when a program is initiated. Disorders of learning and memory may also prevent a patient from seeing his/her progress. Thus, helping the patient to develop trust in the staff by providing frequent feedback on progress is important. Additionally, sequential videotapes over the course of treatment can help the patient to become more aware of changes made, especially when she or he is frustrated by what is perceived to be a lack of progress.

## FINAL CONSIDERATIONS FOR TREATMENT DESIGN

As stated earlier, neuropsychological evaluation is an essential component of the treatment planning process. Results of evaluation can be used to design treatments which are consistent with the patient's strengths, but which do not stress his/her deficits. For example, programs for dysphasic patients must maximize the use of nonverbal instructions and behavior–reinforcer associations; actions, rather than words, should be emphasized. In contrast, programs for patients with visuospatial disorders must maximize the use of verbal materials. Reinforcers for patients with hemi-inattention should always be presented in the nonneglected visual field, or they will not be effective. One must also determine whether a patient learns best through the auditory modality, visual modality, or a combination of both.

The neuropathological effects of TBI dictate certain constant types of cognitive deficits. These deficits, in turn, determine the types of behavioral disorders commonly seen following TBI. Having a good understanding of a patient's cognitive strengths and deficits will help maximize the success of any behavioral program developed. This knowledge will also help to troubleshoot and modify programs when difficulties arise.

ACKNOWLEDGMENTS.    This chapter was first presented in April 1988 as a lecture at the conference Head Injury: An Integrated Approach to Behavioral Rehabilitation, Boston, Massachusetts. Preparation of this chapter was supported, in part, by Greenery Rehabilitation and Skilled Nursing Center, Boston, Massachusetts, and by American Neuroscience Centers, Gaithersburg, Maryland. Many people at Greenery contributed to the development of these ideas. Roger F. Cohen, Ph.D., and Laurence Levine, Psy.D., introduced me to ideas about the relationship between cognitive deficits and behavioral disorders. Ronye Cornblatt, M.S., CCC, helped to refine many of the examples discussed. John Whyte, M.D., Ph.D., Dan Eubanks, Ph.D., and Jack Spector, Ph.D., provided helpful comments during preparation of this chapter, and Drs. Eubanks and Spector contributed several case examples.

DISCLAIMER.    The views and opinions expressed are those of the author and do not purport to be those of the Henry M. Jackson Foundation for the Advancement of Military Medicine.

## REFERENCES

Auerbach, S. H. (1986). Neuroanatomical correlates of attention and memory disorders in traumatic brain injury: An application of neurobehavioral subtypes. *Journal of Head Trauma Rehabilitation*, *1*(3), 1–12.

Barkley, R. A. (1989). Attention. In M. G. Tramontana & S. G. Hooper (Eds.), *Assessment issues in child neuropsychology* (pp. 145–176). New York: Plenum Press.

Ben-Yishay, Y., & Diller, L. (1983). Cognitive deficits. In M. Rosenthal, E. R. Griffith, M. R. Bond, & J. D. Miller (Eds.), *Rehabilitation of the head injured adult* (pp. 167–183). Philadelphia: Davis.

Brooks, N. (1984). Cognitive deficits after closed head injury. In N. Brooks (Ed.), *Closed head injury: Psychological, social, and family consequences* (pp. 44–73). New York: Oxford University Press.

Cope, D. N. (Ed.). (1987). Psychopharmacology [Topical issue]. *Journal of Head Trauma Rehabilitation, 2*(4).

Crosson, B. (1987). Treatment of interpersonal deficits for head trauma patients in inpatient rehabilitation settings. *The Clinical Neuropsychologist, 1*, 335–352.

Crosson, B., Barco, P. P., Velozo, C. A., Bolesta, M. M., Cooper, P. V., Werts, D., & Brobeck, T. C. (1989). Awareness and compensation in postacute head injury rehabilitation. *Journal of Head Trauma Rehabilitation, 4*(3), 46–54.

Evans, R. W., Gualtieri, C. T., & Patterson, D. (1987). Treatment of chronic closed head injury with psycho-stimulant drugs: A controlled case study and an appropriate evaluation procedure. *Journal of Nervous & Mental Disease, 175*, 106–110.

Glenn, M. B. (1986). CNS stimulants: Applications for traumatic brain injury. *Journal of Head Trauma Rehabilitation, 1*(4), 74–76.

Glenn, M. B. (1987a). A pharmacologic approach to aggressive and disruptive behaviors after traumatic brain injury (Part 1). *Journal of Head Trauma Rehabilitation, 2*(1), 71–73.

Glenn, M. B. (1987b). A pharmacologic approach to aggressive and disruptive behaviors after traumatic brain injury (Part 2). *Journal of Head Trauma Rehabilitation, 2*(2), 80–81.

Glenn, M. B. (1987c). A pharmacologic approach to aggressive and disruptive behaviors after traumatic brain injury (Part 3). *Journal of Head Trauma Rehabilitation, 2*(3), 85–87.

Goldstein, F. C., & Levin, H. S. (1987). Disorders of reasoning and problem-solving ability. In M. Meier, A. Benton, & L. Diller (Eds.), *Neuropsychological rehabilitation* (pp. 327–354). New York: Plenum Press.

Gualtieri, C. T. (1987). *Pharmacotherapy and the neurobehavioral sequelae of traumatic brain injury.* Unpublished monograph, North Carolina Memorial Hospital, Chapel Hill, NC.

Jennett, B., & Teasdale, G. (1981). *Management of head injuries.* Philadelphia: Davis.

Levin, H. S., Benton, A. L., & Grossman, R. G. (1982). *Neurobehavioral consequences of closed head injury.* New York: Oxford University Press.

Levin, H. S., Grafman, J., & Eisenberg, H. M. (Eds.). (1987). *Neurobehavioral recovery from head injury.* New York: Oxford University Press.

Lezak, M. D. (1983). *Neuropsychological assessment* (2nd ed.). New York: Oxford University Press.

Luria, A. R. (1980). *Higher cortical functions in man* (2nd ed.). New York: Basic Books.

McGlynn, S. M., & Schacter, D. L. (1989). Unawareness of deficits in neuropsychological syndromes. *Journal of Clinical & Experimental Neuropsychology, 11*, 143–205.

Malec, J. (1984). Training the brain-injured client in behavioral self-management skills. In B. A. Edelstein & E. T. Couture (Eds.), *Behavioral assessment and rehabilitation of the traumatically brain-damaged* (pp. 121–150). New York: Plenum Press.

Malkmus, D., Booth, B. J., & Kodimer, C. (1980). *Rehabilitation of the head injured adult: Comprehensive cognitive management.* Downey, CA: Professional Staff Association of the Rancho Los Amigos Hospital, Inc.

Mapou, R. L. (1987, April). *Double-blind study of the effects of Ritalin on arousal and attention after head injury.* Paper presented at the annual meeting of the Massachusetts Psychological Association, Cambridge, MA.

Mapou, R. L. (1988). An integrated approach to the neuropsychological assessment of cognitive function. In J. M. Williams & C. J. Long (Eds.), *Cognitive approaches to neuropsychology* (pp. 101–122). New York: Plenum Press.

Mirsky, A. F. (1987). Behavioral and psychophysiological markers of disordered attention. *Environmental Health Perspectives, 74*, 191–199.

Muir, C. A., Haffey, W. J., Ott, K. J., Karaica, D., Muir, J. H., & Sutko, M. (1983). Treatment of behavioral deficits. In M. Rosenthal, E. R. Griffith, M. R. Bond, & J. D. Miller (Eds.), *Rehabilitation of the head injured adult* (pp. 381–393). Philadelphia: Davis.

Parasuraman, R. (1985). Sustained attention: A multifactorial approach. In M. I. Posner & O. S. M. Marin (Eds.), *Attention and performance XI* (pp. 493–511). Hillsdale, NJ: Lawrence Erlbaum Associates.

Posner, M. I. (1987). Selective attention in head injury. In H. S. Levin, J. Grafman, & H. M. Eisenberg (Eds.), *Neurobehavioral recovery from head injury* (pp. 390–397). New York: Oxford University Press.

Povlishock, J. T. (1989). Structural aspects of brain injury. In P. Bach-y-Rita (Ed.), *Traumatic brain injury* (pp. 87–96). New York: Demos.

Prigatano, G. P., & Fordyce, D. J. (1986). Cognitive dysfunction and psychosocial adjustment after brain injury. In

G. P. Prigatano, D. J. Fordyce, H. K. Zeiner, J. R. Roueche, M. Pepping, and B. C. Wood, *Neuropsychological rehabilitation after brain injury* (pp. 1–17). Baltimore: Johns Hopkins University Press.

Rose, M. J. (1988). The place of drugs in the management of behavior disorders after traumatic brain injury. *Journal of Head Trauma Rehabilitation*, *3*(3), 7–13.

Silver, J. M., Yudofsky, S. C., & Hales, R. E. (1987). Neuropsychiatric aspects of traumatic brain injury. In R. E. Hales & S. C. Yudofsky (Eds.), *Textbook of neuropsychiatry* (pp. 179–190). Washington, DC: American Psychiatric Press.

Stuss, D. T. (1987). Contribution of frontal lobe injury to cognitive impairment after closed head injury: Methods of assessment and recent findings. In H. S. Levin, J. Grafman, & H. M. Eisenberg (Eds.), *Neurobehavioral recovery from head injury* (pp. 166–177). New York: Oxford University Press.

Stuss, D. T., & Benson, D. F. (1986). *The frontal lobes*. New York: Raven Press.

Stuss, D. T., Stethem, L. L., & Poirer, C. A. (1987). Comparison of three tests of attention and rapid information processing across six age groups. *The Clinical Neuropsychologist*, *1*, 139–152.

Stuss, D. T., Stethem, L. L., & Pelchat, G. (1988). Three tests of attention and rapid information processing: An extension. *The Clinical Neuropsychologist*, *2*, 246–250.

Tankle, R. S. (1988). Application of neuropsychological results to interdisciplinary cognitive rehabilitation with head-injured adults. *Journal of Head Trauma Rehabilitation*, *3*(1), 24–32.

Teasdale, G., & Mendelow, D. (1984). Pathophysiology of head injuries. In N. Brooks (Ed.), *Closed head injury: Psychological, social, and family consequences* (pp. 4–36). New York: Oxford University Press.

Van Zomeren, A. H. (1981). *Reaction time and attention after closed head injury*. Lisse, Netherlands: Swets & Zeitlinger.

Van Zomeren, A. H., & Brouwer, W. H. (1987). Head injury and concepts of attention. In H. S. Levin, J. Grafman, & H. M. Eisenberg (Eds.), *Neurobehavioral recovery from head injury* (pp. 398–415). New York: Oxford University Press.

Van Zomeren, A. H., Brouwer, W. H., & Deelman, B. G. (1984). Attentional deficits: The riddles of selectivity, speed, and alertness. In N. Brooks (Ed.), *Closed head injury: Psychological, social, and family consequences* (pp. 74–107). New York: Oxford University Press.

Wood, R. L. (1984). Behaviour disorders following severe brain injury: Their presentation and psychological management. In N. Brooks (Ed.), *Closed head injury: Psychological, social, and family consequences* (pp. 195–219). New York: Oxford University Press.

Wood, R. L. (1987). *Brain injury rehabilitation: A neurobehavioural approach*. Rockville, MD: Aspen Publishers.

# 6

# Using a Model of Cognitive Function to Plan Cognitive Treatment

## An Axial Model of Brain Function

ROBERT L. PUSAKULICH

The practice of neuropsychological assessment routinely calls for the selection of a series or "battery" of psychometric measures of cortical functions. Rehabilitative interventions for cognitive retraining also require assessment and description of debilitated and normal cortical functions. The selection of tests for an assessment battery or any other clinical test aggregate requires either an explicit or implicit model or scheme based upon the kinds or types of cortical functions expected to be assessed and described. However, such models are not plentiful and it is easy for practitioners in such circumstances to fall back upon functional descriptions generated by the "face validities" of the tests themselves or some "folk psychological" list of cortical functions (see Smith Churchland, 1986, for a discussion of "folk psychological" constructs).

### A PROBLEM WITH MODELING CEREBRAL CORTICAL FUNCTIONS

Cerebral cortical functions are often classified according to the results of exploratory factor analyses of neuropsychological test scores; however, such "statistical" models often have a certain amount of logical circularity in that the factors generated by the analysis are

ROBERT L. PUSAKULICH • Department of Psychology, VA Medical Center, Memphis, Tennessee 38104.

*HANDBOOK OF HEAD TRAUMA: Acute Care to Recovery*, edited by Charles J. Long and Leslie K. Ross. Plenum Press, New York, 1992.

dependent on the types of test scores used in the analysis which, in turn, reflect specific test contents. Furthermore, the selection of specific tests for assessment implies at least a crude a priori notion of significant cerebral cortical functions, which adds further to logical circularity. However, any a priori model, however crude, can be tested by confirmatory factor procedures, thus reducing logical circularity. Confirmatory factor analysis reduces circularity by submitting an a priori model to factor confirmation rather than relying on data-generated factors to establish a model (Long, 1983). Obviously, in such cases, models must be initially derived or established by "rational" rather than statistical methods. Deductive–conceptual models are examples of models derived by rational methods.

There are a number of "deductive–conceptual" models, but the most elaborated and inclusive is that of Aleksandr Luria (1973). Luria conceptualized brain functions as being organized around the three brain units: a vertical core providing activation to other brain units in response to external or internal stimulation; a posterior cerebral unit responsive to input from external sources and characterized by modality specificity, hierarchy, and laterality; and an anterior cerebral unit known for its capacity to initiate, regulate, integrate, and verify behavior. Such succinctness does not do justice to the richness of the Luria model, but it does offer an example of a deductive–conceptual scheme that organizes higher cortical functions around basic principles of brain structure and function.

A lesson taught by Luria's example is the importance of modeling cortical function around basic, organizing principles, rather than attempting a mere listing or classification of functions. The pitfall of such lists is that they have no logical organizational boundaries of the sort provided by the Luria tripartite framework; therefore, models can provide a logical framework for cortical functions that mere "lists" cannot.

Fodor's recent remarks about the description of human cognitive functions are applicable here (Fodor, 1983). Fodor suggests that precision regarding descriptions of cognitive functions is only possible in the realm of "neural modules" which have outputs that can be "computationally" predicted from measurable inputs; however, few if any cerebral cortical functions can be operationally defined as the product of a Fodor-type "module." Fodor's examples of modules are sparse. However, most cortical functions typically described by neuropsychologists are not "modular" and are components of a large collection of cognitive functions Fodor refers to as the "central" system. Unfortunately, designations of central system "components" have an arbitrary nature. This results from what Fodor describes as the "Quinenian" properties of the central system. The interrelationship between components of the central system is so intertwined that an effect acting upon any part of the system is sensed by the entire system. Such interactive dependency proscribes any substantial separation of components, according to Fodor, although it does allow operational and heuristic distinctions between them. The entire field of science is an illustrative example. Negation of a scientific principle affects all sciences; moreover, knowledge gained in one field of science has potential application in all fields. Furthermore, the numbers and kinds of different "sciences" or divisions of the broader field of science seem endless (e.g., biology, zoology, ichthyology, mycology, etc.). The operational and somewhat arbitrary nature of the designations for the different fields of science is the same point that Fodor makes regarding distinctions of cognitive function within the "central system." It is suggested that "reasoning," "memory," "pushing blocks around," and "ordering hamburgers" may all be useful descriptions of cognitive functions. However, the term "pushing blocks around" is not recommended by this author for clinical application.

Regardless of the difficulties inherent in deriving something more than an arbitrary list of descriptive labels for cortical functions, the clinical neuropsychologist must do so or be faced with the prospect of providing little more than a list of tests and test scores in a clinical report. Clinical responsibilities do require interpretation of test data as well as making recommendations based upon those data. Therefore, each clinical neuropsychologist requires some kind of conceptual framework around which to organize interpretations and recommendations, be it deductive or otherwise. A deductive model of cortical functions will be offered here.

## A BIOEMERGENT MODEL OF CEREBRAL CORTICAL FUNCTIONS

The model offered here is biopsychological in that it is bioemergent. The model is deductive and conceptual. Its descriptive terms for cortical functions are derived from the major biological or neurophysiological aspects of the functioning cerebral cortex. Its approach is inspired by Luria's approach but elaborates more extensively the products of functional interactions between its "bio-organizational" principles. This model is biological in that basic biopsychological properties of the brain are its point of origin, rather than statistical analysis or some other nonbiological scheme. The model is intended to generate a priori hypotheses about cortical functioning that could, in turn, be subjected to statistical studies such as factor analysis. "Biological" modeling may be one way to go beyond the informal "list models" commonly found in the practice of clinical neuropsychology, avoiding some of the arbitrariness that Fodor implies is used by psychologists to divide the cognitive "pie" of cortical functions.

The bioemergent model derives its impetus from the several major axes of brain phylogenesis. Among those axes is the left–right, verbal–nonverbal axis so prominent in the neuropsychology of the human brain. However, other brain functions clearly precede the manifestation of language in neuroevolutionary history. One of the most basic manifestations of "neural brain" function, one endogenous to the very definition of nervous tissue, is "response to stimuli." The evolutionary elaboration of the capacity to enact a response to environmental events or stimuli has yielded a remarkable sensory–motor division even within very primitive nervous systems (Nauta & Feirtag, 1979). The sensory–motor division has been carried to the highest levels of nervous development and is no less prominent in the human brain than the language–nonlanguage division to which it is related. "Sensory–motor division" is used here to denote what is functionally discrete within the anatomy of nervous systems, although the neuropsychological interaction between sensory and motor systems is often so extensive that their anatomical separation is misleading. However, for present purposes, the emphasis is on functional separation: the simple notion that neural function begins with an input which at some point yields an output; or, in other words, there are traditionally recognized neural systems that are typically either more sensory or more motor in nature. Sensory and motor systems became "vertically" elaborated as central nervous systems evolved in complexity. Sensory systems became more elaborated in their integration of information and in their capacity to "sense" or identify members of perceptual, categorical sets. In its vertical "climb" the motor system gradually assumed a capacity for volitional, rapid, sequential, dexterous movements. The new systems were usually "laid over" the older sensory and motor systems.

Although the evolving vertical structure of the nervous system retained an activational core that aroused neural systems at all levels, the end result of "verticality" was the neocortex and its remarkable cognitive and volitional capacities.

## MAJOR AXES OF BRAIN FUNCTION

The sensory–motor division, the vertical hierarchy, and the more recent verbal–nonverbal dimension of the human brain provide three basic axes of function (Figure 6.1). Cortical functions can be examined in the framework of these three neurobiological dimensions: a transverse, left–right dimension; a longitudinal, anterior–posterior dimension; and a vertical, cortical–subcortical dimension. These three organizational axes also can be characterized as functional dipoles. Figure 6.1 illustrates the two contrasting poles of each axis: left–right, verbal–nonverbal poles; anterior–posterior, sensory–motor poles; and rostral–caudal, cortical–subcortical poles. The three axes can be crossed two at a time yielding a total of twelve functional "quadrants." Each quadrant represents both a general anatomic area as well as specific cortical functions broadly mediated within that area. Brain functions can be described by either combining or contrasting of the functional poles of the axes. Each, two by two, axis combination will be considered individually.

## LEFT–RIGHT AND ANTERIOR–POSTERIOR AXES

Figure 6.2 shows the crossing of the left–right hemispheric axis with the anterior–posterior axis and the four resulting anatomical/functional, cortical quadrants: right/anterior, left/anterior, left/posterior, and right/posterior. Although some of the neuropsychological functions typically associated with the cerebral cortical tissue of a quadrant may not be related to one another, many do appear related, perhaps through basic or "key" functions characteristic of the general nature of the quadrant.

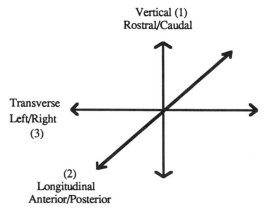

FIGURE 6.1. The three major functional axes of the brain as considered by the axial model.

LONGITUDINAL

|  | Anterior/Motor | Posterior/Sensory |
|---|---|---|
| Left/ Verbal | Expressive Language | Receptive Language |
| Right/ Non-Verbal | Spatial Manipulation | Spatial Analysis |

(left margin, vertical label: **TRANSVERSE**)

FIGURE 6.2. Some functions resulting from a combinational crossing of the transverse (left–right) and longitudinal (anterior–posterior) brain axes.

The best example of a key function is the expressive language or speech that arises from the left anterior quadrant, the verbal motor quadrant. Although both motor and premotor in anatomical locus, the frontal speech zone may have functional extension into prefrontal cortex as well. At some point along its prefrontal extension, speech may become internalized in such a way that "internal speech" becomes an important component in the cognitive activity of the left prefrontal cortex. Thus, even though speech is typically considered a motor output function, its functional nature may include an "internal" aspect that binds together function of the left anterior quadrant. Because prefrontal cortical areas are felt to be probable candidates for mediating the planning of behaviors, as well as mediating the organization and regulation of mental acts, a cognitive framework of internalized speech could easily be integral to such planning, organization, and regulation. Even though the two prefrontal areas may work in tandem in producing behavioral products, such cooperation does not preclude a unique internal verbal contribution from the left anterior cortical quadrant.

When considering the right anterior quadrant, one is confronted with an area that represents the "dark side" of cortical function in that its unique contribution is poorly understood relative to those of other cortical regions. Of course, the right frontal mediation of left body motor functions is well known, but right frontal higher functions remain more mysterious. Although the area represents the combinational intersection of the motor pole of the sensory–motor axis with "nonverbal" aspects of the nondominant hemisphere, its more complex, hierarchical contributions to human cognition can be only guessed at. However, one might at least imagine a nonverbal counterpart to a left, internal linguistic contribution to behavioral planning. Such a nonverbal activity might be a pattern or gestalt of information derived perceptually from both external (environmental) and internal (bodily) sources that enters into the planning and execution of behaviors. Of course, the nonverbal aspect of planning and response selection would very likely work in tandem with its internal verbal counterpart from the left prefrontal cortex. Such a right frontal contribution would be nonverbal in the sense that it would treat perceptual and spatial aspects of the environment in a patterned rather than sequential linguistic fashion. In human behavior much of the nonverbally directed planning may be social, consistent with the notion that much of the functioning of the primate frontal lobes is probably directed toward social acts and their consequences.

Functional crossing of the verbal–nonverbal left–right axis with the posterior cortical sensory poles descriptively yields those well-lateralized perceptual and cognitive functions most familiar to clinical neuropsychologists and behavioral neurologists. The posterior cortical quadrants mediate contralateral body sensation in the three primary senses: vision, audition, and somatosensation. However, those functions quickly change as one proceeds into sensory associational areas, where the full flavor of asymmetrical hemispheric operations becomes apparent. Leading the asymmetry in human brain function is the left posterior quadrant capacity for engaging in linguistic and other symbolically mediated functions, a capacity that extends beyond the boundaries of the three different sensory lobes of the quadrant. The most characteristic functional emanation of this area is receptive or "sensory" language with language comprehension being a special case of auditory comprehension. However, the functional capacity of both posterior cortical lobes also may be understood in their more fundamental capacity to engage in the identification, classification, and categorization of perceptual information, whether it is auditory, visual, or somesthetic. Goldberg (1989) recently described the key function of posterior cortex as "recognizing specific exemplars as members of generic categories." This identification and classification of percepts applies to both verbal and nonverbal materials, but it is most distinct in the perception of auditory phonemes and visual graphemes which strongly characterizes the higher functioning of the left posterior quadrant in its respective temporal and occipital contributions. The left parietal contribution to this quadrant is more obviously "spatial" and treats both environmental and personal spaces in an abstract, symbolic fashion (e.g., it mediates body parts nominally and divides both personal and extrapersonal space into "left" and "right" halves). But the contribution of the left parietal lobe is also clearly linguistic when it contributes to the production of written graphemes. However, even writing may be related to the sensory–motor ability of left parietal lobe to mediate sequences of skilled movement in space, rather than to a fundamental parietal linguistic capacity. Moreover, reading and visuomotor capacity also may be examples of left posterior linguistic capacities related to spatial–motor mechanisms, in this case, eye movements. In fact, control of movement through space may be a fundamental capacity of both left and right parietal areas, especially the superior lobules (Freund, 1987), even though "right posterior, guided movement products" are probably more concrete than reading or writing. Of course, the role of left parietal guided movements in acts of skilled praxis is even more apparent.

Neuropsychologically speaking, the right parietal, temporal, and occipital lobes are the center of "nondominant," nonverbal, perceptual, gestalt brain functions. When neuropsychologists refer to "nondominant hemisphere functions" they are typically implying functions of the right posterior cortical quadrant: the intersection between the nonverbal and sensory poles of the L–R and A–P axes. In that quadrant the cognitive elaboration of auditory, visual, and somesthetic percepts results in complex sensory arrays that represent whole or complete objects; moreover, sense of "object" may apply to the perceiver's body as well. However, the perceptual contribution of the right posterior quadrant may be most obvious in its guidance of motor activities such as during constructions. Such constructions can include drawing, building, or other visuomotor acts, and perhaps even the construction of prose. If it is the function of the right anterior quadrant to use patterned constructions to assist in the selection and evaluation of overt behaviors, it may be the function of the right posterior quadrant to provide those patterned constructions.

Finally, in discussing the general posterior sensory cortex, it would be remiss not to mention more about the extension of secondary sensory processing into the associative realm of multimodal processing, where some of the most "complex" and "highest" human cortical functions probably originate. In the case of both left and right posterior quadrants, the inferior parietal lobules seem to be special centers where auditory, visual, and tactile information are welded into unitary cognitive products. The mechanism of pattern formation may reach its highest level, when different sensory aspects of the same object are joined in a "tertiary," perceptual gestalt. At that level even groups of objects may be perceived as a unitary pattern, or perhaps even as an idea.

## ANTERIOR–POSTERIOR AND CORTICAL–SUBCORTICAL AXES

The results of the intersection or crossing of the L–R and A–P axes have been described as combinational in nature, but the functional result of crossing cortical and subcortical axes seems better described by contrast. Figure 6.3 shows the essential functions of the contrasting sensory and motor components of the vertically examined brain. The first consideration will be the contrasting motor aspects of cortex and subcortex, with cerebral cortex adding to the complexity and plasticity of motor activity.

Human frontal cerebral cortex provides an immense capacity for the preparation and selection of motor responses, as well as the capacity to weigh the behavioral consequences of selected responses. Human cortical motor output is often reflective in origin and, therefore, goal driven in a conscious and deliberate fashion. The cortical contribution to motor activity for most higher organisms is most noticeable in the execution of skilled, dexterous, distal limb movements. But at the human level there is also a tremendous capacity for cortical motoric inhibition that provides an inhibitory "ground" against which

| | | Cortical/Cognitive | Subcortical/Motivational |
|---|---|---|---|
| **LONGITUDINAL** | Anterior/Motor | Motoric Modulation<br><br>Response Selection | Motor Learning |
| | Posterior/Sensory | Sensory Perceptual<br>Objectivity<br>Alloreference | Releaser Perception<br><br>Autoreference |

FIGURE 6.3. Some functions resulting from a combinational crossing of the longitudinal (anterior–posterior) and vertical (cortical–subcortical) brain axes.

the timely contemplation and selection of motoric response "figures" can occur. Cortical motor control characteristically provides a person with a capacity to integrate behavior in a "free-form" manner despite changes in either exogenous or endogenous information. Cerebral motor control apparently allows humans to "willfully" break the bonds of conditioned responses either by not responding to "salient" stimuli, or even by responding in the absence of stimuli. In many routine and typical daily activities the subcortical motor systems provide the substance of motor activities done automatically and without deliberation, although it is probably frontal and prefrontal cortex that initiate those motor activities. Frontal/prefrontal cerebral cortex are also likely to evaluate the continuing effectiveness of the motor activities, as well as guiding their formative stages. In contrast, the subcortical anterior brain may provide for the storage and execution of less deliberate and more "structured" automatic motor skills. (See Freund, 1987; and Miller, Galanter, & Pribram, 1960.)

The world of "structured" motor outputs is probably most familiar to psychologists and others in the form of learned or "overlearned" motor skills, conditioned operants, or just plain "habits." Mishkin (1982) has described a type of memory called "habit learning." Habit learning contrasts the more cognitive, "cortical-limbic" learning. Mishkin's "habit learning" bears a strong similarity to the nondeliberate, nonvolitional motor learning of the human subcortex being considered here. Although the initial acquisition of subcortical types of motor activity may be volitional and cortically guided, once in place they appear to be manifested in an automatic, unconscious fashion often with considerable speed. Such automatic motor skills also may have a "procedural" nature in the sense of current distinctions made between procedural and declarative memories (Cohen & Squire, 1980). The motor activities generated by these anterior subcortical areas, including basal ganglia and related midbrain extrapyramidal structures, have the feedforward quality of released operants: noncognitive, fully integrated, and self-contained. Thus, it seems that the anterior aspect of the vertical axis of the brain mediates motor acts with decreasing volition, as one descends from cerebral cortex to subcortex.

Figure 6.3 also depicts the vertical organizational quadrants of the more posterior and sensory brain regions, descending from cerebral cortex to subcortex. In the area of sensory and perceptual processing, vertical brain organization is conceptualized as yielding a hierarchy of perceptual "objectification" rather than motor control, although motor activity has a clear role in "active perception." Marin, Schwartz, and Saffan (1979) have contrasted cortical and subcortical perceptual processes in their capacity for "allo-reference" or "other reference." Typically subcortical perceptions mimic the perceptual apparatus of more primitive organisms in that the perception of a stimulus and a response to that perception are tightly bound. The organism emits "hardwired" responses to environmental cues in a reflexive or releasor manner. Those authors contrast such "auto-referent" perception with the "allo-referent" perception of organisms with better developed cerebral cortices. Allo-reference allows a response that is more restrained than the behavior automatically elicited by auto-referent perception. In allo-reference there is an objectification of perceptual material that breaks the S–R integrity of the auto-referent system and, thus, clearly establishes both behavioral and cognitive separation of perceived and perceiver. The notion of stimulus objectification also is used by J. Hughlings Jackson (Harrington, 1985) to describe a similar process for the cortical representation of percepts. Jackson maintains that the mental consideration of a percept requires a division of consciousness into two aspects: a perceiving self and a perceived object. According to Jackson, the mental or conscious representation of environmental objects requires the personal awareness of the object as something other than "self." But because the perception of an object requires a perceiving other, it also enhances the sense of self. Thus, Jackson insightfully postulated a mental world in which a perceiving agent is distinct from the representation of objects. In that sense, Jackson anticipated the nature of the allo-reference process later described by Marin: a capacity which may represent the quintessential cortical contribution to sensory processing. Furthermore, an allo-reference capacity would allow effective use of the generic, posterior, perceptual gestalts discussed earlier. Moreover, just as motor responses are tightly bound to sensory perception in the subcortical auto-referent scheme, the objectivity of sensory allo-reference provides an effective complement to cortically deliberated, volitional motor acts. Both capacities add to the effective separation of stimulus and response and, thus, greatly add to the neocortical contribution to adaptive behavioral autonomy and the separation of person and world. The withholding of a response by inhibition permits the organism or person to take advantage of the capacity to objectively perceive and then to weigh the value of the percept prior to responding. Thus, the nature of the vertical hierarchy in the domain of sensation is one of the increasing capacity to release the organism from the behavioral constraints of sensory reflexes. The earliest cortical encephalizations appear to be in the area of sensory rather than motor systems. Such encephalization provided an amplified capacity for more complex perception, not only by enhancing perceptual detail and memory, but also by providing for a conscious sense of perceiver in a world of choices.

## LEFT–RIGHT AND CORTICAL–SUBCORTICAL AXES

The final piece of this scheme of "functional" quadrants is produced by the vertical relationship between the verbal and nonverbal aspects of the left and right hemispheres and a cortical–subcortical dimension. Those quadrants are depicted in Figure 6.4. The current model purports that major components of the left brain, right brain vertical hierarchy also

|  | **VERTICAL** | |
| --- | --- | --- |
|  | Cortical | Subcortical |
| Left/ Verbal | Verbal Cognition | Inhibition of Affect |
| Right/ Non-Verbal | Non-Verbal Cognition | Facilitation of Affect |

FIGURE 6.4. Some functions resulting from a contrasted crossing of the transverse (left–right) and vertical (cortical–subcortical) brain axes.

are best understood in a contrasting rather than combinational fashion. Cortical verbal and nonverbal functions, per se, have only minor representation in subcortical anatomy. Therefore, it will be argued that the major gradient along the "left/right," vertical axes will be one of cognitive–emotional interaction.

The two cortical quadrants in Figure 6.4, those of the left and right hemisphere, and their respective verbal and nonverbal cognitive operations are well known and have been described earlier. The neuropsychological study of cerebral cortical functions has been largely the study of brain based-cognition. The study of brain-based arousal functions such as emotion has been much less frequent; however, there has been increasing effort directed toward understanding the neuropsychology of emotion. (For example, see LeDoux, 1987.) Pribram (1981) organized cortical perceptive functions into two camps, those that process information from the world external to the body and those that process information from the internal milieu of the body. The latter have typically received much less attention in the history of clinical neuropsychology, but nevertheless have been postulated by Pribram to have an important parallel to the cognition that arises from perception and consideration of the external world. The internal sensations trigger arousal systems that have origin in deep subcortical structures; Pribram suggests that such arousal may have origin as the protopathic somatosensations of pain and temperature, sensations that project differently through hypothalamus, amygdala, and corpus striatum, but are ultimately directed to cerebral cortex. Moreover, in addition to Pribram's protopathically based activation, brainstem reticular and limbic activation from both internal and external stimuli also push their type of arousal into the cognitive domain of cerebral cortex. The result is a barrage of at least two different kinds of subcortical activation impinging upon ongoing, left and right cortical processes. But, in the current model, left and right cerebral cortex are postulated as handling that activation or "affect" quite differently.

Clinical neuropsychology has come to regard the nondominant, right hemisphere as the affect hemisphere. Tucker, who has extensively studied the "laterality of emotion," has developed a theory for describing the cortical aspects of emotion or affect (Tucker & Williamson, 1984). Based upon elaboration of earlier suggestions of McGuinness and Pribram (1980), Tucker has described the right hemisphere as most respondent to subcortical systems that provide perceptual mediation of the external world, while the left hemisphere accommodates subcortical systems that assist its internal preparation for action in that external world. Tucker further suggests that the left hemisphere preparation for action may result in the construction of internal models of both world and "action-in-the-world." It is suggested here that a capacity for internal mediation of behavior may have yielded the panoply of left hemisphere cognitive processes, most of which are language assisted or language dependent. The present model also suggests that internal, symbolic, and linguistic mediation of responses to the external world may have a neuropsychological, if not a neurological, incompatibility with cortical processes necessary for the mediation of affect. It may be an incompatibility of either internal states, or even incompatibility of the neuronal architecture needed to provide the inhibition and control and pacing needed for the production of speech and/or sequential, logical thought. In the current model, this incompatibility is hypothesized as creating a general left hemisphere tendency to suppress or dampen the brain arousal related to affect or emotion. Therefore, the interaction between the contrasting verbal cognitive and affective domains of the left cortical and subcortical quadrants is seen as one of suppression. In the case of the right hemisphere, however, the current model accepts that its cortical interaction with affect is facilitative in the manner of current clinical neuropsychological opinion. The finely timed, sequential activities of language seem relatively absent from the right hemisphere, allowing a possible blending of affect and right hemisphere kinds of cognition. Parallel, holistic, and perceptually based cognitions may be more compatible with affect and emotion possibly because of more diffuse and less specific neural organization (Semmes, 1968).

It is interesting to note that one method of fostering control during clinical "crisis intervention" is to urge a patient to verbalize his or her feelings, as if that intervention were designed to take advantage of verbal suppression of affect. Moreover, the belief that directing attention toward the right hemisphere promotes insight and intuitive "feelings" is held by some psychologists and many "laypersons." Also, many of the putative cognitive products of the right hemisphere are commonly regarded as being "feeling based" or to have a "feeling component" (i.e., a gestalt or pattern often "feels right," or certain artistic percepts may generate "aesthetic feelings"). Thus, a right hemisphere, facilitative blending of emotion and "cognition" might be an archetypal brain process that has been unilaterally usurped by the more recent neural demands of speech and language, and the need to cognitively control and/or suppress affect. In summary, the present model offers vertical and left–right brain axes that yield a continuum of affective arousal and cognition, respectively ascending from subcortex to cortex and with emotional inhibition on the left and emotional facilitation on the right.

The preceding discussion has outlined a framework of basic or key cerebral cortical and subcortical functions. It was an attempt to organize the major functional ingredients of human cerebral cortex around the basic biological aspects of brain operation such as sensory, motoric, and activation/arousal capacities. The argument of the bioemergent approach has been that complex brain functions always derive from simpler functions (e.g., language from sensory and motor operations). In the current model the simple principles of sensory, motor, and activation/arousal were elaborated in an axial scheme that has two cortical axes and a single, vertical subcortical axis. Theoretically, one should be able to derive any number of cerebral cortical (and subcortical) functions from one or another quadrant or combination of quadrants.

## A SENSORY COROLLARY

In completing the bioemergent, axial model, it might facilitate application to practical clinical situations (including cognitive retraining) if examples of how some of those cortical functions that appear in everyday clinical problems (such as reading, visuomotor operations, or even environmental sound recognition) might be derived from this 12 "quadrant" scheme. Many so-called higher cortical functions with which clinical neuropsychologists typically deal can be derived from a "corollary" to the model, a corollary that further elaborates the major informational sensory modalities: audition, vision, and somatosensation, across verbal/nonverbal and sensory/motor axes. Figure 6.5 shows some results of that kind of crossing. Those three sensory systems can also be treated as the products of the temporal, occipital, and parietal lobes, the major cortical structures of the posterior cerebrum. The sensory corollary describes both common and less common cortical functions. For example, in the left hemisphere those three modalities yield such functions as

CORTICAL AXES

| | Motor | | Sensory | |
|---|---|---|---|---|
| | Verbal | Nonverbal | Verbal | Nonverbal |
| Auditory<br><br>(Temporal) | Speech Expression<br><br>Oral Reading | Singing<br>Musical Expression<br>Acoustico-motor (Rhythms) | Speech Perception (Comprehension) | Musical Perception<br><br>Environmental Sounds Recognition |
| Visual<br><br>(Occipital) | Writing | Visuomotor Construction | Silent Reading | Visual Object Recognition (Visual Gnosis) |
| Tactile<br><br>Kinesthesia<br>(Parietal) | Writing | Manipulo-Spatial Construction | Graphesthesia | Stereognosis |

MODALITY COROLLARY FUNCTIONS

FIGURE 6.5. Some functions resulting from a sensory modalities corollary for audition, vision, and somato-sensation.

speech comprehension (auditory), silent reading (visual), and graphesthesia (a tactile verbal activity). The sensory, nonverbal line can yield: nonverbal auditory perceptions, such as those of music and environmental sounds; visual object recognition; and stereognosis (tactile object recognition). The "verbal–motor" column, when extended across these three modalities, describes such functions as speech, oral reading, writing, and sequential motor skills. Of course, in this scheme the functions are described under their "endstage" axial pole (e.g., writing or oral reading under verbal–motor), but the implication is that writing, reading, and other "motor products" have a sensory component that is both interactive and concurrent. In this respect the current model follows the descriptive convenience of separating sensory and motor functions, common to neuroscience but probably not true to brain realities.

## A MEMORY OVERLAY

Finally, the absence of memory in the current model is conspicuous. For present purposes, memory is regarded as part of a special class of ubiquitous or generalized brain functions. Such functions permeate widely through vast and different areas of brain structure. Thus, memory is regarded as superordinate to the axial or quadrantal products discussed to this point. However, memory functions can be integrated with the current model as an "overlay" that permeates all levels of cortical function, but is most apparent in those aspects of brain activity that yield the storage and retrieval of sensory/motor or verbal/nonverbal kinds of information. Figure 6.6 suggests a possible memory overlay for cortical

| | Cortical | Subcortical |
|---|---|---|
| Anterior | Retrieval (Cognitive) | Attentional Process and Motor Memory Consolidation/Storage |
| Posterior | Storage (Cognitive) | Consolidation (Cognitive) |

FIGURE 6.6. Some functional aspects of a memory overlay to the axial model.

and subcortical aspects of anterior and posterior cerebral cortex. It is generally considered that subcortical areas (sub-neocortical) mediate the arousal-based aspects of memory, and cortical (neocortical) areas, the content aspects. It is postulated that posterior cortical structures interact with "posterior" subcortical structures to produce respectively long-term memory storage and consolidation; whereas anteriorly, cortical and subcortical structures mediate the retrieval and rehearsal of short-term or "working memory." Posterior "subcortical" structures (e.g., amygdala/hippocampus) provide the arousal base for memory work, in contrast to the neocortical storage base. Of course, subcortical structures like the amygdala/hippocampus must interact with even deeper subcortical structures (e.g., thalamus, hypothalamus, reticular formation) in providing the arousal-based activation for memory processing. The current model does not distinguish between a retrieval-based "working memory" and a consolidation-related "short-term" memory. Both are felt to be closely related to "attentional" processes, and both dependent upon anterior neocortex. Also, anterior cortical/subcortical roles in the storage and consolidation of "motor" memory may not be the same as in posterior "sensory" memory.

In classifying memory "contents" or memory "types," one is again faced with the notion of "non-Quinenian" properties introduced earlier. The number of different types of memories one is willing to describe may be based upon practical need rather than upon empirics. However, among neuropsychologists, memory has some commonly recognized types. Among those, the verbal and nonverbal memories respective to the left and right hemispheres seem the most prominent. Verbal and nonverbal memories can combine in "episodic" recall, a recall that is personal and multifaceted. Language is often considered to have its own objective, semantic, and syntactic memories. The three major sensory modalities might be considered as having their own respective memories: some verbal, others nonverbal. More recently, memory for activity sequences has been treated as a separate type of memory, more "procedural" than "declarative" in nature. Moreover, one might want to distinguish between a more anterior (cortical–subcortical)-related, procedural–motoric memory and more posterior, cortical–limbic, sensory memory. The list can go on, but the open-endedness of such a classification is apparent. Perhaps each type of cortical function has its own respective "memory" to draw upon; and, therefore, memory is in many respects a more generalized than localized brain function. Also, memory is not considered the sole member of the class of generalized brain functions that might be applied as overlays to this model (e.g., activational processes such as directed attention certainly could be, and may be some types of highly integrated, possibly "bilateral" cognitive activities). However, their consideration and elaboration, unfortunately, remain beyond the scope of the present discussion.

## A FINAL COMMENT: FROM FUNCTION TO DYSFUNCTION AND BACK AGAIN

Although any model of "normal" brain function has obvious applications to the rehabilitative retraining of brain functions, the axial model has better potential than some for retraining applications in that the various brain functions of the axial quadrants can be reversed conceptually to yield equivalant brain "dysfunctions." For example, the left posterior, A–P/L–R quadrant, the area that mediates receptive language, could also be considered the primary area for the generation of receptive or Wernicke's aphasia and secondary linguistic disorders such as alexia and agraphia, or even visuokinesthetic disorders such as ideomotor apraxia. The sensory modality overlay chart in Figure 6.6 also could provide a framework for more of the dysfunctions related to various functions. The dysfunctional side of the model could provide a convenient descriptive framework for the impairments a clinical neuropsychologist is likely to encounter during cognitive retraining. Unfortunately, a more thorough discussion of the "dysfunction obverse" of the axial model is also beyond the scope of present considerations, although the reader could generate the various opposing dysfunctions when considering the functions of the model.

## SUMMARY

The preceding work has attempted to develop a model of cortical brain functions around three organizational axes. The three axes range from the primitive, vertical, cortical/subcortical axis to the more recent verbal/nonverbal axis. The model attempts to produce a "list" of specific and general cortical brain functions that have a biological connection and that may help to remedy the "arbitrariness" that often plagues the taxonomy of cortical functions. The entire effort to derive a "cortical functions model" has been directed toward assisting clinical neuropsychologists who must describe the status of cortical brain functions in diagnostic clinical reports and in retraining and rehabilitation therapies. Ultimately, the problem remains one of deciding what is a clinically useful list of cortical functions and having something other than a "folk" or even arbitrary basis for the names of those functions. Hopefully, the present model takes a step in that direction.

## REFERENCES

Cohen, N.J., & Squire, L.R. (1980). Preserved learning and retention of pattern analyzing skill in amnesia: Dissociation of knowing how and knowing what. *Science*, *210*, 207–210.
Fodor, J.A. (1983). *The modularity of mind*. Cambridge, MA: MIT Press.
Freund, H.S. (1987). Abnormalities of motor behavior after cortical lesions in humans. In V.B. Mountcastle, F. Plum, & S.R. Geiger (Eds.), *Handbook of physiology: Sec. 1. The nervous system: Vol. 5. Higher functions of the brain* (Pt. 2, pp. 768–810). Bethesda, MD: American Physiological Society.
Goldberg, E. (1989). Gradiental approach to neocortical functional organization. *Journal of Clinical & Experimental Neuropsychology*, *11*, 489–517.

Harrington, A. (1985). Nineteenth century ideas in hemisphere differences and "duality of mind." *Behavioral & Brain Sciences, 8,* 617–660.

LeDoux, J.E. (1987). Emotion. In V.B. Mountcastle, F. Plum, & S.R. Geiger (Eds.), *Handbook of physiology: Sec. 1. The nervous system: Vol. 5. Higher functions of the brain* (Pt. 2, pp. 768–810). Bethesda, MD: American Physiological Society.

Long, J.L. (1983). Confirmatory factor analysis: A preface to lisrel. In J.L. Sullivan & R.G. Niemi (Series Eds.), Sage University Paper Series: *Quantitative applications in social sciences* (No. 33, pp. 11–17). Beverly Hills, CA: Sage Publications.

Luria, A.R. (1973). *The working brain* (B. Haigh, Trans.). New York: Basic Books.

McGuinness, D., & Pribram, K. (1980). The neuropsychology of attention: Emotional and motivational controls. In M.C. Wittrock (Ed.), *Brain and psychology.* New York: Academic Press.

Marin, O.S.M., Schwartz, M.F., & Saffan, E.M. (1979). Origins and distribution of language. In F.A. King (Ed.), *Handbook of behavioral neurology: Neuropsychology* (M.S. Gazzaniga, Ed., Vol. 2, pp.179–208). New York: Plenum Press.

Miller, G.A., Galanter, E., & Pribram, K.H. (1960). *Plans and structure of behavior* (pp. 81–93). New York: Holt.

Mishkin, M. (1982). A memory system in the monkey. *Philosophical Transactions of the Royal Society of London, Series B, 298,* 85–95.

Nauta, W.J.H., & Feirtag, M. (1979). The organization of the brain. In *The brain: A Scientific American book.* San Francisco: Freeman.

Pribram, K.H. (1981). Emotions. In S.B. Filskov & T.J. Boll (Eds.), *Handbook of clinical neuropsychology* (Vol. 1, pp. 102–134). New York: Wiley.

Semmes, J. (1968). Hemispheric specialization: A possible clue to mechanism. *Neuropsychologia, 6,* 11–26.

Smith Churchland, P. (1986). *Neurophilosophy: Toward a unified science of the mind/brain.* Cambridge, MA: MIT Press.

Tucker, D.M., & Williamson, P.A. (1984). Asymmetric neural control systems in humans: Self-regulation. *Psychological Review, 91,* 185–215.

# 7

# Cognitive Sequelae in Closed Head Injury

## CHARLES J. LONG and MAUREEN E. SCHMITTER

For the past 18 years our laboratory has been conducting neuropsychological assessments on head-injured patients referred by neurosurgeons, neurologists, attorneys, insurance companies, and government agencies. The reports include a complete profile which outlines the patient's strengths and weaknesses, memory quotient, intellectual functions, emotional adjustment, and the examiner's perception of situational factors which may play a role in the patient's difficulties.

Regardless of the amount of test information contained in the neuropsychological report, neither neurosurgeons nor attorneys are concerned about a patient's cognitive function on the particular day he/she is evaluated. Rather, the interest is in what the patient's cognitive functions will be at some specified point in the future and/or what the level of cognitive functioning of the patient was before the trauma. Thus, the primary role of the neuropsychologist is to use neuropsychological data in order to bridge these gaps and to draw inferences with regard to future and/or past cognitive functioning.

In most cases, before entering the neuropsychologist's office, the head-injured patient has undergone a neurological assessment including radiological and/or electrophysiological tests such as the CT scan and EEG. While these tests are sensitive to focal space-occupying lesions or electrophysiological abnormalities, they are, for the most part, insensitive to the neurological effects of closed head injury. In fact, Long and Gouvier (1982) found that CT scan and EEG findings were abnormal in only 25% of mild to moderately impaired head-injured cases, whereas the neuropsychological evaluation revealed that 89% of these same patients were functioning within the impaired range of higher

CHARLES J. LONG • Department of Psychology, Memphis State University, Memphis, Tennessee 38152, and University of Tennessee Center for the Health Sciences, Memphis, Tennessee 38103.     MAUREEN E. SCHMITTER • Department of Psychology, Memphis State University, Memphis, Tennessee 38152.

*HANDBOOK OF HEAD TRAUMA: Acute Care to Recovery*, edited by Charles J. Long and Leslie K. Ross. Plenum Press, New York, 1992.

cortical functions. While the percentages vary depending upon the type of patients referred (severity, age, socioeconomic level, etc.) and/or the referral question, it is clear that the head-injured patient often experiences difficulties which can be assessed more readily by neuropsychological tests. This difference in sensitivity appears to relate to the fact that the neuropsychological battery evaluates the functional consequences of neurological dysfunction; in the case of head injury, the functional consequences are much more pronounced than identifiable focal neurological deficits.

Unfortunately, it is the neurosurgeons' reliance on tests designed to detect structural abnormalities that often forces the neuropsychologist into the role of patient advocate. In those cases where the neurosurgeon relies only on traditional neurological measures that suggest resolution of structural impairment, patients are frequently advised to return to work or school before their cognitive functions have sufficiently recovered.

After conducting a neuropsychological exam, we can often explain why such individuals are experiencing cognitive difficulties which interfere with their work, school, and/or social roles. Nevertheless, the consequences of head trauma cannot be reduced to the patient's performance on neuropsychological tests alone. In order to thoroughly understand the data, it is necessary to both evaluate and integrate information regarding a patient's demographic factors, personality characteristics, and social predictors with their performance on neuropsychological tests.

## DEMOGRAPHIC FACTORS

Data regarding an individual's preinjury level of function play a critical role in understanding the contribution of head injury to the individual's current problems; such information can also serve as a guideline to predictions of recovery. Clinical judgment about a patient's premorbid level of functioning can be made by examining demographic factors such as education, occupation, age, and prior head injuries, as well as familial history, and preexisting diseases. Also, school grades, prior tests of intellectual assessment, and measures of work-related performance, such as stability of employment or a supervisor's rating, may be significant.

Awareness of a patient's premorbid level of functioning is important as research indicates that individuals with above-average IQs, high socio-economic status, and a greater amount of education generally reflect individuals with higher overall cognitive skills prior to trauma; and, with other things being equal, their recovery tends to be greater (Rimel, Giordani, Barth, Boll, & Jane, 1981). In addition, age is often found to be a better predictor of outcome than most medical indicators with studies consistently showing that younger adults recover more rapidly than older adults (Heiskanen & Sipponen, 1970; Overgaard, Hvid-Hansen, Land, Pedersen, Christensen, Haase, Hein, & Tweed, 1973).

The patient's prior medical history is also important because complications related to preexisting disease have been found to result in a five times greater mortality rate. In particular, prior head injuries cause neurological damage that can serve to interact with subsequent injury producing a more pronounced effect. Any preexisting neurological disorder can serve to interact with head injury and augment the behavioral effects. For example, one study reported that 17 out of 135 patients with prolonged coma had a significant history such as previous trauma, epilepsy, alcoholism, or metabolic diseases (Bricolo, Turazzi, & Feriotti, 1980). Of these patients, none made a good recovery, two had moderate disability, and seven were severely disabled. This study also found that 50 patients with angiographic evidence of an intracranial mass lesion showed a lower percentage of satisfactory outcome (22%) than did the 74 patients free of such lesions (30%). Chronic alcohol abuse has been found to interact with the normal process of aging causing a greater decline in cognitive functions (Torres & Long, 1989). Such an interaction may well exist between alcohol abuse and head trauma.

The importance of integrating neuropsychological data with premorbid characteristics is clear in the following example: A lawyer walks into your office complaining of memory deficits following a motor vehicle accident. He reports that the accident occurred one month ago and that he was unconscious for approximately 45 minutes. You give him a complete neuropsychological battery, and he performs in the Average to High Average Range on all tests including the memory tests. Do you then conclude that he has no cognitive dysfunction or weaknesses and discount his memory difficulties as a psychological problem? No, here it is very important to integrate information regarding a lawyer's premorbid characteristics. Obviously, Average to High Average functioning is adequate; but, for someone who was initially functioning at a higher level, this can represent a noticeable deficit.

A reasonably accurate estimate of a patient's premorbid level of functioning is important because it can assist in establishing a reference point with which current performance can be compared in order to estimate the amount of impairment. Furthermore, it indicates general limits with regard to recovery.

## PERSONALITY FACTORS

Personality factors, prior to and following trauma, also significantly influence outcome. While premorbid psychological adjustment is often difficult to assess, clinical experience indicates that it plays an important role in predictions of recovery. Family history of character disorder, retardation, or psychosis has been shown to be related to psychosocial adjustment after injury (Lishman, 1978). For example, postconcussion symptoms are most likely to occur in patients who experience high stress or who have ineffective premorbid coping skills (Long & Novack, 1985; Wood, Novack, & Long, 1984).

Kozol (1946) found that less egocentric, more responsible, socially minded individuals prior to trauma recover best, even though they may have substantial neurotic characteristics, suggesting that brain injury may precipitate the expression of preexisting behavioral aberrations. While brain injury may cause more impulsivity and poor judgment, such tendencies are likely to have been present prior to trauma as evidenced by higher incidence of head injury in young males with low IQ, of low social and occupational status, and with poor social responsibility (Miller, 1961a,b).

Research also indicates that patients who experience significant personality change following head injury have less chance of returning to work, have fewer interests, lower nonverbal IQ, greater memory difficulties, and fewer friends compared to patients who do not experience significant changes in personality (Bond, 1986). Evaluation of a patient's emotional adjustment is important because 25 to 38% of head trauma patients develop some degree of psychiatric disability (Long & Gouvier, 1982). Evaluation of an individual's present emotional level can be obtained through administration of tests like the Minnesota Multiphasic Personality Inventory (MMPI).

For instance, let's use the lawyer in the preceding example. This time he reports that he had a head injury eight months ago and is now beginning to experience memory difficulties. A neuropsychological evaluation again finds that he is functioning within the Average to High Average Range. Personality assessment with the MMPI, however, reveals that he is both very anxious and depressed. In presenting the results of the tests and clarifying the history, he admits to severe financial and marital difficulties. Do you conclude that his memory difficulties are related to his accident? Perhaps, but his memory difficulties may well be secondary to emotional distress. You therefore conclude that the stress that he is experiencing is making it difficult for him to function at his optimal level. Since he is probably preoccupied with other thoughts, he may be finding it difficult to attend to and remember information presented to him. In fact, one study found that patients referred for neuropsychological evaluation more than six months after injury were more emotionally distressed (as assessed with the MMPI) than patients examined six months or less following injury (Fordyce, Roueche, & Prigatano, 1983). In contrast, no significant difference on any of the measures of neuropsychological functioning was found between the two groups. Here, again, one can see the importance of integrating all available information before reaching a conclusion regarding the difficulties of a patient.

## SOCIAL PREDICTORS

Numerous authors have found that psychosocial disabilities account for more of the overall disability than neurological deficits (Bond, 1976; Heaton & Pendleton, 1981; Jennett, Snoek, Bond, & Brooks, 1981; Newcombe, 1982). Studies have also shown that individuals who recover to a higher level, or at a rate faster than would be predicted from general guidelines, are individuals who have extremely strong social support systems (DiMatteo & Hays, 1981; LaRocco, House, & French, 1980); and the primary source of social support comes from the family (Rosenthal & Muir, 1983).

Individuals suffering head trauma vary widely with regard to their social support systems. While children often have the advantage of being dependents in a family structure, many head injury victims are no longer part of an established supportive family/social support system. All too often the young married couple is caught in an extremely difficult situation. Their recently acquired spouse is severely impaired, becomes impulsive, emotionally immature, and/or unable to support the family. If the social support systems were maladjusted prior to trauma, the resulting stress may further undermine the stability of the system and negatively affect the patient's recovery. Because families vary widely with regard to their premorbid stability, an understanding of each patient's social support system is important. A strong social support system can buffer the patient from stress and enhance recovery. Furthermore, family members can be trained to work with the patient and aid during times when memory is impaired and impulsivity is great.

An estimate of a patient's social support system is important because a caring and knowledgeable family member who has the time to work with the recovering patient represents an ideal resource. In some instances, families may be unable to provide the required support, and the patient may be isolated. In other cases, the family may respond excessively and, thus, not function in a manner which will serve to facilitate recovery. Clearly, in cases where good social support is lacking, rehabilitation or day treatment programs can provide a resource essential to recovery. The availability of adequate community and family support has been demonstrated to contribute to eventual functional recovery (Drudge, Williams, Kessler, & Gomes, 1984).

While it is clear that even mild head injury causes cognitive dysfunction for a time, and the focus of neuropsychology is on these cognitive changes, it is hoped that the preceding information and examples illustrate that the impact of head trauma cannot be related either to cognitive dysfunction or to the injury alone. Premorbid factors such as age, IQ, occupation, etc. are very important in determining the impact of the head injury on the individual. In addition, emotional and social/situational factors are important and can interact with the cognitive changes following head injury to greatly influence the impact of head trauma on the individual. While it is clear that other noncognitive factors must be investigated to render a clear picture of the individual's status, there is some question as to the importance of these factors in clinical decision-making. The present research investigates both cognitive and noncognitive factors in order to evaluate the contributions of each toward understanding the patient's status.

Any investigation of the cognitive sequelae following head injury must take the following three variables into account: severity of injury, time since injury, and age. This is because each of these factors has been shown to play a prominent role in the consequences of and the recovery from head injury.

## SEVERITY OF HEAD TRAUMA

Classifying patients according to severity of injury is important when conducting head injury research because severity represents the major factor accounting for impaired cognitive functions and extending the time as well as limiting the level of recovery. Typically, head injury patients seeking medical treatment suffer from at least a brief state of unconsciousness with subsequent amnesia for the traumatic injury and the period immediately following (Parkinson, 1982). This loss of consciousness is thought to be due to (1) rotational sheer stresses when the head is free to move (Denny-Brown & Russell, 1941), (2) centripetal effects (Ommaya & Gennarelli, 1974), and (3) a generalized effect of diffuse injury which is observed most often following brain trauma. Interruption of consciousness, or coma, is indicative of cerebral damage sufficient to impair neuropsychological performance. The resulting injury to the brain varies greatly with regard to severity, which can be estimated by the duration of either coma or posttraumatic amnesia (PTA).

Coma, resulting from head injury, is due to injury involving the brain stem and is most frequently associated with severe bending and stretching of the neck. Such forces may represent the basic mechanism of concussion. However, since sheer stresses are greatest at the cortex and radiate downward, brain stem symptoms are almost always secondary to damage of upper cortical regions (Ommaya & Gennarelli, 1974). Coma duration has been used as a successful indicator of severity of brain damage (Young, Rapp, Norton, Haack, Tibbs, & Bean, 1981; Klonoff, Costa, & Snow, 1986).

Duration of PTA, the period in which the individual loses the ability to store or retrieve new memories, represents another method for estimating the severity of brain injury following trauma. PTA occurs later (including coma but also extending beyond) and lasts a longer period of time than coma (generally four times longer than coma [Guthkelch, 1979]). The presence of PTA suggests that special neural mechanisms in the hippocampus or diencephalon may be impaired. The involvement of these structures may be due to the centripetal effects of injury or may relate to the fact that the medial temporal lobes are more likely to be injured due to the presence of bony structures.

One advantage of using coma as an estimate of severity of injury is that it is not age dependent like PTA. However, the relationship between coma and severity is not linear; only with coma of greater than three months' duration is there a strong correlation with recovery. The major problems with the use of coma as an estimate of severity relate to the fact that it occurs very early following trauma, is often brief in duration, and is seldom adequately measured. In addition, unlike PTA which can be measured at any time after the injury by taking a careful history, the patient typically does not have an awareness of coma duration making this information difficult to estimate at a later time in treatment.

Duration of PTA has been suggested as the best index of severity of injury (Russell & Smith, 1961; Russell, 1971). In fact, it was concluded in *Lancet* in 1961 that PTA was "the best yardstick we have for measuring the severity of blunt head injury." PTA duration has also been found to correlate with IQ level a few months after injury (Mandleberg, 1976). In addition, a relationship between more generalized memory impairment and PTA has been found (Mandleberg & Brooks, 1975).

Jennett (1976) concludes that, while there is no one method for assaying severity that is appropriate for all types of head trauma, reference should always be made to both coma and PTA to distinguish severity from complications. It has been further suggested that PTA is a better predictor in mild/moderate injury and coma is a better predictor in severe injury. However, at least one study found no correlation between deficits following minor head injury and duration of loss of consciousness, PTA, or the presence of sensory and motor deficits. According to Bond (1986), since there is a close correlation between PTA and the amount of brain tissue destroyed or damaged, PTA is a useful guide to certain aspects of later cognitive outcome, particularly memory. In contrast, he states that the Glasgow Coma Scale is useful for predicting early outcome (i.e., within the first few days); however, coma does not tell much about later outcome after the accident.

While most research has indicated that PTA is the most reliable measure of severity for the majority of head injury cases, there remains some disagreement as to the times employed to differentiate between the various classes of severity. Russell (1932) employed the following duration of PTA to differentiate severity: mild < 1 h, moderate 1–24 h, severe 1–7 days, very severe > 7 days. Bond (1983) has suggested that these times should be extended to properly account for variation in recovery from head trauma: mild < 1 day, moderate 1–7 days, severe 7–28 days, very severe > 28 days. Our clinical experience and research has led us to recommend and employ the following classification schema.

Severity Classifications (Table 7.1)

*Minimal (PTA 1–5 min)*

There is some question as to whether brief periods of PTA represent any damage to the brain. Some researchers conclude that if there is structural damage after mild head injury, it generally recovers from the neuropsychological standpoint within one month after trauma (Gentilini, Nichelli, Schoenhuber, Bortolotti, Tonelli, Falasca, & Merli, 1985). Other researchers find that even PTA of a few minutes classifies a patient as having some brain

TABLE 7.1.  Severity Classification Used in This Research
Based upon Duration of Posttraumatic Amnesia[a]

| Severity | PTA | Hospitalized | Recovery | Return to work |
|---|---|---|---|---|
| | | Complete recovery | | |
| Minimal | 1–5 min | | | 1 month |
| Very mild | 5–60 min | 2 days | 1 month | 2 months |
| Mild | 1–24 h | 7 days | 1–3 months | 4 months |
| | | Some impairment | | |
| Moderate | 1–7 days | >7 days | 3–9 months | 6 months |
| Severe | 8–28 days | | 9–12 months | 1 year |
| Very severe | 29+ days | | 24+ months | |

[a]Adapted from Russell (1932) and Bond (1983).

damage (Wrightson & Gronwall, 1980). A potential confound in those studies which found no evidence of impairment after one month may relate to the fact that there could have been impairment that was not measured during retesting due to practice effects (Becker, 1977).

*Very Mild/Mild (PTA 5 min–24 h)*

While patients with very mild head injury should make complete recovery (Lewin, 1968), they have been found to have significant cognitive problems at three days but not at one month (McLean, Temkin, Dikmen, & Wyler, 1983). One study found that although mild head injury patients have significant disruptions of psychosocial functions at one month postinjury (e.g., leisure, work, social interactions, sleep), the reasons were not solely related to head injury but instead to injury of other systems (Dikmen, McLean, & Temkin, 1986). Even in the absence of impairment, difficulties are present in orientation, distractability, memory, and speed of responding. Furthermore, although early neuropsychological sequelae and long-term intellectual deficits are generally related to severity of injury, residual impairment is also found in patients with relatively mild injuries. Longitudinal studies of patients with mild head trauma have documented that most recovery takes place within one to three months (Gentilini *et al.*, 1985; Ruff, Levin, & Marshall, 1986).

*Moderate (PTA 1–7 Days)*

Problems are more pronounced in patients with moderate injury. Approximately 90% of the patients with moderate head injury eventually return to work. Recovery generally occurs within three to nine months.

*Severe (PTA 8–28 Days)*

If PTA exceeds 7 days, 80% of the patients retain neurological deficits, and there remains a slight to severe reduction in mental capacity. One half of these patients are successfully rehabilitated. If PTA exceeds two weeks, 53% remain impaired in cognitive functions after one year (Drudge *et al.*, 1984). Severely injured patients rarely return to work in less than two months and in many there remains a high incidence of hemiparesis, ataxia, dysphasia, and visual defects. Eighty percent eventually return to their former work. In severe head injury cases, VIQ typically recovers within one year and PIQ within three years (Mandleberg & Brooks, 1985). More complex communicative functions may not begin to recover until six months after injury (Brooks, Deelman, Van Zomeren, Van Dongem, Van Hanskamp, & Aughton, 1984).

### Very Severe (PTA > 29 Days and/or Coma > 1 Month)

Research indicates that 38% of these patients die. Mortality increases steadily with age (Bricolo et al., 1980). Statistics also indicate that 15% of those sustaining severe head injuries remain severely disabled, 28% exhibit partial recovery, and only 19% are able to return to their former work. Other researchers have found no improvement in patients with PTA exceeding three months, whereas they observed good recovery with shorter PTA. A 10- to 15-year follow-up of patients suffering severe head injury revealed that no one escaped permanent sequelae. Permanent changes in behavior, personality, and emotion were the most serious burden for the caretakers. It is interesting that, even in cases of very severe head injury, loss of social contacts remained the patients' most disabling handicap (Thomsen, 1984).

### TIME SINCE INJURY

Time since injury must also be taken into account when analyzing head injury data as patients are seen at many different times postinjury and time reflects recovery. That is, the longer the time since injury, the greater the amount of recovery (Dikmen, Temkin, McLean, Wyler, & Machamer, 1987). However, many times patients with mild head injuries who are having difficulties at work or returning to work are referred for a neuropsychological evaluation. In these cases, stress, emotional difficulties, and postconcussion symptoms (such as headaches, dizziness, irritability, etc.) are often more important contributors to their difficulties than actual cognitive impairment.

Recovery is observed as a negatively accelerated curve with recovery occurring rapidly early and leveling off as it reaches asymptote. There is some question as to whether recovery actually conforms to this curve and more specifically whether all cognitive functions conform to such a curve (see Figure 15.1 in chapter by Jones). This curve is based on both clinical experience and research. For instance, recovery has been noted to be quite rapid at first and to level off at 24 months (Leigh, 1979). In addition, most neurological recovery is thought to occur within three to six months. With severe injury some functional recovery may occur up to 10 years following injury (Thomsen, 1984). Furthermore, the evidence supports the assumption that most recovery occurs during the first six months posttrauma in very severely impaired patients (Bond, 1976; Bond & Brooks, 1976).

### AGE

A final factor which must be taken into account when analyzing head injury data is age. While the majority of head injuries occur in young adults (90% below age 45), there is clearly an age effect in recovery. There is a very low prognosis for significant recovery in adults over 60. This relationship may relate to the increased possibility of preexisting neurological damage or it may relate to cell loss with age in the absence of identifiable trauma or disease. A study of 135 patients with coma greater than 2 weeks found that while 16% of the patients in the age group under 20 died, 78% in the age group over 60 died (Bricolo *et al.*, 1980). This study also found that the proportion of satisfactory results decreased gradually with age, from 43% in the age group under 20 years to zero in the age group over 60 years.

In addition, an age–performance relationship on neuropsychological tests has been documented. While this relationship is taken into account on standardized intellectual tests (Wechsler, 1955), it has also been found to hold for most neuropsychological tests (Fromm-Auch & Yeudall, 1983; Long & Klein, 1990; Moehle & Long, 1984).

Performance on complex, timed, and visuospatial tasks were found to decline most with age (Long & Klein, 1987; Moehle & Long, 1984). In addition, they found that, unless an age correction is used, 41% of pseudoneurological controls over 45 would be misclassified as impaired when all other neurological tests revealed no significant neurological damage. The above data suggest the need for standardized age norms in interpreting neuropsychological tests. These data further suggest that with increasing age there is an increase in cognitive weaknesses which will interact with neurological damage thereby augmenting the consequences of such damage on cognitive functions.

The preceding information illustrates how important it is that investigators take into account severity of injury, time since injury, and age when investigating the consequences of head injury. Clearly, all three factors play a prominent role in the consequences of the recovery from head injury.

## OBJECTIVES OF PRESENT RESEARCH

The objectives of the following research were to: (1) investigate the nature of cognitive changes following head trauma in patients referred for neuropsychological evaluation; (2) investigate the contribution of noncognitive factors, such as personality characteristics and premorbid factors, to the overall interpretation of the neuropsychological data; and (3) identify neuropsychological variables which might help differentiate between head-injured and non-head-injured neurologically impaired patients.

The following results were collected using retrospective analysis of data previously collected in our lab. While prospective research is desired to investigate the consequences of head injury in general, it does not answer the question regarding the role of various factors on those patients who are routinely referred for neuropsychological assessment. Furthermore, prospective research is limited by patient attrition regarding follow-up measures, difficulty obtaining adequate controls, practice effects, and it is often very expensive. The problem with practice effects was clearly represented in a study by Becker (1977). He found that after a one-month interval, head trauma patients improved on measures of a neuropsychological battery; however, the control patients also improved, and by a like amount.

While retrospective research avoids many of the problems outlined above, it is very sensitive to the referral question and to the information originally collected. For example, the majority of the patients studied in the research reported here were referred for neuropsychological evaluation by neurosurgeons. The test findings thus do not speak to head injury in general, but rather to the performance of head-injured individuals who had sufficient problems at some point in time following their injury to induce their treating physician to refer them for a comprehensive neuropsychological evaluation.

The data from 585 patients referred for a neuropsychological evaluation were analyzed. In order to control for age effects, all data were converted to standard scores using the mean and standard deviation appropriate for the patient's age group. The results of both analysis of variance and discriminant analysis revealed a wide range of variability among the test scores, indicating that there were a number of factors that influenced the results. Consistent with the variables previously discussed, a review of patient records revealed that patients varied significantly with regard to severity of injury as well as time since injury, which in part reflects the referral question. Therefore, the subjects were categorized into four different severity groups (based on PTA) and five different times since injury (6-month intervals). Both coma duration ($r = 0.28$) and PTA ($r = 0.18$) were found to correlate significantly with the impairment index. The impairment index consisted of the scores on seven tests which included speech perception, rhythm, tapping dominant hand, Trails B, TPT total time, TPT location, and TPT memory. Significant correlations were also noted between the impairment index and memory ($r = 0.36$), and the impairment index and language ($r = 0.22$).

We also sought to identify the pattern of deficits among head-injured individuals which might help differentiate them from other non-head-injured neurologically impaired groups. The other neurologically injured groups analyzed were left anterior, left medial, left posterior, right anterior, right medial, and right posterior.

A discriminate analysis utilizing only the cognitive test data revealed no systematic patterns of specific cognitive deficits which could differentiate head trauma patients from other non-head-injured neurological groups. In order to investigate these data further, the average, age-corrected, standard scores for each test were ranked from most to least impaired. Investigation of this ranking across all head-injured and non-head-injured neurological groups further supported the conclusion that no neuropsychological tests or pattern of test scores were able to reliably differentiate the head injury group from the other non-head-injured lesion groups (Table 7.2a). Based upon these findings, we concluded that there was no systematic pattern of cognitive deficits which differentiated head-injured from other neurologically impaired patient groups. Having reached this point, we sought nonneuropsychological factors that might differentiate between head-injured and non-head-injured, neurologically impaired patients. Other variables of importance might relate to premorbid abilities, personality characteristics, or social variables.

## PERSONALITY VARIABLES

Specifically we analyzed personality characteristics as measured by the MMPI. The following MMPI scales were found to vary significantly across the various head injury severity groups: F, K, D, PD, PT, SC.

When MMPI data were included along with cognitive measures, the ranking revealed that a pronounced number of the MMPI scales showed up at the top of the ranking analysis for the mild and moderate head injury groups, with less in the severe group (Table 7.2b).

TABLE 7.2a. Ranks of Means of Standard Scores for Lesion and Head Injury Severity

| LA[a] | LM | LP | RA | RM | RP | MILD | MOD | SEVERE | V. SEV. |
|---|---|---|---|---|---|---|---|---|---|
| Trails B | % Assoc | AV % | Seq L | AV % | TPT B | WMS M C | Trails B | TPT B | TPT B |
| Aphasia | AV % | % Assoc | Tap L | % Assoc | SEQ L | MQ | TPT B | MQ | MQ |
| Agno R | % L M | % L M | Trails A | % Vis | Graph L | Trails B | MQ | Trails B | Trails B |
| Graph R | % Vis | Trails A | Agno L | % L M | Trails A | Rhythm | TPT Tot | Seq L | WMS Inf |
| Trails A | Trails B | Sup R | AV % | WMS Inf | AV % | WMS Ori | Sp Per | Seq R | WMS P A |
| Word Flu | Aphasia | % Vis | Trails B | MQ | TPT Tot | Word Flu | Graph L | TPT Tot | Trails A |
| MQ | Agno R | Trails B | TPT L | Trails B | Seq R | WMS Inf | WMS M C | WMS Inf | AV % |
| % Assoc | Seq R | Graph R | TPT B | TPT B | Trails B | WMS L M | WMS Inf | Trails A | Seq R |
| Seq R | MQ P A | Agno R | Supp L | WMS Ori | Supp L | AV % | % Log M | TPT L | Graph L |
| MQ P A | Sp Per | Graph L | TPT Tot | WMS Vis | Rhythm | % Log M | Trails A | WMS P A | Seq L |
| AV % | WMS Inf | MQ | Sp Per | Graph L | % Assoc | Graph R | Word Flu | Graph L | TPT L |
| Supp R | Graph R | WMS Vis | Crosses | TPT Tot | % L M | Sp Per | Graph R | % L M | WMS Vis |
| Sp Per | MQ | TPT B | % Assoc | TPT Mem | TPT Mem | Agno R | % Vis | Graph R | % Vis |
| Trails C | WMS L M | TPT Tot | % Vis | Trails A | % Vis | TPT B | TPT L | WMS Vis | Aphasia |

[a]LA = left anterior; LM = left medial; LP = left posterior; RA = right anterior; RM = right medial; RP = right posterior; MILD = mild head injury; MOD = moderate head injury; SEVERE = severe head injury; V. SEV. = very severe head injury.

TABLE 7.2b. Ranks of Means of Standard Scores for Lesion and Head Injury Severity with MMPI and Cornell

| LA[a] | LM | LP | RA | RM | RP | MILD | MOD | SEVERE | V. SEV. |
|---|---|---|---|---|---|---|---|---|---|
| Trails B | % Assoc | AV % | Seq L | AV % | MMPI D | MMPI HS | MMPI D | TPT B | TPT B |
| Aphasia | AV % | % Assoc | Tap L | % Assoc | MMPI HY | MMPI HY | MMPI HY | MMPI SC | MQ |
| Graph R | % L M | % L M | Trails A | Cornell | TPT B | MMPI D | MMPI SC | MQ | Trails B |
| Agno R | Cornell | Trails A | Agno L | % Vis | MMPI HS | Cornell | MMPI HS | MMPI D | WMS Inf |
| Trails A | % Vis | Supp R | AV % | % L M | Seq L | MMPI PT | MMPI PD | MMPI PD | WMS P A |
| MMPI D | MMPI SC | % Vis | Trails B | WMS Inf | Graph L | MMPI SC | MMPI PT | Trails B | MMPI D |
| MMPI HY | MMPI PT | Trails B | TPT L | MQ | MMPI SC | MMPI PD | TPT B | Seq L | Trails A |
| MQ | Trails B | Graph R | TPT B | Trails B | Trails A | WMS M C | Trails B | MMPI HS | AV % |
| Word Flu | MMPI HY | Agno R | Sup L | TPT B | MMPI PT | MQ | MQ | MMPI HY | Seq R |
| % Assoc | MMPI PD | MMPI SC | Graph L | MMPI D | AV % | Trails B | TPT Tot | Seq R | Graph L |
| MMPI HS | Aphasia | Graph L | TPT Tot | WMS Ori | TPT Tot | WMS Inf | Cornell | WMS Inf | MMPI SC |
| AV % | Agno R | MQ | Sp Per | WMS Vis | Seq R | Word Flu | Graph L | TPT Tot | Seq L |
| Seq R | Seq R | WMS Vis | Crosses | MMPI HY | Trails A | WMS L M | Sp Per | TPT L | TPT L |
| WMS P A | WMS P A | TPT B | % Assoc | MMPI SC | Sup L | Rhythm | WMS Inf | WMS P A | WMS Vis |
| Cornell | Sp Per | TPT Tot | % Vis | Graph L | Rhythm | WMS Ori | Trails A | Trails A | Aphasia |
| Sp Per | WMS Inf | MMPI PD | MMPI D | TPT Tot | % Assoc | Sp Per | % L M | MMPI PT | % Vis |
| Supp R | MMPI PA | Aphasia | Word Flu | TPT Mem | % L M | % L M | WMS M C | Graph R | Trails C |

The only other neurological group which revealed a similar ranking was the right posterior group. This group was the most impaired of the six lesion groups. These data clearly indicate that, while much neuropsychological research focuses on cognitive functions, assessment of emotional adjustment is important information which cannot be overlooked.

Further support for these findings can be found by investigating postinjury symptoms. A list of such symptoms is outlined in Table 7.3. As can be seen, only a few of the symptoms represent changes in cognitive functions. The remainder relate to personality variables and postconcussion symptoms. These observations, coupled with our research, further point out the need to expand the analysis of head injury effects and interpret neuropsychological data in this broader context. Particular consideration should be given to patients who, in addition to brain injury, suffer from persistent pain in the head and/or back or other problems secondary to traumatic injury. These consequences may be disabling in a patient who does not display impaired cognitive functions.

Thus, cognitive deficits caused by brain injury play an important role in determining the characteristics of the individual's behavior. However, cognitive deficits are only one factor playing a role with many other factors. These findings suggest that although brain injury plays an important role, it is only one element in a multifactorial etiology involving both neurological and nonneurological variables (Klesges, Fisher, Vasey, & Pheley, 1985).

Since statistical methods were unable to discriminate between head trauma patients and other non-head-injured neurological groups, we are reduced to using descriptive methods. Our data reveal that neuropsychological research might benefit from classifying changes of behavior according to postconcussion symptoms and personality variables such as the individual's stress management skills. Clearly, classification of cognitive deficits such as sensory deficits and memory consolidation weaknesses can only address a small subset of the problem. A full neuropsychological assessment must include not only cognitive measures but also the patient's emotional adjustment and situational factors.

When discussing changes which occur following head trauma, focusing entirely on cognitive deficits will address only one part of the picture. Another part of the picture is the patient's ability to cope with stress, and still a third part is the situational dimension. We are presently working to expand our data base and derive predictive formulas for recovery following head trauma as these formulas cut across (1) occupational status, (2) emotional

TABLE 7.3.   List of Postinjury Symptoms by Category

| Cognitive | Postconcussion symptoms | Personality variables |
|---|---|---|
| Motor retardation | Headache | Anxiety |
| Loss of concentration | Fatigability | Blunted affect |
| Disorientation | Alcohol intolerance | Excitement |
| Conceptual disorganization | Weakness | Depression |
| Hearing defects | Pain | Mental regression |
| Visual defects | Dizziness | Social isolation |
| Anosmia | Irritability | Impaired self-perception |
| Epilepsy | Diplopia | Personality changes |
| Disinhibition | Memory problems | Lack of insight |
| Disorders of perception | | Egocentricity |
| Anticipatory deficit | | Insomnia |
| Memory weakness | | |

adjustment, (3) neurological status as reflected in cognitive function, (4) perceived stress (i.e., change in behavior following neurological trauma and situational factors). In the interim, our approach to evaluating head trauma patients is to take all the factors outlined above into account when formulating hypotheses and making recommendations.

Consideration should also be given to the sensitivity of neuropsychological tests to the effects of head injury. While assessment of cognitive functions by means of neuropsychological tests is more sensitive to the consequences of head injury than other neurological tests, this does not imply that there cannot be cognitive impairment if it is not reflected in the neuropsychological tests. The patient's performance may reflect a change in cognitive functions and yet remain within the average range. Furthermore, deficits may be present that influence the patient's ability to carry out daily activities that are not revealed in the neuropsychological test results. In fact, neuropsychology may only touch tangentially on the problem of behavior disturbances (Weinstein, comments to article by Dikmen & Reitan, 1976).

Although our data revealed that no specific pattern of cognitive deficits appears to represent the head-injured population, there are characteristic changes in behavior that are consistently reported. Behaviors such as slowness of thought, fatigue, poor memory and perceptual memory (Denckler & Lofving, 1958; Ruesch, 1944), inability to maintain sustained effort (Ruesch & Moore, 1943), and impaired ability to deal with complexity (Dikmen, Reitan, & Temkin, 1983) are commonly noted in head-injured patients. While such factors may influence test performance, by their nature, they are likely to influence it in a generalized way. In fact, most workers state that after concussion there is no consistent abnormality in standard psychometric tests (Gronwall & Wrightson, 1974). Future research should direct attention to the following cognitive variables: (1) increased information processing time (RT, timed tasks), (2) impaired processing of complexity (Trails B, TPT), (3) degraded perception (Sensory), (4) impaired attention (Speech, Rhythm), and (5) impaired memory (Memory Quotient and Percent Recall). In addition, research which also takes emotional and situational factors into account will greatly aid in understanding and assisting head-injured patients.

# REFERENCES

Becker, B. (1977). Intellectual changes after closed head injury. *Journal of Clinical Psychology, 47,* 307–309.

Bond, M. R. (1976). Assessment of the psychosocial outcome of severe head injury. *Acta Neurochirurgica, 34,* 57–70.

Bond, M. R. (1986). Psychobehavioral consequences of severe brain injury. *Trends in Rehabilitation,* Summer, 2–8.

Bond, M. R. (1983). Standardized methods of assessing and predicting outcome. In M. Rosenthal, E. Griffith, M. Bond, & J. Miller (Eds.), *Rehabilitation of the head injured adult,* (pp. 97–113). Philadelphia: Davis.

Bond, M. R., & Brooks, D. N. (1976). Understanding the process of recovery as a basis for the investigation of rehabilitation for the brain injured. *Scandinavian Journal of Rehabilitation Medicine, 8,* 127–133.

Bricolo, A., Turazzi, S., & Feriotti, G. (1980). Prolonged posttraumatic unconsciousness. *Journal of Neurosurgery, 52,* 625–634.

Brooks, D. N., Deelman, B. G., Van Zomeren, A. H., Van Dongem, H., Van Haiskamp, F., & Aughton, M. E. (1984). Problems in measuring cognitive recovery after acute brain damage. *Journal of Clinical Neuropsychology, 6*(1), 71–85.

Denckler, S. J., & Lofving, B. A. (1958). A psychometric study of identical twins discordant for closed head injury. *Acta Psychiatrica et Neurologica Scandinavica, 33*(Suppl. 122), 119–126.

Denny-Brown, D., & Russell, W. R. (1941). Experimental cerebral concussion. *Brain*, *64*, 93–164.

Dikmen, S., & Reitan, R. M. (1976). Psychological deficits and recovery of function after head injury. *Transactions of the American Neurological Association*, *101*, 72–77.

Dikmen, S., Reitan, R. M., & Temkin, N. R. (1983). Neuropsychological recovery in head injury. *Archives of Neurology*, *40*, 333–338.

Dikmen, S., McLean, A., & Temkin, N. (1986). Neuropsychological and psychosocial consequences of minor head injury. *Journal of Neurology, Neurosurgery, & Psychiatry*, *49*, 1227–1232.

Dikmen, S., Temkin, N., McLean, A., Wyler, A., & Machamer, J. (1987). Memory and head injury severity. *Journal of Neurology, Neurosurgery, & Psychiatry*, *50*(12), 1613–1618.

DiMatteo, M. R., & Hays, R. (1981). Social support and serious illness. In B. H. Gottlieb (Ed.), *Social networks and social support*. Beverly Hills, CA: Sage Publications.

Drudge, O. W., Williams, J. M., Kessler, M., & Gomes, F. B. (1984). Recovery from severe closed head injuries: Repeat testings with the Halstead–Reitan neuropsychological battery. *Journal of Clinical Psychology*, *40*(1), 259–264.

Fordyce, D. J., Roueche, J. R., & Prigatano, G. P. (1983). Enhanced emotional reactions in chronic head trauma patients. *Journal of Neurology, Neurosurgery, & Psychiatry*, *46*, 620–624.

Fromm-Auch, D., & Yeudall, L. T. (1983). Normative data for the Halstead–Reitan neuropsychological tests. *Journal of Clinical Neuropsychology*, *3*, 221–238.

Gentilini, M., Nichelli, P., Schoenhuber, R., Bortolotti, P., Tonelli, L., Falasca, A., & Merli, G. A. (1985). Neuropsychological evaluation of mild head injury. *Journal of Neurology, Neurosurgery, & Psychiatry*, *48*, 137–140.

Gronwall, D., & Wrightson, P. (1974). Delayed recovery of intellectual function after minor head injury. *Lancet*, *2*, 605–609.

Guthkelch, A. N. (1979). Assessment of outcome: Post-traumatic amnesia, post concussional symptoms, and accident neurosis. *Acta Neurochirurgica Suppl.*, *28*, 120–133.

Heaton, R. K., & Pendleton, M. G. (1981). Use of neuropsychological tests to predict adult patients' everyday functioning. *Journal of Consulting & Clinical Psychology*, *49*(6), 807–821.

Heiskanen, O., & Sipponen, P. (1970). Prognosis of severe brain injury. *Acta Neurologica Scandinavica*, *46*, 343–348.

Jennett, B. (1976). Assessment of the severity of head injury. *Journal of Neurology, Neurosurgery, & Psychiatry*, *39*, 647–655.

Jennett, B., Snoek, J., Bond, M. R., & Brooks, M. (1981). Disability after severe head injury: Observations on the use of the Glasgow Outcome Scale. *Journal of Neurology, Neurosurgery, & Psychiatry*, *44*, 285–293.

Klesges, R. C., Fisher, L., Vasey, M., & Pheley, A. (1985). Predicting adult premorbid functioning levels: Another look. *International Journal of Neuropsychology*, *7*(1), 1–3.

Klonoff, P. S., Costa, L. D., & Snow, W. G. (1986). Predictions and indicators of quality of life in patients with closed head injury. *Journal of Clinical & Experimental Psychology*, *8*(5), 469–485.

Kozol, H. L. (1946). Pretraumatic personality and psychiatric sequelae of head injury. *Archives of Neurology & Psychiatry*, *56*, 245–275.

*Lancet*. (1961). The best yardstick we have. *Lancet*, *2*, 1445–1446.

LaRocco, J. M., House, J. S., & French, J. R. (1980). Social support, occupational stress, and health. *Journal of Health & Social Behavior*, *21*, 202–218.

Leigh, D. (1979). Psychiatric aspects of head injury. *Psychiatry Digest*, *40*, 21–33.

Lewin, W. (1968). Rehabilitation after head injury. *British Medical Journal*, *1*, 465–470.

Lishman, W. A. (1978). Head injury. In *Organic psychiatry* (pp. 192–261). Oxford: Blackwell.

Long, C. J., & Gouvier, W. D. (1982). Neuropsychological assessment of outcome following closed head injury. In R. N. Malatesha & L. C. Hartlage (Eds.), *Neuropsychology and cognition* (Vol. 2). The Hague: Nijhoff.

Long, C. J., & Klein, K. (1987, October). *Analysis of age effects upon neuropsychological functioning and the development of age norms*. Paper presented at the National Academy of Neuropsychology Conference, Chicago.

Long, C. J., & Klein, K. (1990). Decision strategies in neuropsychology II: Determination of age effects on neuropsychological performance. *Archives of Clinical Neuropsychology*, *5*, 335–345.

Long, C. J., & Novack, T. (1985). Interpretation and treatment of post-concussion symptoms following head trauma: Interpretation and treatment. *Southern Medical Journal*, *79*, 728–732.

McLean, A., Temkin, N. R., Dikmen, S., & Wyler, A. R. (1983). The behavioral sequelae of head injury. *Journal of Clinical Neuropsychology*, *2*, 361–376.

Mandleberg, I. A. (1976). Cognitive recovery after severe head injury. 3. Wechsler Adult Intelligence Scale verbal and performance IQs as a function of post-traumatic amnesia and time from injury. *Journal of Neurology, Neurosurgery, & Psychiatry*, *39*, 1001–1007.

Mandleberg, I. A., & Brooks, D. N. (1975). Cognitive recovery after severe head injury: 1. Serial testing on the Wechsler Adult Intelligence Scale. *Journal of Neurology, Neurosurgery, & Psychiatry*, *38*, 1121–1126.

Miller, H. (1961a, April 1). Accident neurosis I. *British Medical Journal*, 919–925.

Miller, H. (1961b, April 8). Accident neurosis II. *British Medical Journal*, 992–998.

Moehle, K. A., & Long, C. J. (1984) *Pattern of decline across neuropsychological measures with aging*. Paper presented at the American Psychological Association Convention, Toronto.

Newcombe, F. (1982). The psychological consequences of closed head injury: Assessment and rehabilitation. *Injury*, *14*, 111–136.

Ommaya, A., & Gennarelli, T. (1974). Cerebral concussion and traumatic unconsciousness. *Brain*, *97*, 633–654.

Overgaard, J., Hvid-Hansen, O., Land, A., Pedersen, K. K., Christensen, S., Haase, J., Hein, O., & Tweed, W. A. (1973, September 22). Prognosis after the injury based on early clinical examination. *Lancet*, 631–635.

Parkinson, D. (1982). The biomechanics of concussion. *Clinical Neurosurgery*, *29*, 131–145.

Rimel, R. W., Giordani, B., Barth, J. T., Boll, J. T., & Jane, J. A. (1981). Disability caused by minor head injury. *Neurosurgery*, *9*, 221–228.

Rosenthal, M., & Muir, C. A. (1983). Method of family intervention. In M. Rosenthal, E. R. Griffith, M. R. Bond, & J. D. Miller (Eds.), *Rehabilitation of head injured adults* (pp. 407–418). Philadelphia: Davis.

Ruesch, J. (1944). Intellectual impairment in head injuries. *American Journal of Psychiatry*, *100*, 480–496.

Ruesch, J., & Moore, B. (1943). Measurement of intellectual functions in the acute stage of head injury. *Archives of Neurology & Psychiatry*, *50*, 165–170.

Ruff, R. M., Levin, H. S., & Marshall, L. E. (1986). Neurobehavioral methods of assessment and the study of outcome in minor head injury. *Journal of Head Trauma Rehabilitation*, *1*(2), 43–50.

Russell, W. R. (1932). Cerebral involvement in head injury: A study based on the examination of 200 cases. *Brain*, *35*, 549–603.

Russell, W. R. (1971). *The traumatic amnesias*. New York: Oxford University Press.

Russell, W. R., & Smith, A. (1961). Post-traumatic amnesia in closed head injury. *Archives of Neurology*, *5*, 4–17.

Thomsen, I. V. (1984). Late outcome of very severe blunt head trauma: A 10–15 year second follow-up. *Journal of Neurology, Neurosurgery, & Psychiatry*, *47*, 260–268.

Torres, I., & Long, C. J. (1989, March). *Relationship between alcohol dependence as defined by DSM-III and its effects on cognitive functions*. Paper presented at the Southeastern Psychological Association Meeting, Washington, DC.

Wechsler, D. (1955). A standardized memory scale for clinical use. *Journal of Neurology, Neurosurgery, & Psychiatry*, *15*, 54–58.

Welford, A. T. (1962). On changes of performance with age. *Lancet*, *1*, 335–339.

Wood, F., Novack, T. A., & Long, C. J. (1984). Post-concussion symptoms: Cognitive, emotional, and environmental aspects. *International Journal of Psychiatry in Medicine*, *14*(4), 277–283.

Wrightson, P., & Gronwall, D. (1980). Time off work and symptoms after minor head injury. *Injury*, *12*, 445–454.

Young, B., Rapp, P. D., Norton, J. A., Haack, D., Tibbs, P. A., & Bean, J. R. (1981). Early predictions of outcome in head-injured patients. *Journal of Neurosurgery*, *54*, 300–303.

# III

# Inpatient and Outpatient Rehabilitation

# 8

# Acute Rehabilitation of the Head-Injured Individual

## Toward a Neuropsychological Paradigm of Treatment

DANIEL E. STANCZAK and W. L. HUTCHERSON

Rehabilitation is the applied use of technology and scientific principles to assist individuals in returning to the greatest possible functional autonomy following severe illness or injury. During the past quarter century the field of rehabilitation has undergone tremendous growth. This growth stems partly from consumer demand and the concomitant development of support organizations such as the National Head Injury Foundation and similar groups which seek to improve the lot of their constituents. The growth in rehabilitative services also stems from technological advances which have improved survival rates from serious illness and injuries, and which have led to the development of more practical and functional adaptive devices. To a large degree, the growth of rehabilitation as a health care specialty has paralleled the development of clinical neuropsychology as a behavioral science. The philosophical tenets of neuropsychology—with its emphasis on brain–behavior relationships, behavioral scaling and analysis, microbehavioral chains, empirical validation of treatment effects, and environmental determinants—created a fertile soil from which many innovations in rehabilitation were to sprout.

Despite these behavioral influences, the field of rehabilitation, as it exists today, evolved primarily from physical medicine, and much of the philosophy underlying services

DANIEL E. STANCZAK • Neuropsychology Department, Baylor University Institute for Rehabilitation, Dallas, Texas 75246.    W. L. HUTCHERSON • The Rehab Hospital in Mechanicsburg, Mechanicsburg, Pennsylvania 17055.

*HANDBOOK OF HEAD TRAUMA: Acute Care to Recovery*, edited by Charles J. Long and Leslie K. Ross. Plenum Press, New York, 1992.

delivery in contemporary rehabilitation stems from a traditional "biomedical paradigm." The adaptation of the biomedical paradigm to the field of rehabilitation brought continuity of care and a rich clinical tradition to rehabilitative service delivery. However, as a greater diversity of health care professionals became involved in the rehabilitative process, it became apparent that the biomedical paradigm of service delivery possessed a number of inherent philosophical weaknesses. With the rapid growth of rehabilitative services during the past quarter century, however, there has been precious little time to stop and reflect on the philosophy of rehabilitative treatment or to ponder the possible conflicts between biomedical and alternative paradigms of service delivery. Unfortunately, as Giles and Fussey (1988) observe, it is this absence of a fundamental, shared philosophy which results in fragmented disjointed delivery of rehabilitative services.

Our goal, in this chapter, is to enumerate what we perceive to be some of the inherent philosophical weaknesses of the traditional biomedical paradigm of rehabilitative service delivery and to propose an alternative model, which we will refer to as a neuropsychological or neurobehavioral paradigm. In the process of comparing these paradigms, we will examine specific assumptions which typically follow from each. It is important for the reader to understand that neither paradigm exists today in its pure form, that most contemporary head injury rehabilitation programs will exhibit characteristics of both paradigms, and that the dichotomization of the biomedical and neuropsychological paradigms of rehabilitation is undertaken to more clearly explicate the philosophical issues under examination.

## ASSUMPTION #1—AN ORGANISMIC LOCUS OF DYSFUNCTION

Fundamental to the biomedical paradigm is the notion of disease (i.e., some pathogen or pathological process which causes discomfort or loss of function). Such a disease model is materialistic, assuming that patients are physical beings whose functions can be explained solely on the basis of physical laws. Moreover, a disease model is reductionistic and presumes that patients can best be understood through an examination of their constituent parts. In a disease model it is assumed that the patient's deficits are the consequence of some deviation from biological norms and that if one only examines the patient at an increasingly microscopic level—moving from system to organ, from organ to tissue, from tissue to cell, from cell to cellular structures, etc.—an appropriate intervention will be found (Snyder, 1989).

This linear notion of disease carries with it a requirement for diagnosis and treatment. Thus, in a traditional biomedical paradigm, the rehabilitation specialist first tries to determine the basis for the patient's problems (diagnosis) and then attempts to establish a plan to remedy or ameliorate the disease process (treatment). Inherent in such a disease model is the assumption that the disease process dwells within the patient either as a direct result of tissue damage or as the combined result of tissue damage and a premorbid psychological abnormality. Simply put, the biomedical paradigm presumes an organismic locus of dysfunction. As a consequence of such reasoning, forms of treatment are sought which can effect change within the patient (i.e., the rehabilitation specialist attempts to "cure" the "disease"). While some complications of head injury such as deep vein thrombosis, heterotopic ossification, or fractured bones yield to traditional medical interventions such as medications, surgery, immobilization, etc., the most disabling sequelae of cerebral trauma do not.

At a minimum, the biomedical paradigm of rehabilitation presumes plasticity of neural tissue, and a number of elaborate theories—such as denervation supersensitivity (Cannon & Rosenblueth, 1949), reactive synaptogenesis (Lly & Chambers, 1958), and neural equipotentiality (Tizard, 1959)—have been proposed to explain the observed recovery of function following central nervous system insult. However, such theories have been of little heuristic value and have provided little in the way of direct treatment approaches (Craine, 1982). Clearly, such theories offer no methodology either for "healing" a chronic central nervous system lesion or for correcting maladaptive, premorbid traits. Thus, the biomedical paradigm, with its assumption that the "disease process" lies within the patient, leads essentially to a "dead end" from a treatment perspective.

The neuropsychological paradigm of rehabilitation is a nonlinear one which does not assume a direct causal relationship between cerebral trauma and subsequent behavioral disturbances. The paradigm recognizes that, unlike other organs, the brain is an organ of interface between the patient and his/her external environment. Damage to the brain produces consequences which are unlike those of damage to any other organ. Damage to other organs affects the internal workings of the patient's body, but damage to the brain affects the ability of that person to function within an environment. Thus, a brain injury is not perceived as just causing an aphasia but, rather, is viewed as disrupting communication between the patient and others. Likewise, brain damage does not just cause a hemiparesis but, rather, impairs the patient's mobility within his or her environment. While such arguments may seem to represent a splitting of hairs, the treatment implications of such a view are substantial.

Instead of presenting an organismic view of neuropathology, the neuropsychological paradigm presents an interactive, emergent, holistic, and environmental one. The patient is no longer seen as a hierarchical collection of molecules and tissues but, rather, is viewed as a whole being whose emergent properties are greater than the summed properties of its constituent parts (Sperry, 1969). The problems are no longer seen as dwelling within the patient but, rather, as occurring in the interface between the patient and his/her environment. This, of course, is one of the basic tenets of Behaviorism (i.e., that behavior is a function of the person and environment) (Lewin, 1935).

Given this tenet, the linear notion of a disease, with its demand for diagnosis and treatment, is no longer a viable one. Instead, the neuropsychological paradigm emphasizes the nonlinear notions of assessment and adaptation. Assessment is the identification and measurement of variables which affect the patient's performance. Adaptation is the systematic control of those variables to maximize the patient's functional autonomy. But assessment and adaptation are continuous processes which, in practice, occur concomitantly and repetitively. Instead of searching for "treatments" which effect change just within the head injury victim, rehabilitation specialists seek to maximize adaptation in two ways: (1) by altering the manner in which the patient interacts with his/her environment, and (2) by altering the way the environment affects the patient. Thus, within the neuropsychological paradigm, the range of possible "treatments" is limited only by the number of relevant variables identified and by the training and creativity of the health care provider. Assumptions of neural plasticity or system substitution are not as important in the neuropsychological paradigm as in the well-founded, simple assumption that the patient and significant others in his/her environment are capable of learning. In contrast to the theoretical foundation of the biomedical paradigm, the neuropsychological paradigm is supported by elaborate theories of learning which have great heuristic value and which have been subjected to rigorous testing in both experimental and applied settings.

The differences between the two treatment paradigms are probably nowhere better illustrated than in their approach to the so-called "agitation" that is commonly observed following cerebral trauma (Corrigan & Myslw, 1988; Levin, 1985; Wesolowski & Burke, 1988; Wood, 1987). During this period, patients appear disoriented, confused, restless, fearful, and apprehensive. Their thought processes may be disordered, and they may become aggressive and combative. Socially inappropriate behavioral displays are common. As one might expect, this stage of recovery is very stressful for the patient and family, and particularly for the staff, who are frequently undertrained in "behavioral management." It is not unusual, therefore, for health care professionals to view posttraumatic agitation as a negative experience which only interferes with rehabilitative treatment. Indeed, some rehabilitative specialists are actually afraid of the agitated patient, since they cannot predict the patient's behavior with any degree of reliability.

In response to such agitated patients, biomedically minded providers often employ a variety of psychotropic drugs, such as benzodiazepines, butyrophenones, phenothiazines, tricyclics, or other antidepressant agents, and request a "behavioral treatment plan" from the psychologist. The problem with such a treatment regimen is obvious. First, there is no consistent, replicated evidence that any class of psychotropics is effective in alleviating posttraumatic agitation without causing significant concomitant sedation. Second, "behavioral treatment plans" have come to be viewed as some sort of "psychological neuroleptic" which will somehow effect change within the patient's psyche regardless of whether or not the contingencies of reinforcement are consistently applied. The consulting psychologist is often put in a role similar to that of a consulting cardiologist or internist (i.e., as someone who will treat a specialized problem), thereby relieving the staff of any further responsibility for that problem. In a sense then, the notion of a "behavioral treatment plan" only underscores the assumption that the source of the agitation lies within the patient and that the psychologist alone can somehow effect change within the patient. Another problem is that the "behavioral treatment plan" will be carried out primarily by those personnel least qualified by training and experience to do so. While these personnel typically demonstrate consumate devotion to their patients and are highly motivated to acquire new skills, many have difficulty transcending their medically oriented backgrounds and experience considerable difficulty thinking in terms of a learning model. Most physicians are aware of these limitations, and many will readily admit that they are prescribing such a treatment regimen more to alleviate the staff's anxieties than for any anticipated benefit to the patient.

Unfortunately, medicating the patient to cure the staff's deficiencies creates its own set of problems. First, psychotropics have long-term side effects, can exacerbate existing mental confusion, and can potentially produce paradoxical reactions (Bontke, Brockman, Cilo, Robert, & Worthington, 1988). Second, baseline data are rarely recorded to determine whether or not such drugs are indeed producing a therapeutic effect. This, of course, leads to an attribution error, wherein any change in a positive direction, even spontaneous remission of symptoms or altered staff perceptions of the patient's performance, is attributed to the drug's action. Third, since the patients may receive "prn" medications during periods of confusion or agitation, they may then come to associate their own disruptive behavior with attention from the nursing staff (social reinforcement of inappropriate behavior). The net effect, then, is that the staff's behavior paradoxically serves to maintain or even exacerbate the patient's behavioral disturbances. As noted in a psychiatric setting by Rosenhan (1973), heavy reliance upon psychotropic medication contributes to depersonalization of the patient by giving staff the inaccurate impression that active treatment is indeed under way and that no further intervention on the part of the staff is warranted. As a consequence, the staff is deprived of an opportunity to develop alternative treatment strategies.

In direct contrast to the apprehension experienced by the biomedically oriented practitioner, the neuropsychologically oriented provider views the agitated phase of recovery with optimism and anticipation. To this practitioner, the emergence of agitation signals an expanded behavioral repertoire for the patient, even if such behaviors appear random or disorganized. This background of seemingly random behavior is a prerequisite for operant learning to occur (Miller, 1981). Through operant learning, the staff shapes such random behavior into more functional activity through the process of successive approximation. The last thing the neuropsychologically minded practitioner would want to do would be to diminish this behavioral repertoire through the use of psychotropics. Rather than ordering psychotropics and a "behavioral treatment plan," the neuropsychological practitioner recognizes that he or she cannot independently effect change within the patient. Instead, the provider implements an "environmental modification plan" designed to identify and control those variables which affect the patient's behavior. Such environmental engineering demands that all staff be skilled in the application of learning principles and that such principles be consistently applied across settings and providers. In this model, the psychologist serves a role similar to that of an architect or engineer, designing a "behavioral blueprint" which is then implemented by a staff of skilled behavioral technicians.

There are positive and negative consequences to such a treatment regimen. On the negative side, implementation of such a plan requires a staff highly trained in a learning model of rehabilitation (Grimm & Bleiberg, 1986), thus possibly increasing the cost of service delivery. On the positive side, there is a reduced need for the use of chemical restraints. As the staff becomes more skilled in modifying environmental variables, there is a lower probability that they will unwittingly reinforce maladaptive behaviors. Additionally, rather than feeling helpless, afraid, or useless, the staff acquires feelings of efficacy and confidence as they successfully manage agitated patients and help those patients move from random to purposeful behavior patterns. Finally, the moral/ethical dilemma of medicating the patient to cure the staff's anxieties is avoided.

## ASSUMPTION #2—A PROVIDER LOCUS OF POWER

Inherent in the biomedical paradigm of rehabilitation is the notion that the power to effect change or "cure" the patient lies within the health care provider. Clearly health care professionals, in rehabilitation and other specialties, are afforded considerable status in our society because of the expertise they acquire through years of study and clinical experience. However, this status often becomes distorted when expertise is mistaken for "power." Such a mistaken assumption may be held by patients and providers alike, especially the less experienced providers who, after passing highly competitive entrance examinations, enduring a grueling regimen of graduate training, and being inculcated with a sense of elitism by their graduate faculty and peers, enter the health care arena with a desire to prove their mettle. Such providers often become distressed and begin to question their own competence when they discover that their sense of power was only an illusion. Similarly, many patients become disillusioned upon discovering that the provider is lacking in this mythical power. Such disillusionment typically leads to suspicion which, in turn, leads to a weakening of the therapeutic relationship.

In a neuropsychological paradigm of rehabilitation, illusions of power are disavowed. Providers recognize that they receive temporary authority, from the patient and/or family, to proceed with "treatment." Providers also recognize that the patient or the family can rescind this authority at any time, either directly by withdrawing from treatment or indirectly by failing to comply with treatment suggestions. Patients are no longer viewed as passive recipients of services, but rather are seen as active and equal participants in the process of adaptation. The health care professional presents him- or herself as a consultant and offers to establish a cooperative working relationship with the patient and family, thereby using his or her power toward therapeutic ends. The provider recognizes that disputes between the patient and the treatment team will always be won by the patient and, thus, takes great care in explaining the rationale for treatment decisions to the patient and in involving the patient and family in the treatment planning process.

Such a paradigm is very difficult for inexperienced providers and for providers heavily steeped in a traditional biomedical paradigm to accept. These providers are often shocked by the mere suggestion that their authority is only temporary and derived from the patient. They experience considerable difficulty recognizing that the patient is responsible for his or her own recovery and that patients may choose to be sick or disabled. At the extreme, some providers go so far as to view acceptance of such a model as somehow an abdication of some social/professional "manifest destiny" bestowed upon them by their graduate training facility or the state licensing board. Others may attempt to force the patient into a more traditional biomedical relationship by telling the patient in effect, "You are too disabled or impaired to make decisions for yourself right now" or "I want you to be responsible and autonomous, so you must do everything I tell you to do." By failing to recognize the true locus of power in the therapeutic relationship, such providers are unfortunately setting themselves up for failure, considerable frustration, and are inadvertently doing their patients a disservice.

While in the traditional medical paradigm health care providers are assumed to have the power to effect change in the patient's condition, it is interesting to note the process that occurs when the patient fails to demonstrate expected progress. In these cases, responsibility for the lack of progress is attributed to the patient or, more precisely, to some variable within the patient such as tissue damage, a lack of motivation, depression, and/or premorbid maladaptive personality traits. In other words, the biomedical paradigm assumes that health care providers have the power to cure, but patients have the power to be sick. Such thinking inevitably leads to conflict between the patient and the treatment team, since patients seldom view themselves as choosing to be disabled and thus attribute their own lack of progress to some deficiency in the treatment regimen. Each party then blames the other for the lack of progress, and further treatment efforts are marked by confrontation rather than cooperation.

In contrast, in the neuropsychological paradigm, health care providers take a hypothesis-testing approach when confronted with a lack of patient progress. They reexamine the environmental variables known to effect change to determine whether or not their treatment regimen is sufficient. They eschew intrapsychic pathologizing until all possible alternative hypotheses have been ruled out. Even if it is determined that intrapsychic factors are influencing the course of the patient's rehabilitation, the rehabilitation specialist is likely to seek environmental interventions which could ameliorate the problem. Above all else, patients are seen as dynamic individuals who demonstrate variation in behavior across time and situations. Such variation is seen as normal and healthy so long as it remains subchaotic. Dysphoric mood and affective variability following cerebral trauma are viewed as normal consequences of the human experience, and, unless such mood and affective variations reach extreme proportions which significantly interfere with the rehabilitation process, the health care professional is loath to deprive his or her patients of such normal human emotional experiences through the naive use of psychotropics. "Premorbid maladaptive personality traits" are seen as learned behaviors which can be modified through manipulation of environmental contingencies rather than as some innate set of limitations which govern the amount of functional return patients can experience.

In such a paradigm, patients perceive that the health care professional accepts responsibility for the efficacy of his or her treatment decisions and do not feel "blamed" for a lack of progress. Rather than feeling that they are being forced into a mold created by the service delivery system, patients perceive that services are being custom designed to meet their unique rehabilitative needs. Furthermore, seeing that the health care professional is willing to alter his or her approach to the problem, the patient becomes increasingly willing to rethink his or her own contributions to the rehabilitative process. Such flexibility of thinking on the parts of both the patient and the rehabilitation specialist provides a fertile ground from which a cooperative rehabilitative effort can grow, particularly if the patient is informed of, and involved in, the treatment planning process.

As a corollary of the presumption of a provider locus of power, it is important, in the biomedical paradigm, that treatments have meaning for the health care professional. This only follows, since it is the provider who possesses the relevant technical expertise and since the patient is a naive recipient of services. In order to collect the data necessary for diagnosis and treatment, the provider must require the patient to undergo procedures which, on the surface at least, appear meaningless. For example, patients may wonder why a venipuncture is necessary when they have sustained a blow to the head. Similarly, they may question the practical value of putting colored pegs into a pegboard or of playing board games. In response to such perceived meaninglessness, the patient is then forced to: (1) submissively yield to the "infinite wisdom" of the provider, or (2) question the meaningfulness of the treatment and risk being labeled as a "difficult patient," as "lacking insight," as "mentally incompetent," as "rebellious," or as "characterologically disturbed". Neither option, it would appear, increases the probability that the patient will perform in a functionally autonomous manner.

Moore (1980) emphasizes that treatment must have some degree of meaning or importance to the patient in order for learning to occur. Since the neuropsychological paradigm rests on the presumption that rehabilitation is a learning process, providers take care to present treatments in a manner which has maximum meaning for the patient. If such meaning is not clearly inherent in the task itself, the provider either explains the rationale behind the task, presents the task in a more meaningful form, or seeks more ecologically valid methods for collecting the necessary information. For example, instead of assessing fine motor skills by having the patient place small objects in containers or by having the patient perform rapid finger oscillations, the provider may simply observe the patient executing more functional tasks such as adjusting the fine tuning on a television, assembling mechanical components, or typing a letter. Additionally, patients are encouraged to question the provider's methods and to take an active role in designing their own rehabilitative regimen. Treatment is viewed as a collaborative venture in which the provider, over time, weans him- or herself out of the process as the patient becomes more independent in pursuing his or her life goals. In the neuropsychological paradigm there are no "difficult," "incompetent," "rebellious," or "characterologically disturbed" patients, only naive or ill-conceived treatment regimens. Such a philosophy, on the part of the health care professional, promotes thorough assessment and adaptation, reinforces the therapeutic relationship, and fosters patient autonomy.

## ASSUMPTION #3—MEDICALLY BASED SERVICE DELIVERY

Yet another difference between the biomedical and neuropsychological paradigms is the manner in which rehabilitative services are delivered. Biomedically oriented programs are hospital based. Patients typically enter a specialized unit where they are provided approximately 120 square feet of space in a double room and where they essentially are architecturally isolated from the rest of the world. Often, avocational resources are scarce, and patients spend an inordinate amount of time laying in bed viewing a television, physically and psychologically isolated from each other. Typically, there is an isolation room where agitated individuals can be continuously observed by nursing personnel. However, methods for varying environmental stimuli are conspicuous only in their absence. As in an acute care facility, doors to patient rooms are usually left open depriving patients of privacy and allowing environmental distractors to permeate each and every room. Staff enter patient rooms at will to administer medications, assist the patient in toileting, or prepare the patient for therapy. Individual meals are prepared for each patient and served on a bedside table thereby maintaining the patient's isolation. While such a service delivery system may be efficient, economical, and comfortable for the staff, it is depersonalizing and does little to accomplish the goal of rehabilitation which is to reintegrate the patient into the social fabric from which he or she came.

The neuropsychological paradigm of service delivery requires a rethinking of the design of rehabilitation facilities. The authors know of no existing facility that is architecturally suitable for the acute rehabilitation of the head injury victim. Obviously, such a facility would need a variety of patient accommodations ranging from an isolation room to a two-bedroom transitional apartment with shared cooking and toileting areas that could be utilized by two patients at once. Such accommodations would require mechanisms for systematically varying the type, amount, and intensity of environmental stimuli the patient receives. Privacy would be maximized while ambient distractors would be minimized. Accommodations would have adequate space for the patient to experiment in the activities associated with a normal lifestyle, would have ample communal recreational resources, and would be furnished according to the specific needs of the patient. Meals would be communally prepared and consumed in a family-style setting. Decisions regarding meals and the use of recreational resources would be made by the patients. Patient accommodations would not contain passive recreational devices such as televisions and telephones, thereby forcing patients to interact and plan the sharing of such communal resources, much as they would in a real home setting. In summary, rehabilitative services would be provided in a setting which successively approximates as closely as possible the community to which the patient is to return. Rather than contributing to depersonalization and social isolation, the presence of adequate facilities would likely increase the patients' degree of social interaction, provide opportunities to develop social skills, and facilitate the transition between the hospital and the real world.

The biomedical and neuropsychological paradigms also differ in terms of organizational structure. The biomedical model follows a traditional pyramidal organizational structure headed by an authoritarian leader such as a physician or program manager. In such a model, communication and conflict resolution tends to proceed on isolated vertical lines rather than on consolidated horizontal ones (Howard, 1988). While in terms of time expenditure and the preservation of professional egos of those at the apex of the organization this is an efficient process, the lack of horizontal communication between treating professionals tends to foster multidisciplinary treatment teams and what we call the "one-patient-with-one-therapist-behind-a-closed-door" phenomenon (i.e., a proliferation of individual treatment sessions with each professional vying against the other for his or her "piece" of the patient and working toward discipline-specific goals which may or may not be appropriate given the entire spectrum of the patient's problems). At best, such competition between therapists creates staff splitting and interdisciplinary rivalry at the expense of a rational and integrated treatment regimen for the patient. At worst, this competition fosters the development of antagonistic and mutually exclusive goals thereby compromising the patient's recovery. Additionally, because of the pyramidal organizational structure inherent in the biomedical paradigm, those professionals who spend the least amount of time with the patient (i.e., the team leaders) make most of the treatment decisions regarding the patient. We think the fallacy in such a process is readily apparent.

With the neuropsychological paradigm comes an entirely different organization of service delivery. Rather than following a static pyramidal organizational structure, the neuropsychological paradigm fosters a flexible, systemic view of service delivery. While there is still a team leader, that leader derives his or her authority from the professionals with whom he or she works rather than from an arbitrary hierarchical structure. Authority in this system is commensurate with the degree of training, experience, and expertise demonstrated by the health care professional rather than being awarded solely on the basis of the type of degree the professional possesses. The team leader, because he or she spends proportionally less time in direct patient contact, does not manage treatment by fiat. Rather, the team leader's job is to foster horizontal communication between the various disciplines, to ensure a rational and integrated treatment regimen by coordinating the activities of the various therapists, and to facilitate group decision making and conflict resolution. While the physician may or may not be the team leader, his or her primary role is to bring a medical perspective to the group decision making process. This is a very difficult role for most physicians to assume, and it indeed takes a very special, insightful, and dedicated professional to sacrifice status for improved service delivery.

The neuropsychological paradigm with its flexible organizational structure facilitates the development of transdisciplinary teams. Goals are formulated on the basis of a common definition of the patients' needs rather than on the basis of exclusive disciplinary philosophies. Goals are then pursued by all team members. In such a paradigm it is not uncommon for a speech and language therapist to be addressing physical therapy goals in the course of his or her treatment and vice versa. The one-patient-with-one-therapist-behind-a-closed-door phenomenon is supplanted by greater numbers of "combined therapies" and group therapy sessions facilitated by members of different disciplines. Rather than fostering interdisciplinary rivalry, staff splitting, fragmented service delivery, and professional frustration, the neuropsychological paradigm promotes interdisciplinary cooperation and respect, horizontal communication, integrated service delivery, and professional autonomy. Most importantly, the neuropsychological paradigm facilitates the delivery of highly effective and efficient services to the patient.

Finally, the biomedical paradigm is a deficit management or reconstructive one which focuses on the tertiary and, to some extent, the secondary rehabilitation of the individual patient at the biological and organismic level. As such, it is very narrow in scope and very inefficient. By tertiary rehabilitation, we refer to the reduction of the physical and cognitive sequelae of an injury. Secondary rehabilitation refers to prophylactic measures designed to prevent complications or the development of additional sequelae (Grimm & Bleiberg, 1986). While no one will deny the importance of secondary and tertiary rehabilitation, it seems clear that such a service delivery model is inefficient in that it addresses problems only after the fact with greater costs in terms of health care expenditures, human suffering, and societal ramifications.

In contrast, the neuropsychological paradigm is a health promotion or prophylactic one. In addition to its innovations in tertiary rehabilitation, this paradigm places great emphasis on secondary and primary rehabilitation (primary rehabilitation being the prevention of head injuries). Moreover, its scope is broader than that of the biomedical paradigm in that interventions may be conducted at the environmental, familial, and societal levels as well as at the biological and organismic ones. By virtue of this broader scope, the neuropsychological paradigm opens the question of efficiency of resource allocation to empirical examination.

## SUMMARY

In this chapter we have identified three philosophical weaknesses of the traditional biomedical paradigm of acute head injury rehabilitation. The biomedical paradigm assumes that the locus of dysfunction lies within the individual patient, that the locus of power to effect change lies within the provider, and that the traditional pyramidal organizational structure is the best for delivery of rehabilitative services. In addition to elucidating the fallacy behind these rarely examined assumptions, we have proffered an alternative paradigm, the neuropsychological paradigm, for consideration (Table 8.1). Again, we wish to emphasize that neither paradigm exists today in its purest form. Furthermore, ours is certainly not an exhaustive list of the difference between the two paradigms.

Certainly, the neuropsychological paradigm, in its pure form, would be very difficult to implement. This paradigm calls for more intensive staffing during a time of critical staff shortages in virtually every discipline. Additionally, it demands that such staff regularly undergo intensive training when there are already too numerous demands on their profes-

TABLE 8.1.   A Comparison of the Biomedical and Neuropsychological Paradigms
of Rehabilitation Service Delivery

|  | Biomedical paradigm | Neuropsychological paradigm |
|---|---|---|
| Philosophy | Materialistic, reductionistic | Emergent, holistic |
| Primary model | Disease model | Dysfunction model |
|  | Linear diagnosis & treatment | Nonlinear assessment & adaptation |
| Theories | Little heuristic value | Proven heuristic value |
|  | Lacks empirical support | Supported by large body of research |
|  | Brain viewed as an internal organ | Brain viewed as an organ of interface |
|  | Presumes plasticity of neural tissue | Presumes learning occurs |
| Locus of dysfunction | Organismic | In the interface between the individual and the environment |
| Role of provider | Healer | Consultant |
| Locus of power | Provider | Patient and family |
|  | Patient blamed for lack of progress | Treatment blamed for lack of progress |
| Intrapsychic pathologizing | Accepted | Eschewed |
| Premorbid factors | Secondary importance | Primary importance |
| Role of patient | Passive recipient of services | Equal and active participant |
| Treatment options | Nil set | Unlimited |
| Behavioral disturbances | Viewed negatively | Viewed positively |
|  | Treated by chemical restraints and behavioral treatment plans | Treated by environment modification plans and operant learning |
| Staff | Passive | Active |
| Meaning | For provider | For patient |
| Service delivery | Traditional static pyramidal model | Flexible systems model |
|  | Authoritarian leadership | Authoritative leadership |
|  | Vertical communication | Horizontal communication |
|  | Leader decision making and conflict resolution | Team decision making and conflict resolution |
|  | Focuses on tertiary and secondary interventions | Focuses on primary and secondary interventions |
|  | Narrow scope | Broad scope |
|  | Inefficient | Efficient |
|  | Relatively inexpensive | Relatively expensive |
|  | Architectural isolation | Architecture promotes resocialization |
|  | Multidisciplinary | Transdisciplinary |
|  | Fragmented treatment plans | Integrated treatment plans |
|  | Staff competition | Staff collaboration |
|  | Professional frustration | Professional autonomy |
|  | Deficit mangement model | Health promotion model |

sional time. Moreover, it calls for physical plants which do not yet exist. All of these factors must ultimately lead to increased rehabilitation costs during a time when funding for rehabilitation is scarce and when competition between rehabilitation programs is fierce. But probably the most formidable obstacles to the implementation of such a paradigm are the traditions and philosophies of biomedically minded providers. There is no doubt in our mind that many physicians would find our paradigm objectionable since, on the surface at least, it appears to deprive them of considerable status and influence. However, we are equally certain that dispassionate reflection on the part of these providers will lead to a recognition that the traditional paradigm is anachronistic and limited and that alternative service delivery models have much to offer in terms of professional rewards. In the end, the needs of the patients must be paramount and must supersede professional rivalries.

Our bias is clear: we espouse the notion that the neuropsychological paradigm is clearly superior to the traditional biomedical one. However, we do not claim to monopolize wisdom, nor do we wish to portray the neuropsychological paradigm as the end product of some teleological process. This discussion, rather, was motivated by what appears to be a generalized complacency in the field of acute head injury rehabilitation. Our purpose is to arouse skepticism, to have rehabilitation providers question their fundamental assumptions regarding care delivery, and to generate debate regarding alternative service delivery paradigms. Along those lines, our goal was less to propose specific content as to initiate a process of professional introspection.

## REFERENCES

Bontke, C. F., Brockman, N., Cilo, M. P., Robert, V., & Worthington, L. (1988). Acute care and rehabilitation. In P. M. Deutsch & K. B. Fralish (Eds.), *Innovations in head injury rehabilitation* (pp. 4-1–4-23). New York: Bender.

Cannon, W. B., & Rosenblueth, A. (1949). *The supersensitivity of denervated structures.* New York: Macmillan Co.

Corrigan, J. D., & Myslw, J. M. (1988). Agitation following traumatic head injury: Equivocal evidence for a discreet stage of cognitive recovery. *Archives of Physical Medicine & Rehabilitation, 69,* 487–492.

Craine, J. F. (1982). Principles of cognitive rehabilitation. In L. E. Trexler (Ed.), *Cognitive rehabilitation: Conceptualization and intervention* (pp. 83–98). New York: Plenum Press.

Giles, G. M., & Fussey, I. (1988). Models of brain injury rehabilitation: From theory to practice. In I. Fussey & G. M. Giles (Eds.), *Rehabilitation of the severely brain-injured adult: A practical approach* (pp. 1–29). London: Croom Helm.

Grimm, B. H., & Bleiberg, J. (1986). Psychological rehabilitation in traumatic brain injury. In S. B. Filskov & T. J. Boll (Eds.), *Handbook of clinical neuropsychology* (Vol. 2, pp. 495– 560). New York: Wiley.

Howard, M. E. (1988). Interdisciplinary team treatment in acute care. In P. M. Deutsch & K. B. Fralish (Eds.), *Innovations in head injury rehabilitation* (pp. 3-1–3-26). New York: Bender.

Levin, H. S. (1985). Neurobehavioral recovery. In D. Becker & J. Povlishock (Eds.), *Central nervous system trauma status report* (Pt. II, pp. 281–299). Bethesda, MD: NINCDS, National Institutes of Health.

Lewin, K. (1935). *A dynamic theory of personality.* New York: McGraw–Hill.

Llu, C. N., & Chambers, W. W. (1958). Intraspinal sprouting of dorsal root axons. *Archives of Neurology & Psychiatry, 79,* 46–61.

Miller, R. (1981). *Meaning and purpose in the intact brain: A philosophical, psychological, and biological account of conscious processes.* New York: Oxford University Press.

Moore, J. C. (1980). Neuroanatomical considerations relating to recovery of function following brain lesions. In P. Bach-y-Rita (Ed.), *Recovery of function: Theoretical considerations for brain injury rehabilitation* (pp. 9–90). Baltimore: University Park Press.

Rosenhan, D. L. (1973). On being sane in insane places. *Science, 179,* 250–258.

Snyder, J. J. (1989). *Health psychology and behavioral medicine.* Englewood Cliffs, NJ: Prentice–Hall.

Sperry, R. W. (1969). A modified concept of consciousness. *Psychological Review, 76,* 532–536.

Tizard, B. (1959). Theories of brain localization from Flourens to Lashley. *Medical History, 3,* 132–145.

Wesolowski, M. D., & Burke, W. H. (1988). Behavior management techniques. In P. M. Deutsch & K. B. Fralish (Eds.), *Innovations in head injury rehabilitation* (pp. 11–43). New York: Bender.

Wood, R. L. (1987). *Brain injury rehabilitation: A neurobehavioral approach* (chap. 5). Rockville, MD: Aspen.

# 9

# The Use of Pharmacology in the Treatment of Head-Injured Patients

## LESLIE K. ROSS

It is common for cognitive, emotional, and behavioral deficits to occur following head injury. However, research reveals that head-injured individuals are more seriously handicapped by emotional and associated behavioral disturbances (e.g., agitation) than by residual cognitive or physical disabilities (Lezak, 1987). These emotional disturbances may impede their overall recovery from the head trauma (Dikeman & Reitan, 1977; Jackson, Corrigan, & Arnett, 1985; Levin, Grossman, Rose, & Teasdale, 1979; Lishman, 1973; Prigatano, 1986; Stern, 1978; Thomsen, 1984). A frequently exhibited problem in up to 33% of patients recovering from significant head-injury is agitation, characterized by cognitive disorganization, interpersonal isolation, combativeness, and affective disturbance (Jackson *et al.*, 1985). Additionally, 67% of patients post-head injury experience anxiety, regressive manifestations, and frontal lobe syndromes (e.g., flattened affect, apathy, loss of inhibitions, disturbance in judgement) (Lishman, 1973; Stern, Najenson, Grosswasser, Mendelson, & Davidson, 1976). Also, emotional and behavioral disturbances are not limited to moderately and severely impaired patients. Patients attaining good cognitive recovery often exhibit significant anxiety and depression as well. It is not uncommon for emotional and behavioral impairments to develop into significant psychiatric disorders of psychotic proportions that can require inpatient treatment.

Furthermore, these impairments do not resolve quickly. Several studies have found that dysfunction pertaining to anger, anxiety, depression, initiative, significant relationships, social contact, work/school, and social appropriateness may persist 12 to 60 months following head injury in 40 to 66% of patients (Brooks, Campsie, Symington, Beattie, & McKinlay, 1986, 1987; McKinlay, Brooks, Bond, Martinage, & Marshall, 1981; Lezak, 1987; Stern *et al.*, 1976). The emotional and behavioral impact of head injury may persist or

---

LESLIE K. ROSS • Department of Psychology, Memphis State University, Memphis, Tennessee 38152, and University of Tennessee Center for the Health Sciences, Memphis, Tennessee 38103.

*HANDBOOK OF HEAD TRAUMA: Acute Care to Recovery*, edited by Charles J. Long and Leslie K. Ross. Plenum Press, New York, 1992.

worsen for as long as 10–15 years posttrauma (Fordyce, Roueche, & Prigatano, 1983; Thomsen, 1984). One survey found that head-injured patients seek help an average of 7.3 years following head injury concerning cognitive, job/school, medical, and emotional problems (Karol, 1989).

Currently, the primary focus of rehabilitation for emotional and concomitant behavioral sequelae following head injury is to train the patient to use alternative behavioral strategies and to develop more effective coping strategies. Although research on recovery of functions via structural and neurochemical reorganization has been sparse, there is evidence of pharmacological modification of the central nervous system following brain injury. However, most of this research has been conducted using animal models (Finger & Stein, 1982; Glick & Zimmerberg, 1978; Luria, Naydin, Tsvetkova, & Vinarskaya, 1969). An exception to this predominance of animal research is Luria and colleagues' (1969) early work with humans that strongly suggests central nervous system reorganization and restoration of function can be augmented by the use of pharmacologic agents.

The rationale for drug therapy following head injury is based on clinical reports and experimental data regarding the success of pharmacologic agents in treating emotional and behavioral changes seen in other neurologic and psychiatric disorders, such as classical psychiatric syndromes, post-cerebrovascular accidents, and minimal brain dysfunction. Although some behavioral and emotional sequelae exhibited in head injury correspond to psychiatric syndromes, psychiatric pharmacologic guidelines are not necessarily applicable to head injury. For example, administering neuroleptics to manage the "organically" agitated patient would be contraindicated in head injury since these medications may impair functional recovery and lower seizure thresholds (Cope, 1987a; Feeney, Gonzalez, & Law, 1982; Feeney, Sutton, Boyeson, Hovda, & Dail, 1985; Glenn, 1987b; O'Shanick, 1987; Prigatano, 1987; Rao, Jellinek, & Woolston, 1985).

Post-cerebrovascular accident depression has also contributed to the rationale for pharmacologic treatment of brain-injured individuals (Jackson et al., 1985; Lipsey, Robinson, Pearlson, Rao, & Price, 1984; Pearlson & Robinson, 1981; Reding, Orto, Winter, Fortuna, Di Ponte, & McDowell, 1986; Robinson, 1979). Antidepressant therapy (trazodone) has enhanced rehabilitation outcome by increasing a patient's motivation to participate in rehabilitation programs (Reding et al., 1986).

Lastly, research on the pharmacotherapeutic management of minimal brain dysfunction further supports the use of pharmacotherapy after head injury. Certainly, many post-head injury symptoms are similar to those exhibited in minimal brain dysfunction. These symptoms include: poor impulse control, disordered attention, aggression, low frustration tolerance, and distractibility (Richmond, Young, & Groves, 1978). Treatment of minimal brain dysfunction using d-amphetamine, methylphenidate, and imipramine have been found to be effective (Arnold, Strobl, & Weisenberg, 1972; Mann & Greenspan, 1976).

Although pharmacologic treatment is beneficial in disorders demonstrating similar symptoms to those seen after head injury, the relationship between pharmacologic agents and changes in neurotransmitter levels, neuroanatomical damage, and recovery following head injury is unclear (Muir, Haffey, Ott, Karaica, Muir, & Sutko, 1983). Since no drug acts selectively on specific behavioral syndromes, the precise mechanism of the role of pharmacologic agents in influencing recovery is unknown. Also, no drug has reliably demonstrated an improvement in memory, attention, or general cognitive functioning in a clinically useful manner (Reisberg, Ferris, & Gershon, 1981). However, research suggests that the effects of these agents can lead to quantitative and qualitative changes in the improvement of functioning (Brailowsky, 1980). Instead of acting on specific cognitive processes, per se, pharmacologic agents probably enhance functioning by attenuating the emotional and behavioral disturbances frequently exhibited by head-injured individuals.

In spite of the suggested usefulness of pharmacologic management for head-injured patients, this treatment option has not received as much attention in the literature as behavioral and social rehabilitation strategies. This is probably attributable to two reasons: (1) diagnostic and treatment guidelines specific to the pharmacologic treatment of head injury are almost nonexistent, and (2) a lack of well-designed pharmacologic studies in the literature (Cope, 1987a). Most information concerning pharmacologic treatment of head injury is based upon numerous case reports and nonexperimental studies that are scattered among various medical, psychiatric and psychological journals. In addition, many of the available studies suffer from methodological difficulties. That is, they did not use controls, medication comparisons, and/or double-blind experimental designs (Cope, 1987a; Haas & Cope, 1985). However, this deficiency in the literature is changing and recently special issues regarding the use of pharmacology in head injury (e.g., appropriate dosage and side effects) are being addressed (Cope, 1987b). Consequently, pharmacology is emerging as an effective and important rehabilitative treatment modality.

With the increasing use of pharmacologic treatment as an adjunct therapy option to traditional rehabilitation approaches for head-injured individuals, it is important for the rehabilitation team members to be aware of drugs that may prove beneficial and those that may impede a patient's recovery. In addition, a better understanding of the factors confronting the prescribing physician's administration of pharmacologic agents will enhance communication between the rehabilitation team and prescribing physician. Through their daily contact with the patient, the rehabilitation team can supply the prescribing physician with important feedback concerning the behavioral effects the medication is having on the patient. For example, drugs prescribed to treat specific disorders may, themselves, induce unwanted side effects such as delirium or an increase in hostility/ aggression. This situation is not uncommon in the acute stage of head injury treatment. The important interaction between the rehabilitation team and prescribing physician is facilitated by having some familiarity with pharmacologic terminology and effects.

The focus of this chapter is on the use of pharmacology to facilitate and manage the recovery/rehabilitation process of the head-injured individual. A discussion of research concerning disrupted neuroanatomical and neurochemical systems following head injury is followed by a discussion of side effects and other factors to be considered in drug selection. Last to be addressed are specific areas in which pharmacologic treatment may be appropriate and beneficial.

## NEUROPHYSIOLOGICAL AND NEUROTRANSMITTER SYSTEMS AFFECTED BY HEAD INJURY

Head injury consists of many components, such as diffuse axonal tear injuries, focal contusions, hypoxic injuries, and damage from increased intracranial pressure. Lesions are frequently found in the frontotemporal regions (frontopolar, orbitofrontal, anterior temporal lobes, and Sylvian fissure) and are commonly bilateral, but asymmetrical. Furthermore, diffuse axonal injury leads to focal changes in the corpus callosum and dorsolateral quadrant of the rostral brain stem, and diffuse microscopic damage to axons (Adamovich, Henderson, & Auerbach, 1985).

Neurophysiologic damage can result in extensive neurobehavioral changes (Adamovich *et al.*, 1985; Hayden & Hart, 1986; Levin & Grossman, 1978; Livingston & Escobar, 1972, 1973; Ross & Rush, 1981). Lesions involving the medial limbic system can be characterized by psychic and motor hypoactivity resulting in clinical syndromes of akinesia, mutism, and apathy. Interpretation of these changes may be thought to reflect a "depressed" state. Contrary to lesions, stimulation or irritative disorders of the medial limbic system are characterized by restlessness, anxiety, irritability, and obsessive compulsive behavior. Orbitofrontal–insular–anterior temporal (basolateral) lesions usually result in disinhibition and hyperactivity. Damage to the anterior temporal lobes may be involved in the altered sensory perception that might be encountered in many psychiatric disorders. Other site-specific syndromes include: (1) attentional deficits associated with frontotemporal lesions and/or diffuse axonal injuries, (2) affective blunting seen in major affective disorders because of white matter degeneration in the corpus callosum, and (3) labile mood due to a disruption of hypothalamic interconnections with the pituitary, thus producing various endocrinopathies (Annegers, Grabow, Kurtland, & Laws, 1980; Blumer & Benson, 1975; O'Shanick, 1986; Peterson & O'Shanick, 1985).

The relationship between neurophysiologic and neurotransmitter systems further complicates the understanding of behavioral and emotional changes following head injury. Altered neurotransmitter metabolism and neuroendocrine disturbances (related to pituitary involvement) contribute to the behavioral changes exhibited by head injury patients (Levin *et al.*, 1979; O'Shanick, 1986). For example, the mesencephalon is a specific site of injury in severe head injury from which many dopaminergic neurons originate. Damage to this area may lead to attentional deficits (Adamovich *et al.*, 1985). Therefore, deficits seen after head injury will frequently arise from both neurophysiologic damage and alterations in neurotransmitters.

Specific neurotransmitter changes have been noted during the acute period after head injury (1–9 days following hospital admission). Frontotemporal lobe contusions result in a decrease in dopamine and serotonin activity, whereas diffuse cerebral contusions produce an increase in serotonin activity (van Woerkom, Teelken, & Minderhoud, 1977). Behaviorally, animal experiments have demonstrated that severe decrements in serotonergic innervation of limbic system structures lead to hyperreactivity and increased locomotor response (Geyer, Puerto, Menkes, Segal, & Mandell, 1976; Jacobs, Trimbach, Eubanks, & Trulson, 1975).

Other researchers, not distinguishing between focal and diffuse damage, found a decrease in catecholamine concentration following head injury (Feeney *et al.*, 1982). Based on neuroanatomical correlations of noradrenergic projections, it is hypothesized that damage to the frontal cortex or rostral anterior cingulate cortex could deprive the entire medial cortex of noradrenergic innervation. Behaviorally, ascending noradrenergic projections from the locus coeruleus and lateral tegmental nuclei are implicated in attention, mood, and vigilance (Morrison, Molliver, & Grzanna, 1979). Therefore, a decrease in norepinephrine may, in part, contribute to a patient's agitation and disinhibitory behavior. Depression has also been associated with norepinephrine deficiency, whereas mania occurs secondary to an excess of norepinephrine (Mysiw & Jackson, 1987).

The muscarinic cholinergic system is another neurotransmitter system associated with long-term behavioral deficits following mild and moderate head injury (Lyeth, Dixon, Jenkins, Hamm, Alberico, Young, Stonnington, & Hayes, 1988). These deficits may result from an excessive release of acetylcholine and possibly other neurotransmitters that lead to widespread, pathological excitation of neurons. The role of acetylcholine in recovery of function is complex. While some researchers have demonstrated improved functioning by administering anticholinesterase drugs, others suggest that muscarinic cholinergic antagonists may prove beneficial in treatment of moderate head injury (Cooper, 1984; Luria *et al.*, 1969; Lyeth *et al.*, 1988).

Alterations in cortisol levels provide additional evidence of neurotransmitter imbalances following head injury. Cortisol secretion abnormalities of the hypothalamo–pituitary–adrenal axis are used as a biological marker of psychopathological states. Cortisol levels are associated with the functioning of the limbic system, which through the neurotransmitters norepinephrine, serotonin, and acetylcholine maintain a functional relationship with the hypothalamo–pituitary–adrenal axis. While norepinephrine exerts tonic inhibition in this axis, acetylcholine and serotonin stimulate corticotropin-releasing factor and adrenocorticotropin release. Therefore, abnormalities in the regulation of the hypothalamo–pituitary–adrenal axis might reflect imbalances in neurotransmitters that are potentially associated with limbic system dysfunction. Since norepinephrine and serotonin fibers course through the frontal lobes, damage to this area would likely cause an imbalance in the norepinephrine and serotonin systems. As measured by the dexamethasone suppression test, cortisol levels are found to be abnormal in more than 70% of head injury patients (Jackson & Mysiw, 1989).

Given the widespread changes in neurotransmitter systems, the use of neuropharmacologic agents may help to rebalance these systems and augment recovery in a head injury patient. The benefits of such therapy may be demonstrated by improvements in cognitive functions such as memory or attention, motor skills, and enhanced emotional functioning. As previously mentioned, it is often the emotional disorders that hinder a patient's progress in rehabilitation. Therefore, appropriate pharmacologic treatment may render the patient more amenable to treatment and rehabilitation by diminishing emotional dysfunction, thus permitting the patient to improve on cognitive tasks (Jackson *et al.*, 1985; Reding *et al.*, 1986; Stern, 1978).


## DRUG SELECTION

The final clinical effect of any neuroactive drug following head injury depends on a complex interaction between neuropathology, primary and secondary drug actions, and various patient variables. Neuropharmacologic agents differ in their effects and act selectively depending on the neurophysiologic and neurotransmitter systems affected by the injury (Olds, 1958). Even though evidence exists that most neuroactive agents reflect a particular agonist or antagonist action within a specific neurotransmitter system, the precise mechanisms leading to a drug's effect are unknown, nor is it known how a change in one neurotransmitter affects other neurotransmitters (Cooper, Bloom, & Roth, 1982). For example, neuroleptics used in the treatment of schizophrenia are understood to block dopamine transmission. However, neuroleptics through their metabolites also affect neuro transmitter systems other than dopamine and frequently elicit secondary symptoms (Tune, Damlouji, Holland, Gardner, Folstein, & Coyle, 1981). Psychotropic medications also may operate through different treatment mechanisms in various neuropathological conditions. For example, the use of tricyclic antidepressants to treat pathologic laughing and crying probably affects different pharmacologic mechanisms from that of depression since the benefits are apparent within 48 hours (Schiffer, Cash, & Herndon, 1983).

Furthermore, all medications may negatively exacerbate a head-injured patient's symptoms (e.g., lowering seizure threshold, increasing confusion, and impairing functional recovery) and may preclude efficient rehabilitation (Adamovich *et al.*, 1985; Feeney *et al.*, 1982, 1985; Gardos, 1980; Glenn, 1987b; Glenn & Joseph, 1987; Griffith, 1983; Healey, Pickens, Meisch, & McKenna, 1983; Jabbari, Bryan, Marsh, & Gunderson, 1985; O'Shanick, 1987; Prigatano, 1987; Rao *et al.*, 1985; Ross & Rush, 1981; Tune *et al.*, 1981; Yudofsky, Williams, & Gorman, 1981). Since psychotropic side effects are related to interactions with histaminic, acetylcholinergic, alpha-adrenergic, and dopaminergic receptors, they may be accentuated because of existing non-CNS organ impairments. Therefore, care must be taken when using these drugs to diminish behavioral problems. Table 9.1 presents some common side effects of frequently cited pharmacologic agents in the head injury literature. While this is not an exhaustive list of medications currently in use, it serves to highlight the importance of being aware of the side effects that any pharmacologic agent can produce.

TABLE 9.1.   Side Effects of Commonly Prescribed Medications

| Medication: generic name (brand name) | Side effects |
| --- | --- |
| Tricyclic antidepressants Amitriptyline (Elavil) Imipramine (Tofranil) | Anticholinergic (e.g., urinary retention, dry mouth, blurred vision, dysphagia, delayed gastric emptying, constipation), delirium, confusion, impaired cognitive functioning, fatigue/sedation, mania, lowered seizure threshold |
| Neuroleptics Haloperidol (Haldol) Thioridazine (Mellaril) | Anticholinergic, extrapyramidal symptoms (e.g., tremor, dyskinesia, ataxia), delirium, confusion, impaired cognitive functioning, lowered seizure threshold, malignant neuroleptic syndrome |
| Benzodiazepines [1]Diazepam (Valium) [2]Chlordiazepoxide (Librium) [3]Lorazepam (Ativan) | [1,2,3]Increased hostility/aggression, [1,2]lowered seizure threshold on withdrawal, [1]anticholinergic, [1]extrapyramidal symptoms, [1]muscle weakness, [1]hypotension, [1]respiratory depression, [1]dizziness, [1]delirium, [1]fatigue/sedation, [3]impaired cognitive functioning |
| Anticonvulsants Phenytoin (Dilantin) Phenobarbital Carbamazepine (Tegretol) | Fatigue/sedation, impaired cognitive function, anticholinergic |
| Antispasticity medications [1]Dantrolene [2]Baclofen | [1,2]Anticholinergic, [1,2]fatigue/sedation, [1]liver toxicity, [1]gastrointestinal complaints, [1]muscle weakness, [1]respiratory depression, [2]anorexia, [2]nausea/vomiting, [2]dizziness |
| Lithium | Extrapyramidal symptoms, confusion, impaired cognitive functioning, lowered seizure theshold, increased hostility/aggression |
| Stimulants *d*-Amphetamine (Dexedrine) Methylphenidate (Ritalin) | Lowered seizure threshold |
| Beta-blocker Propranolol (Inderal) | Bradycardia, hypotension, ventricular failure/cardiac shock, bronchial asthma, fatigue/sedation |

Drug interactions are another possible complication that necessitates evaluation in pharmacologic selection. Through shared metabolic pathways or because agents compete for the same therapeutic locus, the action of psychotropic medications may be altered (O'Shanick, 1987). For example, amphetamines have been shown to accelerate the recovery of function by enhancing dopamine activity, whereas these same functional benefits are blocked by the administration of haloperidol (Feeney et al., 1982). Drug interactions also may change pharmacokinetic properties of medication. An example of this situation occurs when anticonvulsants and antispasmodics interact with psychotropic agents and impair the absorption of the psycho-tropic medication. Similarly, the concomitant administration of drugs that depress the central nervous system (e.g., phenobarbital, diazepam, and meperidine hydrochloride) may substantially depress respiration and worsen cognitive abilities. Also, the simultaneous administration of agents that block muscarinic cholinergic receptors has been shown to have an additive effect and may induce an anticholinergic delirium (Tune et al., 1981). Additional agents that compete for the same metabolic pathways, thus altering drug availability, include: phenytoin and antidepressants, carbamazepine and trazodone, and neuroleptics and antidepressants.

Methodologically flawed research further complicates drug selection concerning behavioral management following head injury (e.g., lacking controls, paucity of double-blind control studies) (Evans, Gaultieri & Patterson, 1987; Haas & Cope, 1985; Mattes, 1986). Interpretation of the results of these studies is confounded by the natural evolution of recovery from head injury (Adamovich et al., 1985; Haas & Cope, 1985).

Currently, accurately predicting which patient will respond to a given neuropharmacologic agent is difficult, if not impossible; and diagnostic and treatment guidelines are almost nonexistent (Cope, 1987a). Although specific treatment guidelines are unavailable, several aspects warrant consideration prior to the initiation of pharmacotherapy. Behavioral changes following head injury may be caused by a variety of different events, such as: (1) the neurological trauma itself, (2) psychological factors, (3) the condition of the central nervous system prior to injury, (4) metabolic and endocrine changes, (5) concomitant medical problems (e.g., sepsis), (6) medications (e.g., Tagamet), and (7) the hospital environment (e.g., ICU psychosis) (O'Shanick, 1987). All of these events contribute to cognitive and emotional changes following head injury. Evaluation of these variables may either influence the drug that is first prescribed, contraindicate the use of a particular pharmacologic agent, or suggest the discontinuation of specific medications. Therefore, a thorough psychological and neuropsychological assessment of the problem behavior should be made in order to sort out contributing factors and possibly facilitate the intervention.

Consideration of psychological factors associated with behavioral problems following head injury should include: (1) the preinjury level of psychological functioning, (2) the level of psychosocial development, (3) cognitive development, and (4) the individual's previous experiences with stress and its resolution (O'Shanick, 1987; Stern et al., 1976). Also, knowledge of a patient's previous response to stressors and/or therapeutic interventions can help predict the efficacy of using similar approaches following head injury. That is, the behaviors following head injury may be a normal extension of the patient's typical coping style to the stresses encountered during hospitalization. In addition, social parameters should be assessed such as original family constellation and status of interpersonal relationships.

The condition of the central nervous system prior to the injury must be evaluated. This would include an assessment of: age, prior head injury, prior toxic exposures, metabolic abnormalities (e.g., diabetes mellitus), structural abnormalities of the brain (e.g., arteriovenous malformation, hydrocephalus). The severity of neuroanatomic, neurochemical, and neuroelectrophysiologic dysfunction, and primary and secondary brain lesions should be examined in order to understand the brain–behavior correlates of resulting dysfunction. Associated physical trauma (e.g., abdomen, chest, spinal cord) is important to evaluate since it may contribute to mental aberrations following head injury. Psychotropic agents require an intact gastrointestinal system, normal functioning renal system, normal hepatic function, normal blood pH, and normal respiratory functioning for optimal dosing. Consequently, impairments in any one of these organ systems can influence the amount of drug in the system. For example, diffuse hypomotility of the gastrointestinal tract will generally decrease the availability of the psychotropic drug in the bloodstream. The blockade of alpha-adrenergic receptors by some neuroleptics and antidepressants will be accentuated in patients who sustained spinal cord injuries or other disuse atrophic states. Postural hypotension, in particular, will be problematic in these patients. Therefore, the physician should be guided toward agents that are relatively less alpha-blocking. Furthermore, drug side effects may be accentuated in patients with non-CNS organ impairment or pharmacologic agents may worsen the dysfunction already present.

Metabolic and endocrine changes can induce significant behavioral disturbances with possibly fatal complications. Since vitamin and mineral cofactors are essential for optimal neurotransmitter functioning, nutritional status pre- and postinjury is an important consideration. Abstinence patterns involving alcohol, benzodiazepines, or opiate abuse also can contribute to behavioral and emotional changes seen following head injury.

Another consideration of drug selection is that pharmacologic interventions used in the acute stage may induce behavioral syndromes. Opiates and synthetic narcotic analgesics may produce hallucinations or dysphoria. Glucocorticoids (e.g., dexamethasone) at high doses are associated with psychotic behavior that can be mistaken for affective disorder. Medication used to increase blood pressure or control cardiac arrhythmias also may create hallucinosis in individuals without a previous psychiatric history.

Individuals also vary in their sensitivity to neurotoxic effects of medication, and side effects are often dose dependent. Pharmacologic intervention should be based on specific indications, such as depression or severe aggression. In general, drugs as the sole treatment modality are not useful in managing long-term behavioral disturbances (Cope, 1987a). They should be part of a comprehensive behavioral, cognitive, and physical rehabilitation program with counseling because the benefits of pharmacologic intervention will be severely limited if not part of a comprehensive approach to the patient and his/her rehabilitation (Feeney *et al.*, 1982, 1985; Glenn, 1987b; Luria *et al.*, 1969; Meyer & Meyer, 1977; Sutton, Weaver, & Feeney, 1987). Similarly, the effectiveness of behavioral, cognitive, and physical rehabilitation may be compromised if the possibility of pharmacologic intervention is not explored.

Pharmacologic agents will affect and change a head-injured patient's symptoms, whereas a comprehensive rehabilitation program that includes counseling will be aimed at the development of new coping skills and at the underlying perceptions involved in the behavioral and emotional disturbances. It is not uncommon for depressive symptoms, such as anergia, to interfere with a patient's progress in rehabilitation. Motivation and participation in rehabilitative activities are important components for recovery following head injury.

Lastly, it should be remembered that a significant effect of drugs is an altering of a patient's state of arousal. Subsequent disordered behavior may be the result of sedation, disinhibition, or a paradoxical response (Gardos, 1980; Glenn, 1987b; Jackson *et al.*, 1985). Therefore, control of dysfunctional behavior may be achieved at the expense of adaptive, as well as dysfunctional, behaviors and may result in the loss of valuable recovery time.

## SPECIFIC AREAS FOR PHARMACOLOGIC TREATMENT

Several situations in which pharmacologic treatments are used include: (1) acute care, (2) emotional changes (e.g., rage and violent behavior, pathologic laughing and crying, depression, secondary mania, bipolar disorder, sexual dysfunction), (3) disturbances associated with organic brain syndrome, (4) headache (as part of the postconcussional syndrome), (5) memory impairments, (6) motor skill dysfunction/spasticity, and (7) hypertension (Table 9.2). Table 9.2 does not represent a comprehensive listing of medications in use for these situations, but cites only those that have been cited in the literature for each situation. For example, there are several medications that are commonly prescribed, such as flouxetine (Prozac) for depression, but research has not been published concerning their effectiveness in a head-injured-population. This does not preclude their possible effectiveness for head injured individuals. In addition, these situations are not clearly delineated aspects of the recovery process; but, rather, they overlap (e.g., emotional disturbances, memory deficits, and organic brain syndrome). Furthermore, since head injury encompasses a multitude of emotional and behavioral deficits that are intertwined, specific disorders commonly seen following head injury are discussed within these general categories. For example, pharmacologic treatment of impairments in attention/concentration and hyperactivity are reviewed in the sections dealing with acute care, emotional changes, disturbances associated with organic brain syndrome, and memory impairments. The following sections will outline the considerations and applicability of initiating pharmacologic treatment and the rationale underlying the efficacy of certain medications.

### Acute Care

During the period of acute care (the immediate period following injury to the end of hospitalization), changes in mental status may produce a wide variety of psychiatric symptoms that range from anxiety and depression to delirium and psychosis. These alterations in mental status may be secondary to several causes: (1) drug effects, (2) drug withdrawal, and (3) metabolic disturbances (Peterson, 1986). Drug effects include the effects of narcotic analgesics, anesthetics, steroids, and other medications that alter the level of consciousness, disturb memory, and alter behavior. The effects of drug withdrawal may appear from the time of admission to 2 weeks later and occur most commonly from alcohol (32% of head injury patients are intoxicated at admission [O'Shanick, 1986]), sedative hypnotics, and anxiolytic agents (e.g., benzodiazepine abstinence phenomenon [O'Shanick, 1986]). Common metabolic disturbances include electrolytic imbalances, liver or kidney malfunction, disturbances attributable to poor nutritional status with resultant deficiencies of trace metals (Mg, Zn, Cu), vitamins (B complex and especially thiamine), and folate. Combinations of these etiologies are common and a careful review of the

TABLE 9.2.   Situations for Pharmacologic Management of the Head-Injured Patient

| Situation | Medication: generic name (brand name) |
| --- | --- |
| Acute care | |
| 1. Drug withdrawal<br>   Anxiety<br>   Sleep disturbances | Patients without cognitive deficits: chlordiazepoxide (Librium), diazepam (Valium)<br>Patients with cognitive deficits: neuroleptics |
| 2. Delusions or hallucinations | Haloperidol (Haldol), trifluoperazine (Stelazine) |
| 3. Agitation and confusion | Tricyclic antidepressants: amitriptyline (Elavil)<br>Beta-blockers: propranolol (Inderal), pindolol |
| 4. Sleep disturbances | Tricyclic antidepressants: amitriptyline (Elavil), trazodone (Desyrel) |
| 5. Posttraumatic stress disorder<br>   (e.g., symptoms of anxiety or<br>   sleep disorder) | Imipramine (Tofranil), phenelzine (Nardil) |
| Intermediate care and beyond | |
| 1. Rage and violent behavior (if<br>   behavior recurs in stereotyped<br>   manner with periods of unre-<br>   sponsiveness or paroxysmal<br>   confusional states) | Lithium, haloperidol (Haldol), amphetamines, benzodiazepines, amitriptyline (Elavil)<br>Anticonvulsant: carbamazepine (Tegretol) |
| 2. Pathologic laughing and crying | Dopamine agonists: amantidine (Symmetrel), levodopa<br>Tricyclic antidepressants: amitriptyline (Elavil), doxepin (Sinequan), imipramine (Tofranil), nortriptyline (Aventyl) |
| 3. Depression | Tricyclic antidepressant: amitriptyline (Elavil)<br>Monoamine oxidase inhibitor: phenelzine (Nardil) |
| 4. Secondary mania | Lithium, carbamazepine (Tegretol) |
| 5. Bipolar disorder | Lithium, carbamazepine (Tegretol), valproate (Depakene) |
| 6. Sexual dysfunction | Medroxyprogesterone acetate |
| 7. Disturbances associated with<br>   organic brain disorder | Methylphenidate (Ritalin), d-amphetamine (Dexedrine) + amitriptyline (Elavil), carbamazepine (Tegretol), trazodone (Desyrel) |
| 8. Headache | Amitriptyline (Elavil), propranolol (Inderal), acetaminophen, butalbital + aspirin |
| 9. Memory | Physostigmine, stimulants, tricyclic antidepressants, benzodiazepines, carbamazepine (Tegretol) |
| 10. Motor skills/spasticity | Diazepam (Valium), baclofen, dantrolene |
| 11. Hypertension | Beta-blockers: propranolol (Inderal), atenolol |

patient's history, medications, and laboratory data is warranted in order to reveal the causes of an alteration in mental status (Peterson, 1986).

Management of mental status changes during this period consists of: (1) treating the underlying medical problem, (2) neuropharmacologic intervention for immediate relief of the behavioral/cognitive disturbance, (3) discussing with the family and hospital staff the expected course of recovery, and (4) the use of environmental manipulations to minimize symptomatology (e.g., night light, frequent reorientation cues by nurses and family, and familiarization of the patient's environment) (Peterson, 1986).

The two primary pharmacologic drugs administered during this phase are benzodiazepines and neuroleptics. Chlordiazepoxide or diazepam are useful in drug withdrawal and with symptoms of anxiety or sleep disturbance in patients without cognitive deficit. Short-acting benzodiazepines should be avoided since they may produce withdrawal symptoms unless carefully titrated. If the patient has an unrecognized organic deficit, he/

she may have a paradoxical reaction and exhibit increased agitation or psychotic behavior. In this case the patient should be switched to a neuroleptic (O'Shanick, 1986; Peterson, 1986). Neuroleptics are advocated if a cognitive deficit or significant delusional or hallucinatory experience is present. Haloperidol and trifluoperazine are most useful because of their minimal anticholinergic effects. Therefore, they will not interact with anticholinergic agents used to potentiate narcotics or anticholinergic drugs used preoperatively. However, some researchers indicate that neuroleptics need to be given in large doses. If so given, sedation will ensue along with a general suppression of cognitive function (Hayden and Hart, 1986). Previous research concerning the detrimental effect of haloperidol on cognitive functioning has demonstrated that the side effects of this drug may hinder the patient's recovery (Feeney et al., 1982, 1985).

An additional concern for a patient receiving neuroleptics, particularly during acute care, is a toxic reaction known as neuroleptic malignant syndrome. This disorder consists of fever, muscular rigidity, altered consciousness, autonomic dysfunction, and occasionally respiratory distress (Gelenberg, 1983). Patients with organic brain disease have been observed to be at higher risk for developing this syndrome. Higher drug doses increase the likelihood of developing neuroleptic malignant syndrome. Careful observation of the patient who is receiving neuroleptics is warranted since the symptoms of this syndrome may be obscured by concomitant medical disease.

The period of posttraumatic amnesia is frequently complicated by agitated behavior that interferes with traditional rehabilitative approaches. Agitation and confusion are characterized by cognitive disorganization, interpersonal isolation, combativeness, and affective disturbance. It is estimated that 30% of head injury patients experience agitation of sufficient severity to require intervention (Levin & Grossman, 1978). Agitation is typically managed by conservative behavioral techniques such as structured environments and/or the removal of any known arousing stimulus. Pharmacological interventions, such as central nervous system depressants, are discouraged as the primary treatment for agitation because of sedative side effects and diminished cognitive capacity, which can result in increased agitation and a possible delay in rehabilitation. However, in cases where medications are required to protect the patient's safety, tricyclic antidepressants, particularly amitriptyline, are generally effective in attenuating agitation (Jackson et al., 1985; Mysiw & Jackson, 1987; Mysiw, Jackson, & Corrigan, 1988). Mysiw et al. (1988) compared a nonpharmacologically treated patient group with an amitriptyline-treated patient group and concluded that amitriptyline successfully treated agitation without adversely affecting cognition or rate of improvement in cognitive functioning.

Amitriptyline's proposed mechanism of action involves its ability to potentiate activity of the biogenic amines, norepinephrine and serotonin, by preventing reuptake. The biogenic amines' projections course through the frontal lobes, a common site of injury in head trauma (Morrison et al., 1979). There is evidence of significant depletion of serotonin following severe frontotemporal injury (van Woerkom et al., 1977). Behaviorally, norepinephrine and serotonin have been implicated in aggressive behavior. Besides amitriptyline's potentiation of the biogenic amines, it has strong anticholinergic properties. The cholinergic system is associated with violent behavior in animals; therefore, amitriptyline's anticholinergic activity may contribute to a diminution of agitation in head injury patients (Mysiw et al., 1988).

Sleep disturbances may become manifest in the intermediate phase of acute care. Sleep initiation is associated with serotonin activity; therefore, low-dose tricyclic antidepressant medication (e.g., amitriptyline) or trazodone may improve sleep and allow better verbalization of grief (O'Shanick, 1986; Peterson, 1986). If amitriptyline is prescribed, the anticholinergic side effects of this drug may complicate medication compliance (O'Shanick, 1986). The use of trazodone may be preferable because of its minimal anticholinergic effects.

Also, during the intermediary phase, and at anytime during recovery from head injury, symptoms of posttraumatic stress disorder (PTSD) may emerge. These symptoms need to be distinguished from anxiety, depression, or psychotic states. The patient with PTSD will report dreams and/or daytime hallucinatory experiences in which they relive the accident. This includes not only seeing the accident happen, but a simultaneous confrontation with overwhelming emotions (e.g., fearfulness, anxiety, rage, and helplessness). The patient should be reassured about the normalcy of their response to the event. The use of a short-term low-dose antidepressant (imipramine) or a monoamine oxidase inhibitor (phenelzine) may help to alleviate anxiety and sleep disturbance associated with PTSD (Peterson, 1986). If monoamine oxidase inhibitors are administered, the patient should avoid foods with high tyramine content to prevent a hypertensive reaction.

During acute care, and recovery in general, it is important to avoid medications that may impair arousal. Some widely used medications with sedative properties are: (1) anticonvulsants—phenytoin, phenobarbital, (2) antihypertensives—propranolol, metoprolol, methyldopa, (3) antispasticity medication—baclofen, diazepam, and (4) psychotropics— neuroleptics, amitriptyline, doxepin, imipramine (Whyte & Glenn, 1986). When drug therapy includes sedative drugs, it might be prudent to attempt periodic drug withdrawals to assess changes in the underlying arousal level. If medications cannot be withdrawn, switching to a less sedating equivalent drug is an option.

## Emotional Changes

### Rage and Violent Behavior

Rage and violent behavior are the primary problems post-head injury requiring pharmacologic management (Cope, 1987a). Disruptive behavior is usually characterized by agitation, hyperarousal, and aggression. Frequently these symptoms are in response to an overly stimulating, physically painful, or frustrating environment. Nonpharmacologic interventions, such as behavioral management, may be the preferable first approaches in order to avoid drug side effects. However, 30% of patients exhibiting agitation are unresponsive to behavioral techniques (Jackson et al., 1985). Presently, several medications are used to treat disruptive behavior; however, there is no medication of choice.

Prior to initiating behavioral or pharmacologic treatment, neuropsychological contributions to disruptive behavior should be evaluated. Neuropsychological complications may include: (1) complex partial seizures, (2) disorders of arousal, attention, and initiation, and (3) other disorders resulting in loss of impulse control. Temporal lobe epilepsy is cited as the most common organic condition associated with rage. These seizures are often attributable to sclerosis of the medial part of the temporal lobe (Elliot, 1976; Mattes, 1986). Preictal, ictal, and postictal phenomenon can be responsible for behavioral disturbances in patients following head injury. A trial of anticonvulsants (carbamazepine) may be warranted if disruptive behaviors recur in a stereotyped manner or are associated with periods of unresponsiveness or paroxysmal confusional states (Elliot, 1976). Carbamazepine is effective in decreasing irritability and other interictal personality difficulties often associated with chronic epilepsy and in diminishing violent behavior in patients without overt epilepsy (Mattes, 1986).

Rage associated with the emergence from coma is hypothesized to be more effectively controlled by large doses of an adrenergic blocking agent such as propranolol, which may act centrally or peripherally by diminishing somatic responses to frustrations, fear, or panic (Elliot, 1976; Yudofsky et al., 1981). Other researchers believe propranolol's effectiveness is unrelated to its beta blocking activity and that it works via an anticonvulsant mechanism of its metabolites which diminishes seizure discharge in areas of the brain involved in aggression (Elliot, 1977; Mattes, 1986). In terms of its side effects, propranolol produces no change in the patient's level of disorientation or memory impairment (Yudofsky et al., 1981). However, propranolol may produce hypotension or bradycardia. Pindolol, another beta blocker that maintains a better resting sympathetic tone than propranolol, significantly decreases the number of assaultive episodes without producing sedation, bradycardia, or hypotensive episodes (Greendyke & Kanter, 1986). Additional research is needed to compare treatment efficacy of these two beta blockers, as well as the effectiveness of propranolol and carbamazepine, given propranolol's anticonvulsant properties.

Contradicting Elliot's and Yudofsky's results concerning the effectiveness of propranolol in managing rage and assaultive behavior, Haas and Cope (1985) found that propranolol did not produce a change in disruptive behavior. Their study was a single case design using a sedative (diazepam), two antipsychotic agents (haloperidol and thioridazine), methylphenidate, propranolol, and lithium, for the management of confusion, agitation, and belligerence in a head injury patient. The sedative, antipsychotics, and propranolol did not alter the patient's behavior, but methylphenidate increased agitation. Lithium produced significant calming in the patient, enabling the patient to complete rehabilitation and be discharged home. However, other researchers have found lithium ineffective in the management of aggressive behavior (Mattes, 1986; Williams & Goldstein, 1979). Williams and Goldstein propose a hypothesis to help account for these conflicting results by suggesting that patients with severe and diffuse brain damage may not be good lithium responders, whereas patients with static lesions of the central nervous system who show a combination of dementia and agitated depression will respond well to lithium. Aside from the equivocal results using lithium, a possible side effect of this drug to be concerned about is an exacerbation of aggressive behavior (Mattes, 1986).

While extreme belligerence often occurs as the patient emerges from coma, it also may occur many months after head injury (Elliot, 1976). Therefore, different mechanisms may underlie early versus late agitation/belligerence. The former is hypothesized to be caused by a breach of the blood–brain barrier, enabling catecholamines to gain access to limbic system structures and stimulate the alpha and beta receptors involved in rage. Rage occurring many months following head injury may be associated with temporal lobe contusions, specifically involving the amygdala (Elliot, 1976). Current research has not specifically investigated the time period in which disruptive behavior first emerges to warrant a distinction in the specific medication prescribed.

Disorders of arousal, attention, and initiation are associated with symptoms of increased irritability, restlessness, and combativeness. A pharmacologic approach to this complex of symptoms would necessitate evaluating whether current medications are compounding or possibly causing these problems. Based on this evaluation, medications should be withdrawn or replaced with pharmacologic agents that are less likely to cause cognitive disturbances (Gardos, 1980; Glenn, 1987a). For example, phenobarbital or phenytoin can be replaced with carbamazepine, an anticonvulsant less likely to cause cognitive disturbances. Likewise, baclofen might be withdrawn and the patient's spasticity managed without medications or by nerve blocks. Sedating medications given for behavioral management, such as neuroleptics or benzodiazepines, may contribute to the patient's behavioral problems (Ross & Rush, 1981). Central nervous system stimulants and some antidepressants with low anticholinergic properties (e.g., trazodone [Brogden, Heel, Speight, & Avery, 1981] and desipramine) can be used to improve alertness, attention, and initiation, and may have a secondary calming effect.

However, there is no guarantee of these positive benefits since as alertness or initiation increase, both desirable and undesirable behaviors become more frequent. One possible approach to obtaining greater control of a pharmacologic agent's effect is to consider factors which may influence the patient's response to the medication, such as the patient's environment. For example, using a stimulant to improve arousal might be more effective in an environment with minimal stimuli, but disruptive in an environment having a multitude of distracting stimuli. The reverse may be true for depressants. An additional caveat is that some undesirable side effects cannot be controlled, such as the lowering of seizure threshold by certain psychostimulants (O'Shanick, 1986).

Other medications prescribed to control agitation and aggressive behavior include haloperidol, amphetamines, benzodiazepines, and amitriptyline. Haloperidol's effectiveness in lessening extreme agitation is hypothesized to be caused by its disruption of the dopamine receptors implicated in general arousal. In a study comparing two groups of patients, one treated with haloperidol and the other untreated, there were no significant differences between the groups in rehabilitation outcome (Rao et al., 1985). However, because of the previously mentioned serious side effects when using this drug, haloperidol probably should not be the drug of choice when initiating pharmacologic management of disruptive behavior. Results using amphetamines and benzodiazepines have been equivocal, decreasing agitation/hostility in some patients while increasing these behaviors in other patients (Rao et al., 1985).

In a case study evaluating amitriptyline for treating agitation in a patient with primarily frontal lobe damage, agitation was effectively decreased and attention span increased (Jackson et al., 1985). The proposed rationale for the usefulness of this drug involves the ascending noradrenergic projections from the locus coeruleus which may mediate attention, mood, and vigilance (Morrison et al., 1979). Damaging the rostral anterior cingulate cortex would deprive the entire medial cortex of noradrenergic innervation. However, it is more likely that the full syndrome of agitated behavior reflects the relative concentration of several neurotransmitters, such as norepinephrine and dopamine, rather than the level of any one specific biogenic amine (van Woerkom et al., 1977). Tricyclic antidepressants appear to affect agitated behavior through their ability to block reuptake of catecholamines in the central nervous system.

*Pathologic Laughing and Crying*

Pathologic laughing and crying are inappropriate laughing and crying unrelated to surrounding circumstances or stimulation, with no accompanying emotions (Udaka, Yamao, Nagata, Nakamura, & Kameyama, 1984). This syndrome occurs in a variety of neurological disorders including cerebrovascular accidents, multiple sclerosis, tumors, and trauma. The proposed lesion involves the basal ganglia or internal capsule, substantia nigra, cerebral peduncle, hypothalamus, bilateral thalamus, bilateral pyramidal tract, and/or extrapyramidal systems. Schiffer *et al.* (1983) hypothesize that this syndrome is the result of a disconnection of subcortical effector systems subserving emotional expression from their cortical inhibition.

Successful treatment has employed dopamine agonists (amantidine or levodopa) and tricyclic antidepressants (amitriptyline, doxepin, imipramine, nortriptyline). However, levodopa is less effective if the lesion is diffuse (Lawson & MacLeod, 1969; Ross & Rush, 1981; Schiffer *et al.* 1983; Schiffer, Herndon, & Rudick, 1985; Udaka *et al.* 1984). The underlying pharmacologic mechanism of tricyclic antidepressants' effect on pathologic laughing and crying probably differs from the mechanism involved in the treatment of depression. Unlike depression, patients treated for pathologic laughing and crying respond rapidly (within 48 hours) to the administration of tricyclic antidepressants (Schiffer *et al.*, 1983, 1985). Another possible explanation for the efficacy of tricyclic antidepressants as a treatment of pathologic laughing and crying is that these drugs partially restore inhibitory transmission by potentiating the transmission of the inhibitory neurotransmitter dopamine in the caudate nucleus (Bevan, Bradshaw, & Szabadi, 1975). This would be consistent with the observation that dopamine agonists are effective treatments for this disorder.

*Depression*

The incidence of depression following head injury is estimated to be between 15 and 25% (Levin *et al.*, 1979). The symptoms of head injury depression may resemble those of major depression. Possible neuropathological changes triggering affective symptoms include: (1) disruption of brain catecholamines and cholinergic metabolism, (2) neuroendocrine disturbances associated with pituitary involvement, and (3) disruption of arousal associated with the mesencephalic reticular formation. Head injury frequently affects the frontal poles and may cause neurotransmitter changes, such as catecholamine decrements, that are similar to those postulated in poststroke depression (Feeney *et al.*, 1982; Morrison *et al.*, 1979; Mysiw & Jackson, 1987). Another similarity with poststroke depression is the higher incidence of acute aphasia in head injury patients who experience anxiety and depression, thus suggesting greater left hemisphere involvement (Levin & Grossman, 1978).

Administering tricyclic antidepressants for treating depression in brain damage individuals has been predicated on their usefulness in poststroke depression (Lipsey *et al.*, 1984; Mysiw & Jackson, 1987; Reding *et al.*, 1986). However, in a study that included a control group diagnosed with major depression without a history of head injury, amitriptyline and phenelzine (a monoamine oxidase inhibitor) were found to be of limited use in treating major depression following minor head injury (Saran, 1985). Prior to treatment, these two groups differed in their depressive symptomatology. Unlike the control group, the head-injured group's depression was not worse in the morning, they did not exhibit significant weight loss, anorexia, psychomotor retardation or agitation, and their dexamethasone suppression test was normal. While additional research is needed, Saran's study suggests that head injury individuals might benefit from different antidepressant medications than those commonly prescribed for depression in non-head injury individuals or in those used to treat poststroke depression.

While cognitive impairment may contribute to depression, it is not a prerequisite for depression. A case report describes a head injury patient, without residual cognitive sequelae, who began experiencing depression soon after returning to work. His depression continued for three years until treated successfully with amoxepine (Zeff & Chung, 1987).

*Secondary Mania*

Secondary mania is the occurrence of manic symptoms produced by toxic, metabolic, or neurologic disorders without a previous history of affective disturbance (Krauthammer & Klerman, 1978). Most cases of secondary mania have involved lesions of the basal forebrain region with specific pathological changes to the basal ganglia, thalamic and midbrain nuclei, and limbic portions of the frontal and temporal lobes (Cummings & Mendez, 1984). These structures have been implicated in the modulation of emotion and neurovegetative functions (Alpers, 1937). Radiological evidence suggests that it is the extent of subcortical damage and not cortical involvement that is directly related to the magnitude of neuro-behavioral deficits (Levin, Handel, Goldman, Eisenberg, & Guinto, 1985). Also, if secondary mania is associated with lateralized lesions of the diencephalic structures and adjacent areas, the lesion is more often on the right than the left (Cummings & Mendez, 1984).

Whether secondary mania is a legitimate sequela to head injury is an issue of recent origin (Schneider & Kaplan, 1989). Schneider and Kaplan reviewed the literature and found 22 reported cases of mania following head injury; of these, only 6 met Krauthammer and Klerman's (1978) criteria for secondary mania. They present an interesting point to account for the lack of literature on secondary mania compared with the wealth of information linking depression with head injury. That is, because approximately 50% of head injuries occur between the ages of 6 and 44, cases of secondary mania are often not reported because the head injury is considered to be coincidental with the idiopathic development of psychological disorders. Schneider and Kaplan suggest that it is prudent to consider secondary mania as a useful and treatable diagnostic entity.

Secondary mania may spontaneously resolve or pharmacologic intervention may be necessary. Effective treatment has included the use of lithium and carbamazepine (Cummings & Mendez, 1984; Joshi, Capozzoli, & Coyle, 1985; Mattes, 1986). Joshi *et al.* report a case study of a 10-year-old girl who experienced a head injury at the age of 4. She showed progressive deterioration in her behavior since the injury. A behavioral management system and methylphenidate were not effective in resolving the behavioral disturbances. Trials of carbamazepine and sodium valproate were unsuccessful. After she began taking lithium, there was a decrease in hyperactivity, impulsivity, lability of mood, and socially intrusive behavior. However, the lithium did not alter the EEG that demonstrated petit mal activity.

*Bipolar Disorder*

Head injury may precipitate cases of bipolar disorder that can be indistinguishable from the more common form of bipolar disorder which is presumed to have a hereditary component (Pope, McElroy, Satlin, Hudson, Keck, & Kalish, 1988). Pharmacologic treatment has included valproate, carbamazepine, and lithium (Hale & Donaldson, 1982; Pope *et al.*, 1988; Stewart & Hemsath, 1988). The mechanism of action of each of these medications is difficult to define, as is the treatment of choice. This is partly attributable to the fact that studies reporting successful treatment are case reports and they rarely compare medication effectiveness. One case study reported that lithium by itself was only partially effective but when carbamazepine was added to the treatment regimen, the bipolar disorder was successfully treated (Pope *et al.*, 1988). Another anticonvulsant, valproate, has also successfully treated bipolar disorder following head injury. Stemming from these results, it was suggested that head injury may trigger ictal activity that manifests as bipolar symptom and therefore responds to anticonvulsants (Stewart & Hemsath, 1988). However, this does not account for the effectiveness of lithium in other cases of bipolar disorder secondary to head injury (Hale & Donaldson, 1982).

## Sexual Dysfunction

Most commonly, brain damage attributed to disease or trauma is associated with hyposexuality. Lehne (1984–1986) cited the work of other researchers who estimated the incidence of hyposexuality as ranging between 58 and 71% (Kosteljanetz, Jensen, Nrgard, Lunde, Jensen, & Johnsen, 1981; Meyer, 1955). Less common is atypical hypersexuality combined with paraphilia that has been reported in cases of temporal lobe epilepsy, temporal lobectomy, brain tumors, and brain trauma.

Medroxyprogesterone actetate has been used successfully to treat temporal lobe epilepsy in males. In addition, it has an erotically calming effect for those patients who evidenced symptoms of hypersexuality (Blumer & Migeon, 1975). Lehne reported the successful treatment, with medroxyprogesterone acetate, of paraphilic sexual disorder in a man with a history of frontal brain damage. Soon after his emergence from a coma of one month's duration, this individual evidenced deviant sexual behavior that was resolved through intensive rehabilitation. Five years after the injury, the deviant sexual behavior reappeared and was unsuccessfully treated with carbamazepine. Even though this patient suffered from a seizure disorder, which was successfully controlled with anticonvulsants, the inappropriate sexual behavior appeared to be distinct from the seizure disorder. Medroxyprogesterone actetate successfully treated the paraphilic sexual disorder in this individual.

The mechanism for medroxyprogesterone acetate's effectiveness in treating paraphilic symptoms is not fully understood. However, treatment effectiveness is hypothesized to be associated with medroxyprogesterone acetate's influence on calming seizure activity, and not simply by a lowering of plasma testosterone levels (Lehne, 1984–1986).

## Disturbances Associated with Organic Brain Dysfunction

Organic brain dysfunction is a broad term encompassing changes in personality, behavior, and thinking. Even though each of the areas of pharmacologic management already discussed deal with aspects of behavioral, personality, and cognitive changes, several researchers cite organic brain dysfunction as a specific area of pharmacologic intervention for head injury patients.

The organic basis of this disorder may be overlooked and mistakenly attributed to a functional process, especially if the cognitive deficits are not apparent and if the head injury occurred several years prior to the presenting disorder (Weinstein & Wells, 1981). Weinstein and Wells reported a case study of a 24-year-old individual, 5 years post-head injury, who presented with a history of problems in living, four psychiatric hospitalizations, and trouble with law enforcement authorities dating back to the time of his head injury at age 19. His symptoms of lack of judgment and insight, paranoia, impaired inhibitions, resentment of authority, poor impulse control, and superficial relationships were interpreted as indicative of personality disorder. After reviewing neuropsychological test results and neuroradiological tests at the time of the final psychiatric admission, it was concluded that the patient's psychiatric disorder was secondary to brain damage involving the left frontal, temporal, and parietal lobes. Treatment was begun with methylphenidate and almost immediately the patient's behavior improved. Although his IQ increased by ten points, deficits in attention span, language use, speech perception, and the capacity to change perceptual sets remained. Weinstein and Wells note that this case highlights a reluctance of physicians to attribute behavioral abnormalities to brain damage unless they are accompanied by a distinctive cognitive loss. They further suggest that the likelihood of overlooking the organic contribution to the overall clinical picture will predominantly occur in frontal lobe lesions. This is particularly significant in head trauma since head injury typically involves damage to the frontal lobes. The importance of correctly attributing a patient's psychiatric dysfunction to head injury can have ramifications concerning how a patient views himself/herself, how others view the patient, and in the outcome of recovery.

Lipper and Tuchman (1976) also report a case in which a patient was diagnosed with organic brain dysfunction secondary to head injury. The patient's symptoms, 16 months post-head injury, included confusion, paranoia, short-term memory deficit, and depression. The patient was treated with $d$-amphetamine that resulted in a decrease in confusion and paranoia, and improved affect and short-term memory. Amitriptyline was also prescribed which enhanced the effects of $d$-amphetamine. The improvement in memory was probably not related to the medication, per se, but rather, attributable to the patient's improved emotional functioning.

Bouvy, van de Wetering, Meerwaldt, and Bruijn (1988) present another case of organic brain dysfunction following head injury in which a 21-year-old male, approximately 2 years following head injury, developed an acute psychosis following a period of acute psychological stress. The psychosis was treated effectively with carbamazepine, whereas haloperidol was ineffective. Although the patient did not evidence signs of epilepsy and the EEG was normal, Bouvy et al. hypothesized the patient's acute psychosis was due to a kindling phenomenon on a biological level and a behavioral sensitization from stress on a psychological level. They proposed that the coexistence of organic vulnerability from the head injury along with psychological stressors had resulted in the development of psychosis. Bouvy et al. do not mention whether this patient had received behavioral or cognitive therapy to help him cope with the change in his functional status following his injury. A comprehensive therapeutic intervention directed toward alleviating some of the psychological stressors this patient experienced (e.g., numerous failures) might have prevented the development of the acute psychosis.

While trazodone has been demonstrated to be effective in treating organic brain dysfunction, its use has been restricted to a geriatric population (Nair, Ban, Hontela, & Clarke, 1973; Simpson & Foster, 1986). It is hypothesized that an increase in information input (arousal), coupled with a slow pace of information processing (integration), produces an imbalance between arousal and integration, which results in cognitive impairment and functional symptoms associated with organic brain dysfunction (Nair et al., 1973). It is suggested that trazodone's effectiveness in treating this disorder is due to its having a positive influence on integrative functions and thereby restoring the balance between arousal and cognitive integration.

## Headache

Headache, a common complaint beyond six to eight weeks after head injury, has an incidence that varies between 30 and 76% (Bray, Carlson, Humphrey, Mastrilli, & Valko, 1987; Saran, 1988). Both incidence and severity of headaches do not necessarily correlate with the severity of the injury. The resulting consequences of headaches may range from an occasional inconvenience to near-total incapacitation for several days or weeks. Headaches following head injury are characterized as diffuse in origin, dull ache, throbbing pain, knifelike pain, and/or burning sensation (Bray *et al.*, 1987). Headaches are often accentuated by emotional and physical distress (i.e., tension), and cluster or migraine headaches may be superimposed on tension headaches. The relationship between headaches and depression in minor head injury is not well established; however, there is a significant prevalence of depressive headaches in the general population that ranges from 49 to 94% (Saran, 1988).

Effective treatment often consists of relaxation therapy, biofeedback training, acupuncture, and medication (e.g., amitriptyline, nortriptyline, clonazepam, propranolol, acetaminophen, and a combination of butalbital and aspirin). Serotonin deficiency has been linked with depression and headaches. A decrement in serotonin or catecholamines may make the patient more vulnerable to chronic pain. Using tricyclic antidepressants, especially amitriptyline, has been effective in treating chronic headache with or without underlying depression. Amitriptyline has also been recommended for posttraumatic headache (Tyler, McNeely, & Dick, 1980). However, another study concluded that amitriptyline is unsuccessful for treating headaches and associated depression in patients with minor head injury (Saran, 1988). The conflicting results between these two studies might be accounted for by differences in methodology. Saran used a control group, had specific selection criteria, and specific measurements to assess improvement. Time postinjury might be an additional factor in successful treatment. Tyler *et al.* report that those patients successfully treated were seen approximately 13 weeks sooner after their injury than patients with unfavorable outcome. It is possible that Tyler and colleagues began treatment earlier than Saran. Therefore, they may have been aided by the "natural" head injury recovery process, or the early intervention may have prevented the development of associated emotional and/ or behavioral symptoms (e.g., depression, anxiety) which would make treatment more difficult.

## Memory

More effort has gone into the pharmacologic treatment of memory than any other neuropsychological impairment (Miller, 1984). Memory depends on the patient's arousal and alertness, and an ability to choose selectively and discriminate among multiple stimuli. Pharmacologic manipulation of attention often involves agents that affect basic arousal mechanisms, thereby making it difficult to delineate drugs that act purely upon processes of memory or attention (Cope, 1986). Also, much of the work attempting to diminish memory deficits has not been done with head-injured patients, but rather with dementia of the Alzheimer type, attention deficit disorder in childhood and adulthood, other psychiatric conditions (e.g., schizophrenia, manic–depressive disorder), and in animals (Cope, 1986; Jackson *et al.*, 1985; Meyer & Meyer, 1977). Presently, no drug has reliably demonstrated an improvement in memory, attention, or general cognitive function in a clinically useful manner (Reisberg, Ferris, & Gershon, 1981).

Based on a literature review, Cooper (1984) draws several conclusions concerning the effectiveness of pharmacologic treatment of memory and the neurochemical systems involved in memory. In general, experiments strongly suggest that cholinergic neuro-transmission is involved in some way in learning and memory processes in animals and humans. Amnesia, or the capacity to form new memories, may be a consequence of a loss of cholinergic activity within the brain. Therefore, facilitating cholinergic activity may lead to improvement on memory tasks, whereas antagonism of cholinergic activity might result in significant impairments (Luria *et al.*, 1969). However, it is not known if all or only a proportion of cholinergic neurons are involved. The ambiguity of this area of research leads Cooper to surmise that no strong conclusion can be drawn to relate cholinergic activity to one or several of the many stages or levels of processing believed to be involved in what is described as memory.

Another line of memory research concerns the role of catecholamines in memory. Catecholamines have a general arousal function and are implicated in reinforcement and reward systems, stress, aggression, feeding behavior, and overall activity level (Cope, 1986). Specifically, the norepinephrine projections of the locus coeruleus are implicated in the regulation of selective attention (Morrison *et al.*, 1979). In head-injured patients, pharmacologic agents that enhance catecholamine function (e.g., stimulants, tricyclic antidepressants) tend to facilitate attention and learning, whereas catecholamine antago-nists (e.g., haloperidol) impair learning and memory (Evans *et al.*, 1987; Feeney *et al.*, 1982, 1985; Higashi, Sakata, Hatano, Abiko, Ihara, Katayama, Wakuta, Okamura, Ueda, Zenke, & Aoki, 1977; Jackson *et al.*, 1985; Lipper & Tuchman, 1976; Meyer & Meyer, 1977; Rao *et al.*, 1985). Several researchers administering stimulants to head injury patients have found a beneficial effect on multiple cognitive functions, including short-term memory (Evans *et al.*, 1987; Lipper & Tuchman, 1976; Weinberg, Auerbach, & Moore, 1987). Weinberg *et al.* concluded that patients with diffuse axonal injury involving the reticular activating core would be better candidates for catecholamine agonist treatment than would patients with more focal lesions. This rationale is based on studies that have demonstrated decreased levels of dopamine and norepinephrine after severe closed head injuries (Feeney *et al.*, 1982).

In general, any medication that alters arousal and attention will affect cognitive functioning. Benzodiazepines cause deficits of attention and concentration and will inter-fere with memory consolidation processes (Healey *et al.*, 1983; Kleindienst-Venderbeke, 1984; Pomara, Deptula, Medel, Block, & Greenblatt, 1989; Vogel, 1979). However, if attention or learning is impaired by excessive anxiety or arousal, benzodiazepines may improve performance. The anticonvulsants phenytoin and phenobarbital have negative effects on arousal and general cognitive processing (Trimble & Thompson, 1983). There-fore, carbamazepine is preferred in the management of seizures because of its minimal effect on cognition and the possibility that it may improve alertness and arousal (Evans &

Gualtieri, 1985). When administering any medication, it is important to monitor a patient's behavior and performance on daily tasks in order to assess whether the level of arousal is optimal or detrimental to the patient's cognitive functioning.

Currently, there is no specific pharmacologic treatment of choice for the enhancement of memory and attention. Although drugs have multiple effects, both beneficial and adverse, guidelines have been suggested to help minimize potential negative pharmacologic effects. These guidelines include clearly identifying and defining target behaviors. Furthermore, the patient's overall functioning should be monitored so that improvement in behavior is not at the expense of overall adaptive behavior. A specific drug choice should attempt to minimize side effects. For example, high-potency neuroleptics are less sedating but produce more acute extrapyramidal reactions. A low-potency drug might be indicated for a fully aroused patient with a memory deficit, such as a tricyclic with minimal anticholinergic properties. Carbamazepine should be considered as an alternative to either phenobarbital or phenytoin (Cope, 1986).

## Motor Skills/Spasticity

Spasticity has been defined as a state of hypertonicity of striated muscle as manifested by increased resistance to passive stretch due to increased response of static and often phasic stretch reflexes (Griffith, 1983). That is, there is an increased resistance to passive movement. Spasticity can be caused by any neurologic condition that damages upper motor neuron pathways. These pathways, the corticospinal tract and corticobulbar tract, have as their major function the initiation and control of skilled voluntary activity.

Pharmacologic approaches to motor deficits and spasticity should be made after attempting treatment through educational and physical modalities. Alternatively, pharmacologic treatment can be viewed as an adjunct to these other therapies and may be established in the early stages of rehabilitation (Bray et al., 1987; Griffith, 1983). Common antispasticity drugs are diazepam, baclofen, and dantrolene. These drugs must be carefully monitored because their side effects may create greater problems than the spasticity itself. Also, in many cases the improvement in spasticity may not correlate with improved function (Griffith, 1983).

Diazepam exerts its action in three sites: (1) inhibition of the contraction mechanism of skeletal muscles, (2) increasing gamma-aminobutyric acid (GABA), enhancing inhibitions mediated at the spinal cord and brain stem levels, and (3) depressing the reticular activating system. Besides the major side effects noted in Table 9.1, there may be a severe intensification of spasticity if diazepam is abruptly withdrawn. Also, the management of seizure activity might be complicated since diazepam interacts with anticonvulsants to cause a change in seizure activity or frequency (Griffith, 1983).

Baclofen, a derivative of the neurotransmitter GABA, acts at the same sites in the brain stem and spinal cord as does diazepam. Baclofen is most effective for spasms that impede voluntary effort. It may prove beneficial alone or in combination with dantrolene. Although baclofen often causes sedation, it is not as severe as diazepam. Similar to diazepam, there may be an intensification of spasticity upon withdrawal of baclofen. Also, after baclofen is discontinued, the patient might experience hallucinations.

Dantrolene has as its main site of action striated muscles. The possible side effects of this agent are listed in Table 9.1. Dantrolene is contraindicated when liver disease and dysfunction is present because of rare fatalities associated with liver disease. It is most effective in combination with the other two antispasticity drugs (Griffith, 1983).

## Hypertension

Hypertension following head injury is not uncommon and is usually treated with a thiazide diuretic or a beta-blocker (Glenn, 1987c). There are several cautions associated with the use of each of these pharmacologic treatments in hypertension. For those patients with increased urinary frequency or incontinence, the diuretics may exacerbate the problem. Also, diuretics may not be as effective as other antihypertensives (Glenn, 1987c).

One hypothesis accounting for hypertension following head injury implicates excessive catecholamine release from a hyperactive sympathetic nervous system. Therefore, beta-blockers are considered to be the drug of choice because of their catecholamine antagonist action. However, the side effects caused by a further decrement in catecholamine levels following head injury may prove detrimental to rehabilitation efforts. Propranolol, a commonly used beta-blocker, has side effects that include depression, memory impairments, attentional problems, sexual dysfunction, and physical symptoms (e.g., lethargy, nightmares, dry mouth, and loss of taste). These undesirable effects may be due to propranolol's ability to cross the blood–brain barrier in high concentrations. Therefore, a beta-blocker that is less likely to cross the blood–brain barrier, such as atenolol, may be preferable (Glenn, 1987c).

Although rehabilitation team members will not treat a patient for hypertension, per se, this condition emphasizes the need for the rehabilitation team to be cognizant of all medications taken by a head injury patient. Side effects from medications taken for physical disorders can impede a patient's progress in a rehabilitation program.

## CONCLUSION

After reviewing the literature on pharmacologic management of head-injured patients, it is proposed that pharmacologic interventions can be an effective treatment modality following head injury. However, the obtained benefits cannot be attributed to a single mechanism but, rather, several that may operate separately or together.

First, given the widespread changes in neurotransmitter systems following head injury, many behavioral and emotional symptoms arise. The use of neuropharmacologic agents may help to rebalance these systems and augment recovery in a head-injured patient. The benefits of such therapy may be demonstrated by changes in cognitive functions, such as memory or attention, motor skills, and enhanced emotional functioning. As previously mentioned, it is often the emotional disorders that hinder a patient's progress in rehabilitation. Therefore, appropriate pharmacologic treatment may render the patient more amenable to treatment and rehabilitation (Jackson et al., 1985; Reding et al., 1986; Stern, 1978).

Second, pharmacologic intervention would be effective in those cases in which cognitive impairment precludes psychological treatment, such as counseling. This type of intervention would attenuate some of the emotional and/or behavioral difficulties and permit the patient to work with the rehabilitation team on behavioral strategies of coping.

Third, pharmacologic management of the head-injured individual by alleviating emotional disorders that limit therapeutic progress can be beneficial as an adjunct rehabilitation treatment approach (Adamovich *et al.*, 1985; Jackson *et al.*, 1985; Reding *et al.*, 1986; Stern, 1978; Sundet, Finset, & Reinvang, 1988). Sundet *et al.* found emotional disturbances in a stroke population to contribute significantly to the prediction of rehabilitation outcome. It would not be unreasonable to expect similar results within a head-injured population. For example, throughout the time of agitation and decreased attention span, treatment goals cannot be directly addressed, and secondary goals aimed at decreasing agitation must be substituted for traditional multidisciplinary rehabilitation. Therefore, emotional disorders need to be actively treated along with supplying cognitive therapy to facilitate rehabilitation progress.

Maximal benefits of pharmacologic intervention will not be seen unless behavioral and other rehabilitation management efforts are optimal (Glenn, 1987b). Presently, no drug by itself significantly improves cognitive functioning. Rather, pharmacologic agents make available "lost" functions which are then strengthened by rehabilitative efforts. Therefore, experience or appropriate rehabilitation is an important component in the recovery of functions (Feeney *et al.*, 1982, 1985; Luria *et al.*, 1969; Meyer & Meyer, 1977; Sutton *et al.*, 1987).

Furthermore, due to potential side effects of many drugs, a behavioral program should usually be attempted prior to pharmacologic treatment. Because of negative side effects, it is important not only to monitor the drug response but also to define the parameters of the therapeutic trial (e.g., dosing, target symptoms, and drug response should be rated by raters who are blind on whether the patient is receiving the drug or a placebo). Therefore, it is suggested that at no time should a neuropsychotropic agent be used as a substitute for good behavioral programming.

Currently, decisions concerning the best pharmacologic agent to use for a specific disorder are difficult due to a considerable overlap among the various agents used in behavioral disturbances. The medications cited in this chapter only represent those agents which have been mentioned in the literature for use with brain-injured individuals. Therefore, there are many other pharmacologic agents being used to effectively treat emotional and behavioral disturbances which have not been included in this chapter. Furthermore, new medications are being tested and approved for clinical use, and their appropriateness for head-injured individuals has yet to be assessed. Lastly, the lack of well-designed studies published in the literature contributes to the difficult decision in selecting an appropriate drug to facilitate rehabilitation. Therefore, the choice of pharmacologic intervention should be guided by such considerations as medication side effects and psychological factors.

No member of the rehabilitation team will be directly responsible for decisions related to pharmacologic intervention, per se. However, they should know when pharmacologic management would be appropriate and how these agents may impact on the head-injured patient's progress in rehabilitation. It is also important to be cognizant of the consequences a patient's medication regime will have on their advancement in a rehabilitation program. Pharmacologic treatment of disorders not directly addressed in head injury programs, such as hypertension, can influence the head-injured individual's recovery. Consequently, there are a multitude of avenues in which pharmacologic intervention can affect head injury rehabilitation, both positively and negatively. The most efficacious head injury treatment approach is dependent on the rehabilitation team to choose among all available intervention options, which includes pharmacologic management.

## REFERENCES

Adamovich, B. B., Henderson, J. A., & Auerbach, S. (1985). *Cognitive rehabilitation of closed head injured patients: A dynamic approach.* San Diego: College-Hill.

Alpers, B. J. (1937). Relation of the hypothalamus to disorders of personality. *Archives of Neurology & Psychiatry, 38,* 291–303.

Annegers, J., Grabow, J., Kurtland, L., & Laws, E. (1980). The incidence, causes, and secular trends of head trauma in Olmstead County, Minnesota. *Neurology, 30,* 912–919.

Arnold, L. E., Strobl, D., & Weisenberg, A. (1972). Hyperkinetic adult: Study of the "paradoxical" amphetamine response. *Journal of the American Medical Association, 222,* 693–694.

Bevan, P., Bradshaw, C. M., & Szabadi, E. (1975). Effects of desipramine on neuronal responses to dopamine, noradrenaline, 5-hydroxytryptamine and acetylcholine in the caudate nucleus of the rat. *British Journal of Pharmacology, 54,* 285–293.

Blumer, D., & Benson, D. (1975). Personality changes with frontal and temporal lobe lesions. In D. Benson & D. Blumer (Eds.), *Psychiatric aspects of neurologic disease* (pp. 151–170). New York: Grune & Stratton.

Blumer, D., & Migeon, C. (1975). Hormone and hormonal agents in the treatment of aggression. *Journal of Nervous & Mental Disease, 160,* 127–137.

Bouvy, P. F., van de Wetering, B. J. M., Meerwaldt, J. D., & Bruijn, J. B. (1988). A case of organic brain syndrome following head injury successfully treated with carbamazepine. *Acta Psychiatrica Scandinavica, 77,* 361–363.

Brailowsky, S. (1980). Neuropharmacological aspects of brain plasticity. In P. Bach-y-Rita (Ed.), *Recovery of function: Theoretical considerations for brain injury rehabilitation* (pp. 187–224). Baltimore: University Park Press.

Bray, L. J., Carlson, F., Humphrey, R., Mastrilli, J. P., & Valko, A. S. (1987). Physical rehabilitation. In M. Ylvisaker & E. M. R. Gobble (Eds.), *Community re-entry for head injured adults* (pp. 25–86). Boston: Little, Brown.

Brogden, R. N., Heel, R. C., Speight, T. M., & Avery, G. S. (1981). Trazodone: A review of its pharmacological properties and therapeutic use in depression and anxiety. *Drugs, 21,* 401–429.

Brooks, N., Campsie, L., Symington, C., Beattie, A., & McKinlay, W. (1986). The five year outcome of severe blunt head injury: A relative's view. *Journal of Neurology, Neurosurgery, & Psychiatry, 49,* 764–770.

Brooks, N., Campsie, L., Symington, C., Beattie, A., & McKinlay, W. (1987). The effects of severe head injury on patient and relative within seven years of injury. *Journal of Head Trauma Rehabilitation, 2,* 1–13.

Cooper, J. R., Bloom, F. E., & Roth, R. H. (1982). *The biochemical basis of neuropharmacology* (4th ed.). New York: Oxford University Press.

Cooper, S. J. (1984). Drug treatments, neurochemical change and human memory impairment. In B. A. Wilson & N. Moffat (Eds.), *Clinical management of memory problems.* Rockville: Aspen Publications.

Cope, D. N. (1986). The pharmacology of attention and memory. *Journal of Head Trauma Rehabilitation, 1,* 34–42.

Cope, D. N. (1987a). Psychopharmacologic considerations in the treatment of traumatic brain injury. *Journal of Head Trauma Rehabilitation, 2,* 1–5.

Cope, D. N. (1987b). Psychopharmacology [Special issue]. *Journal of Head Trauma Rehabilitation, 2*(4).

Cummings, J. L., & Mendez, M. F. (1984). Secondary mania with focal cerebrovascular lesions. *American Journal of Psychiatry, 141,* 1084–1087.

Dikeman, S., & Reitan, R. M. (1977). Emotional sequelae of head injury. *Annals of Neurology, 2,* 429–494.

Elliot, F. A. (1976). The neurology of explosive rage: The dyscontrol syndrome. *The Practitioner, 217,* 51–60.

Elliot, F. A. (1977). Propranolol for the control of belligerent behavior following acute brain damage. *Annals of Neurology, 1,* 489–491.

Evans, R. W., & Gualtieri, C. T. (1985). Carbamazepine: A neuropsychological and psychiatric profile. *Clinical Neuropharmacology, 8,* 221–241.

Evans, R. W., Gualtieri, C. T., & Patterson, D. (1987). Treatment of chronic closed head injury with psycho-stimulant drugs: A controlled case study and an appropriate evaluation procedure. *Journal of Nervous & Mental Disease*, *175*, 106–110.

Feeney, D. M., Gonzalez, A., & Law, W. A. (1982). Amphetamine, haloperidol, and experience interact to affect rate of recovery after motor cortex injury. *Science*, *217*, 855–857.

Feeney, D. M., Sutton, R. L., Boyeson, M. G., Hovda, D. A., & Dail, W. G. (1985). The locus coeruleus and cerebral metabolism: Recovery of function after cortical injury. *Physiologic Psychology*, *13*, 197–203.

Finger, S., & Stein, D. G. (1982). *Brain damage and recovery: Research and clinical perspectives*. New York: Academic Press.

Fordyce, D. J., Roueche, J. R., & Prigatano, G. P. (1983). Enhanced emotional reactions in chronic head trauma patients. *Journal of Neurology, Neurosurgery, & Psychiatry*, *46*, 620–624.

Gardos, G. (1980). Disinhibition of behavior by antianxiety drugs. *Psychosomatics*, *21*, 1025–1026.

Gelenberg, A. J. (1983). Psychoses. In E. L. Bassuk, S. C. Schoonover, & A. J. Gelenberg (Eds.), *The practitioner's guide to psychoactive drugs* (2nd ed.) (pp. 115–165). New York: Plenum Press.

Geyer, M. A., Puerto, A., Menkes, D. B., Segal, D. S., & Mandell, A. J. (1976). Behavioral studies following lesions of the mesolimbic and mesostriatal serotonergic pathways. *Brain Research*, *106*, 257–270.

Glenn, M. B. (1987a). A pharmacologic approach to aggressive and disruptive behaviors after traumatic brain injury (Part 1). *Journal of Head Trauma Rehabilitation*, *2*, 71–73.

Glenn, M. B. (1987b). A pharmacologic approach to aggressive and disruptive behaviors after traumatic brain injury (Part 3). *Journal of Head Trauma Rehabilitation*, *2*, 85–87.

Glenn, M. B. (1987c). Chronic hypertension after traumatic brain injury: Pharmacologic options. *Journal of Head Trauma Rehabilitation*, *2*, 71–73.

Glenn, M. B., & Joseph, A. B. (1987). The use of lithium for behavioral and affective disorder after traumatic brain injury. *Journal of Head Trauma Rehabilitation*, *2*, 68–76.

Glick, S. D., & Zimmerberg, B. (1978). Pharmacological modification of brain lesion syndromes. In S. Finger (Ed.), *Recovery from brain damage: Research and theory* (pp. 281–296). New York: Plenum Press .

Greendyke, R. M., & Kanter, D. R. (1986). Therapeutic effects of pindolol on behavioral disturbances associated with organic brain disease: A double-blind study. *Journal of Clinical Psychiatry*, *47*, 423–426.

Griffith, E. R. (1983). Spasticity. In M. Rosenthal, E. R. Griffith, M. R. Bond, & J. D. Miller, (Eds.), *Rehabilitation of the head injured adult* (pp. 125–141). Philadelphia: Davis.

Haas, J. F., & Cope, D. N. (1985). Neuropharmacologic management of behavioral sequelae in head injury: A case report. *Archives of Physical Medicine & Rehabilitation*, *66*, 472–474.

Hale, M. S., & Donaldson, J. O. (1982). Lithium carbonate in the treatment of organic brain syndrome. *Journal of Nervous & Mental Disease*, *170*, 362–365.

Hayden, M. E., & Hart, T. (1986). Rehabilitation of cognitive and behavioral dysfunction in head injury. *Advances in Psychosomatic Medicine*, *16*, 194–229.

Healey, M., Pickens, R., Meisch, R., & McKenna, T. (1983). Effects of clorazepate, diazepam, lorazepam, and placebo on human memory. *Journal of Clinical Psychiatry*, *44*, 436–439.

Higashi, K., Sakata, Y., Hatano, M., Abiko, S., Ihara, K., Katayama, S., Wakuta, Y., Okamura, T., Ueda, H., Zenke, M., & Aoki, H. (1977). Epidemiological studies on patients with a persistent vegetative state. *Journal of Neurology, Neurosurgery, & Psychiatry*, *40*, 876–885.

Jabbari, B., Bryan, G. E., Marsh, E. E., & Gunderson, C. (1985). Incidence of seizures with tricyclic and tetracyclic antidepressants. *Archives of Neurology*, *42*, 480–481.

Jackson, R. D., & Mysiw, W. J. (1989). Abnormal cortisol dynamics after traumatic brain injury: Lack of utility in predicting agitation or therapeutic response to tricyclic antidepressants. *American Journal of Physical Medicine & Rehabilitation*, *68*, 18–23.

Jackson, R. D., Corrigan, J. D., & Arnett, J. A. (1985). Amitriptyline for agitation in head injury. *Archives of Physical Medicine & Rehabilitation*, *66*, 180–181.

Jacobs, B. L., Trimbach, C., Eubanks, E. E., & Trulson, M. (1975). Hippocampal mediation of raphe lesion- and PCPA-induced hyperactivity in the rat. *Brain Research*, *94*, 253–261.

Joshi, P., Capozzoli, J. A., & Coyle, J. T. (1985). Effective management with lithium of a persistent post-traumatic hypomania in a 10-year-old child. *Developmental and Behavioral Pediatrics*, *6*, 352–354.

Karol, R. L. (1989). The duration of seeking help following traumatic brain injury: The persistence of nonneurological symptoms. *The Clinical Neuropsychologist*, *3*, 244–249.

Kleindienst-Venderbeke, G. (1984). Informational processing and benzodiazepines. *Neuropsychobiology*, *12*, 238–243.

Kosteljanetz, M., Jensen, T. S., Nrgard, B., Lunde, I., Jensen, P. B., & Johnsen, S. G. (1981). Sexual and hypothalamic dysfunction in the postconcussional syndrome. *Acta Neurologica Scandinavica, 63*, 169–180.

Krauthammer, C., & Klerman, G. L. (1978). Secondary mania. *Archives of General Psychiatry, 35*, 1333–1339.

Lawson, I. R., & MacLeod, R. D. M. (1969). The use of imipramine ("Tofranil") and other psychotropic drugs in organic emotionalism. *British Journal of Psychiatry, 115*, 281–285.

Lehne, G. K. (1984–1986). Brain damage and paraphilia: Treated with medroxyprogesterone acetate. *Sexuality & Disability, 7*, 145–158.

Levin, H. S., & Grossman, R. G. (1978). Behavioral sequelae of closed head injury: A quantitative study. *Archives of Neurology, 35*, 720–727.

Levin, H. S., Grossman, R. G., Rose, J. E., & Teasdale, G. (1979). Long-term neuropsychological outcome of closed head injury. *Journal of Neurosurgery, 50*, 412–422.

Levin, H. S., Handel, S. F., Goldman, A. M., Eisenberg, H., & Guinto, F. C. (1985). Magnetic resonance imaging after diffuse nonmissile head injury—A neurobehavioral study. *Archives of Neurology, 42*, 963–968.

Lezak, M. D. (1987). Relationships between personality disorders, social disturbances, and physical disability following traumatic brain injury. *Journal of Head Trauma Rehabilitation, 2*, 57–69.

Lipper, S., & Tuchman, M. M. (1976). Treatment of chronic posttraumatic organic brain syndrome with dextroamphetamine: First reported case. *Journal of Nervous & Mental Disease, 162*, 366–371.

Lipsey, J. R., Robinson, R. G., Pearlson, G. D., Rao, K., & Price, T. R. (1984). Nortriptyline treatment of post-stroke depression: A double-blind treatment trial. *Lancet, 1*, 297–300.

Lishman, W. A. (1973). The psychiatric sequelae of head injury: A review. *Psychological Medicine, 3*, 304–318.

Livingston, K. E., & Escobar, A. (1972). The continuing evolution of the limbic system concept. In E. Hitchcock, L. Laitinen, & K. Vaernet (Eds.), *Psychosurgery* (pp. 25–33). Springfield, IL: Thomas.

Livingston, K. E., & Escobar, A. (1973). Tentative limbic system models for certain patterns of psychiatric disorders. In L. V. Laitinen & K. E. Livingston (Eds.), *Surgical approaches in psychiatry* (pp. 245–252). Lancaster, Great Britain: Medical & Technical Publishing.

Luria, A. R., Naydin, V. L., Tsvetkova, L. S., & Vinarskaya, E. N. (1969). Restoration of higher cortical function following local brain damage. In P. J. Vinken & G. W. Bruyn (Eds.), *Disorders of higher nervous activity* (Vol. 3, pp. 368–433). New York: American Elsevier.

Lyeth, B. G., Dixon, C. E., Jenkins, L. W., Hamm, R. J., Alberico, A., Young, H. F., Stonnington, H. H., & Hayes, R. L. (1988). Effects of scopolamine treatment on long-term behavioral deficits following concussive brain injury to the rat. *Brain Research, 452*, 39–48.

McKinlay, W. W., Brooks, D. N., Bond, M. R., Martinage, D. P., & Marshall, M. M. (1981). The short-term outcome of severe blunt head injury as reported by relatives of the injured persons. *Journal of Neurology, Neurosurgery, & Psychiatry, 44*, 527–533.

Mann, H. B., & Greenspan, S. I. (1976). The identification and treatment of adult brain dysfunction. *American Journal of Psychiatry, 133*, 1013–1017.

Mattes, J. A. (1986). Psychopharmacology of temper outbursts: A review. *Journal of Nervous & Mental Disease, 174*, 464–470.

Meyer, D. R., & Meyer, P. M. (1977). Dynamics and bases of recoveries of functions after injuries to the cerebral cortex. *Physiological Psychology, 5*, 133–165.

Meyer, J. E. (1955). Die sexuellen storungen der hirnverletzten. *Archives of Psychiatry, 199*, 449.

Miller, E. (1984). *Recovery and management of neuropsychological impairments*. New York: Wiley.

Morrison, J. H., Molliver, M. E., & Grzanna, R. (1979). Noradrenergic innervation of cerebral cortex: Widespread effects of local cortical lesions. *Science, 20*, 313–316.

Muir, C. A., Haffey, W. J., Ott, K. J., Karaica, D., Muir, J. H., & Sutko, M. (1983). Treatment of behavioral deficits. In M. Rosenthal, E. R. Griffith, M. R. Bond, & J. D. Miller (Eds.), *Rehabilitation of the head injured adult* (pp. 381–393). Philadelphia: Davis.

Mysiw, W. J., & Jackson, R. D. (1987). Tricyclic antidepressant therapy after traumatic brain injury. *Journal of Head Trauma Rehabilitation, 2*, 34–42.

Mysiw, W. J., Jackson, R. D., & Corrigan, J. D. (1988). Amitriptyline for post-traumatic agitation. *American Journal of Physical Medicine & Rehabilitation, 67*, 29–33.

Nair, N. P. V., Ban, T. A., Hontela, S., & Clarke, M. A. (1973). Trazodone in the treatment of organic brain syndromes, with special reference to psychogeriatrics. *Current Therapeutic Research, 15*, 769–775.

Olds, J. (1958). Self-stimulation of the brain. *Science, 127*, 315–324.

O'Shanick, G. J. (1986). Neuropsychiatric complications in head injury. *Advances in Psychosomatic Medicine*, *16*, 173–193.

O'Shanick, G. J. (1987). Clinical aspects of psychopharmacologic treatment in head-injured patients. *Journal of Head Trauma Rehabilitation*, *2*, 59–67.

Pearlson, G., & Robinson, R. (1981). Suction lesions of the frontal cerebral cortex in the rat induce symmetrical behavioral and catecholaminergic responses. *Brain Research*, *218*, 233–242.

Peterson, L. (1986). Acute response to trauma. *Advances in Psychosomatic Medicine*, *16*, 84–92.

Peterson, L., & O'Shanick, G. (1985). Endocrine diseases presenting with psychiatric symptoms. *Postgraduate Medicine*, *77*, 233–239.

Pomara, N., Deptula, D., Medel, M., Block, R. I., & Greenblatt, D. J. (1989). Effects of diazepam on recall memory: Relationship to aging, dose, and duration of treatment. *Psychopharmacology Bulletin*, *25*, 144–148.

Pope, H. G., McElroy, S. L., Satlin, A., Hudson, J. I., Keck, P. E., Jr., & Kalish, R. (1988). Head injury, bipolar disorder, and response to valproate. *Comprehensive Psychiatry*, *29*, 34–38.

Prigatano, G. P. (1986). Personality and psychosocial consequences of brain injury. In G. P. Prigatano, D. J. Fordyce, H. K. Zeiner, J. R. Roueche, M. Pepping, & B. C. Wood (Eds.), *Neuropsychological rehabilitation after brain injury* (pp. 29–50). Baltimore: Johns Hopkins University Press.

Prigatano, G. P. (1987). Recovery and cognitive retraining after craniocerebral trauma. *Journal of Learning Disabilities*, *20*, 603–613.

Rao, N., Jellinek, H. M., & Woolston, D. C. (1985). Agitation in closed head injury: Haloperidol effects on rehabilitation outcome. *Archives of Physical Medicine Rehabilitation*, *66*, 30–34.

Reding, M. J., Orto, L. A., Winter, S. W., Fortuna, I. M., Di Ponte, P., & McDowell, F. H. (1986). Antidepressant therapy after stroke: A double blind trial. *Archives of Neurology*, *43*, 763–765.

Reisberg, B., Ferris, S. H., & Gershon, S. (1981). An overview of pharmacologic treatment of cognitive decline in the aged. *American Journal of Psychiatry*, *138*, 593–600.

Richmond, J. S., Young, J. R., & Groves, J. E. (1978). Violent dyscontrol responsive to d-amphetamine. *American Journal of Psychiatry*, *135*, 365–366.

Robinson, R. (1979). Differential behavioral and biochemical effects of right and left hemispheric cerebral infarction in the rat. *Science*, *205*, 707–710.

Ross, E. D., & Rush, A. J. (1981). Diagnosis and neuroanatomical correlates of depression in brain-damaged patients. *Archives of General Psychiatry*, *38*, 1344–1354.

Saran, A. S. (1985). Depression after minor closed head injury: Role of dexamethasone suppression test and antidepressants. *Journal of Clinical Psychiatry*, *46*, 335–338.

Saran, A. S. (1988). Antidepressants not effective in headache associated with minor closed head injury. *International Journal of Psychiatry in Medicine*, *18*, 75–83.

Schiffer, R. B., Cash, J., & Herndon, R. M. (1983). Treatment of emotional lability with low-dosage tricyclic antidepressants. *Psychosomatics*, *24*, 1094–1096.

Schiffer, R. B., Herndon, R. M., & Rudick, R. A. (1985). Treatment of pathologic laughing and weeping with amitriptyline. *The New England Journal of Medicine*, *312*, 1480–1482.

Schneider, S. K., & Kaplan, S. M. (1989). Secondary mania resulting from a closed-head injury. *The Clinical Neuropsychologist*, *3*, 230–234.

Simpson, D. M., & Foster, D. (1986). Improvement in organically disturbed behavior with trazodone treatment. *Journal of Clinical Psychiatry*, *47*, 191–193.

Stern, J. M. (1978). Cranio-cerebral injured patients. *Scandinavian Journal of Rehabilitation Medicine*, *10*, 7.

Stern, J. M., Najenson, T., Grosswasser, Z., Mendelson, L., & Davidson, S. (1976). Psychiatric aspects of the rehabilitation of the severely brain injured. *Israel Annals of Psychiatry & Related Disciplines*, *14*, 333–344.

Stewart, J. T., & Hemsath, R. H. (1988). Bipolar illness following traumatic brain injury: Treatment with lithium and carbamazepine. *Journal of Clinical Psychiatry*, *49*, 74–75.

Sundet, K., Finset, A., & Reinvang, I. (1988). Neuropsychological predictors in stroke rehabilitation. *Journal of Experimental Neuropsychology*, *10*, 363–379.

Sutton, R. L., Weaver, W. S., & Feeney, D. M. (1987). Drug- induced modification of behavioral recovery following cortical trauma. *Journal of Head Trauma Rehabilitation*, *2*, 50–58.

Thomsen, I. V. (1984). Late outcome of very severe blunt head trauma: A 10-15 year second follow-up. *Journal of Neurology, Neurosurgery, & Psychiatry*, *47*, 260–268.

Trimble, M. R., & Thompson, P. J. (1983). Anticonvulsant drugs and cognitive function and behavior. *Epilepsia*, *24*(Suppl. 1), 555–563.

Tune, L. E., Damlouji, N. F., Holland, A., Gardner, T. J., Folstein, M. F., & Coyle, J. T. (1981). Association of postoperative delirium with raised serum levels of anticholinergic drugs. *Lancet*, *2*, 651–652.

Tyler, G. S., McNeely, H. E., & Dick, M. L. (1980). Treatment of post-traumatic headache with amitriptyline. *Headache*, *20*, 213–216.

Udaka, F., Yamao, S., Nagata, H., Nakamura, S., & Kameyama, M. (1984). Pathologic laughing and crying treated with levodopa. *Archives of Neurology*, *41*, 1095–1096.

van Woerkom, T. C. A. M., Teelken, A. W., & Minderhoud, J. M. (1977). Difference in neurotransmitter metabolism in frontotemporal-lobe contusion and diffuse cerebral contusion. *Lancet*, *1*, 812–813.

Vogel, J. R. (1979). Objective measurement of human performance changes produced by antianxiety drugs. In S. Fielding & H. Lal (Eds.), *Anxiolytics* (pp. 343–374). Mount Kisco, NY: Futura Publishing.

Weinberg, R. M., Auerbach, S. H., & Moore, S. (1987). Pharmacologic treatment of cognitive deficits: A case study. *Brain Injury*, *1*, 57–59.

Weinstein, G. S., & Wells, C. E. (1981). Case studies in neuropsychiatry: Post-traumatic psychiatric dysfunction—diagnosis and treatment. *Journal of Clinical Psychiatry*, *42*, 120–122.

Whyte, J., & Glenn, M. B. (1986). The care and rehabilitation of the patient in a persistent vegetative state. *Head Trauma Rehabilitation*, *1*, 39–53.

Williams, K. H., & Goldstein, G. (1979). Cognitive and affective responses to lithium in patients with organic brain syndrome. *American Journal of Psychiatry*, *136*, 800–803.

Yudofsky, S., Williams, D., & Gorman, J. (1981). Propranolol in the treatment of rage and violent behavior in patients with chronic brain syndromes. *American Journal of Psychiatry*, *138*, 218–220.

Zeff, K., & Chung, R. (1987). Traumatic brain injury as an etiology of organic affective syndrome. *Military Medicine*, *152*, 529–530.

# 10

# Cognitive Rehabilitation after Head Trauma

## Toward an Integrated Cognitive/Behavioral Perspective on Intervention

LINDA WARREN DUKE, SHERRY L. WEATHERS, SANDRA G. CALDWELL, and THOMAS A. NOVACK

Cognitive interventions are increasingly used and accepted as components of rehabilitation programs after head trauma. A number of recent reviews assess the general effectiveness of cognitive retraining in general (Butler & Namerow, 1988; Gouvier, Webster, & Blanton, 1986; Rimmele & Hester, 1987). Others have reviewed the effectiveness of particular cognitive rehabilitation programs (Ben-Yishay, Rattok, Lakin, Piasetsky, Ross, Silver, Zide, & Ezrachi, 1985; Prigatano, 1987; Williams, 1987) and of retraining in specific cognitive domains, such as attention (Sohlberg & Mateer, 1987; Wood, 1986) and memory (Glisky & Schacter, 1986). Despite varying perspectives among practitioners, a general consensus appears to be evolving regarding effective intervention strategies, and this consensus is reflected in current cognitive rehabilitation texts (Adamovich, Henderson, & Auerbach, 1985; Najenson, Rahmani, Elazar, & Auerbach, 1984; Sohlberg & Mateer, 1989; Szekeres, Ylvisaker, & Holland, 1985; Trexler, 1982).

The consensus of opinion regarding effective intervention strategies includes consideration of the stage of recovery and the nature of the cognitive deficit. Further, general agreement has been reached regarding the typical course of recovery. The ability to perform

LINDA WARREN DUKE, SHERRY L. WEATHERS, SANDRA G. CALDWELL, and THOMAS A. NOVACK • Spain Rehabilitation Center, Department of Rehab Medicine, University of Alabama at Birmingham School of Medicine, Birmingham, Alabama 35294.

*HANDBOOK OF HEAD TRAUMA: Acute Care to Recovery*, edited by Charles J. Long and Leslie K. Ross. Plenum Press, New York, 1992.

many cognitive tasks recovers spontaneously after head trauma, with the most rapid recovery within the first 6 months after injury. Unfortunately, there frequently are residual cognitive deficits that do not spontaneously recover. The speed of spontaneous recovery and the nature of the residual cognitive deficit typically depend on the severity of the injury. When appropriate cognitive interventions are administered concurrent with spontaneous recovery, cognitive recovery can be facilitated (Rimmele & Hester, 1987). Cognitive interventions can also reduce residual cognitive deficits that remain after spontaneous recovery reaches asymptote (Sohlberg & Mateer, 1987). Practitioners further agree that intervention strategies must be matched appropriately to cognitive tasks. Cognitive tasks may require repeated practice of stimulus-initiated response sequences to improve performance (stimulation or rote rehearsal techniques), training in task-appropriate problem-solving skills and strategies to improve performance (reorganization techniques) and/or restructuring of the environment so that external sources of information supplement or support deficient internal information processing (external aids).

This evolving consensus regarding the course of recovery and effective cognitive interventions has not yet been related to a coherent cognitive theory which can guide practice and generate relevant research. The purpose of this chapter is to present a theoretical perspective, drawn from cognitive psychology, that offers a potential basis for development of a cognitive theory of intervention.

## CURRENT THEORETICAL INFLUENCES AND APPROACHES

The dominant theoretical influence on the development of cognitive rehabilitation has clearly been the work of Luria (1963, 1980). His ideas regarding the basic organization of the brain into functional cortical systems are reflected in the current practice of targeting specific clusters of cognitive behavior (language, attention, memory) for rehabilitation and also in the assumption that behavior within these domains can be reorganized to allow recovery of function after injury. Luria's ideas regarding the hierarchy of processing within each system, from arousal units to sensory-input units to organization and planning units, offer a model of the hierarchical course of spontaneous recovery, as well as a justification for a hierarchical intervention program within domains of cognitive behaviors (Sohlberg & Mateer, 1989). A similar approach is advocated by the developmental perspective in which recovery of function following injury is assumed to follow the course of original development (Bolger, 1982; Craine, 1982).

Another important influence on cognitive rehabilitation is learning theory, particularly as reflected in the application of behavior therapy to the remediation of cognitive deficits (Goldstein, 1979). Cognitive rehabilitation is grounded in the key assumption that the injured brain (and the brain-injured person) can continue to learn. The principles of learning theory dictate the form of therapy. The task of the rehabilitation therapist is to identify the cognitive behavior that is deficit, to target specific behavior for change, to elicit and reinforce targeted behaviors using appropriate environmental manipulations, and to monitor the effectiveness of the interventions using appropriate research designs.

A final theoretical influence on treatment is rooted in a more psychodynamic tradition and, as advocated by practitioners (Adamovich *et al.*, 1985; Prigatano, Fordyce, Zeiner, Roueche, Pepping, & Wood, 1986; Trexler, 1982), emphasizes the importance of psychosocial variables and the need to view cognitive remediation in the broader context of interpersonal adjustment. In particular, self-awareness, motivation for change, and an interpersonal and community focus are viewed as essential for any practical generalization of newly trained and newly reorganized cognitive behaviors.

## A COGNITIVE BEHAVIORAL PERSPECTIVE

Lacking from current theoretical influences on cognitive rehabilitation is a truly *cognitive*, as opposed to a neurological, behavioral, or psychodynamic, perspective (Gross, 1982; Piasetsky, 1982). Cognitive psychologists and cognitive neuroscientists attempt to study and model human cognition in both normal and brain-injured individuals by focusing on the information processing characteristics of the cognitive system (Gazzaniga, 1984; Semenza, Bisiacchi, & Rosenthal, 1988). The cognitive perspective has been introduced as a theoretical basis for remediation of disorders of attention (Sohlberg & Mateer, 1989) and memory (Baddeley, Harris, Sunderland, Watts, & Wilson, 1987; Grafman, 1984) and has been applied more broadly as a theoretical basis for behavioral self-management (Carver & Scheier, 1983; Malec, 1984) and psychotherapy (Kendall & Bemis, 1983). The lack of a general cognitive theory of cognitive rehabilitation has led to shortcomings in current clinical practice. These shortcomings include an inadequate rationale for matching intervention strategy to deficit, a lack of appreciation of which cognitive behaviors are most readily changed and why, and an often misguided belief that limited amounts of cognitive training will yield lasting change.

In this section we shall attempt to integrate current conceptions of cognitive functioning derived from a variety of sources. These conceptions include the work of Shiffrin and Schneider (1977) on automatic and controlled processes, the work of Baddeley (Baddeley & Hitch, 1974; Baddeley, 1987) on working memory, and elaborations and extensions of this general view of information processing by others (Norman, 1981; Norman & Shallice, 1980; Reason, 1984; Shallice, 1982). While acknowledging that this attempt will borrow freely from these and other authors, our perspective may not in all respects be consistent with their views. The goal is to present a working conceptualization of cognitive functioning that is derived from current cognitive theory and that can guide the development and evaluation of cognitive rehabilitation procedures.

### Automatic Processes

A number of theorists have proposed a distinction between automatic and controlled cognitive processing. Many cognitive processes occur relatively automatically, without direct conscious control. Such processes, while initiated by the current external or internal stimulus environment, are carried out by "hard-wired" or highly overlearned cognitive systems. Once an automatic process has been initiated, it runs to completion and cannot be consciously inhibited or changed. Automatic processes are minimally affected by attentional and intentional processes (Shiffrin & Schneider, 1977). Because automatic processes do not require conscious attention, they do not demand processing resources, nor do they benefit from practice or feedback. Examples of cognitive activities which are largely dependent on automatic processes are ordinary orienting and perceptual processes and the accessing of general semantic knowledge, including many language processes and motor programs for familiar activities. Many aspects of other complex cognitive behaviors also rely on automatic mechanisms. In particular, memory encoding of contextual aspects of perceptually based information (such as spatial location, time of occurrence, and frequency of repetition) may be relatively automatic, as are the operations that store and retrieve information in the memory systems. Automatic processes, once established, are believed to be unaffected by developmental changes (Hasher & Zacks, 1979). In the face of nonfocal neurological disease or injury, it has also been proposed that automatic processes may be the "last to go" (Johnson, 1977).

## Controlled Processes

Many cognitive operations are under direct conscious control and, therefore, are optional and effortful. These operations do depend on attentional and intentional processes and do require processing resources. Since the processing capacity available for such activities is assumed to be limited, only a limited amount of mental "work" can be carried out at a time. Thus, controlled processing operations are typically conducted sequentially (Shiffrin & Schneider, 1977). Although restricted in terms of cognitive work accomplished per unit of time, controlled processes are maximally flexible. Controlled processes can be initiated, modified, or abandoned at will, and are highly responsive to practice and feedback. Controlled processes allow us to plan, monitor, and change our behavior.

Within this framework, learning is accomplished through the development of new controlled processing sequences. New controlled processing sequences will often incorporate previously acquired information or modify old controlled processing sequences. The ability to both adapt and generalize behavior to new situations is largely a function of controlled processing. Under certain circumstances, a controlled processing sequence may be activated so often under similar conditions that it becomes "automatized" (Schneider, 1985). With extensive repetition such processes may become automatic in the sense of "highly overlearned." Examples of effortful-turned-automatic processes include many of the cognitive and motor programs involved in speech comprehension and production.

The controlled processing system can be viewed in terms of three sub-systems: an executive system, an attentional system, and a memory system. The executive component initiates and monitors the outcome of ongoing controlled processes. The function of the executive system is to plan internal and external behaviors, to activate the appropriate memory information necessary to carry out those plans, and to monitor whether behavioral goals or objectives are being met. The controlled processing system is hierarchical, in that the executive allocates attentional resources and selects information to be stored or retrieved from memory. As a cognitive system, the executive system functions in relation to the motivational and emotional agenda of the organism (Roth & Tucker, 1986). Thus, it is the cognitive mechanism through which we attempt to get what we want. The success of the executive system depends upon the attention system.

The attention system is the guidance or energy system which provides the cognitive resources necessary for carrying out the executive system's plans. If attention is not sufficient for carrying out a cognitive plan, or if attention is prematurely distracted from a controlled processing sequence, then potentially successful plans for processing information will fail. In a normal person, the amount of attentional capacity available for controlled processing is a relatively fixed resource; minor fluctuations in capacity may occur as a function of arousal level, but in general, processing efficiency will depend upon the deployment of the fixed attentional resource.

Both automatic and controlled cognitive operations are assumed to access a common permanent memory store. The implementation of memory storage and retrieval operations and the resulting structure of the contents of memory are all assumed to be automatic operations not subject to conscious control. The units of information stored in permanent memory are frequently referred to as schema. Possibly everything we perceive or think about is stored automatically and relatively permanently in such memory schemata (Johnson, 1983; Posner, 1984). However, the controlled processing system determines, in part, what the *content* of those perceptions and thoughts will be. Selective processing and elaboration upon one's perceptions and thoughts is a form of controlled processing referred to as memory encoding. Although memory storage and retrieval can occur automatically, to be an effective component of cognition, memory must be accessed under controlled processing. Access by the consciously controlled processing system to information in memory depends upon the generation of effective retrieval cues which will activate the desired schemata. What retrieval cues are effective will depend upon how the memory was originally encoded. Thus, one function of controlled processing is to *encode* information for memory in a way that makes the second function, *retrieval* of information, possible. Encoding and retrieval strategies are selected by the executive system and are carried out in real time and mental "space" by the controlled processing component of the memory system called working memory.

The conceptualization of working memory presented here is considerably broader than that proposed by Baddeley (1987) but includes many of the features of his model. Working memory consists of the cognitive systems responsible for maintaining the current contents of consciousness. Working memory is controlled by the executive system, requires attentional resource allocated by the attention system, and briefly retains the immediate mental products of these systems. These products include current perceptual awareness; information retrieved from permanent memory; the current cognitive plan; and a limited amount of information selected from just-completed controlled processing operations. It is this latter residual information that is referred to as "working memory" by Baddeley and is assumed to be contained in specialized memory buffers. He assumes that one of these memory buffers is designed for the maintenance of verbal articulative information and another is specialized for the maintenance of visuospatial information. All information in working memory is potentially available for memory encoding, but most of it occupies working memory only briefly and may never be retrievable. Controlled processing is required to select salient information in working memory and initiate encoding operations so that it can subsequently be retrieved from permanent memory. (A brief theory of how memory retrieval works and how to select optimal encoding strategies will be presented in the memory intervention section.)

## POSSIBLE IMPLICATIONS FOR THE COURSE OF RECOVERY

During the acute phases of recovery from head injury (0–6 months postonset), both automatic and controlled cognitive processes are expected to show rapid spontaneous recovery due to a variety of mechanisms of neurological recovery (Marshall, 1984). Whether or not preceded by coma, the initial phases of cognitive recovery, marked by emotional lability, inattention, confusion, disorientation, and communication disorders, are assumed to be dependent on the course of recovery of both the controlled and automatic processing mechanisms. As neurological recovery in the automatic processing mechanisms begins to slow, recovery of automatic systems is assumed to reach asymptote. Deficits in automatic processing mechanisms which persist after the acute phase of neurological recovery would be assumed to be difficult and slow to remediate.

Recovery of controlled processing mechanisms is expected to follow a hierarchical course similar to the proposed hierarchy of cognitive control. First to recover should be conscious sensitivity to sensory stimulation in the form of a return of conscious awareness. Next to recover would be executive control of attentional mechanisms along with the attentional capacity necessary to carry out any controlled processing operations. The ability to manipulate information in working memory via shifts of attention from perceptual input to associated thoughts and memories would be expected to recover next. The ability to plan and execute more complex sequences of thought and behavior should recover last, due to the reliance of these executive functions on sufficient attentional control and capacity, as well as on the simultaneous maintenance and use of several forms of information in working memory buffers. As higher levels of executive functions improve, the efficiency of lower levels will also increase. For example, as the ability to reliably shift attention from one source of information to another recovers, the ability to monitor a single source should also continue to improve. Or as the ability to develop a plan for solving a problem recovers, the ability to scan and identify relevant features of a task should also benefit from the higher level of executive control. Thus, executive control of information processing mechanisms may continue to spontaneously recover over prolonged periods which extend well beyond the period of active neurological recovery.


## POSSIBLE IMPLICATIONS FOR
## COGNITIVE REHABILITATION INTERVENTIONS

### Rehabilitation of Automatic Processes

A general implication of the cognitive model presented here is that the opportunity for restitution of function of automatic processes should be greatest during the active or acute phases of neurological recovery which typically occur during 0–6 months postinjury. According to this model, the initial phases of cognitive rehabilitation should focus on assessment of the integrity of sensory-perceptual and language functions. If deficits in these processes are identified, attempts to stimulate the appropriate automatic processes in the deficient systems should be the initial focus of cognitive intervention. Because the automatic processes are needed to provide a "data base" for controlled cognitive processes, it may not make sense to address deficits in cognitive control until recovery of automatic systems has reached either a functional level or asymptote. To facilitate recovery of the automatic cognitive processes, stimulation or "exercise" interventions that make limited demands on attentional capacity and executive control are indicated. Exposure to music, television, and social conversation, as well as moving around in the environment are all excellent sources of such stimulation. Possibly the presence of a normally stimulating environment, even during coma, would enhance recovery of automatic processing mechanisms. Attempts to enhance the typically bland and potentially sensory-deprived hospital environment with familiar sights and sounds would be consistent with the model. Since automatic motivational and emotional systems may also be undergoing active neurological recovery, creating a positive and supportive emotional environment during cognitive stimulation might also enhance recovery.

Obviously much is to be gained from maximizing the recovery of the automatic, stimulus-driven processes during the acute stages of recovery from head injury. Not only are such processes assumed to be difficult to alter in postacute phases of recovery, but any persistent deficits in automatic processes will place increased long-term demands on the controlled processing mechanisms (Hirst, 1982). Because automatic processes are initiated by stimulus events and are not under direct conscious control, stimulation interventions are theoretically appropriate and potentially beneficial. In attempting to stimulate automatic processes during acute phases of recovery, the goal is not relearning or generalization. Rather, the rehabilitation goal is the activation and maintenance of automatic processing skills during the period of active neurological healing. Whether such activation is beneficial remains an empirical question.

Any damage to automatic processing systems which remains after acute neurological recovery is complete would be assumed to be both difficult and slow to remediate via cognitive rehabilitation procedures. If the deficient automatic processes depend upon damaged "hard-wired" neurological systems, recovery may not occur at all. If the automatic processes depend upon highly overlearned information processing sequences, relearning might be expected to take at least as long as the original acquisition process. For example, many of the cognitive operations of the skilled adult reader are assumed to be automatic (Flores d'Arcais, 1988). Some reading skills depend upon "hard-wired" perceptual analysis while others are obviously learned over a period of years. If reading is deficient following the acute phase of recovery after head injury, it may potentially be returned to a functional level via improvement in controlled processing mechanisms. Recovery of premorbid proficiency after the acute phase of recovery, although theoretically possible, would be assumed to depend on amounts of practice at least comparable to that required for original learning. As another example, recent studies (Levin, Goldstein, High, & Williams, 1988; Goldstein & Levin, 1988; Tweedy & Vakil, 1988) report that head-injured individuals are deficient both in their memory for frequency of occurrence information, which is assumed to be encoded automatically (Hasher & Zacks, 1984), and in their performance on more effortful memory tasks. It would be expected that after acute phases of recovery, effortful memory tasks are more likely to benefit from cognitive interventions than are more automatic aspects of memory performance. Thus, after the acute phases of recovery, automatic processes are not likely to benefit from limited training over weeks or months, and should not typically be targeted for such treatment. Patients with persistent sensory-based perceptual deficits, most language deficits, and certain memory deficits should be counseled realistically about the probable slow, long-term basis of their recovery in these areas.

## Rehabilitation of Controlled Processes

According to the model presented here, the most effective form of intervention to improve controlled processing is to restore executive skills which are appropriate for a particular domain of cognitive functioning. Intervention at the highest possible level of executive control should be most effective because it is assumed that improvement of higher-level controlled processing skills will simultaneously improve lower-level ones. Depending on the extent of controlled processing deficits and the stage of recovery, intervention might focus on the executive control of attention, the executive control of memory, or the executive control of reasoning. During the acute phases of recovery the goal is *restitution* of controlled processing functions (Rothi & Horner, 1983). Thus, interventions should follow the proposed hierarchical course of recovery. Intervention should attempt to stimulate the reemergence of functional executive control without placing excessive demands on working memory and available processing capacity until those subsystems have sufficiently recovered. During postacute phases of recovery, the goal is either true *retraining* or *substitution* of function. It is assumed that controlled processing skills that have not spontaneously recovered to functional levels during the active phase of neurological recovery should be treated as persistent, but not necessarily permanent, deficits. Because learning occurs via the development of new controlled processing sequences, deficits in controlled processing can potentially be reduced or compensated for with appropriate training. For progress to occur, such deficits need to be addressed by both patient and therapist as cognitive problems which may be solved in a variety of ways (Miller, 1980).

The most appropriate intervention program will attempt to remediate deficits of executive control by using any residual problem-solving skills. Depending on an individual's condition and needs, this approach includes three alternative strategies. The therapist can attempt to actively *retrain* those information processing strategies assumed to have been available premorbidly. Second, the therapist can select and train new *substitute* information processing strategies adapted to the individual's current limitations of cognitive control, memory, or attentional capacity. Third, the therapist can train the individual to use external prosthetic supports to *supplement or replace* deficient information processing mechanisms. Regardless of the strategy selected, the emphasis in all three alternatives should be to restore functional executive control in such a way that problem-solving skills or external aids will generalize beyond the training task. In the following sections specific examples of how interventions at the executive/intentional level might effect recovery in various domains of cognitive behavior will be described.

## Executive Control of Attention

Rehabilitation of controlled processing during acute phases of recovery typically begins with assessing and remediating deficits in the control of attention. A variety of neuropsychological tests can be used both to assess deficits of attentional control and to monitor progress (Sohlberg & Mateer, 1989; Gronwall, 1987). Training materials, such as the Attention Process Training (APT) approach advocated by Sohlberg and Mateer (1986), and those available in software packages (Sandford & Browne, 1988) can be used for both assessment and intervention. Much of the published literature is based on attention training with patients in the postacute phase of recovery (Sohlberg & Mateer, 1987). The cognitive model proposed here, however, suggests that attention interventions should begin as early as possible following injury. The model suggests, as do Sohlberg and Mateer (1989), that effective training of attentional control (1) begin with easy tasks that make minimal demands on attentional capacity, working memory, and the planning and monitoring functions of the executive and (2) progress to more difficult tasks only when some criterion level of performance has been achieved. Beginning with automatic responses, such as orienting to stimuli, may be necessary, with the progression to more controlled, effortful processing awaiting improvement in more basic areas. To effect recovery, training of attention tasks is expected to result in more effective controlled processing sequences for the intentional control of attentional resources. Also, each attention training task would ideally use a variety of sensory-perceptual modalities (visual, auditory, tactile) and response methods (speech, key pressing, tapping, writing, etc.) to ensure maximum generality and to identify deficient subsystems.

## Executive Control of Attitude, Mood, and Anxiety

Before systematic progress can occur in remediation of more complex controlled processing skills, the motivational and emotional systems must recover sufficiently to allow acknowledgment of deficits, the setting of goals, and the regulation of fluctuations in mood and anxiety (Trexler, 1982). This interdependence of motivational, emotional, and cognitive systems is consistent with the cognitive model, in that all levels of executive control operate in relation to feedback from the current motivational and emotional agenda. Patients who are too depressed, anxious, or angry literally cannot focus on other aspects of cognition. The general psychotherapeutic techniques of cognitive–behavioral therapy (Rimm & Masters, 1974), such as relaxation techniques, positive self-statements, thought stopping, modeling, role playing, and assertiveness training, may succeed with head-injured patients. The challenge involves getting a person to use psychotherapy techniques outside the structured therapy session, at a stage of recovery when intentional control of behavior is typically deficient. Thus, the focus of *cognitive* rehabilitation is to devise techniques that result in a person being able to self-administer psychotherapy instructions or to provide psychotherapy reminders when fluctuations in motivational or emotional state are likely to occur. Depending on the individual's condition and needs, appropriate psychotherapeutic instructions may be prerecorded on tape, written in memory notebooks, incorporated into other prosthetic devices, or learned. Head-injured persons may be taught to manage fluctuations in motivation or emotion by taking brief psychotherapy breaks in which they self-administer therapy using aids to psychotherapeutic intervention designed for them. The goal is to reestablish the link between motivational/emotional states and the executive–intentional control of behavior. An example of the application of these techniques is the case of a person who spent most of her time in stubborn resistance or angry outbursts during cognitive and physical therapy. She was encouraged to listen to an imagery, self-efficacy relaxation tape daily for a week. She liked the tape and felt it helped her to relax. Thereafter, she was encouraged to take a "psychotherapy break" and listen to the tape when angry feelings surfaced. The negative emotional expressions decreased, while self-initiated use of the tape gradually increased, resulting in a significant step in the self-management of her emotional behavior.

## Executive Control of Verbal Reasoning

Verbal reasoning skills can be assumed to provide the mental tools for many controlled processing operations. Verbal reasoning skills are thought to underlie a variety of executive functions such as planning, organizing, and solving problems, as well as language and communications skills (Ben-Yishay & Diller, 1983a). Thus, improving verbal reasoning is a natural target for intervention when any of these executive functions are deficient (Ben-Yishay & Diller, 1983b). Normal verbal reasoning relies heavily on association strategies (Ben-Zur, 1989) which, in turn, require the activation of a rich associative network. While such activation is, in part, an automatic process which occurs without conscious intent once the problem is presented, retrieval of appropriate semantic knowledge can also be guided by appropriate controlled processing strategies, such as rule-oriented or partial rule strategies (Embretson, Schneider, & Roth, 1986). Thus, most verbal reasoning tasks can be approached using a variety of general problem-solving skills (Goldstein & Levin, 1987). Lezak (1983) divides problem solving into four stages: (1) goal formulation (realization and statement of an objective—"What do I want or need?"); (2) planning (analysis of the situation—"How will I get what I need?"); (3) carrying out activities (actual behavior— "Am I doing things to attain my objective?"); and (4) effective performance (feedback and self-correction—"Are my activities fulfilling my objective?"). These executive skills can potentially be improved via training and practice. Problem-solving skills are also potentially generalized to a wide variety of other cognitive tasks.

A variety of materials are available which are useful in training verbal reasoning (Holloran & Bressler, 1983; Carter, Caruso, & Languirard, 1984; Craine & Gudeman, 1981; Smith, 1986) and structured interventions to address reasoning deficits have been proposed (Ben-Yishay, Lakin, Ross, Rattok, Cohen, & Diller, 1980; Sohlberg & Mateer, 1989). However, a need continues in this area for standardized assessment devices that assess reasoning deficits and that can be used repetitively to evaluate a person's progress resulting from intervention procedures.

In our preliminary attempts to develop an intervention program to improve executive skills in verbal reasoning tasks, it proved necessary to address the need for such assessment and evaluation devices. Eight comparable forms of an assessment instrument containing five separately scored subsections were developed. Two forms of the test, with a guide for scoring, are presented in Appendix A. Most test items were taken directly from Holloran and Bressler (1983) with a few items from other sources (Brown, Sherbenow, & Johnsen, 1982; Ben-Yishay *et al.*, 1980; Carter *et al.*, 1984) plus comics taken from daily newspapers. The five test subsections are intended to correspond roughly to: (I) simple convergent reasoning, (II) simple sequential reasoning, (III) simple divergent reasoning, (IV) complex convergent reasoning, and (V) combined convergent and sequential reasoning.

In order to obtain normative data on the test, the eight forms of the instrument were administered to 147 normal controls (mean age 21.3 years [17-47], 61% female). Test results for this normal sample are presented in Table 10.1. Mean performance on the overall instrument was 74% correct (45.9 out of 62). The mean total scores on the eight alternate forms were found to be statistically equivalent. Attempts to establish reliability and validity of the test are still in progress.

The lowest scoring 10% of the normal sample was retested on the same form of the initial test and improved from 51% to 67% correct. This result likely represents a practice effect. Each of these low-scoring persons then received approximately 30 minutes of intense instruction with regard to strategies and practice on reasoning tasks with feedback from the trainer, closely approximating the interventions we have used with head-injured individuals. At the end of the training session, subjects were tested on an alternate form of the test, with a mean performance of 76% correct. These results indicate that initially deficient

TABLE 10.1.   Development of Verbal Reasoning Test:
Performance of a Normal Young Adult Group

| Test section | Maximum score | Form I n = 20 | | Form II n = 17 | | Total group n = 147 | |
|---|---|---|---|---|---|---|---|
| | | Mean (S.D.) | % | Mean (S.D.) | % | Mean (S.D.) | % |
| I. Convergent | 18 | 13.60 (3.5) | 76 | 14.35 (1.7) | 78 | 14.01 (2.6) | 78 |
| II. Sequential | 12 | 9.50 (2.1) | 79 | 9.82 (1.1) | 82 | 8.86 (2.3) | 74 |
| III. Divergent | 10 | 6.95 (1.7) | 70 | 8.18 (1.2) | 82 | 6.96 (2.1) | 70 |
| IV. Complex 1 | 12 | 9.30 (1.9) | 78 | 9.12 (2.4) | 76 | 9.16 (2.0) | 76 |
| V. Complex 2 | 10 | 7.25 (2.1) | 72 | 6.41 (1.3) | 64 | 6.86 (1.9) | 69 |
| Test total | 62 | 47.40 (9.4) | 76 | 47.82 (4.8) | 77 | 45.88 (7.4) | 74 |

performance in the reasoning skills represented by this instrument can be improved through practice and instruction.

While the assessment instruments were being standardized as described above, four head-injured individuals were undergoing cognitive rehabilitation focusing on problems with reasoning abilities. All had sustained a severe closed head injury (posttraumatic amnesia > four weeks) and were approximately six months postinjury at the initiation of treatment. Prior to injury, one was a high school sophomore and the others were college students. Compared to the normative sample, two individuals were impaired on the Verbal Reasoning Test and the other two were not. Even in the latter two cases, however, one of the persons (a former college scholarship student) had obvious deficits in study skills compared to premorbid abilities. Evaluation was followed by participation in 15 biweekly 30-minute sessions (with some rescheduling due to vacations) of cognitive remediation using an ABA design. Each of the first five sessions consisted of training on verbal reasoning problems similar (but not identical) to those in one of the five subsections of the assessment instrument. The training procedures were adapted from Ben-Yishay et al. (1980) and Lezak (1983). These focused on teaching the person to ask and answer the following questions, with feedback from the therapist, during the training on each subsection: (1) What is the task? (2) What do I need to do? (3) Is this a good answer? Performance on each subsection was evaluated before and after each session using alternate forms of the test. The next five sessions (B) were memory training sessions, with testing on one of the alternate forms of the verbal reasoning subtests pre and post each session. The final five sessions (A) focused on more verbal reasoning problems, including examples of everyday problem-solving tasks (Denney, 1988), with pre- and posttests on alternate forms of the appropriate subsections of the assessment instrument. Unfortunately, one subject dropped out of treatment at the end of the eighth session (partially through memory training). The other three subjects completed the treatment program. Results for the four patients are presented in Table 10.2.

Analysis of the data thus far indicates modest, statistically nonsignificant improvement for the group (from 72% correct on the first pretests to 81% correct on the final posttests) but with considerable individual variability in performance. As might be expected, the two individuals who were initially deficient on the Verbal Reasoning Test demonstrated more quantitative benefit from the treatment than the two individuals whose Verbal Reasoning Test scores were at normal levels prior to treatment. Three individuals,

TABLE 10.2.   Development of Verbal Reasoning Treatment:
% Correct Responses on Verbal Reasoning Test

| Verbal reasoning | Pretest | A Reasoning (5 sessions) | | B Memory strategy (5 sessions) | | A Reasoning (5 sessions) | | Follow-up (no treat) (mos) |
|---|---|---|---|---|---|---|---|---|
| | | Pre | Post | Pre | Post | Pre | Post | |
| Deficient | | | | | | | | |
| CH | 60 | 66 | 69 | 70 | 82 | *a* | | 68 (1) |
| JC | 65 | 67 | 70 | 71 | 64 | 74 | 80 | 71 (1) |
| Mean (*n* = 2) | 63 | 66 | 70 | 70 | 73 | | | 70 |
| Normal | | | | | | | | |
| PM | 84 | 77 | 82 | 77 | 87 | 84 | 88 | 77 (5) 94 (9) |
| SW | 81 | 73 | 81 | 84 | 76 | 90 | 76 | 80 (2) |
| Mean (*n* = 2) | 82 | 75 | 82 | 80 | 82 | 87 | 82 | 79 |
| Total mean (*n* = 4) | 72 | 71 | 76 | 76 | 77 | 80 | 81 | 79 |

*a*Dropped out of treatment.

one deficient and two normal in verbal reasoning at the start of treatment, have returned to school and have functioned adequately, although below premorbid levels. The fourth person has not returned to either school or employment.

In summary, this preliminary study provides evidence that a remediation program focusing on improving verbal reasoning is feasible with head-injured individuals when the program is presented under the protocol described. Obviously, a larger sample of head-injured individuals, all of whom complete the full training protocol, will be necessary to adequately evaluate the effectiveness of the remediation approach. More intensive training, such as more frequent appointments of longer duration, may be necessary. Nevertheless, the present study does provide a conceptual framework and an adequate basis for evaluating a training program.

## Executive Control of Memory

Considerable dissatisfaction with previous approaches to the remediation of memory deficits has been expressed by practitioners (Glisky & Schacter, 1986; Poon, 1980), and a variety of alternative memory remediation paradigms and conceptualizations are beginning to appear in the literature (Baddeley *et al.*, 1987; Duke, Haley, & Bergquist, 1991; Hirst & Volpe, 1988; Parente & Anderson-Parente, 1989; Mateer & Sohlberg, 1988; Tulving, 1987). The cognitive/behavioral approach to memory disorders, presented by Duke *et al.* (1991), will be addressed here. This approach focuses on the development of specific executive skills to improve memory functioning.

Common conceptions of memory problems as difficulty in retaining information are somewhat misleading. As suggested by the cognitive model presented here, memory storage is a potentially automatic process and information stored in memory is relatively permanent. However, even when memory functioning is normal, retrieval may fail. Thus, memory functioning must be thought of as an interactive process of encoding and retrieving information. Information must be *encoded* in a way that makes it more readily *retrieved*. Ideally, information in memory should become available to the working memory system when needed and stay unobtrusively in storage when not needed. The memory system manages this problem of information access by requiring that a memory cue be present in working memory in order for a target memory to be activated or retrieved. A *memory cue* is some piece of information that was a part of, or connected with, the target information at the time of storage *and* that would have been effective at activating or retrieving the target information at that time. Memory *encoding* is the process of establishing such memory cues. Potential memory cues occur constantly in the environment. We notice them and automatically memories are activated. We enter a building and the location of the elevator springs spontaneously to mind. At times, one memory serves as a cue for another, and we relive past events. And at other times, these automatic retrieval processes fail. We see a familiar person and his name does *not* spring to mind. We consciously, and often with great effort, control the search for an effective memory cue, trying one thing and then another, until the sought-for information finally comes to mind—or we give up.

The fundamental mechanism for improving memory is to encode more effective memory cues, via effortful, controlled processing. The only direct way we can influence memory storage and retrieval is (1) by controlling our thoughts, i.e., using executive mechanisms to attend to, or think of, effective memory cues during storage and at retrieval, and (2) by controlling the environment so that external memory cues will be attended to as needed.

What makes a piece of information an effective memory cue other than its presence at both storage and retrieval? Considerable research and current theoretical debate focuses on this issue (Humphreys, Bain, & Pike, 1989). Duke *et al.* (1990) argue, based on a similar analysis by Morris (1978), that memory skills training may fail to generalize to everyday memory because individuals are often trained to use "mnemonic" devices that are not appropriate encoding strategies for many common memory problems. These authors suggest that most patients complain of memory problems that fall into three broad areas: remembering autobiographical information, remembering factual information, and remembering intentional information. Each of these types of information requires somewhat different encoding strategies to generate effective memory cues. Thus, individuals must be taught to match an appropriate encoding strategy to a particular memory problem.

Table 10.3 is a summary of information that we provide to patients to help in the analysis of memory problems and in the teaching of relevant encoding strategies in each of these broad categories of memory functioning.

## Autobiographical Information

Autobiographical memory refers to memory for the events and activities of one's daily life. Autobiographical memory is clearly a form of episodic memory (Tulving, 1983, 1987), but the distinction that we propose here between autobiographical and factual memory is based on its practical utility in memory intervention training. It does not in every respect parallel the theoretical distinction between episodic and semantic memory as proposed by Tulving (1983). Here, autobiographical memory refers to memory for events in a particular perceptual context. Memory problems will often relate to remembering what happened, where it happened, when it happened, or whether it happened. Retrieval of this type of

TABLE 10.3.  Cognitive/Behavioral Approach to Solving Specific Memory Problems

| Type of memory problem | Resulting behavior | Required mediating cues | Strategies |
|---|---|---|---|
| Autobiographical | Forgetting past experience | Perceptual cues<br>Sensations<br>Images | —Attention and concentration on who, what, when, where<br>—Keep things the same<br>—Use external storage |
| Factual | Forgetting a piece of information | Structure cues<br>Grouping<br>Associating | —Work on organizing and associating<br>—Use mnemonics<br>—Use external storage |
| Intential | Forgetting to do something | Trigger cues | —Think ahead<br>—Plant an external cue: it must be timely, active, task-specific |

information typically involves the self-presentation of imagery cues as one tries to mentally relive bits of a past experience. Thus, memory training focuses on: (1) teaching encoding strategies that ensure that relevant aspects of one's environment and activities are encoded during the experience (attention, concentration, keeping things the same); (2) external storage of information (note taking, photo taking, tape recording); and (3) use of the memory cues generated during encoding to aid memory retrieval. For example, problems with misplacing personal articles are best addressed by keeping things the same, by concentrating on putting things in a particular well-known place and thus retrieving the "thing," rather than the memory. Problems of losing one's way, forgetting locations, or where the car is parked, involve training a strategy of "checking," i.e., actively looking around and attending to landmarks, verbalizing those landmarks, making appropriate written or taped notes or maps, and mentally rehearsing one's planned return using the landmarks. Confusion about people, who they are, what they do, what they said, can be addressed in a similar way.

## Factual Information

Factual information always occurs initially in some autobiographical–episodic context, but factual information is considered to be relevant as *knowledge*, independent of a particular perceptual context. If the factual information is organized or meaningfully related, the best memory cues will be those which relate to that structure or organization, or to the relation of the new information to prior knowledge. Memory training will focus on using or enhancing these cues. Because analyzing factual information in order to identify its structure and meaningful relations typically requires verbal reasoning skills, learning to encode factual information is relevant training for improving executive functioning in both domains. For example, formal study techniques, such as those suggested by Rowntree (1970) under the acronyms SQ3R (survey, question, read, recall, review) and PQRST (preview, question, read, state, test) are explicit guides to forming an executive plan for organizing, encoding, and retrieving factual information. Less formal organizational techniques, such as giving a title, a one-sentence summary, or a simple outline of information, also work well. If the factual information is arbitrary or less meaningful, such as names, dates, phone numbers, lists of shopping or chores, etc., the classic "mnemonic" techniques for encoding such information (Moffat, 1984) may be effective. However, in general, the most effective and practical memory strategy for remembering such information is to use external rather than internal storage, i.e., write it down. Which memory strategy is most appropriate will typically depend on when and how often the arbitrary factual information must be retrieved. It is important to remember one's own name, address, and phone number. On the other hand, a grocery list should probably be written down.

## Intentional Information

Intentional memory is also referred to as prospective memory. It refers to remembering one's plans for future activities and behaviors. Forgetting of one's intentions typically involves some negative consequence or inconvenience. Hence, most people can be easily motivated to attempt to improve intentional memory, making it an excellent source of target memory problems for the initial stages of memory training. An additional training advantage of intentional memory problems is that they require a person to develop a plan to remember. The key to remembering intentions is identifying a memory cue that will be effective at cuing recall of the intention at the intended future time and place. An effective memory cue for remembering to stop at the store for milk on the way home must not only remind you of the content of the intention (stop for milk) but must also capture your attention at the right place and time (two blocks before you get to the store rather than as you approach your home driveway). Thus, the unique aspect of strategies for remembering intentions is the focus on a trigger cue or reminder that will capture attention at the intended time and place. Such trigger cues will typically be external, and at best, should be active, timely, and task-specific (Harris, 1984). Active means the trigger cue captures attention, that is, it is difficult to ignore. Timely means it captures attention at the intended time and place. Task-specific means the trigger cue will tend to activate the appropriate intention. The general strategy for training intentional memory is to identify the future time and place where the intention needs to be retrieved. The trigger must be placed *now* so that it cannot be ignored at the *later* intended time. Placing an umbrella by the door is a good trigger cue, but placing the umbrella on the door handle, so that the door cannot be opened until the umbrella is removed, is better (Skinner & Vaughn, 1983). In attempting to identify and use a good trigger cue, a person learns general self-management skills for remembering. Such skills are essential for improving intentional memory, but also may result in improved strategy use in other domains of executive behavior.

## General Strategies for Improving Memory Function

The most important goal in any rehabilitation program is to transfer treatment gains into daily life situations. Patients must be taught appropriate and practical strategies for remembering. But such training will be of no practical benefit unless it is used at the appropriate time and place. Thus, the focus of memory training is on anticipating memory problems and teaching techniques to prevent them. Either the therapist or the patient must "plan to remember." A natural way to develop a "plan to remember" is as a by-product of the behavioral assessment technique known as functional analysis (Meichenbaum, 1977).

Using this approach, memory training starts with targeting of a real world memory problem, individually selected and elaborated upon by the patient. The therapist then guides the analysis of the problem, focusing on: (1) *motivation* (why is it important to improve this memory-related behavior?), (2) *strategy selection* (what type of strategy is most likely to help?), and (3) *strategy use* (what is the best way to get the use of the strategy incorporated into the behavioral repertoire?). When memory rehabilitation is approached in this way, it becomes clear that selecting and teaching an appropriate memory strategy is only part, usually the easier part, of memory training. Learning when to use a strategy is a much greater challenge for the head injured. Virtually no research exists on the application of self-management techniques (self-monitoring, self-cuing, self-instructions, self-reinforcement) to assist memory functioning. However, such techniques have been used effectively to improve problem-solving ability in the elderly (Labouvie-Vief & Gonda, 1976; Meichenbaum, 1974) and offer a possible way to teach the head-injured individual effective use of memory strategies. For example, after the individual is taught a strategy for solving a particular target memory problem, he can then be guided through active overt and covert planning for its use. This planning can include identifying situations in which the memory problem occurs, visualizing the relevant situations; experiencing an actual environment in which the problem occurs; rehearsing the motivation for improving the memory problem; talking through the planned use of the strategy; anticipating how the strategy might work, including imagining successful remembering; and reinforcement for success. Obvious advantages of this type of training are that it focuses on self-initiated memory-related behaviors and that these behaviors are more readily generalized than are particular memory aids or strategies to new target memory problems. This approach also helps both patient and family to move from global complaints about memory to concrete plans to solve the specific daily memory problems encountered.

## SUMMARY

The effective rehabilitation of cognitive deficits from head injury presents a tremendous clinical challenge that can only be addressed with appropriate research programs to define effective treatment. Unfortunately, during the past decade the development of overly specific techniques and programs with limited rationale for application has led to a narrow and inconsistent approach to cognitive remediation. Despite the work of Luria and colleagues (1963, 1980), only recently have theoretical frameworks been generated for cognitive remediation activities which provide a conception of why interventions at particular levels may be helpful and how improvement might relate to overall cognitive skills. The frameworks which have been developed, such as by Sohlberg and Mateer (1989) and in this chapter, recognize that cognitive deficits do not occur in isolation. Cognitive functioning overall can be viewed in a hierarchical and interdependent fashion. Where in the hierarchy the intervention is to take place is extremely important and the treatment may have a mushrooming effect into other areas. In assuming a cognitive perspective on recovery from head injury, it is apparent that there are automatic and controlled processing mechanisms which likely recover at different rates. During early recovery a focus on automatic processing, such as basic attention, perception, and language skills, is appropriate. Once these skills have recovered (and perhaps *only* if they have recovered), it is appropriate to proceed to controlled processing tasks that are built on a substructure of automatic processing. Within the area of controlled processing, a focus on executive functions may have the greatest impact on overall recovery of cognitive skills. For instance, the ability to adequately organize material (an executive function) will have an impact on the ability to retrieve information from memory as well as on the ability to plan an appropriate course of action. In this chapter basic protocols for remediation of deficits in executive functioning in the areas of verbal reasoning and memory have been presented with an emphasis on developing controlled processing skills that have the greatest likelihood of generalization to everyday functioning. The protocols presented are obviously tentative, and their effectiveness will have to be evaluated objectively with further research. However, if this presentation serves to generate thoughts concerning the application of a cognitive framework to remediation activities and increases the evaluation of those remediation activities, then a purpose has been served.

ACKNOWLEDGEMENT. The authors thank John A. Caldwell, Robert L. Duke, Jr., and Nancy Marshall for reviews and editorial comments on this manuscript.

## APPENDIX A

### Verbal Reasoning Test—Form I

I. Convergent
  1. Fill in the missing word: Sky is to blue as fire is to _____ .
  2. Fill in the missing word: Blueprints is to draftsman as dress is to _____ .
  3. Fill in the missing word: Dwarf is to giant as Rhode Island is to _____ .
  4. What category do **cup, bowl, saucer** belong to? _____
  5. What category do **clubs, tee, cart** belong to? _____
  6. What category do **elevator, escalator, stairs** belong to? _____
  7. What do **rug, tile, wax** have in common? _____
  8. What do **ants, basket, lunch** have in common? _____
  9. What do **vineyard, cellar, bottles** have in common? _____

II. Sequential
  1. Put these four words in order:
     _____ mother _____ great grandfather _____ grandmother _____ son
  2. Put these four words in order:
     _____ eagle _____ sparrow _____ parrot _____ bluejay
  3. List two words in order that belong between **tent** and **skyscraper**.
     _____  _____
  4. List three words in order that follow or come before **elephant**.
     _____  _____  _____
  5. Put the events in order by numbering them 1, 2, 3.
     _____ Anna put the letter in an envelope, addressed it, and put a stamp on it.
     _____ Anna put on her coat and went to mail the letter.
     _____ Anna wrote her daughter a letter.

6. Put the events in order by numbering them 1, 2, 3, 4, 5.
   _____ Realizing that the car would not start, Dan caught a bus.
   _____ Dan woke up late.
   _____ Dan made it to work just in time, and promised himself to get up earlier in the future.
   _____ Jumping into his car, Dan found that it simply would not start.
   _____ Alarmed, Dan showered and dressed quickly, and ran out to his car.

III. Divergent
   1. Name three things that are long and thin_____ _____
      _____.
   2. Name three things that are soft and sticky_____ _____
      _____.
   3. You forget to turn off the running bath water. Describe two outcomes of that situation.
   4. You leave on vacation and don't cancel the newspaper. Describe two outcomes of that situation.
   5. What would you do to find out why yeast is used in breads and pastries?

IV. Complex 1
   1. Circle the one that does not belong: **APPLE ORANGE CELERY PEACH**
   2. Circle the one that does not belong: **ARIZONA CONNECTICUT TEXAS SAN FRANCISCO**
   3. How are **chair** and **bed** similar?
   4. How are **seal** and **whale** similar?
   5. How are **microscope** and **binoculars** similar?
   6. Use the code to figure out the message:

| A | B | C | D | E | F | G | H | I | J | K | L | M | N | O | P | Q | R | S | T | U | V | W | X | Y | Z |
|---|---|---|---|---|---|---|---|---|---|---|---|---|---|---|---|---|---|---|---|---|---|---|---|---|---|
| 1 | 2 | 3 | 4 | 5 | 6 | 7 | 8 | 9 | 10 | 11 | 12 | 13 | 14 | 15 | 16 | 17 | 18 | 19 | 20 | 21 | 22 | 23 | 24 | 25 | 26 |

```
  9  6     25 15 21    8  1  22 5     23 9  20     21 19 5      9  20
  __ __    __ __ __    __ __ __ __    __ __ __     __ __ __     __ __

  16 12 5  1  19 5     1  14 4     14 15 20    20 15     8  21 18 20
  __ __ __ __ __ __    __ __ __    __ __ __    __ __     __ __ __ __
```

7. a. One of the boxes on the right, lettered A, B, C, or D, is related to the ones on the left. Choose the correct one.

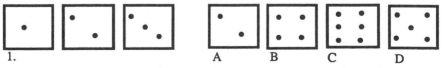

   1.                              A        B        C        D

   b. One of the boxes on the right, lettered A, B, C, or D, is related to the 3 boxes on the left. Choose the correct one.

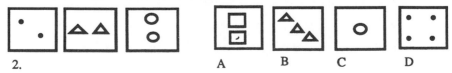

   2.                              A        B        C        D

V. Complex 2
1. You need to send out invitations to a wedding on October 15, but you want the invitations to arrive a month in advance. If they take three days to mail, when should you put them in the mail? _____
2. Dinner needs to bake for 90 minutes. If you put it in the oven at 5:15, when will dinner be ready? _____
3. Read the following paragraph. It describes a person who must send a telegram. In 12 words or less, how should the telegram read?

Paul was unable to make his plane which had just departed for Boston. He had finished his last business meeting in Los Angeles, but his taxi was delayed in heavy traffic on the way to the airport. The next available flight was not leaving until the middle of the night. His schedule had been very hectic for three days and he was quite exhausted. The idea of having to get up in the middle of the night to catch the flight was not very appealing to him. He decided to telegram his wife to tell her that he would take the 8:00am flight the next morning and would arrive at 8:00pm Eastern time. Since he would be arriving at night, he also planned to tell her that she need not pick him up at the airport, as he would take a taxi home.

_____ _____ _____ _____ _____ _____ _____ _____ _____ _____ _____ _____

4. Arrange these pictures in the right order so that they make the most sensible story. Insert four-panel comic here
5. Arrange these pictures in the right order so that they make the most sensible story. Insert nine-panel comic here

Verbal Reasoning Test—Form II

I. Convergent
1. Fill in the missing word: Calf is to cow as cub is to _____.
2. Fill in the missing word: Grape is to vineyard as corn is to _____.
3. Fill in the missing word: Democrat is to donkey as Republican is to _____.
4. To what category do **pie, cake, brownies** belong? _____.
5. To what category do **prescription, appointment, lab coat** belong? _____.
6. To what category do **hen, rooster, Cornish game hen** belong? _____.
7. What do **chills, fever, aches** have in common? _____.
8. What do **dice, cards, risk** have in common? _____.
9. What do **metal, dollar, precious** have in common? _____.

II. Sequential
1. Put these four words in order:
   _____ ocean _____ stream _____ river _____ lake
2. Put these four words in order:
   _____ airplane _____ car _____ bicycle _____ motorcycle
3. List two words in order that belong between **word** and **book**:
   _____ _____
4. List three words in order that follow or come before **watermelon**:
   _____ _____ _____

5. Put the events in order by numbering them 1, 2, 3.
   \_\_\_\_\_ The rain soaked the laundry Helen had put on the line to dry.
   \_\_\_\_\_ As Helen put her laundry on the clothesline she noticed some clouds in the sky.
   \_\_\_\_\_ An hour later the clouds grew thick and it began to rain.
6. Put the events in order by numbering them 1, 2, 3, 4, 5.
   \_\_\_\_\_ She wanted a very special gown, so she went to one of the best stores in town.
   \_\_\_\_\_ The green gown fit her better, but the blue was more suitable.
   \_\_\_\_\_ Alice wanted to buy a new dress for her son's wedding.
   \_\_\_\_\_ Alice could not decide between a blue gown and a green one.
   \_\_\_\_\_ The saleslady promised that the store could easily alter either dress, so Alice bought the blue gown.

III. Divergent
   1. Name three things that are round and hard.
      _____  _____  _____
   2. Name three things that are small and expensive.
      _____  _____  _____
   3. You lock your keys in your car. Describe two outcomes of that situation.
   4. You buy a pair of shoes but decide at home that they do not fit. Describe two outcomes of that situation.
   5. If you misplaced your driver's license what should you do?

IV. Complex 1
   1. Circle the one that does not belong: **Joe Pete Sarah Sam**
   2. Circle the one that does not belong: **pepper oregano sugar dill**
   3. How are **finger** and **toe** similar? _____
   4. How are **cucumbers** and **radishes** similar? _____
   5. How are **amount** and **sum** similar? _____
   6. Use the code to figure out the message:

| A | B | C | D | E | F | G | H | I | J | K | L | M | N | O | P | Q | R | S | T | U | V | W | X | Y | Z |
|---|---|---|---|---|---|---|---|---|---|---|---|---|---|---|---|---|---|---|---|---|---|---|---|---|---|
| + | - | X | ÷ | l | ll | ≡ | Z | $ | \ | \\ | / | ▯ | ▱ | 0 | — | 8 | ◐ | ◑ | ⌣ | ⅋ | ) | ( | U | ∩ | * |

Z l   — / + ∩ ◗   ll 0 0 ⌣ - + / /   / $ \\ l   +   - ⅋ / /

$ ▯   +   x z $ ▯ +   ◗ z 0 —

7. a. One of the boxes on the right, lettered A, B, C, or D, is related to the three boxes on the left. Choose the correct one.

1.                                    A        B        C        D

b. One of the boxes on the right, lettered A, B, C, or D, is related to the 3 boxes on the left. Choose the correct one.

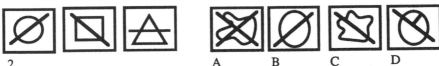

2.                                    A        B        C        D

V. Complex 2

1. If a 12-hour drive is equivalent to a 90-minute flight, how long would it take to drive a distance equivalent to a 2-hour flight? _____

2. An appetizer takes 15 minutes to prepare and 30 minutes to bake. Your guests will arrive at 7:30. What time should you put the appetizer in the oven? _____

3. Read the following paragraph. It describes an author who must write a telegram to his publisher regarding a missed deadline. In 12 words or less, how should the telegram read?

Yesterday there was some excitement here at the cottage. A fire broke out in my study as a result of a faulty electrical heater which shorted. Being all alone in the house at the time, I became somewhat panicky and did a very clumsy fireman's job. I managed to destroy the completed last chapter of the manuscript. Now I must go back to the typewriter and start from scratch. It is quite obvious that I am unable to meet the deadline. I will of course be responsible for the added expenses. Please call me.

____ ____ ____ ____ ____ ____ ____ ____ ____ ____ ____ ____

4. Arrange these pictures in the right order so that they make the most sensible story. Insert four-panel comic here

5. Arrange these pictures in the right order so that they make the most sensible story. Insert eleven-panel comic here

## Verbal Reasoning Test

*Scoring Guidelines*: Most questions have more than one answer. Try to figure out why and how subjects came up with an obscure answer. If it has any rule governed connection with the questions, partial credit should be given. If there is no logic at all, it's a zero score. If the answer makes the best sense possible, it is full credit.

I. *Convergent*—18 total points possible

0, 1, 2 possible points for each item (0 = bad answer, 1 = fair answer, 2 = best answer)

**Sample question:**

What do the following words have in common?

*lift poles mountains*

**Sample answers:**

*outside*—very general connection with words; too general for partial credit; 0 score

*snow skiing*—some relationship with all words but "not necessarily" connected; partial credit; score of 1

*elevation*—this word relates to all three words no matter what the circumstances; full credit; score of 2

II. *Sequential*—12 total possible points

0, 1, 2 possible points for each item (0 = bad answer, 1 = fair answer, 2 = best answer) and 4 possible points for number four.

**Sample question:**

List three words that come before or after: inch _____ _____ _____

**Sample answers:**

    *ing worm two*—no consistency between the three words in relation to inch; all could connect but there is no flow of thought; zero score

    *jungle key monkey*—person is thinking alphabetically with first letter of each word; there is consistency between all four words; partial credit; score of 1

    *foot yard mile*—person is using the meaning of inch; logical thought and the words are correct in all cases; full credit; score of 2

III. *Divergent*—10 total possible points

0, 1, 2 possible points for each item (0 = bad answer, 1 = fair answer, 2 = best answer).

**Sample question:**

Name three things you wear found in boxes _____ _____ _____

**Sample answers:**

    *watches shirts ties*—these things aren't necessarily bought or stored in boxes; 0 score

    *shirts shoes hat*—hats and shoes are good answers but not shirts; partial credit; score of 1

    *shoes hats cuff links*—these are generally bought or stored in boxes; full credit; score of 2

IV. *Complex 1*—12 total possible points

0, 1, 2 possible points for each item (0 = bad answer, 1 = fair answer, 2 = best answer) and 0, 1 possible points for other items that are either right or wrong (see score sheet).

**Sample question:**

How are contaminated and polluted similar?

**Sample answers:**

    *You can't drink either of them:* this is too general and the object need not be liquid; 0 score

    *Both can make you sick:* this probably is true but is too specific; person is thinking too narrowly; partial credit; score of 1

    *Both contain an unwanted substance in it:* this answer is true and identifies similarity of meaning; full credit; score of 2

V. *Complex 2*—10 total possible points

Certain answers in this section can only have one correct answer such as the math questions with possible points of 0, 1. For the telegram questions, four points are scored if the telegram gives *all* the necessary information correctly. 1, 2, or 3 points can be given for near perfect telegrams. A zero score is for meaningless telegrams.

The cartoons are worth two points if pictures are arranged in perfect order. If there is one mistake but it still makes sense, give 1 point. Give zero if cartoon is numbered wrong and does not make sense.

*Calculating final score*

After calculating score on individual sections, add up total from all sections. Total score will be out of 62.

*Note*

Items I. 1-9, II. 1-4, III. 1-4, IV. 1-5, and V. 1-2 are reprinted with permission from Holloran and Bressler (1983). Items II. 5-6, and V. 3 (Form I) are reprinted with permission from Carter *et al*. (1984). Item V. 3 (Form II) is reprinted with permission from Ben-Yishay *et al*. (1980). Item IV. 7 (Form II) is reprinted with permission from Brown *et al*. (1982). Copyright permission to reproduce the comics in items V. 4-5 is pending. Copies of the comics are available upon request from the authors.

## REFERENCES

Adamovich, B. B., Henderson, J. A., & Auerbach, S. (1985). *Cognitive rehabilitation of closed head injured patients: A diagnostic approach*. San Diego: College-Hill.

Baddeley, A. (1987). *Working memory*. New York: Oxford University Press.

Baddeley, A., & Hitch, G. J. (1974). Working memory. In G. Bower (Ed.), *Recent advances in learning and motivation* (Vol. 18). New York: Academic Press.

Baddeley, A., Harris, J., Sunderland, A., Watts, K. P., & Wilson, B. A. (1987). Closed head injury and memory. In H. S. Levin, J. Grafman, & H. M. Eisenberg (Eds.), *Neurobehavioral recovery from head injury* (pp. 295–317). New York: Oxford University Press.

Ben-Yishay, Y., & Diller, L. (1983a). Cognitive deficits. In E. A. Griffith, M. Bond, & J. Miller (Eds.), *Rehabilitation of the head injured adult* (pp. 167–183). Philadelphia: Davis.

Ben-Yishay, Y., & Diller, L. (1983b). Cognitive deficits. In E. A. Griffith, M. Bond, & J. Miller (Eds.), *Rehabilitation of the head injured adult* (pp. 367–380). Philadelphia: Davis.

Ben-Yishay, Y., Lakin, P., Ross, B., Rattok, J., Cohen, J., & Diller, L. (1980). A modular approach to training (verbal) abstract reasoning in traumatic head-injured patients: Revised procedures. In Y. Ben-Yishay (Ed.), *Working approaches to remediation of cognitive deficits in brain damaged*. New York University Monographs. New York: New York University.

Ben-Yishay, Y., Rattok, J., Lakin, P., Piasetsky, E. B., Ross, B., Silver, S., Zide, E., & Ezrachi, O. (1985). Neuropsychologic rehabilitation: Quest for a holistic approach. *Seminars in Neurology*, *5*, 252–259.

Ben-Zur, H. (1989). Automatic and directed search processes in solving simple semantic-memory problems. *Memory and Cognition*, *17*, 617–626.

Bolger, J. P. (1982). Cognitive retraining: A developmental approach. *Clinical Neuropsychology*, *4*, 66–70.

Brown, L., Sherbenou, R. J., & Johnsen, S. K. (1982). *Test of nonverbal intelligence (TONI)*. Austin: Pro-Ed.

Butler, R. W., & Namerow, N. S. (1988). Cognitive retraining in brain-injury rehabilitation: A critical review. *Journal of Neurological Rehabilitation*, *2*, B1–B5.

Carter, L. T., Caruso, J. L., & Languirard, M. A. (1984). *The thinking skills workbook*. Springfield, IL: Thomas.

Carver, C. S., & Scheier, M. F. (1983). A control-theory approach to human behavior, and implications for problems in self-management. *Advances in cognitive-behavioral research and therapy*. New York: Academic Press.

Craine, J. F. (1982). Principles of cognitive rehabilitation. In L. E. Trexler (Ed.), *Cognitive rehabilitation: Conceptualization and intervention* (pp. 83–97). New York: Plenum Press.

Denney, N. W. (1988). Everyday problem solving. *Gerontology Review*, *1*, 67–74.

Duke, L. W., Haley, W. E., & Bergquist, T. F. (1991). Cognitive/behavioral interventions for age-related memory impairment. In P. A. Wisocki (Ed.), *Handbook of clinical behavior therapy with the elderly patient*. New York: Plenum Press.

Flores d'Arcais, G.B. (1988). Automatic processes in language comprehension. In G. Denes (Ed.), *Perspectives on cognitive neuropsychology* (pp. 91–114). Hillsdale, NJ: Erlbaum.

Gazzaniga, M. S. (1984). Advances in cognitive neurosciences: The problem of information storage in the human brain. In G. Lynch, J. L. McGaugh, & N. M. Weinberger (Eds.), *Neurobiology of learning and memory* (pp. 78–88). New York: Guilford Press.

Glisky, E. L., & Schacter, D. L. (1986). Remediation of organic memory disorders: Current status and future prospects. *Journal of Head Trauma Rehabilitation, 1,* 54–63.

Goldstein, F. C., & Levin, H. S. (1987). Disorders of reasoning and problem-solving ability. In M. J. Meier, A. L. Benton, & L. Diller (Eds.), *Neuropsychological rehabilitation* (pp. 327–354). New York: Guilford Press.

Goldstein, F. C., & Levin, H. S. (1988). Automatic processing of frequency information in survivors of severe closed injury. In H. A. Whitaker (Ed.), *Neuropsychological studies of nonfocal brain damage: Dementia and trauma.* Berlin: Springer-Verlag.

Goldstein, G. (1979). Methodological and theoretical issues in neuropsychological assessment. *Journal of Behavioral Assessment, 1,* 23–41.

Gouvier, D., Webster, J. S., & Blanton, P. D. (1986). Cognitive retraining with brain-damaged patients. In D. Wedding, A. M. Horton, Jr., & J. Webster (Eds.), *The neuropsychology handbook: Behavioral and clinical perspectives* (pp. 278–324). Berlin: Springer-Verlag.

Grafman, J. (1984). Memory assessment and remediation in brain-injured patients: From theory to practice. In B. A. Edelstein & E. T. Couture (Eds.), *Behavioral assessment and rehabilitation of the traumatically brain-damaged* (pp. 151–188). New York: Plenum Press.

Gronwall, D. (1987). Advances in the assessment of attention and information processing after head injury. In H. S. Levin, J. Grafman, & H. N. Eisenberg (Eds.), *Neurobehavioral recovery from head injury* (pp. 355–371). New York: Oxford University Press.

Gross, Y. (1982). A conceptual framework for interventive cognitive neuropsychology. In L. E. Trexler (Ed.), *Cognitive rehabilitation: Conceptualization and intervention* (pp. 99–113). New York: Plenum Press.

Harris, J. E. (1984). Remembering to do things: A forgotten topic. In J. E. Harris & P. E. Morris (Eds.), *Everyday memory, actions, and absent-mindedness* (pp. 71–92). New York: Academic Press.

Hasher, L., & Zacks, R. T. (1979). Automatic and effortful processes in memory. *Journal of Experimental Psychology, 108,* 356–388.

Hasher, L., & Zacks, R. T. (1984). Automatic processing of fundamental information: The case of frequency of occurrence. *American Psychologist, 39,* 1372–1388.

Hirst, W. (1982). The amnesic syndrome: Descriptions and explanations. *Psychological Bulletin, 91,* 435–460.

Hirst, W., & Volpe, B. T. (1988). Memory strategies with brain damage. *Brain and Cognition, 8,* 379–408.

Holloran, S. M., & Bressler, E. J. (1983). *Cognitive reorganization: A stimulus handbook.* Austin, TX: Pro-ed.

Humphreys, M. S., Bain, J. D., & Pike, R. (1989). Different ways to cue a coherent memory system: A theory for episodic, semantic, and procedural tasks. *Psychological Review, 96,* 208–233.

Johnson, M. K. (1977). What is being counted nonetheless? In I. M. Birnbaum & E. S. Parker (Eds.), *Alcohol and human memory* (pp. 43–58). Hillsdale, NJ: Erlbaum.

Johnson, M. K. (1983). A multiple-entry, modular memory system. In G.H. Bower (Ed.), *The psychology of learning and motivation: Advances in research theory* (Vol. 17, pp. 81–124). New York: Academic Press.

Kendall, P. C., & Bemis, K. M. (1983). Thought and action in psychotherapy: The cognitive-behavioral approaches. In M. Herson, A. E. Kazdin, & A. S. Bellack (Eds.), *The clinical psychology handbook* (pp. 565–592). New York: Pergamon Press.

Labouvie-Vief, C., & Gonda, J. N. (1976). Cognitive strategy training and intellectual performance in the elderly. *Journal of Gerontology, 31,* 327–332.

Levin, H. S., Goldstein, F. C., High, W., Jr., & Williams, D. (1988). Automatic and effortful processing after severe closed head injury. *Brain & Cognition, 7,* 283–297.

Lezak, M. D. (1983). *Neuropsychological assessment.* New York: Oxford University Press.

Luria, A. R. (1963). *Restoration of function after brain injury.* New York: Macmillan Co.

Luria, A. R. (1980). *Higher cortical functions in man.* New York: Basic Books.

Malec, J. (1984). Training the brain-injured client in behavioral self-management skills. In B. A. Edelstein & E. T. Couture (Eds.), *Behavioral assessment and rehabilitation of the traumatically brain damaged* (pp. 121–150). New York: Plenum Press.

Marshall, J. F. (1984). Brain function: Neural adaptations and recovery from injury. *Annual Review of Psychology, 35,* 277–308.

Mateer, C. A., & Sohlberg, M. M. (1988). A paradigm shift in memory rehabilitation. In H. A. Whitaker (Ed.), *Neuropsychological studies of nonfocal brain damage* (pp. 202–225). Berlin: Springer-Verlag.

Meichenbaum, D. (1974). Self-instructional strategy training: A cognitive prosthesis for the aged. *Human Development*, *17*, 273–280.

Meichenbaum, D. (1977). *Cognitive-behavior modification: An integrative approach*. New York: Plenum Press.

Miller, E. (1980). Psychological intervention in the management and rehabilitation of neuropsychological impairment. *Behavioral Research & Therapy*, *18*, 527–535.

Moffat, N. (1984). Strategies of memory therapy. In B. Wilson & N. Moffatt (Eds.), *Clinical management of memory problems*. London: Aspen.

Morris, P. E. (1978). Sense and nonsense in traditional mnemonics. In M. M. Gruneberg, P. E. Morris, & R. N. Sykes (Eds.), *Practical aspects of memory* (pp. 155–163). New York: Academic Press.

Najenson, T., Rahmani, L., Elazar, B., & Auerbach, S. (1984). An elementary cognitive assessment and treatment of the craniocerebrally injured patient. In B. A. Edelstein & E. T. Couture (Eds.), *Behavioral assessment and rehabilitation of the traumatically brain-damaged* (pp. 313–338). New York: Plenum Press.

Norman, D. A. (1981). Categorization of action slips. *Psychology Review*, *88*, 1–15.

Norman, D. A., & Shallice, T. (1980). *Attention to action. Willed and automatic control of behavior*. University of California, San Diego CHIP Report 99.

Parente, R., & Anderson-Parente, J. K. (1989). Retraining memory: Theory and application. *Journal of Head Trauma Rehabilitation*, *4*, 55–65.

Piasetsky, E. B. (1982). The relevance of brain–behavior relationships for rehabilitation. In L. E. Trexler (Ed.), *Cognitive rehabilitation: Conceptualization and intervention* (pp. 115–130). New York: Plenum Press.

Poon, L. W. (1980). A systems approach for the assessment and treatment of memory problems. In J. M. Ferguson & C. B. Taylor (Eds.), *The comprehensive handbook of behavioral medicine* (pp. 191–212). New York: Spectrum.

Posner, M. I. (1984). Selective attention and the storage of information. In G. Lynch, J. L. McGaugh, & N. M. Weinberger (Eds.), *Neurobiology of learning and memory* (pp. 89–101). New York: Guilford Press.

Prigatano, G. P. (1987). Neuropsychological rehabilitation after brain injury: Some further reflections. In J. M. Williams & C. J. Long (Eds.), *The rehabilitation of cognitive disabilities* (pp. 29–42). New York: Plenum Press.

Prigatano, G. P., Fordyce, D. J., Zeiner, H. K., Roueche, J. R., Pepping, M., & Wood, B. C. (1986). The outcome of neuropsychological rehabilitation efforts. In G. P. Prigatano (Ed.), *Neuropsychological rehabilitation after brain injury* (pp. 119–133). Baltimore: Johns Hopkins University Press.

Reason, J. T. (1984). Absent-mindedness and cognitive control. In J. E. Harris & P. E. Morris (Eds.), *Everyday memory, actions, and absent-mindedness* (pp. 113–132). New York: Academic Press.

Rimm, D.C., & Masters, J. C. (1974). *Behavior therapy: Techniques and empirical findings*. New York: Academic Press.

Rimmele, C. T., & Hester, R. K. (1987). Cognitive rehabilitation after traumatic head injury. *Archives of Neuropsychology*, *2*, 353–384.

Roth, D. L., & Tucker, D. M. (1986). Neural systems in the emotional control of information processing. In R. E. Ingram (Ed.), *Information processing approaches to clinical psychology* (pp. 77–94). New York: Academic Press.

Rothi, L. J., & Horner, J. (1983). Restitution and substitution: Two theories of recovery with application to neurobehavioral treatment. *Journal of Clinical Neuropsychology*, *5*, 73–81.

Rowntree, D. (1970). *Learn how to study*. London: MacDonald.

Sandford, J. A., & Browne, R. J. (1988). *Captain's Log Cognitive Training System*. Richmond, VA: Network Services.

Schneider, W. (1985). Toward a model of attention and the development of automaticity. In M. Posner & O. S. Marin (Eds.), *Attention and performance XI* (pp. 475–492). Hillsdale, NJ: Erlbaum.

Semenza, C., Bisiacchi, P., & Rosenthal, V. (1988). A function for cognitive neuropsychology. In G. Denes, C. Semenza, & P. Bisiacchi (Eds.), *Perspectives on cognitive neuropsychology* (pp. 3–30). Hillsdale, NJ: Erlbaum.

Shallice, T. (1982). Specific impairments in planning. In D. E. Broadbent & L. Weiskrantz (Eds.), *The neuropsychology of cognitive function* (pp. 199–209). London: The Royal Society.

Shiffrin, R. M., & Schneider, W. (1977). Controlled and automatic human information processing: II. Perceptual learning, automatic attending, and a general theory. *Psychology Review*, *84*, 127–190.

Skinner, B. F., & Vaughn, M. E. (1983). *Enjoy old age: A program of self-management*. New York: Norton.

Smith, J. (1986). *Cognitive rehabilitation*. Dimondale, MI: Hartley Courseware.

Sohlberg, M. M., & Mateer, C. A. (1986). *Attention process training (APT)*. Puyallup, WA: Association for Neuropsychological Research and Development.

Sohlberg, M. M., & Mateer, C. A. (1987). Effectiveness of an attention training program. *Journal of Clinical & Experimental Neuropsychology*, *9*, 117–130.

Sohlberg, M. M., & Mateer, C. A. (1989). *Introduction to cognitive rehabilitation: Theory and practice*. New York: Guilford Press.

Szekeres, S. F., Ylvisaker, M., & Holland, A. L. (1985). Cognitive rehabilitation therapy: A framework for intervention. In M. Ylvisaker (Ed.), *Head injury rehabilitation: Children and adolescents* (pp. 219–246). San Diego: College-Hill.

Trexler, L. E. (Ed.). (1982). *Cognitive rehabilitation: Conceptualization and intervention*. New York: Plenum Press.

Tulving, E. (1983). *Elements of episodic memory*. London: Oxford University Press (Clarendon).

Tulving, E. (1987). Memory experiments: A strategy for research. In H. S. Levin, J. Graffman, & H. M. Eisenberg (Eds.), *Neurobehavioral recovery from head injury* (pp. 341–351). New York: Oxford University Press.

Tweedy, J. R., & Vakil, E. (1988). Evaluating evidence for automaticity in frequency of occurrence judgments: A bias for bias? *Journal of Clinical & Experimental Neuropsychology*, *10*, 664–674.

Williams, J. M. (1987). The role of retraining in comprehensive rehabilitation. In J. M. Williams & C. J. Long (Eds.), *The rehabilitation of cognitive disabilities* (pp. 43–56). New York: Plenum Press.

Wood, R. L. (1986). Rehabilitation of patients with disorders of attention. *Journal of Head Trauma Rehabilitation*, *1*, 43–53.

# 11

# Memory Rehabilitation

## GERALD GOLDSTEIN

I would first like to propose a distinction between memory rehabilitation and recovery from organic memory disorders. The literature on recovery is well summarized by O'Connor and Cermak (1987) and will not be re-reviewed here. The material presented here will focus on memory rehabilitation. Efforts at designing, applying, and evaluating various memory rehabilitation methods have become a growth industry in recent years and merit separate discussion. Furthermore, I would propose the position that memory rehabilitation cannot be unequivocally evaluated while natural recovery is or is likely to be ongoing. Such evaluations may only confirm the view of our more cynical critics that rehabilitation is what one does while the patient gets better by herself or himself. It may actually be the case that systematic rehabilitation efforts potentiate natural recovery, but there is an obvious indeterminacy problem here from the standpoint of scientific evaluation. Thus, the ideal subject for rehabilitation research is a patient with a stable but nonprogressive condition.

The medical definition of rehabilitation involves restoration of function following illness or injury to a normal or near-normal state. However, the definition contained in a psychiatric dictionary (Hinsie & Campbell, 1960) begins with the following sentence: "The use of all forms of physical medicine in conjunction with psychosocial adjustment and vocational retraining in an attempt to achieve maximal function and adjustment, and to prepare the patient physically, mentally, socially, and vocationally for the fullest possible life compatible with his abilities and disabilities" (p. 639). It would appear that the rehabilitation of patients with substantial structural brain damage would be more compatible with the psychiatric than with the general medical definition. Restoration to a normal or near-normal state is rarely seen among seriously brain-damaged patients, but the efforts described in the psychiatric definition may lead to an improved quality of life that is optimal for the patients' abilities and disabilities. We would be inclined to accept this psychiatric definition as the more appropriate one for memory rehabilitation. Thus, rehabilitation is

GERALD GOLDSTEIN • VA Medical Center, Pittsburgh, Pennsylvania 15206.

*HANDBOOK OF HEAD TRAUMA: Acute Care to Recovery*, edited by Charles J. Long and Leslie K. Ross. Plenum Press, New York, 1992.

conceptualized as a worthwhile effort rather than as perfect or near-perfect attainment of a goal.

Memory disorders associated with different kinds of brain damage are of different types, varying qualitatively and quantitatively (Butters, 1984). Rehabilitation strategies may be oriented toward developing different programs for the different types of disorder or toward the development of a generic system that is effective regardless of type of disorder. One method of achieving the latter alternative would consist of developing a system that is so basic that it can be applied effectively to patients with global and extremely severe amnesia. The difficulty with that approach is that while it may be effective, it may not be optimal for less impaired patients since their capabilities for restoration of function may be greater than what is required by the program. The achievement of maximal restoration of function would appear to require development of programs that relate to the characteristics of the memory disorder, with regard to both pattern and level. In that sense, we would view memory rehabilitation as similar to rehabilitation of aphasia, since aphasia is such a diverse condition that it would be inconceivable that there could be one treatment method for it that may be applied regardless of type or severity.

Memory rehabilitation or training has historical roots in the writings of the mnemonists: those individuals who could perform such astounding feats of memory that their demonstrations had entertainment value. There have also been books written and schools established to teach normal people to improve their memories (Lorayne & Lucas, 1974). While the mnemonists have described methods that have been applied to rehabilitation of brain-damaged patients, notably those utilizing visual imagery, those methods cannot be productively applied to brain-damaged patients without some consideration being given to the neuropsychological status of those patients. Even the venerable method of loci, that O'Connor and Cermak (1987) attribute to the ancient Greek poet Simonides, has been called into service for rehabilitation of brain-damaged patients (Wilson, 1987). While the methods of the mnemonists certainly provide valuable tools for rehabilitation of memory, it should be understood that any particular method is no more likely to be effective with all patients than any particular method of language therapy is likely to be effective for all aphasic patients. For example, methods based upon visual imagery are unlikely to be effective with patients who have neurological deficits that compromise imagery abilities.

For practical purposes, we have found it useful to distinguish among three types of memory impairment. The first type is the patient with modality-specific amnesia. Such cases are relatively rare but have been reported in the literature. The condition is generally seen in patients with unilateral brain damage. In general terms, the memory disorder only involves either verbal or nonverbal content. Thus, the patient may be able to remember names, but not faces or locations, or vice versa. The widely cited study of Gasparrini and Satz (1979) describes a treatment program for left hemisphere stroke patients with modality-specific memory difficulties. The strategy in such methods is generally that of using an intact modality to support an impaired modality. The second type, which is less rarely seen, is the patient with severe and permanent amnesia. Alcoholic Korsakoff's syndrome is the most well-known subtype of this group, but some patients with severe trauma, aneurysms of the anterior communicating artery, cerebral infections, or cerebral anoxia may also develop very severe chronic amnesia. Patients with progressive dementias such as Alzheimer's disease also become very amnesic, but here the amnesia is combined with communicative and intellectual disorders, making the rehabilitation situation far more complex.

The third type is seen most frequently among patients with histories of severe closed head injury. Levin, Benton, and Grossman (1982) have reported that a substantial proportion of these patients have persistent memory difficulties that go beyond the period of posttraumatic amnesia. There is an extensive research literature devoted to description of the characteristics of this memory disorder, but here we will only attempt to characterize it clinically. These patients cover a range of severity of amnesia but typically do not have the dense, global amnesia of the Korsakoff patient. More typically, we see a picture that can probably be better described in terms of memory difficulties than as an amnesia. Often these patients have a combined attention and memory disorder such that failure to learn new information may relate to concentration difficulties experienced when the material is initially presented or taught. However, we have seen many patients with no evidence of significant attentional dysfunction who nevertheless had significant difficulties with new learning. As a general descriptive term, *forgetfulness* is probably more appropriate than *amnesia*. Clinical experience with these patients often teaches us that they forget to keep appointments or arrive for them at the wrong time. While they may be working or in school, they have difficulties in functioning because they forget instructions or do not retain as much of what was learned in class as the non-head-injured student. In general, one can say that their capacity to remember, or to encode, store, and retrieve new information, is not as efficient as it was prior to brain injury.

This distinction among three kinds of memory disorder has proven to be useful to my colleagues and myself in rehabilitation planning. In the case of the patient with a modality-specific disorder, the implication is clear that one might attempt to exploit the resources of the preserved modality. In the case of the severely and globally amnesic patient, one would attempt to find some aspect of memory that is preserved, perhaps in the manner that one would attempt to find a channel of communication with the severely aphasic patient. Forgetful head injury patients may benefit most from educational approaches that attempt to teach efficient methods of learning new information. I believe that the methods of the mnemonists are of most use in this latter case.

## THE MATTER OF REHABILITATION GOALS

It is particularly important to consider the goals of memory training for many reasons. Training is generally lengthy, taxing on the patient, and could be costly. The experience of loss of memory is generally frightening and extremely distressing to the patient and his or her family and associates. Therefore, it becomes particularly important to formulate reasonable goals that on the one hand don't promise more than can be delivered and on the other, don't unnecessarily reflect an attitude of gloomy pessimism. I would like to propose sets of what I would consider to be reasonable goals for densely amnesic and for forgetful patients, as described above.

The densely amnesic or Korsakoff-type patient is typically not involved in active rehabilitation programs. These patients are typically found in nursing homes or in veterans or state hospitals that care for chronically mentally ill patients. Because of the severity of the memory disorder, these patients typically require custodial care, mainly to avoid wandering. They are generally ambulatory and may perform routine work assignments at their institution. Medication is usually quite limited, but alcoholic Korsakoff patients are typically maintained on thiamine. The pathologies upon which these disorders are based are generally irreversible, and there is no spontaneous recovery from the amnesic component of Korsakoff's syndrome. In the past, goals for these patients have usually involved optimal adjustment to an institutional setting and prevention of further pathology. In the case of the alcoholic Korsakoff's patient, abstinence from alcohol, adequate nutrition, and supplemental thiamine are major considerations. However, research with these patients has shown that there is preservation of certain aspects of memory. Following several reformulations of the nature of the pattern of impaired and preserved abilities, investigators appear to have accepted the view that these patients have relatively preserved implicit memory or knowledge. That is, they can learn without awareness that they are learning. Numerous demonstrations have been made indicating that densely amnesic patients can produce objective evidence of learning new skills, but without any awareness that the learning is taking place. The evidence for this phenomenon is reviewed in several places (e.g., Schacter, 1990) and will not be repeated here. The only point we would make here is that if very amnesic patients can acquire implicit knowledge, then that suggests a rehabilitation goal. That is, the learning capabilities that these patients have demonstrated in the laboratory may be utilized to achieve rehabilitation-related ends. We will shortly illustrate this point in a description of one of our own studies. Beyond that, the capability of severely amnesic patients to acquire skills based upon simple conditioning may provide opportunities for prosthetic or "smart technology" approaches to the rehabilitation of these patients. Thus, any suggestion that one can restore normal or near-normal memory to Korsakoff-type patients through memory training techniques would be an overly optimistic goal and would indeed suggest quackery. However, the pessimism that has traditionally surrounded this disorder may have been somewhat alleviated by the identification of an at least partially preserved memory system.

In the case of the head-injured patient with persistent forgetfulness, the situation is quite different. As indicated above, these patients are frequently not globally amnesic, but are inefficient with regard to acquiring and retaining information. Such a condition might lead to the inference that improvements might be made by educating patients to learn more efficiently. The methods taught might be viewed as restoring, perhaps to only a limited extent, the learning capabilities available to an individual with an intact brain. Thus, various mnemonic devices, such as those involving imagery, can possibly be taught to head-injured patients with that goal. Possibly, the devices used by the mnemonists to perform extraordinary feats of memory can be used by brain-injured people to support more conventional memory functions. Indeed, many of the published studies concerning memory training for brain-damaged patients did just that. While Simonides used the method of loci to perform the feat of identifying a number of unrecognizable bodies crushed to death by a building cave-in, brain-damaged patients may be able to use the same method to achieve more modest goals.

Educational goals generally have two components. One has to do with the extent to which the student learned what was taught, and is usually evaluated with a final examination or some other assessment procedure that occurs immediately following the teaching sessions. The second component involves the extent to which the material taught is applied outside of the learning situation. This latter component is commonly known as transfer of learning or generalization. Since rehabilitation means restoration of function, one would think that generalization is an absolute necessity for concluding that a rehabilitation goal has been achieved. After all, it is of little consequence if the athlete's injured knee shows improved function in the physical therapy clinic but not on the football field. In the case of cognitive rehabilitation, the problem becomes more complex because of several considerations. First, the matter of generalization is not of major consequence when prosthetic or "smart technology" approaches are used. The function in question should be performed at goal level as long as the prosthetic is present. In the case of the work we did with our Korsakoff-type patients, there was no anticipation of generalization since the goal was only that of having the patients learn specifically what was taught. When generalization is proposed as a goal, we should take note of a distinction made by Seron (1987) among three types of transfer of learning. In the first type, there is transfer to nontrained, identical structural responses. In the second type, there is transfer to different behaviors; and, in the third type, there is transfer to daily life situations. Thus, with regard to memory training, one may set as goals the following kinds of alternatives: (1) teaching a patient to recall a shopping list of particular items will increase learning efficiency on subsequent lists containing different items, (2) teaching a patient to recall a shopping list of particular items will increase ability to recall locations or names of new acquaintances, and (3) teaching a patient to recall a shopping list of particular items will decrease forgetting to purchase items, purchasing the wrong items, or other memory-related errors that occur when the patient actually goes shopping. The failure to meet any of these criteria, even though the patient learns the specific materials taught, would suggest absence of transfer of any sort (i.e., learning without generalization). While most of us might select the third alternative as the most desirable one, the other alternatives could be of some clinical value in certain situations. For example, there may be some particular need for a patient to learn some specific information. If it is learned, one's goal may be achieved with no transfer of learning at all.

## TWO RESEARCH STUDIES

The following material provides summaries of two studies accomplished in our laboratory. Both studies are published, and the reader may refer to the original articles for details (Goldstein & Malec, 1989; Goldstein, McCue, Turner, Spanier, Malec, & Shelly, 1988). The major points to be made here are that memory training methods can be quite diverse, depending upon the condition of the patient, and that different goals may be appropriate for different kinds of patients.

The first study was an evaluation of a memory training program for six patients with Korsakoff or Korsakoff-type amnesias. These patients were hospitalized at a Veterans Administration facility on a long-term care basis primarily because of the severity of their amnesias. They averaged 55 years in age and had a mean WAIS IQ of 86. Their mean Wechsler Memory Scale Memory Quotient (MQ) was 70.5, with none of them having an MQ higher than 84. Thus, they all demonstrated severe memory impairment on an absolute basis or relative to their general level of intelligence. They were disoriented with regard to time and place, and had little if any accurate recall of recent events.

The essential idea we had about memory training for these patients was that despite their severe, global amnesias, if they in fact had relatively intact implicit memory systems, they might be able to learn new information, albeit without awareness. If that were the case, then the information taught could be of adaptive significance because it might involve orientation, safety, and related matters. For example, a densely amnesic patient could be taught the name of his or her medicine, which the patient would then have available in emergency situations. After preliminary explorations of how to teach this material, we arrived at a rote rehearsal method utilizing a multiple baseline design.

The procedure began by selection of a set of no more than five items. An item could be the name of a person, the name of a place or object, a date, or a location. Most commonly, we used the doctor's and head nurse's name and the name of the hospital. It was first determined through a series of baseline probes that the patient did not have the information available. We then started teaching the first item on the list. The training was conducted at daily sessions during which the patient was probed on all of the items on the list but was asked to repeat the trained item twenty times after being told the correct response. For example, the patient might be told that his doctor's name was Dr. Harris. Immediately after that, the trainer would ask, "What is your doctor's name?" and the patient would answer. The question and answer were repeated twenty times at each daily session. Training on an item was discontinued when the patient gave the correct response during the probe period on six out of seven consecutive days. We discontinued training the item after ten days, regardless of whether or not the patient met criterion. In either event, training on a new item was started. Thus, the design was of the multiple baseline across items type in which all items were probed at each session but only one item was trained.

Utilizing this procedure, all six patients learned and retained at least some of the items. When we had the opportunity to do follow-ups, we found that some patients retained the learned items for up to a month following training. Further follow-up was not feasible and so retention time might have been even longer. We did not inquire systematically, but the impression was clear that the learning was taking place without awareness, with the patients having no recollection of previous sessions at the current one. Furthermore, for material other than what was trained, they remained as amnesic and disoriented as they were prior to training.

With regard to the matter of goals, hopeful expectations were met in this case. Patients learned and retained the materials taught, despite the severity of their memory disorders. Had we formulated unrealistic goals for these patients, we would have been disappointed and perhaps discouraged from going further. On the other hand, had we been unduly pessimistic, we would not have accomplished what we did. We would add that this project might not have been attempted were it not for the basic research done with Korsakoff and other severely amnesic patients that demonstrated the existence of a preserved memory system. It may also be noted that the view that rote rehearsal or repetition is not an effective or efficient method of memory training is not warranted. In the case of these patients, repetition worked when our preliminary explorations using imagery and related mnemonics in memory training with similar patients did not yield comparably encouraging findings.

The second study was accomplished with ten young patients with histories of closed head injury. Their average age was 27 years, and they were all past the posttraumatic period. Their number of months postinjury ranged from 12 to 137. They all had serious head injuries with neurosurgical or radiological evidence of brain damage. Aside from the history of closed head injury, patients were selected for the study because of persistence of memory difficulties. Despite the average level of general intelligence in this group (mean IQ = 97), they all complained of memory dysfunction and the group as a whole had a mean MQ of 82.

Our expectation for these patients was that, although they had significant memory dysfunction, they might benefit from training in which the goal was to teach them some systematic, effective methods of learning new information. Two programs were conducted, one involving free recall of lengthy lists of nouns and the other associating names with faces. For the list learning program we used the ridiculously imaged-story technique that was shown in two studies (Kovner, Mattis, & Goldmeier, 1983; Kovner, Mattis, & Pass, 1985) to dramatically promote free recall in very amnesic patients. Our adaptation of the technique involved the following steps. Patients received a pretraining evaluation during which their free recall capacity was tested using the Buschke (1973) selective reminding technique. This procedure involves having the subject recite a list of words over a series of trials. The subject is reminded of missed words after each trial. Free recall and free recall with selective reminding levels were used as baselines against which to evaluate the efficacy of the program. The ridiculously imaged-story technique consists of embedding the word list into a bizarre humorous story. For example, if the first three words of the list were *shirt*, *palace*, and *grass*, the first sentence of the story might be: "The magic shirt sought by the prince was located in a palace made of grass." We presented the stories on a computer screen with the to-be-learned words printed in bold type. Subjects were oriented to the story method and were taken through a story containing a 20-word list at each session. The training itself involved three repetitions of the story at each session accompanied by providing cues consisting of the element of the story in which the word appeared (e.g., something about a prince) and then by providing an appropriate category (e.g., an article of clothing). A free recall trial was held at the end of this procedure, and the number of words correctly recalled was used as the score for the session. Since we wanted to build generalization into the program, following several sessions with the same lists, a different list and different story were given at each session. In order to encourage patients to use the method spontaneously, they were asked to bring in their own lists and stories. By the end of the training, all of the material used consisted of lists and stories provided by the patients. Following pretraining evaluation, the program consisted of fifteen triweekly sessions.

The face–name association training was done in conjunction with the list learning. The goal of the program was to enhance the ability of subjects to associate names with photographs of unfamiliar people's faces. A visual imagery technique borrowed from Lorayne and Lucas (1974) and Moffat (1984) was used, which is described as formation of a link in the form of an image made between a distinctive feature of the face and the name.

Following obtaining baseline data, the training initially consisted of encouraging subjects to assign a name to each face based upon some distinctive characteristic of the face. For example, someone with a white, pearly complexion could be named Pearl, or someone with a great deal of facial hair could be called Harry. Of course, we do not assign names of our choice to our acquaintances, and so the training gradually shifted to trainer-provided names, and the subject had the more difficult task of forming an association between a given name and face. As the training proceeded, we noted that subjects used two apparently effective strategies. One was linking a feature of the face with the name, as illustrated above, and the other was linking the picture with a person familiar to the subject, either a celebrity or a personal acquaintance. For example, if the name was John, the subject might indicate that the man in the photograph looked like John Wayne. Alternatively, the subject may have indicated that the man in the photograph looked like a friend of his in high school, whose name was John. During training, a great deal of coaching was done to get the subject to provide reasons for the assignments. For example, if the subject indicated that the face looked like a friend in high school, the trainer would inquire about what characteristics of the face reminded him of his friend. The subject might have then gone on to say that the person in the photograph had red hair and big ears, and so did his friend.

In order to encourage generalization, a different set of faces was used at each training session. The proportion of subject-provided to trainer-provided names was changed in the direction of increasing the percentage of trainer-provided names. By the last sessions, all names were trainer-provided. Cuing was accomplished during training, consisting of giving the subjects' own associations to the face (e.g., "You said he had red hair and big ears"). The score for each session was the number of photographs correctly named following cuing.

The results for the list learning training are presented in Figure 11.1. The mean recall score went as high as 17.5 out of 20 words during training. It was particularly interesting to note that the mean scores went up during the generalization trials since the lists and stories were changed at each of these trials. We appear to have accomplished transfer of learning of the first type, but we don't know whether this form of training helped our subjects learn types of material other than word lists, nor do we know whether it helped them in remembering in their everyday lives.

The results for the face–name learning are not as clear-cut since subjects tended to produce high scores from the beginning of training, correctly naming an average of 6 to 7 of the 8 faces over trials. It is interesting to note, however, that they maintained a stable performance level despite the fact that the proportion of examiner-provided names continuously increased. Further analysis of the learning data also indicated that there was a decrease in trials needed to learn a complete list of eight names. Prior to training, it took an average of 5.9 trials to learn a complete set of names, while after training, using a different set of photographs, it took an average of 3 trials. This difference was statistically significant ($t(9) = 3.27$, $p < .01$). We viewed this improvement in learning efficiency as

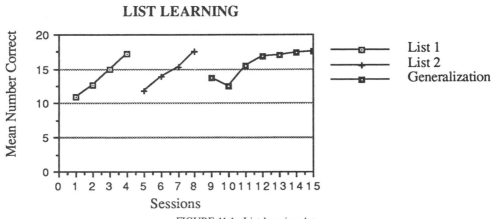

FIGURE 11.1. List learning data.

probably being the most important finding. One often doesn't learn the name of a new acquaintance after the first introduction, but normally does so after a few meetings. Perhaps we helped our subjects in normalizing the number of meetings needed before a name is learned and retained.

## CONCLUSIONS

We have reviewed these two studies primarily for making two points. First, different types of training are appropriate for different types of memory disorder. Application of an inappropriate training either may be too elementary for the patient and produce little functional change, even if technically successful, or may be too complex for the patient and lead to disappointing failure. Admittedly, finding out what is appropriate and inappropriate may have to be determined on a trial-and-error basis, but we have suggested that recourse to the scientific literature on neuropsychological aspects of memory can be quite helpful. The second, but highly related, point is that rehabilitation goals can be set most realistically when the neuropsychological situation of the patient is well understood. The neurology and the memory structure of patients with Korsakoff's syndrome is quite different from what is the case for closed head injury patients. We have tried to show that rehabilitation goals can be reasonably successfully achieved when these considerations are utilized in program planning.

If we had used the rehearsal-oriented program with the closed head injury patients, my guess is that we would have succeeded, but we would not have accomplished much. These patients were probably already quite capable of learning individual items by rote. On the other hand, had we tried to use the ridiculously imaged-story and face–name association methods with the Korsakoff patients, we probably would have failed. That is at least in part because the learning required for those tasks requires access to declarative memory, which may be impaired but still existent in closed head injury patients, but is essentially totally obliterated in Korsakoff patients. While we cannot be absolutely certain about this matter, in a previous study (Goldstein, Ryan, Turner, Kanagy, Barry, & Kelly, 1985) we reported on the cases of two densely amnesic patients using training methods in which generalization could be evaluated. In the first case, we used a paired-associate learning technique with verbal elaboration as the mnemonic device. While some improvement was noted over sessions with the same list of paired associates, when previously unstudied paired associates were used, the patient showed no evidence of improvement over sessions. It will be recalled that the closed head injury patients did continue to improve when item content was changed from session to session. In the second case, we taught the patient to respond correctly to the items contained in the Luria–Nebraska Neuropsychological Battery Memory Scale (Golden, Hammeke, & Purisch, 1980) through daily administration of the scale over a series of 29 sessions. Starting with a very poor performance, he eventually performed quite normally, mastering 10 of the 13 items on the scale. However, when we shifted to an alternate form of the scale consisting of 13 items corresponding in form but with different content from the original items, he showed absolutely no generalization or savings. The learning curves for the two forms were essentially identical. Indeed, it was our experience with these patients that led us to develop the rehearsal method for Korsakoff patients described above.

In the case of the severely amnesic patient, it may be possible to go one step further. I have argued that these patients have the capability of learning specific items of new information through repetition, but they do not have access to memory systems that support transfer of learning, even to similar materials. I have also observed that they do not benefit from the commonly used practice of having patients carry lists of items or tasks they need to remember. They forget the lists and, when reminded, may have no awareness that they ever had a list. A possible next step, then, might be to develop a type of list that these patients will remember to use. If they have and remember to use a list, then it becomes unnecessary to train recall of the items on it. We are currently working on a program in which we plan to incorporate information lists into a simple prosthetic device carried by the patient. It will probably look like a small pocket calculator with a few buttons and a window for displaying information. Once the device is developed, the plan is to implement a training program based upon what we learned from the rehearsal study. Thus, through a conditioning procedure based upon repetitive trials, we hope to teach patients to remember to use the device. If we are successful, then patients can carry around a limited "memory prosthesis" which can be accessed when needed. With regard to the conditioning, we are now considering a "vanishing cue" method (Glisky, Schacter, & Tulving, 1986) in which a signal will be emitted by the device periodically. The signal will initially remind the patient of the presence of the device. Through rehearsal, we hope to form an association between the signal and taking out the device in order to use it to answer a question. If we reach that goal, we will fade the signal by only using it intermittently. Hopefully, the signal can be completely dispensed with eventually, and the patient will use the device spontaneously when in need of information.

Memory dysfunction is sometimes seen as a relatively isolated syndrome, but is more often associated with other neuropsychological deficits. We don't have much information about how memory training programs of the type discussed here work with patients with multiple deficits. Obviously, patients with aphasia and other language-related disorders would have difficulties with programs of the list learning type. However, a far more common problem involves the patient with memory dysfunction as part of a more general dementia. Even during the early stages of Alzheimer's disease, individuals may have significant memory dysfunction. However, associated problems with conceptualization and communication are also present, or appear eventually. There is some reasonably considered debate in our field concerning whether or not one should attempt cognitive rehabilitation with patients suffering from progressive, degenerative diseases. Often, the progress of the disease gradually cancels out any rehabilitation-related improvements. One solution may involve adopting a continuum of prosthetic methods such that the environment increasingly supports a progressively failing memory. The technological and experimental neuropsychological work needed for the development of these patient–environment linkages would appear to be a highly worthwhile task for the future.

## REFERENCES

Buschke, H. (1973). Selective reminding for analysis of memory and learning. *Journal of Verbal Learning & Verbal Behavior*, *12*, 543–550.

Butters, N. (1984). The clinical aspects of memory disorders. Contributions from experimental studies in amnesia and dementia. *Journal of Clinical Neuropsychology*, *6*, 17–36.

Gasparrini, B., & Satz, P. (1979). A treatment for memory problems in left-hemisphere CVA patients. *Journal of Clinical Neuropsychology*, *1*, 137–150.

Glisky, E.L., Schacter, D.L., & Tulving, E. (1986). Learning and retention of computer-related vocabulary in memory-impaired patients: Method of vanishing cues. *Journal of Experimental & Clinical Neuropsychology*, *8*, 292–312.

Golden, C.J., Hammeke, T.A., & Purisch, A.D. (1980). *The Luria–Nebraska Battery manual*. Los Angeles: Western Psychological Services.

Goldstein, G., & Malec, E.A. (1989). Memory training for severely amnesic patients. *Neuropsychology*, *3*, 9–16.

Goldstein, G., Ryan, C., Turner, S.M., Kanagy, M., Barry, K., & Kelly, L. (1985). Three methods of memory training for severely amnesic patients. *Behavior Modification*, *9*, 357–374.

Goldstein, G., McCue, M., Turner, S.M., Spanier, C., Malec, E.A., & Shelly, C. (1988). An efficacy study of memory training for patients with closed-head injury. *The Clinical Neuropsychologist*, *2*, 251–259.

Hinsie, L.E., & Campbell, R.J. (1960). *Psychiatric dictionary* (3rd ed.). New York: Oxford University Press.

Kovner, R., Mattis, S., & Goldmeier, E. (1983). A technique for promoting robust free recall in chronic organic amnesia. *Journal of Clinical Neuropsychology*, *5*, 65–71.

Kovner, R., Mattis, S., & Pass, R. (1985). Some amnesic patients can freely recall large amounts of information in new contexts. *Journal of Clinical & Experimental Neuropsychology*, *7*, 395–411.

Levin, H.S., Benton, A.L., & Grossman, R.G. (1982). *Neurobehavioral consequences of closed head injury*. New York: Oxford University Press.

Lorayne, H., & Lucas, J. (1974). *The memory book*. New York: Stein & Day.

Moffat, N. (1984). Strategies of memory therapy. In B.A. Wilson & N. Moffat (Eds.), *Clinical management of memory problems* (pp. 63–88). Germantown, MD: Aspen Systems Corporation.

O'Connor, M., & Cermak, L.S. (1987). Rehabilitation of organic memory disorders. In M.J. Meier, A.L. Benton, & L. Diller (Eds.), *Neuropsychological rehabilitation* (pp. 260–279). Edinburgh: Churchill Livingstone.

Schacter, D.L. (1990). Toward a cognitive neuropsychology of awareness: Implicit knowledge and anosognosia. *Journal of Clinical & Experimental Neuropsychology*, *12*, 155–178.

Seron, X. (1987). Operant procedures and neuropsychological rehabilitation. In M.J. Meier, A.L. Benton, & L. Diller (Eds.), *Neuropsychological rehabilitation* (pp. 132–161). Edinburgh: Churchill Livingstone.

Wilson, B.A. (1987). *Rehabilitation of memory*. New York: Guilford Press.

# 12

# The Efficacy of Attention-Remediation Programs for Traumatically Brain-Injured Survivors

ROBERT J. McCAFFREY and DAVID A. GANSLER

## HISTORY OF ATTENTION DEFICITS SECONDARY
## TO TRAUMATIC BRAIN INJURIES

Meyer (1904) was the first to report slowness of thought and an inability to concentrate as sequelae of traumatic brain injury (TBI). It has been recognized for over 45 years that TBI can result in disorders of attention. Pioneering studies by Conkey (1938) and Ruesch (1944) noted the presence of deficits in mental speed and the inability to sustain attention in patients who had suffered a TBI. Following these initial reports, investigators focused their efforts on other sequelae of TBIs, such as memory, language, perception, and "intelligence." The apparent neglect of attentional deficits by investigators working in the field of TBI appears to have occurred for several reasons. First, deficits in memory, perception, language, and other factors were more closely tied to the mainstream of experimental psychology in non-TBI populations. Thus, a literature based on nonneurologically impaired individuals was present for clinicians attempting to deal with the sequelae of TBI. Unfortunately, basic experimental research on the concept of attention and into the mechanisms of attention has lagged behind. One major reason for this is that attention is

ROBERT J. McCAFFREY • Department of Psychology, State University of New York at Albany, Albany, New York 12222.    DAVID A. GANSLER • Boston Veterans Medical Center, Boston, Massachusetts 02130.

*HANDBOOK OF HEAD TRAUMA: Acute Care to Recovery*, edited by Charles J. Long and Leslie K. Ross. Plenum Press, New York, 1992.

not a unitary concept. As such, attempts at operationally defining attentional difficulties posed a considerable obstacle.

In the 1970s, there was a growing body of literature suggesting that attentional deficits almost invariably follow a TBI (Miller, 1970; Van Zomeren, 1981; Van Zomeren, Brouwer, & Deelman, 1984). As noted by Lezak (1987), deficits in attention are likely to underlie many other cognitive difficulties experienced by TBI survivors and may require amelioration prior to commencing other forms of rehabilitative interventions. In fact, the impact of attentional deficits in situations in which patients are exposed to new material, with the goal of having them acquire compensatory skills and/or strategies, cannot be overstated.

In the last decade, there have been experimental attempts both to design and to evaluate attentional remediational strategies for TBI patients. This, in part, stems from the realization that attentional deficits are likely to underlie other cognitive deficits (Lezak, 1983). The pioneering work by the cognitive psychologist, Michael Posner (Posner, 1975; Posner & Boies, 1971; Posner, Snyder, & Davidson, 1980), has provided the experimental backdrop against which to begin to conceptualize attentional deficits in the TBI patient.

There have been several recent studies designed to evaluate the ability of treatment programs to remediate attentional deficits in TBI patients. Not surprisingly, the studies have shown mixed results. The purpose of the present chapter is to review the existent treatment outcome studies for the remediation of attentional deficits in TBI patients, provide a critical analysis of these studies, and offer possible reasons for the differences in the outcome across studies.

## PIONEERING TREATMENT PROGRAM

There is little question that the New York University Medical Center group working under the direction of Yehuda Ben-Yishay has been the pioneers in the application of a systematic method for the amelioration of basic attentional disorders. The work by this group dates back to the early 1970s. These investigators have developed an Orientation Remedial Module (ORM) consisting of five procedures which involve the reception of visual and/or auditory stimuli and require a series of simple, visuomotor responses with an emphasis on not requiring higher levels of information processing by the TBI patient.

In a recent review of work in their laboratory, Ben-Yishay, Piasetsky, and Rattok (1987) present data on the first 40 patients who underwent the attention-remediation program based on the ORM. The patients included in the Ben-Yishay *et al.* (1987) review were all at least one year post-TBI and reportedly typically between two and four years post-TBI. The authors provide pretraining and posttraining scores on the various components of the ORM to document the changes in the patients as a function of the program. The patients appear to improve on psychometric tests used as measures of attentional abilities in TBI patients from pre-ORM training to post-ORM training.

In terms of the maintenance of treatment effects, the authors report data on a subgroup of 11 patients who were followed serially and evaluated on all five of the ORM tasks. Criteria for the selection of this group of 11 patients were not specified. Overall, the data indicate the maintenance of the treatment-related effects at three months ($n = 11$) and for up to six months posttraining ($n = 5$).

As is often the case in clinical research, the authors indicate quite correctly that the larger objectives of their studies, plus the special structure of the treatment program, created limitations regarding their ability to adhere to rigorous scientific methods of research design in evaluating the ORM program. Nonetheless, the data presented by the authors are suggestive of a treatment-related effect.

The authors also include several qualifications regarding the positive changes observed in their TBI patient population. First, the patients themselves were not a homogeneous sample since the magnitude of functional changes was reported to vary considerably from patient to patient. Second, due to the holistic nature of the treatment program, the exact source of improvement on the ORM cannot be ascertained. Third, the magnitude of functional changes, the course of improvement on tasks, and the carryover affects of training were reported to vary considerably across patients.

In summary, the ORM training program developed by Ben-Yishay and his colleagues has served as a catalyst for other investigators interested in cognitive remediation in general and attention-remediation in particular.

## VIDEO GAME PRACTICE

The potential utility of video game practice in the remediation of attentional deficits in TBI patients was evaluated by Malec, Jones, Rao, and Stubbs (1984). The patients in this study were selected based on the following criteria: medically stable, 16 years of age or older, greater than 24 hour duration of coma, corrected visual acuity in one eye of at least 20/30, and the use of at least one upper extremity. The later two inclusion criteria assured that the patients could participate meaningfully in the video game program. The sample consisted of a total of 13 consecutive TBI patients. Two patients did not meet the inclusion criteria while another left the hospital against medical advice.

A total of eight male and two female patients completed the program. Table 12.1 contains a summary of relevant patient characteristics. All patients entered the study within six months post-TBI. The measures of sustained attention included the Stroop Test (Stroop Word, Stroop Color, and Stroop Color/Word Indices), two cancellation tasks, one involving letters of the alphabet and another involving symbols, and a reaction time task that utilized

TABLE 12.1.  Summary of Patient Characteristics
for the Malec *et al.* (1984) Study

| Characteristic | Malec *et al.* sample |
| --- | --- |
| $N$ | 10 |
| Age | 17–48 years ($M = 30$; $SD = 10.5$) |
| Sex | 8M, 2F |
| Education (years) | N.R.[a] |
| Time since injury (months) | <6 months ($M = 80$ days; $SD = 42$) |
| Etiology | TBI |
| Coma duration | $M = 14.5$ days; $SD = 13$ |
| GOAT | 50–100 (3 patients < 66) |
| Handedness | N.R. |

[a]N.R., not reported.

a verbal warning which preceded each stimulus presentation. Patients participated in either an A-B-A-B or B-A-B-A treatment design (Hersen & Barlow, 1984) with each phase being one week in duration. The treatment phase (A) consisted of playing video games for 30 minutes twice a day, Monday through Thursday, with Friday reserved for obtaining the measures of sustained attention. Throughout the study, the authors attempted to keep the patient–therapist interaction to a minimum, in order to control for this variable. The results of this study were reported as a percentage improvement and indicated that the only outcome measure which *approached* statistical significance was reaction time. In general, the authors caution clinicians against assuming that video game practice alone will be useful in terms of generalizing to improvement in patients' attentional abilities.

The findings in this study are difficult to interpret for two reasons. First, the authors evaluated patients who were all within six months of their TBI. Given the time since TBI, it is not unreasonable to expect to obtain changes in cognitive factors (e.g., reaction time) attributable to spontaneous recovery of function. Second, the data analyses were conducted on percentage improvement scores and not the actual scores. In summary, the study by Malec *et al.* (1984) cannot be considered an appropriate evaluation of the efficacy of video game practice as a technique to assist in the remediation of sustained attentional deficits in TBI patients.

## COMPUTER-ASSISTED PROGRAM

A controlled study of computer-based remediation of psychomotor performance and vigilance in TBI patients was undertaken by Wood and Fussey (1987). A sample of 20 TBI patients were assigned to either an active treatment condition or a wait-list control. A nonneurologically impaired control group was also included to assess for pre- to posttreatment practice effects. Table 12.2 contains a summary of patient characteristics. As indicated in Table 12.2, the TBI patients were well beyond the period where the process of spontaneous recovery of function would be expected to be present.

The computer-assisted remediation training was aimed at information processing in the

TABLE 12.2.   Summary of Patient Characteristics
for the Wood and Fussey (1987) Study

|  | Patient group | | Nonpatient group |
|  | Controls | Treatment | Controls |
|---|---|---|---|
| Age | $M = 24.8$ | $M = 27.2$ | $M = 29.4$ |
| Sex | 3M, 7F | 10M, 0F | 5M, 5F |
| Education | N.R.[a] | N.R. | N.R. |
| Time since injury (months) | $M = 27.5$ | $M = 36.5$ | — |
| Etiology | 6 TBI | 4 TBI | — |
|  | 4 TBI/skull fx. | 3 TBI/skull fx. | — |
| Coma duration | N.R. | N.R. | N.R. |
| Handedness | N.R. | N.R. | — |

[a]N.R., not reported.

visual modality. The computer task involved visual screening, perceptual discrimination, judgment and anticipation, and a motor response.

Patients underwent training daily for 60 minutes, Monday through Friday, for 20 days with posttreatment follow-up at Days 35 and 63. The outcome measures included: pursuit motor, digit symbol, choice and simple reaction time, a visual vigilance test, and a continuous performance task. Two behavioral indices of attention in daily functioning were also included: attention to the therapist during a therapy task and an attention rating scale completed by the nursing and therapy staff.

The results provided no evidence to indicate that the computer-based attention-remediation task improved psychomotor or vigilance performances, as indexed by the outcome measures. Wood and Fussey (1987) report a significant improvement from baseline to posttreatment only for the attention to the therapist. Why patients would demonstrate improvement on this task and none of the others is unclear. Perhaps the experimenters were not blind as to the patients' condition and an observer-expecting factor was operating.

A recent study by Gray and Robertson (1989) evaluated the efficacy of a computer-assisted attention-remediation program. Three severely TBI adult males were employed as subjects. Table 12.3 contains a summary of relevant patient factors. The single case experimental design utilized in this study involved a multiple baseline across behaviors design (Hersen & Barlow, 1984). The dependent variable was a composite score based on the sum of the digit span forward and digit span backward (form of the WAIS not specified) and performance on a simple arithmetic task. The control variable differed across the three TBI cases with no justification: Case 1 utilized a discriminate reaction time task, Case 2 used the Buschke Selective Reminding Test (numbers of items in long-term storage) while Case 3 utilized a delayed recall measure of an unspecified instrument.

The training used in all three cases involved computer-assisted attention-remediation programs. Case 1 was trained using a rapid number comparison and a digit symbol transfer test. Case 2 was trained using an alternating Stroop program while Case 3 underwent the alternating Stroop program plus the Symbol Digit Transfer and an arcade game known as *Breakout*. The justification for utilizing different training tasks and sets of tasks was not presented.

TABLE 12.3. Summary of Patient Characteristics
for Gray and Robertson (1989)

|  | Patient | | |
|---|---|---|---|
|  | 01 | 02 | 03 |
| Age | 20 | 30 | 19 |
| Sex | M | M | M |
| Education (years) | N.R.[a] | N.R. | N.R. |
| Time since injury (months) | N.R. | 36 | 6 |
| Etiology | TBI | TBI | TBI |
| Coma duration | N.R. | N.R. | N.R. |
| Handedness | N.R. | N.R. | N.R. |

[a]N.R., not reported.

The duration of baseline for Case 1 was six sessions with nine sessions of treatment over a period of approximately two months. The total duration of baseline for Case 2 appears to have been three sessions with only one data point for the control variable during baseline. During the subsequent seven treatment sessions, data were missing for two of the control variable sessions. For Case 3, the baseline period was four sessions and treatment consisted of eight additional sessions. During the active treatment phase, the data for two of the control variable sessions are missing. The authors made no mention as to the factors contributing to the missing data. The graphic presentation of the data by Gray and Robertson is based on interpolated values for the missing data.

The Gray and Robertson study also presented pre- and posttreatment data on selected measures of attentional functioning. The data are presented for Cases 2 and 3 only with no explanation as to the absence of data for Case 1. The variables evaluated include the digit span performance of the WAIS, the Wisconsin Card Sorting Test (Errors and Perseverative Responses), and patients' performance on the Paced Auditory Serial Addition Test (PASAT—4 seconds). The pre- to posttraining improvement on the WAIS Digit Span is confounded with the fact that this pre- to posttreatment variable may have been a dependent variable during the course of treatment. Thus, it is possible that the improvement noted on the WAIS Digit Span is due to familiarity with this dependent variable. The data presented by Gray and Robertson make it impossible to determine whether or not the improvement was related to familiarity with this task since the target variables (digits forward and digits backward and arithmetic task) were presented as a single cumulative score. For Case 2, performance on the Wisconsin Card Sorting Test improved by more than one standard deviation unit relative to available norms from pretreatment to posttreatment. No changes were noted on perseverative errors on the Wisconsin Card Sorting Test or on percent correct on the PASAT. For Case 3, there were no reported improvements for the Wisconsin Card Sorting Test, although errors went from 9 to 3. The pre- to posttraining PASAT scores showed improvement greater than one standard deviation relative to available norms.

The Gray and Robertson study (1989) purports to show improvement in attentional functions of severely TBI adults who underwent approximately eight weeks of computer-assisted remediation. The results of the remediation task were most evident in the data for Case 1. Unfortunately, the time since the TBI was not specified for Case 1. Thus, the degree to which spontaneous recovery of function was operating cannot be ascertained. Cases 2 and 3 were three years and six months post-TBI, respectively. Another factor worthy of consideration is that the definition of severe TBI was apparently made by the authors using some unspecified criteria. Specifically, no Glasgow Coma Scale scores or other routine severity indices of TBI are reported.

While Gray and Robertson (1989) conclude that the results of their study support the efficacy of computer-assisted attention-remediation programs in severely TBI subjects, a number of methodological factors suggest otherwise. Specifically, the authors failed to provide sufficient information on the characteristics of their sample to allow for a clearer interpretation of their data. Moreover, there is no discussion as to why there were so many missing data points. This is particularly important given the small number of cases involved in this study and the relatively short training time. In addition, the baseline for Case 2 was a total of three sessions. There was only one data point for the control variable, and the data on the target variable were highly unstable. Finally, an average of the data points on the target variables for Case 3 reveals little, if any, clear treatment-related effect.

## ATTENTION PROCESS TRAINING PROGRAM

The most successful attention-remediation study reported to date was conducted by Sohlberg and Mateer (1987). This study involved the use of a single subject multiple baseline across behaviors design (Hersen & Barlow, 1984) with four subjects, all of whom demonstrated gains in attention following the initiation of attention training. Relevant patient characteristics are summarized in Table 12.4. The treatment model involved a hierarchical approach on tasks which were orthogonal to dependent variables. The primary dependent variable was the PASAT (Gronwall, 1977). The Spatial Relations Subtest from the Woodcock–Johnson Psychoeducational Battery was included as a control procedure since the Attention Process Training (APT) program, developed by Sohlberg and Mateer (1989), was predicted not to have a significant impact on the spatial relations performance of the patients.

The participants were randomly selected from a series of consecutive admissions to the Center for Cognitive Rehabilitation. Each participant underwent a two-week comprehensive cognitive and psychosocial evaluation assessing attention, visual processing, memory, and reasoning. The results of this testing were then used to determine which cognitive processes should be addressed and at what level within the patient's program. The patients received four to eight weeks of attention training with the length of training being determined by the severity of the attentional deficit. During the course of training, patients received between seven and nine individual cognitive retraining sessions per week which focused specifically on attention, visual processing, or memory, according to the specific treatment phase.

The results of the study revealed that subjects who presented with mild to moderate attention deficits at the pretreatment evaluation, as indicated by PASAT scores within two standard deviations below the normative mean, increased to within normal limits at the

TABLE 12.4.   Summary of Patient Characteristics
for Sohlbert and Mateer (1987)

|  | Patient | | | |
| --- | --- | --- | --- | --- |
|  | 01 | 02 | 03 | 04 |
| Age | 30 | 29 | 28 | 25 |
| Sex | M | M | M | M |
| Education (years) | 13 | 12 | 12 | 11 |
| Time since injury (months) | 14 | 72 | 12 | 48 |
| Etiology | Aneurysm | Gunshot | TBI | TBI |
| Coma duration (weeks) | 7 | 24 h | 5 | 2 |
| Handedness | N.R.[a] | N.R. | N.R. | N.R. |

[a]N.R., not reported.

conclusion of the APT program. Two other participants with severe attention deficits, whose original baseline PASAT scores were greater than three standard deviations below the normative mean, were within the mildly impaired range at the conclusion of the APT program. The improvements in attention in these four cases remained above baseline levels for up to eight months of follow-up. A potential confound is that the participants also received concurrent intervention in the areas of daily living, prevocational skills, and psychosocial skills which may have an impact on the outcome variables.

The results reported by Sohlberg and Mateer (1987) are promising for the remediation of attentional disorders secondary to TBI. More recent empirical research, however, has raised questions regarding the complex nature of treatment approaches to the remediation of attentional deficits.

## EFFECTS OF SPONTANEOUS RECOVERY OF FUNCTION

The report by Van Zomeren *et al.* (1984) that information processing is the most impaired aspect of attentional skills in TBI patients led Ponsford and Kinsella (1988) to design and evaluate a computer-mediated attentional training program focusing on improving the speed of information processing in severely TBI patients.

Ponsford and Kinsella (1988) present data on a total of 10 severely TBI patients ages 17 to 38 who were on average less than 9 months post-TBI with a period of posttraumatic amnesia ranging from 10 days to 12 weeks. The performance of the TBI group was compared to a control group of 16 nonneurologically impaired orthopedically impaired patients from a rehabilitation hospital. The two groups were matched on age, years of education, and neither had a premorbid history of neurological or psychiatric disturbance. A summary of relevant patient characteristics is presented in Table 12.5.

Ponsford and Kinsella (1988) utilized a multiple baseline across patients design (Hersen & Barlow, 1984) to evaluate the effectiveness of their computer-mediated program for the remediation of deficits in speed of information processing in the severely TBI patients. The initial baseline phase was either 3 or 6 weeks and patients were randomly

TABLE 12.5.   Summary of Patient Characteristics for Ponsford and Kinsella (1988)

|  | TBI patients | Orthopedic controls |
|---|---|---|
| Age | 17 to 38 y/o ($M = 24.4$; $SD = 8.7$) | 25.5 (7.8) |
| Sex | 4M, 6F | 13M, 3F |
| Education (years) | 6–13 ($M = 11$; $SD = 1.9$) | $M = 11.8$;$SD = 2.0$ |
| Time since injury (months) | <9 months ($M = 13.8$ weeks; $SD = 9.4$) Range 6–34 weeks |  |
| Etiology | N.R.[a] |  |
| Coma duration | N.R. |  |
| Handedness | N.R. |  |

[a]N.R., not reported.

assigned to either condition. Following the baseline phase, each patient underwent half-hour daily training sessions on the computer-mediated program designed to train speed of visual reaction time, visual search, and selective attention. At each of the daily sessions, the patients completed one set of trials on each of the remediation tasks. During this phase of the study, the therapist gave no feedback or reinforcement to the patient regarding his or her performance. The computer-mediated program did provide feedback on the screen to each patient after the completion of each task. In the third phase of this study, the same training tasks were given for an additional 3 weeks but the therapist became actively involved in providing feedback to each of the patients regarding his or her performance. Praise was given verbally whenever systematic gains were made and the performance was also recorded graphically. Following this combined treatment phase, patients returned to a final 3-week baseline in order to determine whether the gains as indexed by the dependent variables were maintained or lost at the conclusion of treatment.

The authors stated that the computer-mediated attention training tasks were orthogonal to the dependent variables. A total of five tasks were chosen for training purposes. The first two tasks *react* and *search* were designed by Gianutsos and Kintzer (1981). The remaining tasks were designed by the authors. The *react task* is a reaction time task while the *search task* involves a visual search for a shape embedded in an array of shapes which matches the display in the center of the screen. The *red square/green square* task requires the patient to respond differentially to the presentation of a red square versus a green square by depressing a button with the left or right hand, respectively. The patient must also withhold responding if other colored squares are presented. The *spot the letter* task involves presentation of 50 random numbers and letters in an array to which the patient is to respond only to the letters. Finally, the *evens and fives* test involves the presentation of 40 random numbers on the screen to which the patient is to respond as quickly as possible when the number on the screen is *either* an even number *or* a multiple of five. These training tasks were presented exclusively in the visual modality and were aimed at improving speed of information processing.

The dependent variables were grouped into two sets. The first set consisted of psychometric measures of speed of information processing and included the Four Choice Reaction Time Task (Van Zomeren, 1981), the Symbol Digit Modalities Test (Smith, 1973), and a Two-Letter Cancellation Task. These were obtained three times per week throughout the study. The authors included three additional dependent variables which were administered prior to and at the conclusion of each phase in the experimental design. The first was the Wechsler Adult Intelligence Scale/Naylor–Harwood Adult Intelligence Scale (Naylor & Harwood, 1972) similarities subtest which is a measure of a patient's capacity to deal with abstract verbal concepts. This task was included since it did not involve speed or other attentional components and was designed to evaluate generalization of improvement to other cognitive functions. The second variable included a rating scale of attentional behaviors completed by the patient's occupational therapist. This 15-item instrument was designed by the authors to evaluate attentional behaviors observed in day-to-day activities. Finally, a 30-minute video of the patient's performance of a clerical task was obtained and evaluated for the presence of overt-attentional behavior, such as distractibility and inability to sustain attention to a task.

The outcome of this attentional remediation program was evaluated at both an ideographic and a nomothetic level. Regardless of the length of the initial baseline phase, patients showed a gradual improvement across all phases of the study. Ponsford and Kinsella interpreted this as reflecting the ongoing process of spontaneous recovery of function. In order to determine the effectiveness of the various interventions, the authors performed regression analyses based on the slopes of the dependent variables within each of the phases. The slopes were then used in a two-way repeated measures analysis of variance, in order to examine whether or not there were significant changes in the slopes across the various phases. Surprisingly, there were no statistically significant intervention effects on any of the three psychometric measures of attention.

The data for the other three dependent variables obtained pre- and postphases were also analyzed using a two-way repeated measures analysis of variance. The rating scale of attentional behaviors revealed no significant differences between groups and no significant group × phase interaction. The phase effect was statistically significant, indicating improvement in rating scale scores across *all* phases. The authors conclude that in the absence of a significant group effect, the phase effect is most likely attributable to the process of spontaneous recovery of function. On the similarities subtest there was a significant phase effect reflecting either the effects of spontaneous recovery of function or possibly practice effects. The analysis of the 30-minute video recordings revealed no significant effects whatsoever.

Ponsford and Kinsella (1988) concluded that while there were a number of instances of clinically significant improvement in the combined attention-remediation plus feedback phase for three out of the ten cases, it was not possible to differentiate the subjects who responded significantly on the basis of age, sex, educational background, length of posttraumatic amnesia, time since injury, the nature of their neuropsychological deficits, or the severity of their attentional deficits. In summary, Ponsford and Kinsella conclude that once the effects of the process of spontaneous recovery of function and practice effects were controlled for, their remediation program had very little effect.

The Ponsford and Kinsella (1988) study is methodologically superior to the studies reviewed thus far for several reasons. First of all, the authors provide a clear and adequate description of the demographic background of the patients, their time postinjury, length of posttraumatic amnesia, and severity of TBI using established criteria (e.g., Russell, 1971). The total number of TBI patients in this study was significantly larger than those used in prior studies. An appropriate control group was also included. The tasks chosen for the attention-remediation component were orthogonal to the dependent variables. The authors also attempted to monitor the impact of the attention-remediation program on patients' attentional behaviors in their daily lives by using the Rating Scale of Attentional Behaviors and videotapes of patients' behavior on a clerical task. The latter measures are very important since it is possible that patients might show minimal improvement on the selected dependent variables and yet obtain improvement on other aspects of attentional behaviors in their day-to-day life. Moreover, the goal of attention-remediation programs is to improve the quality of the daily living of the TBI patient. In this regard, Ponsford and Kinsella's efforts at obtaining information on this point are a major contribution. Finally, Ponsford and Kinsella demonstrate convincingly that the role of both practice effects and the process of spontaneous recovery of function must be taken into consideration in the design and implementation of attention-remediation programs and other cognitive remediation programs as well.

The study by Ponsford and Kinsella (1988) was the first to attempt to control for the effects due to the process of spontaneous recovery of function using a post-hoc statistical procedure. The result of the Ponsford and Kinsella study casts doubt on the efficacy of prior attention-remediation programs which failed to control for the effects due to the process of spontaneous recovery of function from either an experimental design perspective or a post-hoc data analytic plan. While there are a number of important differences between the attention-remediation studies conducted to date, the overriding issue of the efficacy of these types of programs warrants rigorous scientific investigation.

The work by Sohlberg and Mateer (1987) supports the position that attentional deficits in TBI patients may be remediated through specific intervention programs. On the other hand, the study by Ponsford and Kinsella (1988) casts some doubt on the efficacy of attention-remediation programs, specifically with patients who are less than 9 months post-TBI. Clearly, what is needed are studies evaluating the efficacy of attention-remediation programs which address issues such as spontaneous recovery of function.

## LONG-TERM ATTENTIONAL DEFICITS

A recent study conducted in our laboratory (Gansler & McCaffrey, 1991) addressed the issue of the effects of the process of spontaneous recovery of function by recruiting four patients who ranged from 4 to 27 years post-TBI but who either complained of attentional problems or had members of their family indicate that they had persistent attentional difficulties. Table 12.6 summarizes the characteristics of this sample. This study operationally defined attention according to Michael Posner's (1975) basic work on attention from the cognitive psychology literature. In addition, this study attempted to control for the presence of practice effects and to evaluate both the patients' and significant others' perceptions of the impact of the attention-remediation program on activities of daily living and changes in patients' psychological and neuropsychological status.

Gansler and McCaffrey (1991) utilized an ABA single case design (Hersen & Barlow, 1984). The initial A-phase consisted of a four-week, pretreatment baseline. The attentional remediation program (B-phase) was conducted over the next eight consecutive weeks. Follow-up assessment occurred four weeks following the end of the remediation program (second A-phase). The choice of the four-week baseline and eight-week attention-

TABLE 12.6.   Summary of Patient Characteristics
for Gansler and McCaffrey (1991)

|  | Patient | | | |
| --- | --- | --- | --- | --- |
|  | 01 | 02 | 03 | 04 |
| Age | 35 | 19 | 30 | 37 |
| Sex | M | M | M | M |
| Education (years) | 12 | 12 | 12 | 12 |
| Time since injury (months) | 27 | 4 | 13 | 20 |
| Etiology | TBI | TBI | TBI | TBI |
| Coma duration (weeks) | 2.5 | 6 | 2.5 | 6 |
| Handedness | R | R | L | L |

remediation program was based on matching, as closely as possible, the duration of the remediation component in prior studies (Ponsford and Kinsella, 1988; Sohlberg & Mateer, 1987; Malec *et al.*, 1984). The dependent variables consisted of four attentional capacity variables, patients' subjective rating of their level of concentration, quality of performance and satisfaction with ADLs and ratings of three subjective psychological states: depression, anxiety, and anger. These three groups of variables were collected on a weekly basis throughout the A and B phases of the study, as well as during the second A phase. The ABA design was supplemented with pre- and posttreatment measures of neuropsychological functioning and a significant other's rating of each of the patient's level of independence with activities of daily living.

The dependent variables were chosen to correspond to Posner's (1975) hierarchical component model of attention. Posner's model consists of four levels of attentional processes: tonic awareness, phasic awareness, selective attention, and vigilance/sustained attention. Tonic awareness is conceptualized as an involuntary basal level of arousal which is subject to diurnal variation. Tonic awareness was measured, in this study, using a simple visual reaction time paradigm. Phasic awareness is considered to be under voluntary control and subject to rapid fluctuations in response to environmental demands. Phasic awareness was measured using reaction time to a visual stimulus which was preceded one half second by an auditory stimulus. Selective attention involves the filtering out of irrelevant stimuli in the search for a relevant stimulus. Selective attention was evaluated by using visual reaction time to a specified light in an array of four colored lights which were activated individually by the therapist according to a predetermined random sequence. The final component, vigilance/sustained attention, involves the ability to maintain focused effort for a period of time. Sustained attention/vigilance was assessed utilizing an auditory vigilance task. Patients were instructed to respond to the letter "A" embedded within a two-minute audiocassette tape comprised of a string of letters of the alphabet.

Three psychological variables were also monitored: depression using the Beck Depression Inventory (Beck, Ward, Mendelsohn, Mock, & Erbaugh, 1961), the State–Trait Anxiety Inventory (Speilberger, Gorsuch, & Lushene, 1970), and the State–Trait Anger Inventory (Speilberger, Jacobs, Russel, & Crane, 1983). The Activities of Daily Living were based on patients' self-reported ratings of ability to concentrate on their ADLs, satisfaction in performing their ADLs, and the quality of their performance. In addition, a significant other rated each patient's ability to perform ADLs using the New York University Skilled Checklist (Diller, Fordyce, Jacobs, & Brown, 1979).

The neuropsychological battery was designed to provide a brief assessment of executive functions, verbal and nonverbal memory capacity, verbal fluency, psychomotor functions, verbal and nonverbal problem-solving capacities, and attention/concentration capacity. During the pretreatment phase, the neuropsychological battery was administered twice in order to control for practice effects. Performance on the second pretreatment administration was used as the baseline for comparison with the posttreatment (end of phase B and at follow-up [i.e., end of second A phase]). The battery was comprised of the following instruments: the Wechsler Memory Scale (Form 1)—Russell's Revision (1975), Paired Associate Subtest of the Wechsler Memory Scale, Trail Making Test (Parts A & B), Minute Estimation Test, the Thurston Word Fluency Test, the Grooved Pegboard Test, and the following subtests from the WAIS-R: Picture Arrangement, Block Design, Arithmetic, Digit Span, and Similarities.

The attention-remediation program consisted of four consecutive two-week components organized hierarchically. Each component was conducted daily in two-hour sessions on Monday through Thursday, with Friday devoted to the administration of the attentional and ADL dependent variables.

Component one consisted of basic mental tracking utilizing a passage of time test. Component two consisted of two separate exercises adapted from Craine and Gudman (1983). The first task involved having patients identify letters of the alphabet sequentially (i.e., A, B, C. . .) in an array of randomly presented letters. The second task involved the capacity to switch sets. Specifically, patients were asked to scan rows of digits for odd or even numbers. At specified intervals they were asked to switch from identifying one type of number to identifying the other type of number. Component three consisted of a continuous visual attention/eye–hand coordination task adapted from the previous work of Malec *et al.* (1984). This task consisted of the computer game *Invaders* which contains four levels of difficulty. The fourth component was a divided attention task taken from the work of Hirst, Spelke, Reaves, Caharock, and Neisser (1980) which involved having the patient read for comprehension while simultaneously processing auditorily presented words.

The goal of this study was to evaluate the efficacy of an attention-remediation program in which the potential for the process of spontaneous recovery of function was minimal. Overall, the treatment-related improvements in the measures of attentional abilities were minimal and of questionable clinical significance. While there was a trend for the subjects to rate their own performance on their ADLs during and after the treatment phase as improved, the significant other's rating of the subject's ADLs did not reveal a trend toward improvement. Furthermore, the measures obtained on a neuropsychological battery revealed no significant trends across any of the phases of the study. In summary, the attention-remediation program evaluated in this study failed to demonstrate clearly meaningful change in either the targeted cognitive functions or in patients' general cognitive functioning.

## CONCLUSION

Overall, the data on the efficacy of attention-remediation programs for TBI patients are, at best, divided. The most convincing support for the efficacy of a specific attention-remediation program has been provided by Sohlberg and Mateer (1987). Based upon the results reported by Ponsford and Kinsella (1988) and those of Gansler and McCaffrey (1991), one might be tempted to argue that the improvement noted in the Sohlberg and Mateer (1987) study was due to the process of spontaneous recovery of function independent of the specific attention-remediation program. A close examination of the time post-TBI for the four patients studied by Sohlberg and Mateer (1987) indicates that only two of the four subjects were less than 14 months postinjury. The other two subjects were 48 and 72 months postinjury. The inclusion of two subjects who were postinjury beyond a point where the process of spontaneous recovery of function would be expected to be operating to a clinically significant degree argues against the notion that the results reported by Sohlberg and Mateer (1987) reflect nothing more than spontaneous recovery of function. Nonetheless, the Sohlberg and Mateer (1987) paper evaluates only four subjects with a limited number of dependent variables and no tests of generalization to activities of daily living.

Improved performance on the PASAT has been predictive of an individual's ability to return to work (Lezak, 1983). While suggestive of a treatment remediation effect, the data presented by Sohlberg and Mateer (1987) contain relatively few data points across the phases in the study. In fact, the majority of Sohlberg and Mateer's (1987) claim of a treatment effect is based on two data points obtained during active treatment.

The apparent discrepancy between those studies reporting positive findings and those studies indicating no treatment-related effects appears to be the result of several factors. First, the attention-remediation programs have been based largely on the differing conceptualizations as to what constitutes attentional deficits in TBI patients. As such, it is not surprising that the studies conducted to date have all utilized different paradigms and treatment procedures in their attention-remediation programs. The operational definition of attention also has varied widely across studies. As a result, the selection of attention-remediation outcome variables has not been uniform across studies. This makes meaningful comparisons across studies difficult. A second factor has been the assumption that TBI patients are homogeneous with respect to attention deficits. Finally, the effects of the process of spontaneous recovery of function must be controlled either statistically or in terms of the experimental design of the attention-remediation study.

Clearly, the issue of the efficacy of attention-remediation programs cannot be determined based on the present literature. Further outcome studies are required in order to determine the utility, if any, of attention-remediation programs for TBI survivors.

## REFERENCES

Beck, A. T., Ward, C. H., Mendelsohn, M., Mock, J., & Erbaugh, J. (1961). An inventory for measuring depression. *Archives of General Psychiatry, 4*, 561–571.

Ben-Yishay, Y., Piasetsky, E. B., & Raottok, J. (1987). A systematic method for ameliorating disorder in basic attention. In M. J. Meier, A.J. Benton, & L. Diller (Eds.), *Neuropsychological rehabilitation* (pp. 165–181). New York: Guilford Press.

Conkey, R. C. (1938). Psychological changes associated with head injuries. *Archives of Psychology, 33*, 232.

Craine, J. F., & Gudman, H. E. (1983). *The rehabilitation of brain functions: Principles, procedures, and techniques of neurotraining.* Springfield, IL: Thomas.

Diller, L., Fordyce, W., Jacobs, D., & Brown, M. (1979). *Skill indicators: Skill list.* New York: Rehabilitation Indicators Project.

Gansler, D. A., & McCaffrey, R. J. (1988). Clinical trial of attentional remediation of traumatic brain injured adults. *Journal of Clinical & Experimental Neuropsychology, 10*, 67 (Abstract).

Gansler, D. A., & McCaffrey, R. J. (1991). Remediation of chronic attention deficits in traumatic brain injured patients. *Archives of Clinical Neuropsychology, 6*, 335–353.

Gianutsos, R., & Kintzer, C. (1981). *Computer programs for cognitive rehabilitation* (Computer Programs). Bayport, NY: Life Sciences Associates.

Gray, J. M., & Robertson, I. (1989). Remediation of attentional difficulties following brain injury: Three experimental single case studies. *Brain Injury, 3*, 163–170.

Gronwall, D. (1977). Paced auditory serial addition task: A measure of recovery from concussion. *Perceptual & Motor Skills, 44*, 367–373.

Hersen, M., & Barlow, D. H. (1984). *Single case experimental designs: Strategies for studying behavior change* (2nd ed.). New York: Pergamon Press.

Hirst, W., Spelke, E. S., Reaves, C. L., Caharock, G., & Neisser, U. (1980). Dividing attention without alternation or automaticity. *Journal of Experimental Psychology: General, 109*, 98–117.

Lezak, M. D. (1983). *Neuropsychological assessment.* New York: Oxford University Press.

Lezak, M. D. (1987). Assessment for rehabilitation planning. In N. J. Meier, A. L. Benton, & L. Diller (Eds.), *Neuropsychological rehabilitation* (pp. 41–58). New York: Guilford Press.

Malec, J., Jones, R., Rao, N., & Stubbs, K. (1984). Video game practice effects on sustained attention in patients with craniocerebral trauma. *Cognitive Rehabilitation, 2,* 18–23.

Meyer, A. (1904). The anatomical facts and clinical varieties of traumatic insanity. *American Journal of Insanity, 60,* 373–441.

Miller, E. (1970). Simple and choice reaction time following severe head injury. *Cortex, 6,* 121–127.

Naylor, G. F. K., & Harwood, E. (1972). *Naylor–Harwood Adult Intelligence Scale.* Hawthorn, Victoria: Australian Council for Educational Research.

Ponsford, J. L., & Kinsella, G. (1988). Evaluation of a remedial programme for attentional deficits following closed-head injury. *Journal of Clinical & Experimental Neuropsychology, 10,* 693–708.

Posner, M. (1975). Psychobiology of attention. In M.S. Gazzaniga & C. Blakemore (Eds.), *Handbook of psychobiology* (pp. 441–480). New York: Academic Press.

Posner, M., & Boies, S. J. (1971). Components of attention. *Psychological Review, 78,* 391–408.

Posner, M., Snyder, C., & Davidson, B. (1980). Attention and the detection of signals. *Journal of Experimental Psychology: General, 109,* 160–174.

Ruesch, J. (1944). Dark adaptation, negative after images, tachistoscopic examinations and reaction time in head injuries. *Journal of Neurosurgery, 1,* 243–251.

Russell, W. R. (1971). *The traumatic amnesias.* New York: Oxford University Press.

Russell, W. R. (1975). *Explaining the brain.* New York: Oxford University Press.

Smith, A. (1973). *Symbol digit modalities test manual.* Los Angeles: Western Psychological Services.

Sohlberg, M. M., & Mateer, C. A. (1987). Effectiveness of an attention-training program. *Journal of Clinical & Experimental Neuropsychology, 9,* 117–130.

Sohlberg, M. M., & Mateer, C. A. (1989). *Introduction to cognitive rehabilitation: Theory and practice.* New York: Guilford Press.

Speilberger, C. D., Gorsuch, R. W., & Lushene, R. E. (1970). *State–Trait Anxiety Inventory.* Palo Alto, CA: Consulting Psychologists Press.

Speilberger, C. D., Jacobs, G., Russel, S., & Crane, R. S. (1983). Assessment of anger: The State–Trait Anger Scale. In J. N. Butcher & C. D. Speilberger (Eds.), *Advances in personality assessment* (Vol. 2, pp. 159–187). Hillsdale, NJ: Erlbaum.

Van Zomeren, A. H. (1981). *Reaction time and attention after closed head injury.* Amsterdam: Swets & Zeitlinger.

Van Zomeren, A. H., Brouwer, D. & Deelman, B. G. (1984). Attentional deficits: The riddles of selectivity, speed and alertness. In D. N. Brooks (Ed.), *Closed head injury: Psychological, social and family consequences* (pp. 74–107). New York: Oxford University Press.

Wood, R. L. I., & Fussey, I. (1987). Computer-based cognitive retraining: A controlled study. *International Disability Studies, 9,* 149–153.

# 13

# The Executive Board System

## An Innovative Approach to Cognitive–Behavioral Rehabilitation in Patients with Traumatic Brain Injury

RONALD F. ZEC, RANDOLPH W. PARKS,
JANICE GAMBACH, and SANDRA VICARI

Traumatic brain injuries often result in frontal lobe damage, in addition to diffuse damage, from the impact of the frontal lobes against the protruding frontal bones (Levin, Benton, & Grossman, 1982). Frontal lobe damage produces behavioral, emotional, and cognitive problems, especially impaired executive functioning (Lezak, 1983; Sohlberg & Mateer, 1989). Memory and attentional deficits are also very common long-term sequelae after traumatic brain injuries due to diffuse brain damage that affects both the medial temporal lobe structures and the brain stem. Although impairments in executive functions (e.g., planning, self-monitoring, self-correction) largely determine the extent of psychosocial and vocational recovery following head injury, rehabilitation efforts have been minimal (Sohlberg & Mateer, 1989).

There are few studies in the literature pertaining to the rehabilitation of executive functions (Sohlberg & Mateer, 1989). Cicerone and Wood (1987) reported successful treatment of a patient with traumatic brain injury who displayed both poor planning ability and poor self-control. They used a self-instructional procedure that required the patient to

RONALD F. ZEC • Departments of Psychiatry and Internal Medicine (Division of Neurology), and the Center for Alzheimer Disease and Related Disorders, Southern Illinois University School of Medicine, Springfield, Illinois 62794-9230.    RANDOLPH W. PARKS, JANICE GAMBACH, and SANDRA VICARI • Department of Psychiatry, Southern Illinois University School of Medicine, Springfield, Illinois 62794-9230.

*HANDBOOK OF HEAD TRAUMA: Acute Care to Recovery*, edited by Charles J. Long and Leslie K. Ross. Plenum Press, New York, 1992.

verbalize a plan of behavior before and during execution of the training task—a modified version of the Tower of London Puzzle. Luria (1963) noted the benefits of a behavioral approach for managing executive functioning deficits. Craine (1982) recommended that a routine daily schedule be set up, memorized by the patient and practiced until it becomes automatic, thereby circumventing the executive system. Sohlberg and Mateer (1989) recommend external cuing systems and work involving repetitive structured tasks to facilitate successful functioning despite impaired executive ability. In other words, the environment needs to be modified so that it can compensate for the patient's damaged frontal lobes.

The rehabilitation of impaired executive functions is critically important because they are the major barrier to successful reintegration into the community (Sohlberg & Mateer, 1989). The guiding principle in the rehabilitation of executive functions is organization and structure (Sohlberg & Mateer, 1989). Creation of structure is the key to both retraining executive skills and compensating for deficits in executive functioning. Sohlberg and Mateer (1989) note that although there are a few isolated procedures that have been reported that address specific executive deficits, no comprehensive approach has been developed to address the broad range of executive functioning deficits exhibited by many victims of traumatic brain injury.

The problem is how to provide structure for head injury patients to help them reestablish order in their lives. Both the ability to perform and the motivation to perform are often impaired in victims of traumatic brain injury. The Executive Board System (EBS) was designed to directly, in a simple but elegant fashion, address both the deficits in planning ability and motivation exhibited by patients with closed head injury (Zec, 1985; Zec, Gambach, & Meyers, 1988; Zec & Meisler, 1986). The development of this system was influenced by the principles and techniques associated with the literature dealing with cognitive rehabilitation, cognitive–behavioral modification, behavioral self-regulation, metaintelligence, metacognition, and executive functioning. The EBS involves making a written plan and keeping a written record of one's behavior on index cards called Job Cards. Two key assumptions of this technique are that making plans explicit by writing them down will facilitate planning, and keeping a written record of one's behavior will facilitate the execution of plans. Thus, the EBS can help a person to solve more of his/her daily problems, attain more of his/her goals, and more efficiently and effectively manage more of his/her daily activities. The EBS also addresses the attentional and memory deficits commonly associated with traumatic brain injury in addition to a wide variety of executive functions.

In this chapter, the EBS, an innovative approach to cognitive–behavioral rehabilitation designed to both facilitate everyday functioning and executive skills, will be discussed. In the next section, executive functioning and metacognition will be reviewed.

## EXECUTIVE FUNCTIONING AND METACOGNITION

Executive functioning refers to "those capabilities that enable a person to engage in independent, purposive, self-serving behavior successfully" (Lezak, 1983, p. 28). Metacognition, a closely related concept, is "an awareness of one's own cognitive skills and abilities, and the efficient use of this self-awareness to self-regulate cognitive activity" (Loper & Murphy, 1985, p. 224). Executive functioning is the ability to self-manage one's daily life or in colloquial terms "to be one's own boss" and "to get one's act together."

A person must be able to tell himself what to do and then be able to do it (i.e., to plan and carry out those plans). In other words, one must think (plan) before acting and act (execute or implement) after thinking. Specific executive functions or metacognitive activities include planning, checking, monitoring, testing, evaluating, and revising (Wong, 1985, p. 138). It entails the ability to mobilize, allocate, and coordinate cognitive resources in order to solve problems, achieve goals, and manage one's daily activities.

The concept of "metacognition" developed from the research of John Flavell (1970) on "metamemory" (i.e., knowledge of one's own memory skills and strategies) (Brown, 1978):

> "Metacognition" refers to one's knowledge concerning one's own cognitive processes . . . [and] to the active monitoring and consequent regulation and orchestration of these processes . . . , usually in the service of some concrete goal or objective. (Flavell, 1970, p. 232)

> Metacognitive processes in problem-solving include the following: (1) problem analysis, (2) thinking about what one knows or does not know that may be needed to solve the problem (information gathering), (3) planning, (4) monitoring progress toward a solution. (Miller, 1985, p. 206)

Problem solving can most simply be conceptualized as a two-stage process involving planning and control (i.e., thinking and acting) (Hayes-Roth & Hayes-Roth, 1979). The first step in planning is selecting a goal. However, selecting a goal is a necessary but not sufficient condition to attaining that goal. People often do not follow through on their resolutions. This failure is, in part, due to a lack of planning. "Failing to plan is planning to fail" and "poor planning predicts poor performance." A predetermined course of action is needed (i.e., a person needs to know what he/she is actually going to do to attain that goal).

After setting a goal and formulating a plan to achieve that goal, the plan needs to be implemented. Control processes are necessary to execute a plan. To successfully carry out a plan, one must be able to monitor, evaluate, correct, and reinforce one's own performance. Self-monitoring and self-evaluation are necessary to determine whether the plan being implemented is working or not. If the plan is not working, it must be revised (self-correction).

Lezak (1983) has stated that executive functioning is "the most subtle and central realm of human activity" (p. 508). Lezak identified four major component processes which comprise executive functioning: goal formulation, planning, carrying out goal-directed plans, and effective performance. Each of these is a complex process composed of many subprocesses. Goal formulation requires conceptual and abstraction ability, anticipatory thinking, decision-making, self-awareness, and motivation. Lezak emphasized that "persons who lack the capacity to formulate goals simply do not think of anything to do" (p. 509). Planning involves the ability to conceptualize, abstract, organize steps, generate alternatives, weigh and make choices, and sustain attention. Executing goal-directed plans involves the ability to initiate, maintain, switch, and stop sequences of complex behavior. It also requires flexibility and the ability to shift perceptual, cognitive, and behavioral sets. Effective performance involves the ability to self-monitor, self-correct, and self-regulate.

Stuss and Benson (1986) described executive functioning as the "ultimate mental activity" (p. 246). Executive functioning is "the ability to take the information extracted from other, higher brain systems, verbal and nonverbal, and to anticipate, select goals, experiment, modify, and otherwise act on this information to produce novel responses" (p. 246). Stuss and Benson further explained that "executive control functions" are "called into action in nonroutine or novel situations, and provide conscious direction to the functional systems for efficient processing of information" (p. 244).

The major executive control functions emphasized by Stuss and Benson (1986) are anticipation, goal selection, preplanning, monitoring, and use of feedback (p. 244). Self-awareness is viewed as emerging from the executive functions. Drive (motivation and will) and sequencing (set and integration) are closely related processes controlled by the executive functions. Drive and sequencing regulate the more basic functional systems that include attention, alertness, visuo-spatial skills, autonomic functioning, emotion, memory, sensory/perception, language, motor skills, and cognition.

Lezak (1983), like Stuss and Benson (1986), clearly distinguished between executive functions and more basic cognitive functions. Intact executive functioning is both a necessary and sufficient condition for independent, adaptive behavior (Lezak, 1983):

> So long as the executive functions are intact, a person can sustain considerable cognitive loss and still continue to be independent, constructively self-serving, and productive. When executive functions are impaired, the individual may no longer be capable of satisfactory self-care, of performing remunerative or useful work on his own, or of maintaining normal social relationships regardless of how well preserved are his cognitive capacities-or how high his scores on tests of skills, knowledge, and abilities. (p. 38)

The "behavioral problems arising from impaired executive functions" in patients with brain damage, according to Lezak (1983, pp. 38, 81, 83), include the following: (1) defective capacity for self-control or self-direction (e.g., emotional lability or flattening); (2) heightened tendency to irritability and excitability; (3) impulsivity, disinhibition, overresponsiveness, and problems in modulating and stopping behavior; (4) erratic carelessness; (5) rigidity and difficulty in making shifts in attention and ongoing behavior (e.g., perseveration); (6) deterioration in personal grooming and cleanliness; (7) impaired ability to initiate activity and problems of starting; (8) decreased or absent motivation (anergia); (9) defects in planning; (10) deficits in carrying out goal-directed behavior; (11) defective self-criticism and an inability to perceive performance errors; (12) concreteness and stimulus-bound behavior; (13) poor judgment; (14) poor adaptation to new situations; (15) blunted social responsibility; and (16) impaired mental efficiency.

Impaired executive functions are most closely associated with frontal lobe damage (Lezak, 1983). Stuss and Benson (1986) also closely link executive functioning to the frontal lobes:

> The frontal lobes perform the supervisory, attentional tasks suggested by Shallice, the planning and design formulation proposed by Luria, the establishment of goals postulated by Damasio, and the executive function of Fuster, Lhermitte, Milner, and others (p. 246).

However, Lezak (1983) also pointed out that defective executive functions are also associated with subcortical damage, especially involving limbic structures.

Luria (1973, 1980) refers to the tertiary portions of the frontal lobes (i.e., prefrontal cortex) as the third functional unit of the brain that performs the "universal function of general regulation of behaviour." The prefrontal lobes participate in the integration of conscious activity and organization of complex purposive, goal-directed behavior. When the frontal lobes are damaged there is a "disintegration of goal-directed behavior" (Luria,

1973, 1980) and the "unity of personality is destroyed" (Luria, 1973, 1980). Component prefrontal functions described by Luria include the following executive skills: active anticipation, voluntary attention, abstract thought, initiative, planning, "ability to inhibit irrelevant and inappropriate action," monitoring and checking, and critical judgment. According to Luria (1973, 1980) the prefrontal region is the most important part of "the unit for programming, regulation and verification of activity":

> Man not only reacts passively to incoming information, but creates intentions, forms plans and programmes of his actions, inspects their performance, and regulates his behavior so that it conforms to these plans and programmes; finally he verifies his conscious activity, comparing the effects of his actions with the original intentions and correcting any mistakes he has made. (Luria, 1973, 1980)

In the next section, EBS, a cognitive–behavioral rehabilitation technique designed to promote self-management and improve an individual's executive functioning, is discussed.

## THE RATIONALE AND DESCRIPTION OF THE EBS

> Give a man a fish and feed him for a day; teach a man to fish and feed him for a lifetime. (Chinese proverb)

The EBS or Job Card System is a cognitive–behavioral rehabilitation technique which is designed to both facilitate everyday functioning and improve problem solving or metacognitive skills. It is a simple, versatile method for solving problems, attaining goals, and ordering one's day and life. This method relies upon the use of the "Executive Board" and "Job Cards." A separate Job Card is made up for each task the individual user of the EBS should do during the day, and the cards are assembled into a deck of Job Cards that are organized according to the sequence in which they should be carried out. The Job Card consists of three parts: the task command, the task analysis, and the reinforcement analysis. The task command and task analysis are provided on the front of the Job Card, and the reinforcement analysis is provided on the reverse side (Tables 13.1 and 13.2).

The Executive Board (EB) consists of two rows and two columns of clear plastic pockets (Figure 13.1). The EB comes in two versions to accommodate the two larger

TABLE 13.1.  Anatomy of a Job Card

| | |
|---|---|
| *Front of the Card*: | A PLAN |
| TASK COMMAND: | activity to be done. |
| MATERIALS: | what tools, concrete resources, etc. |
| INFORMATION: | who, when, where, etc. |
| TASK ANALYSIS: | step-by-step plan of action. |
| *Back of the Card*: | BENEFITS |
| REINFORCEMENT ANALYSIS: | a list of the beneficial consequences of successfully doing the activity (WHY). |
| PERSONAL POINT VALUE: | Priority level:A–E (50–10), Difficulty: A–E (50–10). |
| SELF-CONGRATULATIONS: | e.g., health is wealth! |
| CALENDAR FOR THE YEAR: | the date is circled for each day a task is completed. |

TABLE 13.2.    An Example of a Job Card by a TBI Client

---

*Front of the Card*:

TASK COMMAND:    DRIVE SAFELY
MATERIALS:            car in good repair, driver's license, registration, money, gas, map
INFORMATION:        rules of road
TASK ANALYSIS:

(1) Wear seat belts                          (8) Don't drive when fatigued
(2) Use your blinkers                        (9) Pay attention
(3) Do not speed                             (10) Stop on amber
(4) Obey traffic laws                        (11) Drive courteously
(5) Don't cut people off                     (12) Drive defensively
(6) Don't drink and drive                    (13) Leave plenty of time for trip—don't be in a hurry
(7) Keep car in good repair—periodic checks

*Back of the Card*:

REINFORCEMENT ANALYSIS:

(1) Stay alive                               (6) Keep car reliable and durable
(2) Don't hurt someone else                  (7) Avoid losing my license
(3) Avoid giving someone else the hell of head    (8) Avoid injury to myself
    injury                                   (9) It is the right thing to do
(4) Keep insurance rates down
(5) Tickets are expensive/and a waste of money
    and time

AA = 100 points.
"Please don't bump somebody's rump."

---

standard sizes of index cards: 4″ × 6″ or 5″ × 8″. The pockets are mounted on either a 15″ × 15.5″ or a 17″ × 19.5″ piece of poster board (Figure 13.1). The Executive Pocket (EP) is a portable EB which resembles the cover of a checkbook. The deck of Job Cards describing tasks that are to be carried out today are kept in the "Day in Preview" (DIP) pocket in the upper left-hand corner of the EB or EP (i.e., in the Jobs "To Do" column) (Figure 13.1). The user reads the Task Command for the next job, visible through the clear plastic pocket, and proceeds to carry out the task according to the step-by-step instructions provided by the task analysis.

After the task is successfully completed, the user removes the Job Card from the DIP pocket and turns it over, and transfers it to the "Day in Review" (DIR) pocket. The subject

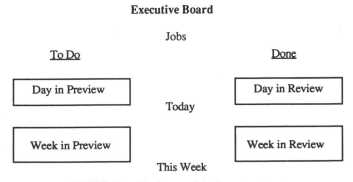

FIGURE 13.1.    The layout of the Executive Board.

then reads the reinforcement analysis consisting of three parts: the reasons why it was important to carry out the task, the personal point value of the task, and the self-congratulations or surrogate social reinforcer. A yearly calendar is provided on the lower right-hand corner of the card. The appropriate date on this calendar should be circled indicating that the task was successfully completed that day. In the process of transferring the completed Job Card to the DIR pocket in the "Done" column on the right-hand side of the EB, the next Job Card in the DIP pocket is revealed. The task command *cues* the user of the EBS about which task is to be carried out next, and the transfer of the completed Job Card and the reading of the reinforcement analysis combine to provide *immediate reinforcement* for having accomplished one's goal.

The EB organizes and advertises the Job Cards. The EB and EP, while useful, are not absolutely necessary in using the EBS. The essential component of the EBS is the "Job Card" that cues and reinforces behavior. The Job Cards organize and advertise the discrete tasks to be done, the steps required to carry out each task, and the task-contingent consequences.

The EBS is designed to improve cognitive and adaptive functioning in both intact and impaired individuals. It is clear from the problems of adaptive functioning displayed by many individuals with traumatic brain injury that these people need some sort of "structure" to put order back into their lives. The EBS is a method of providing "structure" for individuals with traumatic brain injury. The EBS is a *self-help* system that provides both compensation for deficits and retraining of functions. It can be used in the hospital and in the community, and should facilitate the transition from the hospital into the community. Furthermore, using a single technique both in the hospital and in the community should greatly increase the likelihood that the users of the EBS will receive the extensive practice that is necessary for them to learn something well. The more practice and rehearsal in using the EBS, the higher the degree of skill and greater the strength of habit will result. If the use of the EBS becomes a strong *habit and skill*, the user will be able to apply the method to a wide variety of problems over the course of a lifetime.

## Adaptive Skills Improved by the EBS

The EBS helps compensate for deficits and retrain functions in the following *18* adaptive processes: attention, learning, memory, thinking, sequencing, monitoring, motivation, anticipatory thinking (including planning and goal-directed behavior), judging cause-and-effect relationships, novel and complex problem-solving, initiative, maintaining and shifting set, insight, managing information overload and response interference, time management, maintaining an active-independent cognitive and behavioral mode, conditioning, habit and skill development. A brief explanation of how the EBS facilitates each of these functions is provided below:

1. *Attention:* by supplying clear, explicit, salient cues to focus, direct, and sustain attention (thus aiding both selective and sustained attention).
2. *Learning:* by providing repeated rehearsal and practice.
3. *Memory:* by providing written retrieval cues or reminders to jog one's memory; by forcing attention on the to-be-remembered material, by promoting elaborative or deep processing in doing the task analysis, and by promoting repeated rehearsal each time the Job Card is reviewed.

4. *Thinking:* can compensate for paucity of thought and for inappropriate thought by providing self-commands and self-instructions (i.e., raises awareness thus promoting insight).
5. *Sequencing:* by providing an organized sequence of cues or commands (both between tasks and within tasks); by writing steps down in the order they are to be carried out, one is less likely to miss a step or get the steps out of sequence (which will often derail the activity and result in failure to achieve the goal).
6. *Monitoring:* by providing clear, salient, and immediate feedback for behavior when circling the dates on the calendars and calculating and recording one's daily Gross Personal Product.
7. *Motivation:* by providing clear stimulus control and self-reinforcement.
8. *Anticipatory thinking, planning, and goal-directed behavior:* by facilitating forethought and hopefully foresight by preparing for the next day, week, month, etc.
9. *Cause and effect relationships:* related to #8, anticipating consequences.
10. *Novel and complex problem-solving:* by doing a task analysis in which a complex problem or task is broken down into simpler component parts or steps.
11. *Initiative:* by overcoming behavioral inertia in which there is a disinclination to act; this also counters both *procrastination* and avoidant behavior.
12. *Maintaining set and shifting set:* by providing explicit cues about what should be done at a given moment and providing reinforcement for successful task completion.
13. *Insight:* having clear task commands, instructions, and consequences displayed or "in sight" promotes learning and internalization which constitute "insight."
14. *Information overload and response interference:* because of a limited channel capacity and problems with attentional allocation, too much information or too many response choices can lead to being "overwhelmed" and "immobilized," but presenting one clear task command at a time helps prevent stimulus overload and response competition.
15. *Time management:* by budgeting time and scheduling activities to match time demands and resources along with the assignment of priorities.
16. *Passive-dependency:* by instigating, guiding, and motivating self-help behaviors, an individual will become more active, responsible, and independent.
17. *Making and breaking habits:* new and better habits are strengthened by repeatedly practicing an activity, while bad or unwanted habits are broken or extinguished by repeatedly refraining from engaging in an activity in the presence of the situational cues.
18. *Skill development:* new skills can be developed through repeated practice of the step-by-step instructions of an activity along with close self-monitoring, self-assessment, and self-correction.

## Preparing a Job Card

The EBS is an organized way of presenting cues and reinforcement for behavior. The fundamental premise of this approach is the writing of behavioral prescriptions. Behavioral prescriptions are written on index cards called Job Cards that the clients help co-write or write themselves. Each job or activity is written on a separate Job Card that can cue and reinforce specific behaviors. The format of each Job Card consists of a task command and task analysis on the front of the card (i.e., a plan of action) and a reinforcement analysis on the reverse side of the card (i.e., the beneficial consequences).

The task command is the translation of a problem or goal into an operationally defined activity (e.g., "take out the garbage," "take your medication"). The task command consists of a verbal and sometimes visual identification of the task to be carried out (e.g., verbal cue: "brush your teeth"; visual cue: a picture of a toothbrush). The task analysis lists the materials, information, and sequence of steps that are necessary to carry out the task. The task command tells the person *what* to do and the task analysis is the set of instructions that tell the person *how* to do it.

On the back of the card is the reinforcement analysis listing the benefits or consequences of carrying out this task (i.e., tells the person *why* the task should be done)—for example, why take your medication, or why adhere to your diet. People with traumatic brain injury often have difficulty bridging delays of reinforcement or anticipating the distant consequences of their action. The reinforcement analysis consists of a detailed list of the reasons why the task should be done including the intrinsically reinforcing properties of the task (e.g., walking is a relaxing and enjoyable activity), the naturally reinforcing consequences (e.g., walking can improve a person's physical fitness and health), and the extrinsic reinforcing consequences (each mile walked in a day earns a set number of points).

The total personal point value earned for doing a given task is written on the back of the Job Card after the list of reasons for doing the task. The total personal point value for the task is the sum of the personal difficulty level (PDL) and personal priority level (PPL) for the task given in a letter code (A–E) and in points on a scale from 50 to 10 where A or 50 is high priority or difficult, and E or 10 is low priority or easy.

After the priority level and difficulty levels for the task are given, a self-congratulatory statement or a surrogate social reinforcer is provided by a verbal reinforcer (e.g., "well done," "good work," "looking good") or by a memorable saying (e.g., "health is wealth"). Lastly, a calendar for the year is printed in the bottom right-hand corner of the card, and today's date is circled after the task has been successfully completed. At the end of each day the client spends 10 minutes calculating his/her Gross Personal Product (GPP). This involves first circling the date on the calendar on the backs of the Job Cards that were worked on that day (if the circling was not done during the day). Then the client counts the number of Job Cards that were "done" and records that number on the GPP card. This procedure increases the probability that the person will do more of the self-assigned activities over time.

The task and reinforcement analyses should be done by both the client and the case manager working together. It is important that the client—to the extent possible—learn to be a task and reinforcement analyst because this will help stimulate cognitive activity, teach a valuable cognitive skill, and make this a truly self-help system. It will also involve the client more in the rehabilitation program, give the patient a greater sense of control over his/her own life, and lead to a greater commitment to the goals that are set. These task and reinforcement analyses can also be practiced and learned during "think tank" sessions with small groups of clients led by a case manager. As much as possible, however, the analyses should come from the client. The staff functions as consultants, advisors, and coaches to the client by making recommendations and offering encouragement.

In summary, the *Job Card* consists of a *job command*, a *task analysis*, and a *reinforcement analysis*, and *explicitly* answers the questions who, what, when, where, why, and how as they pertain to the job assignment. In other words, the Job Card tells the user *what* to do, *when* and *where* to do it, *who* is involved, *how* to do it, and *why*. This is important because clear and salient cues are needed to help direct and motivate behavior. Unlike mere list-making, Job Cards specify a plan of action and the beneficial consequences for each task to be done. Also, unlike lists, Job Cards can be reused and reorganized on a daily basis and provide a procedure for keeping track of one's performance record.

## Written Plans and Records

There are several advantages to writing plans. First, writing goals and plans on paper can strengthen one's commitment or resolution to act. Second, working problems out on paper facilitates the problem-solving process including both planning and execution. Third, making written notes aids memory. Fourth, writing plans down on Job Cards can help a person keep track of all the tasks that he/she needs to do in a day, a week, a month, etc.

Planning entails the manipulation of many facts or bits of information. Alternative courses of action should be generated, the best course of action needs to be chosen, and step-by-step instructions for carrying out that course of action must be generated and sequenced. Planning can be done more effectively on paper because a person cannot easily do all these operations in one's head. Written notes can help a person manipulate all the relevant facts and to generate and evaluate alternatives. Working problems and plans out on paper can help a person to rearrange, sequence, and juxtapose information. If a plan is written, it is also easier to add a step to the sequence later. In this way, a plan can be revised and improved over time. Thus, writing can facilitate the development of a plan. Also, the more you plan on paper, the more you will also be able to plan in your head due to the frequent rehearsal.

Job Cards facilitate processes that promote memory. Making out a Job Card guarantees that attention (awareness, orientation, registration) has been focused on the to-be-remembered information. Doing a task and reinforcement analysis ensures elaborated encoding of information (depth of processing, elaboration, organization). Repeated exposure to information recorded on Job Cards provides rehearsal (practice, overlearning). Job Cards supply retrieval cues (prompts, reminders) that can "jog" memory.

An example that illustrates the function of reminder cues is what happens when you visit the dentist. The dentist informs you that you are not flossing your teeth adequately and that this will lead to receding gums and the loss of your teeth. Although he/she has not told you anything you did not already know, you are on your best behavior for a few days and floss your teeth. Soon, the regular flossing stops—you have reverted to your old ways. What has happened here is that for a few days you are consciously aware of the dentist's admonishment—his/her words are ringing in your ears but then as these reminder cues fade so does the flossing. Job Cards, by providing written cues, help keep reminders in one's conscious awareness so they can alter behavior.

At the end of the day, the client sorts the deck of Job Cards into a pile of jobs that were done and those that were not done. The date is circled on the calendar on the back of each of the Job Cards that were completed. The number of Job Cards completed is an index of the day's activity or productivity (GPP) and is recorded on another card. Circling the calendars of the Job Cards done that day and calculating the GPP only takes 5–10 minutes. This procedure promotes self-monitoring, self-evaluation, self-correction, and self-reinforcement. It helps reinforce activities successfully completed and reminds you of goals not yet attained.

## Metacognitive Exercise

Each time a client makes out a Job Card, a specific activity of daily living is promoted (e.g., doing the dishes, controlling anger, improving one's diet, studying for an exam, going on a date). In addition, a general metacognitive skill is practiced. The metacognitive skill or problem-solving strategy consists of the following: (1) translating problems/goals into operationally defined activities, (2) writing a self-command (i.e., the task command [e.g., take my medication, take out the garbage, prepare for my job interview]), (3) listing needed materials (e.g., a pen, paper, stamp, envelope, money, shoes, income tax forms, reference book, resume, medication, glass of water), (4) listing needed information (e.g., names, addresses, telephone numbers, cost), (5) listing step-by-step instructions, and (6) listing the consequences of carrying out the plan (health, wealth, accomplishment, helping others, fun). The client learns that any problem, goal, or activity, no matter how simple or complex, can be addressed by using this metacognitive strategy of making out a Job Card. In this way the client learns to generalize this problem-solving and self-management technique to a wide variety of situations. In addition, by making out Job Cards and keeping track of these Job Cards, a person learns to think before he/she acts (plan) and learns to act after thinking (execute). Thus, the EBS not only facilitates daily functioning but teaches a problem-solving technique.

## Problem-Solving Meetings

One of the essential procedural components of the EBS is that the clients attend a weekly 90-minute problem-solving group in which each client makes out a Job Card. The group consists of three to six clients and usually two professional group leaders. Each client goes to the blackboard and works on a problem or goal that they have identified. It does not matter how big or how small the problem/goal may be. It can be something small like going to the movies. Making out a Job Card to go to the movies (i.e., setting a goal, making a plan, and listing the benefits) will increase the probability of actually going to the movies. The client then copies the Job Card on a color-coded index card. Each client's mean GPP (i.e., number of Job Cards and points) achieved that week is calculated and recorded during group.

## CONCLUSIONS

Patients with traumatic brain injury typically have deficits in attention, memory, and problem solving due to diffuse brain damage and prefrontal lobe damage. The impairments in problem solving include difficulty in generating efficient strategies and in monitoring and utilizing feedback. It is necessary to take the long view in working with head injury patients. Conducting brief time-limited training in activities of daily living or social skills is insufficient to assist head injury patients in learning to deal with community life. The EBS provides both compensation for deficits and retraining of functions, including attention, memory, and executive control. In behavioral terms, this method provides clear "reminder cues" and immediate "reinforcing feedback" for productive behavior. It is practical, inexpensive, and easy to use. It can be used in the hospital and the community, and should facilitate transition into the community. Over the past four years we have treated both patients with traumatic brain injury and chronic schizophrenia using the EBS. Our clinical experience and preliminary data indicate that this system is highly successful in gradually improving daily functioning and metacognitive skills in those individuals who consistently apply this technique.

## REFERENCES

Brown, A.L. (1978). Knowing when, where and how to remember: A problem of metacognition. In *Advances in instructional psychology* (Vol. 1, pp. 77–165). Hillsdale, NJ: Erlbaum.

Cicerone, K.D., & Wood, J.C. (1987). Planning disorder after closed head injury: A case study. *Archives of Physical Medicine & Rehabilitation, 68*, 111–115.

Craine, S.F. (1982). The retraining of frontal lobe dysfunction. In L.E. Trexler (Ed.), *Cognitive rehabilitation: Conceptualization and intervention* (pp. 239–262). New York: Plenum Press.

Flavell, J.H. (1970). Developmental studies of mediated memory. In H.W. Reese & L.P. Lipsitt (Eds.), *Advances in child development and behavior* (Vol. 5). New York: Academic Press.

Hayes-Roth, B., and Hayes-Roth, F. (1979). A cognitive model of planning. *Cognitive Science, 3*, 275–310.

Levin, H.S., Benton A.L., & Grossman, R.G. (1982). *Neurobehavioral consequences of closed head injury*. New York: Oxford University Press.

Lezak, M.D. (1983). *Neuropsychological assessment* (2nd ed.). New York: Oxford University Press.

Loper, A.B., & Murphy, D.M. (1985): Cognitive self-regulatory training for underachieving children. In D.L. Forrest-Pressley, G.E. MacKinnon, & T.G. Waller (Eds.), *Metacognition, cognition, and human performance: Vol. 2. Instructional practices* (pp. 223–266). New York: Academic Press.

Luria, A.R. (1963). *Restoration of function after brain injury*. New York: Pergamon Press.

Luria, A.R. (1973). *The working brain: An introduction to neuropsychology*. New York: Basic Books.

Luria, A.R. (1980). *Higher cortical functions in man* (2nd ed.). New York: Basic Books.

Miller, P.H. (1985). Metacognition and attention. In D.L. Forrest-Pressley, G.E. MacKinnon, & T.G. Waller (Eds.), *Metacognition, cognition, and human performance: Vol. 2. Instructional practices* (pp. 181–221). New York: Academic Press.

Sohlberg, M.M., & Mateer, C.A. (1989). *Introduction to cognitive rehabilitation: Theory and practice*. New York: Guilford Press.

Stuss, D.T., & Benson, D.F. (1986). *The frontal lobes*. New York: Raven Press.

Wong, B.Y.L. (1985). Metacognitive and learning disabilities. In D.L. Forrest-Pressley, G.E. MacKinnon, & T.G. Waller (Eds.), *Metacognition, cognition, and human performance: Vol. 2. Instructional practices* (pp. 137–180). New York: Academic Press.

Zec, R.F. (1985). *Working with the psychiatrically disabled: A new approach—The Executive Board System*. Tenth Annual Meeting and Conference of the Illinois Association of Rehabilitation Facilities, Springfield, IL.

Zec, R.F., & Meisler, N. (1986). *Executive Board System: A new approach to cognitive-behavior modification*. Eleventh Annual IAPSRS Conference: International Association of Psychosocial Rehabilitation Services, Cleveland, OH.

Zec, R.F., Gambach, J., & Meyers, R.D. (1988). *Improved adaptive functioning in schizophrenic patients using the "Executive Board System."* Paper presented at the International Neuropsychological Society Meeting, New Orleans, LA.

# Computer-Assisted Cognitive Remediation of Attention Disorders following Mild Closed Head Injuries

## MARVIN H. PODD and DONALD P. SEELIG

Roughly half of the head injuries in this country are of the mild closed head variety, and many victims develop postconcussional syndrome. Attention deficits are almost always present in this syndrome (Jennett & Teasdale, 1981; Sbordone, 1986). The ability to attend and concentrate is a necessary precondition for most higher cognitive functions and should therefore be effectively treated before addressing other cognitive deficits, such as memory impairment, spatial problems, or abstract reasoning difficulties.

Neuropsychological assessment is the best method for evaluating sequelae to mild closed head injuries because routine neurological tests such as CT scan, MRI, and EEG are usually within normal limits, as is the neurological exam. Many postconcussional syndrome patients perform abnormally on tests measuring attention, concentration, immediate visual and/or verbal memory, and processing speed (Gronwall, 1986; Gronwall & Wrightson, 1974; Modlin & Sargent, 1986; Rimel, Giordani, Barth, Boll, & Jane, 1981; Sbordone, 1986). Other specific cognitive difficulties may show up from time to time (e.g., cognitive inflexibility, impaired spatial organization, dyscalculia, perceptual problems, and intellectual deficits).

Lynch (1984) was among the first to use the computer in cognitive remediation efforts, initially with the game Breakout and later with a variety of games available on Atari and Apple computers. Arcade-type games made the treatment challenging and fun but might have been too complex and demanding for many types of brain dysfunction. Gianutsos

MARVIN H. PODD • Department of Psychology, National Navy Medical Center, Bethesda, Maryland 20814-5011.    DONALD P. SEELIG • Psychological Consultation and Treatment Center, Fort Washington, Maryland 20744.

*HANDBOOK OF HEAD TRAUMA: Acute Care to Recovery*, edited by Charles J. Long and Leslie K. Ross. Plenum Press, New York, 1992.

(1981) developed programs specifically for visual perception, attention, and memory disorders. She also included a manual to explain her programs. However, the manual and some of the programs were unclear, and none of the programs were in the form of games. Therefore, motivation may not have been maximized for many of the patients. Bracy (1983) developed a package of computer programs ("Foundations") which included attentional and perceptual, problem-solving, and memory remediation programs. Each area was sold as a separate package, making it more expensive than Gianutsos's remedial package. The graphics were colorful and superior to Gianutsos's programs, but many of the programs were still more like tasks than games. Sbordone (1985) published attentional memory programs and a problem-solving remedial program. The latter program seemed to baffle many psychologists who were therefore unable to use it remedially with their patients. Although it was in a gamelike format, and both interesting and challenging, it was too complex and demanding for a brain dysfunctional population. Ben-Yishay and Piatsky (1985) developed several modules for retraining patients in his head injury program. He concluded that only the attentional programs seemed systematically helpful. Another program, CAPTAIN (Sandford & Browne, 1986), having 21 exercises related to attention, visual–motor, and conceptual skills, required more expensive hardware than most other programs but it had the added dimension of using a "mouse." The "mouse" added interest, and the programs were in a game format.

The computer-based cognitive remediation program (neurXercise™, 1989; Podd & Seelig, 1989) we will discuss in this chapter provides the gamelike format absent in most of the other programs. It covers more cognitive areas and introduces multiple levels of complexity within many of the exercises that permits the patient to begin at a level in which some success can be assured. On most of the exercises feedback appears on the screen following responses, and help screens appear when the patient is experiencing difficulty. These help screens suggest "alternate functional systems" (Luria, 1973) through which the task may be accomplished by bypassing the dysfunctional link. The trainer may at times determine which help screens should appear and in what order, based upon the results of the neuropsychological assessment. There are a total of 31 exercises, several in each of the six modules (Attention, Perception, Memory, Judgment, Reasoning, and Daily Living). Table 14.1 presents the modules and the types of skills included in each. This is the only program to include ecologically valid exercises (i.e., the Daily Living module). It is also the only program to feature social judgment exercises. A manual is provided which teaches the trainer how to use the program in a step-by-step fashion, analyzes the different exercises, and provides guidance in developing a remedial program. Criteria are suggested for each exercise based on the senior author's experience. Normative data are currently being gathered and will take the place of these guidelines. In addition, several research projects are being pursued in order to answer many basic questions about the effectiveness of cognitive remediation and mechanisms underlying successful treatment with a variety of populations.

This chapter will cover remediation of attention/concentration deficits using the Attention module of neurXercise™. The exercises, their neuropsychological makeup, and their appropriate selection for remediation are discussed. A method for enhancing skill generalization, a multicriterion approach for evaluating effectiveness of treatment, and the role of psychotherapy in treating brain dysfunction will also be presented.

## DESCRIPTION OF THE ATTENTION EXERCISES

Darts presents a colorful, stylized dartboard and a slow-moving "dart" that begins traveling horizontally across the bottom of the screen once the trainee presses any key. Another key press projects the dart vertically to the target. Points are awarded for the accuracy of each shot. Printed feedback is provided on screen after each shot. A focused attentional strategy is suggested. If the trainee's attention begins to fade, as reflected by two consecutive shots which miss the target, a help screen presents a strategy for focusing the trainee's attention. Parameters which can be set by the trainer include length of exercise, skill level, amount of information on screen, and whether instructions will be presented.

There are three skill levels in this exercise. Level 1 presents a dartboard with a pair of guidelines leading directly to the bull's-eye. The trainee needs only concentrate on these guidelines to make a perfect shot, thereby minimizing the visual scanning and tracking component and making the exercise almost entirely a visual, focused attention exercise. On Level 2 the dart moves at the same speed as Level 1 but the guidelines are farther apart. The trainee must concentrate on the middle of this wider space to make a perfect shot. Scanning and tracking are still minimized if the trainee focuses on the center of the space between the guidelines. In Level 3 the display is the same as in Level 2 but the dart moves faster. The number of darts used to reach a designated score is displayed at the end of the exercise. This score is automatically recorded and stored on the Master Disk.

Get Q is a discrimination and reaction time exercise which requires the trainee to attend to the screen and press a key whenever a Q appears. Written feedback is presented on screen after each key press. The trainee may adjust instructions, skill level, and immediate feedback on latency of response.

Level 1 of Get Q is a simple Go/No-Go paradigm requiring the trainee to press RETURN as soon as he/she spots a Q and to do nothing when other letters appear. Letters remain on screen for 4.5 seconds. The letters appear initially in center screen but later in different places. Number of correct discriminations and reaction time are the scores recorded for the center and each quadrant. In Level 2 the trainee is asked to press RETURN when seeing a Q and to press the space bar when a different letter appears. In addition to making a letter discrimination, trainees are required to make differential motor responses. Accuracy and latency of response are recorded. Level 3 uses the same format but stimuli are presented more quickly.

Two in One requires the trainee to type an alternating sequence of numbers and letters. While little concentration is needed to type 1 through 26 or A through Z, sustained and divided attention are required to alternate numbers and letters while maintaining the sequence of each. The visual scanning component is limited to finding letters and numbers on the keyboard. Incorrect responses are signaled by a tone; the incorrect answer blinks until it is corrected. Time to complete the exercise and number of errors appear on screen and are recorded on the Master Disk.

Level 1 of Two in One requires trainees to alternate between the numbers 1 through 26 and the letters A through Z. In Level 2 the alternation is double digits and double letters (e.g., 11AA22BB, etc.). Level 3 is a "serial threes" paradigm [i.e., the trainee must perform the alternations task counting by threes (e.g., 1A4D7G, etc.)]. All three levels of this exercise are verbal (i.e., letters and numbers). This exercise requires sustained and

TABLE 14.1. A Descriptive Analysis of neurXercise™

| | Attention | Perception | Memory | Reasoning | Judgment |
|---|---|---|---|---|---|
| Darts | Visual attention on a central spot | Very mild component; visual–motor skill | | | |
| Get Q | Visual attention on a central spot and on random places on the monitor | Scanning; visual–motor; letter discrimination | Mild component: different responses for different stimuli | | |
| Two in One | Concentration on alternation and on which response is next | Scanning keyboard for number and letter location; spatial operations (mental arithmetic) | | | |
| Type it | Concentration | Visual–motor coordination for typing | Slight component on hardest items | Most difficult items require generating members of given categories, performing operations on words, etc. | |
| Flasher | Attention to audiovisual patterns; concentration on the sequence when replicating it | Spatial component and strategies using location | Minimum auditory, visual, and verbal memory, especially on Level 3 | | |
| Shaping Up | Attention to size differences | Visual discrimination of size differences; sequencing | Visual memory on Levels 2 and 3 | | |
| Compare | Attention to size differences | Visual size discrimination | | | Avoid irrelevant distraction |
| Naval Strike | Inhibition of response when timing is unsynchronized | Visual perception and spatial organization in aiming, dropping bombs, and taking changing speeds into account | | Strategy planning for which ships at high speed should be bombed | Make adjustment based on observation of one's own performance |
| Run Silent | Attention on which missile to fire on Level 3 | Spatial planning for accurate aiming and firing | Remember keys for sub and plane; remember to alternate and plot different trajectories on level 3 | | Make adjustment based on observation of one's own performance |
| Invaders | Sustained attention on stimulus location and movement | Right–left discrimination; visual–spatial organization; visual–motor coordination; visual scanning | Remember to move in right angles only; remember key codes | Avoid boxing oneself in; reasoning out when it is not safe to intercept the invader; anticipating where he will probably go | Avoid panicking when invader jumps and leaves a space mine; cognitive flexibility |

| Game | Attention | Perception/Discrimination | Memory | Strategy | Problem Solving |
|---|---|---|---|---|---|
| Bomber | Attention to boundaries within which bomb must be dropped | Visual perception and spatial analysis in aiming and dropping bombs | | | Determine best rocks to bomb toward end of game to get highest score; use feedback from one's performance to adjust and find best strategies toward end of game |
| Dart Board | Attention to speed of dart and bull's-eye target area | Visual scanning of dart and bull's-eye; visual–motor coordination | | | |
| Even Flashier | Same as Flasher | Visual scanning of flashing sequence; auditory perception of pitch pattern | Nonverbal auditory and visual memory (beeps and flashes); spatial and verbal memory strategies | | |
| Symbol Memory | Attention to stimuli appearing on screen | Shape discrimination of stimuli and response choices; visual scanning of response choices to select the ones seen | Recognition and recall of nonverbal material; strategies include verbal memory | Transformation from shape to symbol | |
| Concentration | Attend to stimuli and their location | Visual–spatial organization of where objects are located | Visual and spatial memory; strategies include visuoverbal and audiovisual memory | Strategies include a logical systematic approach to the task | Avoid perseverating on incorrect response |
| Memory Game | Attend to stimuli appearing on screen | Letter discrimination; word discrimination | Verbal encoding on Level 1; memory on Level 2; strategies on Level 2 include audio-associational memory, audioverbal memory, and audiovisual memory | | Sufficient study time must be taken by the player prior to removing stimuli from screen on level 2 |
| Foreign Intrigue | Attention to detail | Letters have similar shapes; the same pictures are shown in different spatial orientations | Recognition of verbal and nonverbal stimuli after a brief study period; visual and audioverbal memory | Strategies include consonant encoding on Level 1 | |
| Line Up | Attention to facial details | Discrimination of subtle facial details | Visual recognition; audioverbal memory strategy can be used | Deduction of which face was not seen on Level 2 | |

(Continued)

TABLE 14.1. (Continued)

| | Attention | Perception | Memory | Reasoning | Judgment |
|---|---|---|---|---|---|
| Super Line Up | Attention to hair color and clothing style | Perception of different colors | Visual recognition; audioverbal memory strategy can be used | | |
| Tower of Hanoi | Concentration for planning and not repeating the same moves | Visual–spatial perception and operations in space both mentally and as seen on screen | | Planning moves in advance | Developing strategies based on recognition of faults on previous moves |
| Vocabulary | Attend to clues | | | Abstraction ability; flexibility in reasoning; deductive powers at beginning (definitions); inductive powers based on subsequent hints | Taking all hints into account and ensuring guesses are consistent with the hints and feedback |
| Number Guesser | Attention to feedback | | | Understanding relationships between numbers | Use of feedback to improve problem solving |
| Strategy | Attend to the computer's moves and to the entire board | Visual scanning; visual–spatial organization of sequences across four grids | | Planning strategy; flexible thinking to modify strategies while blocking computer from winning | Use implications of feedback from computer's move to generate next move |
| Spies | Attention to subtle differences | Visual perception of subtle differences | | Abstract reasoning; categorization | |
| Detective | Attention to letter sequences on some items | Perception of relationships through the visual channel | | Verbal and nonverbal analogies | Implementation of alternate strategies when the old ones fail |
| Golf | Attention to feedback | Working with distances and relationships | Remembering functions served by different clubs and relationship among different numbered clubs | Planning and inductive reasoning | Use of feedback to learn and improve score |
| Mission Decode | Attention to details for generating hypotheses | | | Figure out underlying principle leading to correct answers. Principles become increasingly abstract. Concept formation; flexible thinking | Use of feedback to find correct principle |

| | | | | | |
|---|---|---|---|---|---|
| Hid In The Grid | Attention to feedback | Use of compass directions; spatial analysis | | Understanding implications of feedback | Use of feedback to improve ability in game |
| Silent Talk | Attention to facial expression and body tension on drawings | Perceiving visual–nonverbal cues | | Reasoning out possibilities based on cues | Making judgments based on visual–nonverbal cues and feedback |
| Shopping List | Attention to stimuli on screen | | Visuoverbal memory | Abstract categories used to help organize and remember | Implementation of strategies like categorization |
| Body Language | Same as Silent Talk | Same as Silent Talk | | Same as Silent Talk | Exercising judgment based on implications of visual–nonverbal perceptions. Corrective feedback provided to improve judgment |
| Buying Power | Attention to questions and feedback | | Recalling Level 2 prices when performing Level 3 (short-term memory) | Understanding and using number relationships | Use of monetary system and price information to prevent getting shortchanged or overcharged |
| Map Reading | Attention to map, destination, and instructions | Spatial organizational skills; visual scanning; visual–motor skills when using joystick | | Planning ahead | |
| What's My Name | Attention to names, facial features, and associations suggested on the game | Perceiving a prominent feature and visualizing the face and the feature linked to the name cue | Verbal memory of a name linked to visual–nonverbal memory of face or prominent feature. Strategies include audioverbal–association memory and visuoverbal–association memory | Peg word system provides a logical strategy for recollection | |

divided attention which is different from the focused and selective attention involved in the exercises discussed earlier in this section.

Type It requires the trainee to study written directions as long as he/she wishes, remove them from the screen, and then carry them out. Adjustable parameters include skill level and use of instructions. At levels of greater complexity, additional concentration and study time are required, which increases the use of focused attention. Carrying out the directions on screen requires some degree of visual memory—or audioverbal memory if the trainee repeats the directions aloud. Earlier parts of the exercise are simple, overlearned, and have little or no memory component. The score is the number of commands correctly followed.

Level 1 of Type It utilizes from one to four keys which are numbers and letters. In Level 2 the trainee is directed to type specific combinations of increasing complexity with the right hand and others with the left hand. In Level 3 the amount to be typed increases, verbally emitted responses (e.g., recite the alphabet) are sometimes required, and simple reasoning must at times be performed in carrying out the command (e.g., type the names of four animals). The trainer must be vigilant during this exercise as the computer cannot detect whether the trainee is using the requested hand or properly typing names of family members. The score is the number of correct responses.

Flasher is a computerized version of "Simon Says." It requires the trainee to match the sequence of flashing colors and tones produced by the computer. It is a visual–nonverbal and auditory–nonverbal attention/concentration exercise which requires minimal memory until the trainee approaches the criterion for normal performance, regardless of level of complexity. The trainee responds by typing in sequence the initial letters of each color flashed. These letters remain on screen at all times as reminders. Adjustable parameters include skill level and several alternate strategies (all, some, or none of which can be preprogrammed as help screens). The order in which these strategies appear is also determined by the trainer. These strategies include using the audioverbal channel, visuo-spatial cues, and "chunking" the individual stimuli into groups. All levels present four stimuli of different colors (red, yellow, blue, green), each associated with a different tone.

Level 1 randomly selects two of the four color–tones and randomly produces a sequence using these two color–tones. The series begins with a sequence of two flashes/tones. The number of these increases until the trainee fails to match the sequence. When the help screens fail to improve the trainee's score, or when the trainee correctly matches a sequence of eight or more color–tones, the exercise ends and the score is recorded. Level 2 randomly selects three color–tones and Level 3 randomly selects from among the four color–tones. Thus, concentration demands are made by increasing the number of stimuli involved in the exercise. Because speed of presentation is relatively slow, memory plays a minor role before the trainee approaches criterion.

Thus, the Attention module affords an opportunity to work on simple, focused attention tasks in the verbal sphere using Get Q and the nonverbal sphere with Darts; sustained and divided attention on Two in One; and complex attentional tasks in verbal and nonverbal modalities using Type It and Flasher, respectively. If additional work on divided attention is indicated, this may be accomplished using homogeneous or heterogeneous exercises. For example, working on Get Q while simultaneously performing the Seashore Rhythm Test divides attention between verbal and tonal stimuli. It is even more difficult to perform homogeneous divided attention tasks. Such a task would include two exercises within the same modality, verbal or nonverbal. Examples which might be used include working on Two in One while reciting the names of animals, or working on Darts while naming the colors on page 2 of the Stroop Color Word Test.

With this as background, we can now discuss how to choose from among these exercises in order to develop an individualized plan for remediation of attention deficits.

## SELECTING EXERCISES FOR ATTENTION REMEDIATION

To determine which exercises should be selected, the first step is to identify cognitive strengths and weaknesses based on neuropsychological test interpretation. Figure 14.1 presents a Luria–Nebraska Neuropsychological Battery profile on E.Y., a man who suffered a closed head injury seven months prior to testing. Based on behavioral observation and item analysis, the Rhythm (C2) and Receptive Speech (C6) scales are interpreted as reflecting concentration/attention difficulties and word finding problems, respectively. These are the scales showing the most impairment. Low scores on Visual (C4) and Reading (C8) scales suggest a relative strength in the visual area.

The next step is to select exercises from the neurXercise™ Attention module which emphasize the patient's strengths and minimize the patient's weaknesses. This allows the patient to use areas of strength to bolster the attention remediation effort. There are five different attention/concentration exercises. Each contains three levels of increasing demand or difficulty, making a total of 15 combinations. Nine of the combinations are verbal and six are nonverbal (three are visual and three are audiovisual).

Table 14.2 presents a neuropsychological analysis of each exercise in the Attention module. Darts and Flasher have a strong visual component while minimizing the potential verbal weaknesses uncovered in the neuropsychological testing. Therefore, these appear to be good candidates for E.Y.'s attention retraining program since visual skills are a strength, according to Figure 14.1. E.Y.'s performance on Darts and Flasher are depicted in Figures 14.2 and 14.3, respectively. Figure 14.2 demonstrates that E.Y. meets the criterion for success (two consecutive trials on which he achieved 1000 points in less than 26 shots) but has more difficulty on Level 3. He eventually met the same criterion on Level 3 as well.

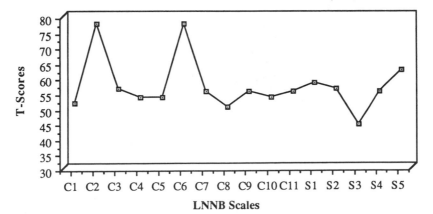

FIGURE 14.1. Pretraining results.

TABLE 14.2.   Neuropsychological Analysis of the Attention Exercises in neurXercise™

| | Attention | Perception | Memory | Reasoning |
|---|---|---|---|---|
| Darts | Visual attention on a central spot | Mild component; visual–motor skill | | |
| Get Q | Visual attention on a central spot and on random places on the monitor | Scanning; visual–motor; letter discrimination | Mild component: different responses for different stimuli | |
| Two in One | Sustained attention for number and letter | Scanning keyboard | | |
| | | Spatial operations in mental arithmetic | | |
| Flasher | Attention to audiovisual patterns; concentration on the sequence when replicating it | Spatial component and strategies using location | Auditory, visual and verbal | |
| Type It | Focused attention | Visual–motor coordination | Recall on hardest items | Generating members of given categories; performing operations on words, etc. |

Figure 14.3 demonstrates steady improvement on Flasher and the criterion for success is eventually met in the fourth training session. Each exercise selected should be performed to criterion at the most demanding level, if possible.

When the trainee has successfully completed work on the attention/concentration exercises, the trainer should next evaluate skill generalization and treatment effectiveness.

## SKILL GENERALIZATION AND TREATMENT EFFECTIVENESS

To increase the likelihood that the target skill will generalize, several attention/concentration exercises should be performed to criterion. In the case of E.Y. we presented him with remedial tasks on both Darts and Flasher; he works on these until he meets the criteria for successful performance. To test for skill generalization, the neuropsychological battery is repeated and his score on the Rhythm scale (C2) is compared with the pretraining score on the same scale. Figure 14.4 reveals a dramatic improvement of two and a half standard deviations.

The question of practice effects accounting for improvement, rather than change resulting from treatment, should be addressed here. The patient had repeated exposure to the computer tasks which were selected because of their theoretical link with attention and concentration. If improvement is related solely to task-dependent effects, no significant changes should be differentially observed on the most attention-dependent scale (Rhythm) of the Luria–Nebraska. However, this was one of the scales that changed the most, although its content bears no similarity to the computer tasks. The Rhythm scale is linked to the remedial exercises only by the a priori theoretical notion that attention underlies ability to perform well on the Attention module. It is unlikely that taking the test a second time made

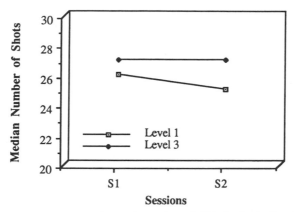

FIGURE 14.2. Attention training on darts—Comparison of difficulty levels (Level 1 vs. Level 3).

a significant difference based on the simplicity of the items to begin with, and because of the high degree of test–retest reliability among neurologic patients (Moses & Maruish, 1987).

In addition to performance on neuropsychological tests and exercises, subjective report is critical for assessing improved functioning. The patient and significant others are important sources of these data. For example, E.Y. initially complained that he could not concentrate on professional journals for more than a minute or two; following attention remediation he complained just as adamantly that he could not concentrate on professional journals for more than an hour or two.

Another measure of treatment effectiveness is job performance ratings, especially if pretreatment and posttreatment comparisons can be made. E.Y. received a rating of "outstanding" after treatment. Another patient, who ran his own business, was initially unable to do so for over a year after his head injury. The head injury had left him not only

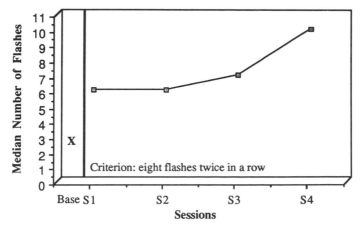

FIGURE 14.3. Performance on flasher—Difficulty Level 3.

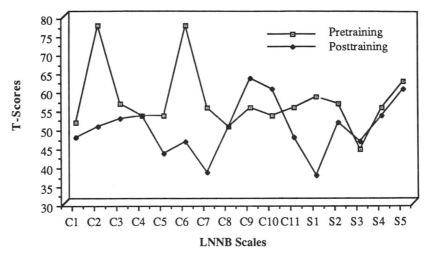

FIGURE 14.4. Pretraining versus posttraining.

with concentration problems but also with visual scanning and spatial difficulties. These precluded his being able to find his inventory on his shelves. Following attention remediation, practice with programs from the Perception module improved his scanning and spatial abilities. He was then able to take control of his business again and expand it.

Lastly, patient follow-up is an important indicator of continued success over time. This should be accomplished by repeat testing and gathering updated information from the patient, significant others, and the job. If performance has deteriorated, determine the cause (e.g., depression, neurological event secondary to or independent of the head injury). Thereafter, institute appropriate interventions such as psychotherapy, medication, neurological evaluation, etc. Figure 14.5 depicts E.Y.'s neuropsychological performance in pretreatment, posttreatment, and follow-up. Attention/concentration gains are maintained 14 months after they were initially documented by testing. A potentially critical, but often overlooked, factor in remedial work with head-injured patients is the inclusion of psychotherapy in the treatment plan.

## THE ROLE OF PSYCHOTHERAPY IN COGNITIVE REMEDIATION

In addition to cognitive remediation, an important part of treatment for patients with head injuries is concurrent psychotherapy. This is often a crucial factor in assisting the patient to become open and emotionally ready to utilize remediation. These patients are often depressed and anxious about their conditions and the effects the injury has had on their job performance and role in the family. If they are not given help with these areas of concern, they will find it difficult to put forth their best effort on the remedial exercises and will benefit little, if at all. Remediation and psychotherapy can be given concurrently. In my experience, those who report that their patients do not improve with cognitive remediation, have not provided concurrent psychotherapy; those who find it successful have

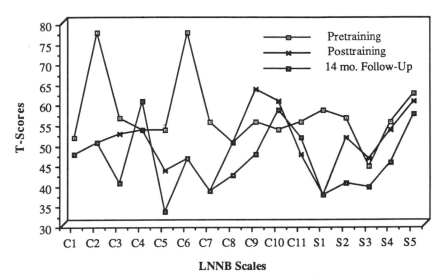

FIGURE 14.5. Stability after 14 months.

included psychotherapy as part of the treatment (Ben-Yishay & Diller, 1981; Goldstein & Ruthven, 1983; Prigatano, 1987; Sbordone, 1986). This may have been a critical factor in Ponsford and Kinsella's study (1988) in which they found that a program for the cognitive remediation of attention deficits was unsuccessful when compared to a control group. We are currently conducting a carefully controlled study that examines the role of psychotherapy in successful cognitive remediation (Podd, House, Miller, Krehbiel, & Reeves, in progress).

## KEYS TO SUCCESSFUL REMEDIATION

To review, the keys to successful cognitive remediation of attention deficits are:

1. Create an individualized treatment program based on the strengths and weaknesses revealed by neuropsychological testing.
2. Provide psychotherapy to optimize emotional readiness for cognitive remediation and to resolve emotional sequelae of the head injury.
3. Use several attention/concentration tasks and exercises to increase the likelihood of skill generalization.
4. Practice each exercise until the criteria for improved or normal performance are met.
5. Increase the attention/concentration demand on each task until improved or normal performance is achieved on the most demanding level.
6. Assess improvement on measures of neuropsychological performance, on reports by the trainee and significant others, and on job performance.
7. Provide periodic follow-up to assure that treatment benefits are maintained over time and provide appropriate intervention when they are not.

## REFERENCES

Ben-Yishay, Y., & Diller, L. (1981). Rehabilitation of cognitive and perceptual deficits in people with traumatic brain damage. *International Journal of Rehabilitation Research*, *4*, 208–210.

Ben-Yishay, Y., & Piatsky, G. (1985, May). *Systematic cognitive retraining following traumatic head injury: Remediation or amelioration?* Paper presented at the National Association of Rehabilitation and Training Centers Conference, Washington, DC.

Bracy, O. L. (1983). Computer based cognitive rehabilitation. *Cognitive Rehabilitation*, *1*, 7–8.

Gianutsos, R. (1981). *Computer programs for cognitive rehabilitation.* Software published by author.

Goldstein, G., & Ruthven, L. (1983). *Rehabilitation of the brain-damaged adult.* New York: Plenum Press.

Gronwall, D. (1986). Rehabilitation programs for patients with mild head injury: Components, problems and evaluation. *Journal of Head Trauma Rehabilitation*, *1*(2), 53–62.

Gronwall, D., & Wrightson, P. (1974). Delayed recovery of intellectual function after minor head injury. *Lancet*, *2*, 605–609.

Jennett, B., & Teasdale, G. (1981). *Management of head injuries.* Philadelphia: Davis.

Luria, A. R. (1973). *The working brain.* New York: Basic Books.

Lynch, W. J. (1984). *A guide to Atari home computer and Apple II+/IIe programs for rehabilitation settings* (6th ed.). (Available from W. J. Lynch, Ph.D., 3801 Miranda Avenue, Palo Alto, CA 94304)

Modlin, H. C., & Sargent, J. (1986). Neuropsychological assessment in a head injury case: The positive value of negative findings. *Bulletin of the Menninger Clinic*, *50*, 50–57.

Moses, J. A., Jr., & Maruish, M. E. (1987). A critical review of the Luria–Nebraska Neuropsychological Battery literature: 1. Reliability. *International Journal of Clinical Neuropsychology*, *9*(4), 149–157.

Podd, M. H., Mills, M. W., & Seelig, D. P. (1989). neurXercise™ cognitive remediation software (available from M. H. Podd).

Podd, M. H., Mills, M. W., & Seelig, D. P. (1989). *A manual for neurXercise™* (available from M. H. Podd).

Podd, M. H., House, J. F., Miller, J., Krehbiel, M., & Reeves, D. (in progress). Neurophysiological changes in the EEG as a function of successful cognitive remediation of attention deficits in postconcussional patients.

Ponsford, J. L., & Kinsella, G. (1988). Evaluation of a remedial programme for attentional deficits following closed head injury. *Journal of Clinical & Experimental Neuropsychology*, *10*(6), 693–708.

Prigatano, G. (1987). Neuropsychological rehabilitation after brain injury: Some further reflections. In M. Williams & C. Long (Eds.), *The rehabilitation of cognitive disabilities.* New York: Plenum Press.

Rimel, R. W., Giordani, B., Barth, J., Boll, T. J., & Jane, J. A. (1981). Disability caused by minor head trauma. *Neurosurgery*, *9*, 221–228.

Sandford, J. A., & Browne, R. J. (1986). *CAPTAIN.* Unpublished manuscript.

Sbordone, R. J. (1985). *Computer-assisted cognitive rehabilitation.* Unpublished manuscript.

Sbordone, R. J. (1986, August). *A neuropsychological approach to cognitive rehabilitation.* Presented at a workshop entitled Neurobehavioral syndromes: Their assessment and treatment, Naval Hospital, Bethesda, MD.

# IV

# Outcome Prediction following Head Injury

# 15

# Recovery from Head Trauma: A Curvilinear Process?

## CHRISTY L. JONES

### INTRODUCTION

Literally millions of Americans suffer from head injury annually (Caveness, 1977), and nearly one half million of these injuries are severe and require medical treatment and possible rehabilitation (Kolb, 1989). Head injuries occur at the highest frequency between the ages of 2 and 6 and again between 15 and 18 years of age (Gordon, 1989). An analysis of trauma victims from two trauma centers indicates that head injury is the most expensive and time-consuming form of medical emergency for the American public (MacKenzie, Siegel, Shapiro, Moody, & Smith, 1988). While advancing medical technology has significantly decreased the number of deaths resulting from these accidents (Levin, Grossman, Rose, & Teasdale, 1979), progress in the areas of outcome prediction and rehabilitation has been slow to follow (Long & Gouvier, 1982). One possible reason for the paucity of progress in these areas is the lack of a well-defined conceptualization of the course of recovery.

The justification of the investment of time into the development of an empirically based recovery curve lies in the curve's potential to increase the understanding of the course of recovery, particularly in four domains. First, such a curve would allow the therapist to answer the question: to what degree will a patient's premorbid level of functioning be restored and how long will this process take? Second, it is likely that a more detailed description of the course of recovery will facilitate insights into the mechanisms of this process (Dikmen, Reitan, & Temkin, 1983). Third, further information concerning the mechanisms as well as a person's position in the recovery process are needed in order to devise the most efficient treatment strategies. Fourth, this curve may serve as an important research tool. If individual cases can be extrapolated to a standard curve, the curve could

CHRISTY L. JONES • Department of Psychology, Memphis State University, Memphis, Tennessee 38152.

*HANDBOOK OF HEAD TRAUMA: Acute Care to Recovery*, edited by Charles J. Long and Leslie K. Ross. Plenum Press, New York, 1992.

provide investigators with a baseline against which the value of various interventions could be evaluated.

Although there are clinicians who implicitly view recovery as a curvilinear function which initially occurs at a fast pace and becomes slower as the time since injury increases, further research is needed in order to substantiate this clinical prediction (Brooks, Deelman, Van Zomeren, Van Dongen, Van Harskamp, & Aughton, 1984; Dikmen *et al.*, 1983). A possible reason for the lack of a clear conceptualization of recovery is that the number of factors affecting the course of recovery is too great to be represented by a single curve (without a large amount of variance). Many factors such as time since injury, complexity of the ability assessed, severity of injury, and the age of the individual at the time of injury have all been posited to influence the clinician's interpretation of an individual's recovery from head trauma. In order to adequately analyze the possibility of the existence of a recovery curve by which clinicians could facilitate communication and understanding of their patients' recovery course to the entire family, these factors must all be incorporated into such a model.

The numerous possible combinations of these factors in any given sample of head-injured individuals, sample heterogeneity, have been coined as the perennial problem of neuropsychological research (Lezak & Gray, 1984). The debate between scientists using single case versus group designs is amplified in populations in which heterogeneity of the data and variance are high. The major argument against those choosing to use group data is the introduction of added variance. Therefore, when using group data, a priori decisions must be made in order to obtain the most homogeneous sample possible. In addition, the interpretation of results with large variances should be treated with suspicion in these instances.

A second alternative is the single case design with repeated testings. The two major shortcomings of this design include limited generalizability to a more heterogeneous population as well as difficulties with the interpretation of practice effects and alternate forms of assessment measures. Others have chosen the middle ground between these two extremes suggesting that a more feasible solution may be to adopt the strategy that chooses the most frequently occurring pattern of individual recovery as the model for the population (Brooks *et al.*, 1984). For example, recovery from injuries resulting in the loss of consciousness has been described in terms of the series of behavioral sequelae through which individuals progress; this is based upon clinical observations of the most frequent patterns in this population. An examination of the designs of the existing empirical research may provide possible explanations for the discrepancies that emerge when describing the course of recovery.

It is the aim of this chapter to investigate the existence of a standard model of recovery by examining the role that individual factors play in the recovery process. This analysis will begin with an overview of the mechanisms involved in acceleration/deceleration injuries across various levels of severity as well as the neuroanatomical correlates of injury and recovery. A summary of a model in the current literature based primarily upon clinical experience will then be presented, followed by the refutation or support of this model through an empirical study that investigates both recovery's course and the factors that make this process unique to each individual.

Data on the recovery of 163 head-injured individuals will be presented in order to test two hypotheses. The first hypothesis postulates that recovery represents a curvilinear function such that the majority of recovery occurs rapidly after which the rate of recovery gradually decelerates in a curvilinear manner. The second hypothesis suggests that the discrepancies in the literature concerning the nature of the recovery curve (linear versus curvilinear) occur because more simple measures of recovery may have reached the asymptote of their curvilinear trajectory by the time patients' performance is assessed, thereby appearing linear. In contrast, the recovery process of more complex skills occurs later; therefore, the entire curve is measurable during the period that neuropsychological batteries are applicable. Finally, the results of these experiments will be compared with those of previous studies and directions for future research will be proposed.

## TRAUMATIC UNCONSCIOUSNESS: ANATOMICAL CORRELATES AND RECOVERY

While there are many forces affecting the brain following closed head injury, these can generally be classified as either rotational (or sheering) forces or acceleration/deceleration forces. Acceleration/deceleration forces usually result from direct blows to the head; rotational forces, however, result when the head is suddenly thrown into motion. As a result of the head's attachment to the body by the neck, the head pivots or rotates toward the force. Although the skull moves, there is resistance in the brain due to inertia. Early studies of the mechanics of head trauma (Letcher, Corrao, & Ommaya, 1973; Ommaya, 1968, 1973) suggest that resistance and damage resulting from these injuries are greatest at the surface of the cortex and decrease in magnitude toward the center of the brain. Thus, smaller acceleration/deceleration forces will result primarily in cortical impairment.

The severity of an individual's injury is commonly classified according to the behavioral correlates of the neuroanatomical damage. The less severe injuries, which affect primarily the cortex and produce cognitive effects, vary according to the location and the force of the impact as well as the structural and material properties of the brain tissue (Ommaya, 1968; Ommaya & Gennarelli, 1974). Damage to deeper structures in the brain (diencephalon) accompanies increasing rotational or sheering forces. Since one important function of this area is memory, the individual will report impaired memory. This is noted by a period following the injury, referred to as posttraumatic amnesia (PTA), in which the individual loses the ability to store and retrieve new memories. Finally, if the rotational forces are severe enough, damage will extend even deeper into the well-protected brain stem and disrupt the reticular activating system. This area of the brain is necessary for consciousness and damage here will consequently produce coma. This periphery-to-center mechanism of injury implies that subcortical damage cannot occur without some insult to cortical areas of the brain as well.

It is intuitive that the recovery of less damaged structures precedes that of more severely damaged structures. Since central structures receive the least amount of force from the impact, it follows that these structures should recover first. The sequence of recovery through which individuals progress supports this hypothesis. Recovery of brain stem functioning, and thus consciousness, usually precedes the recovery of motor and sensory functions. This, in turn, antedates the recovery of memory consolidation which precedes the return of cognitive functions. This suggests that the extent to which internal areas of the brain are damaged may serve as a prognostic tool for the outcome prediction of the eventual level of cognitive functioning.

A plethora of research has been conducted in an attempt to define severity of injury and predict outcome by correlating behavioral features of coma. Although behavioral features characteristic of this first stage of recovery may be difficult to quantify, systematic endeavors such as the Glasgow Coma Scale (GCS) have been made (Teasdale & Jennett, 1974). This scale attempts to predict outcome by numerically rating levels of responsiveness on the basis of eye opening and best verbal and motor responses on a 15-point scale. Not only is this scale easily administered by hospital staff, but it has been demonstrated to be predictive of outcome as well (Jennett & Bond, 1975; Jennett, Snoek, Bond, & Brooks, 1981; Levin et al., 1979). Recent studies have found the GCS to be superior in its ability to predict mortality (Rocca, Martin, Viviand, Bidet, Saint-Gilles, & Chevalier, 1989) and recovery based upon the Halstead Impairment Index (Gensemer, Smith, Walker, McMurry, Indeck, & Brotman, 1989) as compared to other severity rating scales which are based upon physiological and therapeutic intervention scoring systems. The GCS has also been demonstrated to be effective in predicting recovery based upon the Glasgow Outcome Scale in instances where multiple trauma, in addition to head injury, is involved (Pal, Brown, & Fleiszer, 1989).

Research assessing the second phase of recovery, PTA, has also demonstrated a relationship with severity. Studies have found that the incidence of coma, posttraumatic confusion, dementia, memory deficits, and retrograde amnesia increase with the duration of PTA (Brooks, 1976; Von Wowern, 1966). Early longitudinal research demonstrates the prognostic value of PTA duration in terms of neurological and neuropsychological sequelae (Russell & Smith, 1961; Von Wowern, 1966). However, the perennial problem of research employing PTA duration as a measure of severity involves the lack of objective criteria by which these behaviors may be quantified. Unless patients are admitted to research hospitals, records of the individual's behavioral changes are usually sparse and pertain more to the state of consciousness rather than assessing the patient's ability to form continuous memories.

Several strategies for assessing PTA duration are employed in the literature. Some studies question the patients as to when they first obtain a continuous memory for current events; however, some would argue that as time elapses, the reliability of this measure becomes more doubtful (Miller, 1979). Jennett (1976) maintains that when the estimation of PTA duration is categorized within large time spans, it can be reliably equated with different degrees of severity. In an attempt to solve some of the difficulties involved in using PTA as a measure of severity, and thus document its duration in a manner easily assessed by hospital staff, Levin and his colleagues (1979) developed the Galveston Orientation and Amnesia Test (GOAT). This instrument evaluates the patient in the spheres of: (1) orientation of time, place, and person, (2) an estimation of PTA duration, and (3) an estimation of retrograde amnesia (RA) duration.

Once patients have regained the ability to form continuous memories again, and thus have recovered adequate functioning of brain stem structures as well, their cognitive deficits become more apparent. Instruments used to assess previous phases of recovery are no longer sensitive to the deficits which become apparent during this prolonged phase of cognitive recovery. Closed head injury is responsible for more diffuse lesions; therefore, no single measure will adequately assess the functional integrity of the brain. Neuropsychological assessment is more appropriate during this phase of recovery due to its ability to assess intelligence, memory, language, and other higher cortical functions (Long, Gouvier, & Cole, 1984). Long and Gouvier (1982) demonstrated that neuropsychological evaluation is more sensitive in assessing cognitive impairment during this chronic phase than an electroencephalogram, CT scan, or psychological sequelae for patients who had been referred for evaluation after incurring mild to severe head injuries (Table 15.1). This analysis was based upon patients with documented head injuries who were referred for both neuropsychological and standard neurological evaluations. Recovery of overall functioning is an orderly process which progresses through various phases paralleled by the recovery of various anatomical structures. Each phase has instruments which are most efficient for measuring the recovery processes unique to it.

## A MODEL OF RECOVERY

As mentioned previously, individuals suffering from head trauma comprise a rather heterogeneous population, experiencing a wide range of cerebral dysfunction which involves intellectual skills, judgment, reaction time, sensory integration, attention and concentration, language skills, and memory (Long & Gouvier, 1981). In order to incorporate the heterogeneity of the head-injured population into a single, clinically based recovery model, Long *et al.* (1984) utilized the design strategy that is similar to that proposed by Brooks and his colleagues (1984); the pattern that occurs with the greatest frequency is adopted as the model for that population. Their recovery paradigm depicts the overall level of cognitive functioning as it pertains to time since injury (Figure 15.1). It asserts that recovery proceeds through a series of chronological phases that begins with coma or unconsciousness and progresses through PTA and impaired cognitive functions to recovery. Others have proposed models similar to this one in which the majority of recovery occurs shortly after injury with less dramatic recovery as patients approach their premorbid level of functioning (Drudge, Williams, Gomes, & Kessler, 1984).

This model of recovery divides the process into acute and chronic phases. The acute phase represents that time during which the patient is hospitalized and is progressing through PTA. Although the period during which the patient remains unconscious can be prolonged by the severity of the injury, once consciousness is regained, the course of recovery is initially rapid. The cessation of PTA, and usually of the patient's hospitalization, marks the end of the acute phase and the beginning of the chronic phase. This phase involves the recovery of cortical functioning which is reflected in improved cognitive

TABLE 15.1.  Hit Rates of Various Assessment
Techniques as a Function of the Severity
of Head Trauma[a]

| Assessment techniques | Severity of injury | |
|---|---|---|
| | Mild | Severe |
| EEG | 28% | 72% |
| CT scan | 26% | 45% |
| Neuropsychological evaluation | 87% | 89% |
| Psychological sequelae | 60% | 64% |

[a]Modified from Long and Gouvier (1982).

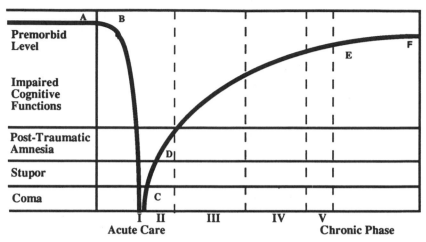

FIGURE 15.1. Head trauma recovery curve.

functions. Implicit in its name, the course of the chronic phase is much more prolonged as its rate of recovery gradually decelerates over time. Physical problems become less obvious, and society expects individuals to return to their premorbid level of functioning during this phase. Cognitive deficits, which are less obvious to others, become significant sources of stress for those trying to return to jobs and other activities requiring them to function at their premorbid level. It is during the chronic phase that complete neuropsychological assessments become relevant and useful. One of the primary functions of the neuropsychological evaluation at this time is to measure weaknesses and plan a course of rehabilitation.

A number of studies exist that examine the recovery process, although few actually examine the proposed differential rate across its various phases as described in Long's model. Instead, many studies examine recovery using a two-point measurement system. Subjects are assessed shortly after injury and some time during the period extending from 6 to 18 months following injury. This method is adequate if the researcher's goal is to quantify the amount of recovery as in a study examining the effects of various interventions. However, if the intent is to examine the rate at which recovery occurs over time, a binary measure using a within-subjects design is insufficient. With only two data points, it is impossible to differentiate linearity from curvilinearity. These studies have, however, contributed to our understanding of the factors that affect the recovery process.

## EMPIRICAL STUDIES EXAMINING THE PROCESS OF RECOVERY AND THE FACTORS THAT AFFECT IT

In order for researchers to formulate a central model of a recovery curve that is applicable to such a heterogeneous population, it is necessary to incorporate those variables that vary significantly within the sample. Based upon the neuroanatomical and clinical literature, factors which should be incorporated into the model, and therefore covaried across time since injury, include the severity of the injury, the complexity of the function being assessed, and the age of the individual. The severity of injury determines when an individual's recovery of cognitive functions begins as well as the degree to which complex cognitive functioning is disrupted. If cognitive abilities requiring more complex and integrative processing recover more slowly than those demanding more simple and distinctive processing, the complexity of the external criterion will affect the rate of recovery as well. Finally, it has been demonstrated that normal nonmedical controls exhibit a trend toward declining cognitive functioning with age (Fromm-Auch & Yeudall, 1983). Even if there were no interaction between age and the rate of recovery, age should be controlled in studies examining the recovery process.

## Time since Injury

Early recovery studies dealt primarily with the issue of time since injury. The results of several of these studies suggest that the majority of recovery occurs within the first two to three months following injury (Head, 1926; Butfield & Zangwill, 1945). A large number of studies from the last two decades report that the majority of recovery occurs within the first six months to a year following injury (Bond, 1975; Brooks & Aughton, 1979; Jennett et al., 1981; Mandelberg, 1975; Mandelberg, 1976; Parker & Serrats, 1976) with recovery being near maximum after two years (Oddy, Coughlan, Tyerman, & Jenkins, 1985). Studies that find a longer recovery period tend to deal with a more severely injured population (Brooks, Hosie, Bond, Jennett, & Aughton, 1986; Oddy & Humphrey, 1980). The discrepancies concerning the time limits in which the majority of recovery occurs are likely a reflection of the heterogeneity of the population and the functions chosen to represent recovery. As Table 15.2 demonstrates, studies base their criteria of recovery upon functions ranging from cognitive to emotional recovery.

Few studies have ventured beyond the clinical impression of a recovery curve and plotted this process using empirical data. Using a single subject design, Newcombe, Marshall, Carrivick, and Hiorns (1975) plotted recovery curves of three patients who experienced language difficulties as a result of head trauma. The patients were tested on multiple occasions during a 70-week period using the same measure of performance at each retest.

The result was a curve for each patient that improved exponentially with time; the initial improvement was rapid with improvement decreasing gradually as the patients reached their premorbid level of functioning. Although the results of this experiment suggest that recovery is curvilinear, a between-subjects design would help to verify that these results were not due to practice effects.

In a study following 27 individuals who sustained a period of posttraumatic unconsciousness, Dikmen et al. (1983) examined the course of recovery using various measures from the Halstead–Reitan Battery. The patients were examined when first alert and then 12 and 18 months following this first examination. This study found that the recovery of most of the individual's functions occurred at a constant rate with no differentiation between various phases. These results would suggest that the process is linear, contrary to the multiphasic, curvilinear model proposed by Newcombe et al. (1975) and Long et al. (1984).

There are several reasons why Dikmen and her colleagues did not find this curvilinear component. First, their subject size was rather small as is typical in most long-term follow-

TABLE 15.2. Studies Examining Recovery from Head Trauma

| Study | N | Severity (PTA in days) | Follow-up (months) | Type of study | Criteria for recovery |
|---|---|---|---|---|---|
| Bricolo et al. (1980) | 135 | Severe, >14 | 1, 3, 6, 12 | Retrospective | Neurological status |
| Brooks et al. (1986) | 42 | Very severe, >48 | 3,6, 12, 60 | Prospective | Self-care, behavioral changes |
| Dikmen et al. (1983) | 27 | Mild to severe | Alert, 12, 18 | Prospective | HNB[a] |
| Dikmen et al. (1986) | 20 | Minor, <1 hour | 1, 12 | Prospective | HNB |
| Dikmen et al. (1987) | 102 | Mild to severe | 1, 12 | Prospective | Memory (WAIS, SRT) |
| Fordyce et al. (1983) | 160 | Not specified | Those before/after 6 | Retrospective | MMPI, Katz |
| Jones et al. (1989) | 163 | Mild to very severe | Between-subjects | Retrospective | Halstead Impairment Index |
| Klonoff et al. (1977) | 117 (final) | Not specified | Alert, every year for 5 years | Prospective | EEG, school progress, neurological status |
| Najenson et al. (1978) | 15 | Severe to very severe | Weekly until stable | Prospective | Locomotion, communication skills |
| Newcombe et al. (1975) | 3 | Not specified | 2–166 weeks | Prospective | Reading errors |
| Oddy & Humphrey (1980) | 54 | Moderate to very severe | 6, 12, 24 | Prospective | Katz Adjustment Scale, motor & sensory |
| Oddy et al. (1985) | 31 | Severe, >7 | 7-year follow-up to above study | Prospective | Raven's Progressive Matrices, work, social |
| Prigatano et al. (1984) | 18 | Moderate to very severe | Mean = 21.6, 27.6 | Prospective | Neuropsychological Battery |
| Thomsen (1984) | 40 | Very severe, 68%, >90 | 4.5, 30, 120–180 | Prospective | Medical, psychosocial, neuropsychological |
| Winogron et al. (1981) | 51 | 17 mild, moderate, severe | Mean = 12 | Retrospective | Knights–Notwood Neuropsychological |

[a]HNB, Halstead Neuropsychological Battery.

up studies. Since the sample was composed of individuals with head trauma that ranged from mild to moderate severity, a large sample would likely be needed in order to find an effect in the midst of such heterogeneity. Due to this heterogeneity of sample severity, they may have found a differential recovery rate if they had used an additional assessment after a period of five to eight months. Second, a gradual deceleration in the recovery rate during the last six months as compared to the first 12 months may have been masked somewhat by practice effects.

## Severity of Injury

Positively correlated with time since injury, the severity of an individual's injury is another factor that displays considerable variability, is involved at some level in all head trauma studies, and has been demonstrated to affect outcome. The outer limits of severity of injury extend from a bump on the head to death. Is the actual course of recovery for severe and minor head injuries different or similar, only characterized by a lower level of postmorbid functioning in the more severely impaired group? Is the recovery of severely injured individuals more constant and prolonged or is there first an apparent delay and then improvement progressing over a curvilinear trajectory? These questions are of importance to therapists as well as clients involved in designing rehabilitation programs and distributing often limited resources.

According to the models presented by both Ommaya and Gennarelli (1974) and Long et al. (1984), the severity of an individual's injury will be an important factor in the determination of his/her course of recovery across time. Clinical research has supported these observations. Najenson, Sazbon, Fiselzon, Becker, and Schechter (1978) have demonstrated that the point at which recovery actually begins is delayed in the more severely impaired which further supports the positive correlation between time since injury and severity of injury. Bond (1983) has demonstrated that mildly impaired individuals (PTA < 24 hours) recover within 4–6 months, moderately impaired individuals (PTA 1–7 days) recover within 6–12 months, severely impaired individuals (PTA 8–28 days) recover within 1–2 years, and very severely impaired persons (PTA > 1 month) have residual damage after a period of 2–3 years. Impairment in rote intellectual functioning after 3 years and in complex integrative functioning after 5 years can be regarded as residual and permanent (Long et al., 1984).

## Complexity

Another factor that has been posited to covary with the recovery of cognitive functions and is related to the severity of injury is the complexity of ability, or function, which is used as a criterion for recovery. Clinical work suggests that the amount of complex skills that are disrupted following head trauma increases with the severity of injury (Miller, 1979). As would be predicted from a neuroanatomical model, more complex functions have been demonstrated to recover more slowly than simple abilities (Brooks et al., 1984; Mandelberg, 1975; van Zomeren & Deelman, 1978). In fact, in a study examining the recovery of speech in aphasics, Najenson et al. (1978) suggested that recovery of more complex integrative functions may have a period of delay before which recovery actually begins. Looking at this from a different perspective, aphasics may not have demonstrated improvement in their communicative abilities until 5 to 7 months, because it was necessary for more fundamental skills to recover before the more complex skills such as language.

A good example of the variations in recovery rates of two functions which differ on a continuum of complexity involves the reaction time studies of van Zomeren and Deelman (1978). They found that if simple reaction time is the measure on which recovery is based, the population will have recovered within the first year, whereas if choice reaction time were used, recovery will not occur until the second year. Another example includes studies that have found improvement on the Verbal Scale of the Wechsler Adult Intelligence Scale (WAIS) continued throughout the first year, whereas improvement on the Performance Scale displayed consistent change for up to 30 months (Mandelberg, 1975; Mandelberg & Brooks, 1975; Miller, 1979). The fact that the Performance Scale is composed of timed tasks is likely to account for the increased difficulty with the brain-injured population. Recovery of more obvious physical deficits occurs rapidly, whereas recovery of more subtle cognitive deficits may be more torpid (Gulbrandsen, 1983).

The possibility that more complex abilities recover after simple and overlearned tasks is intuitive, yet the implications of this are tremendous and are often overlooked. This would suggest that recovery is task-specific, meaning that the task that researchers choose as their measure of recovery may influence their interpretation of the course of recovery. A hypothesis to be tested later in this chapter postulates that all recovery is curvilinear; however, the interpretation of recovery's course for simple and complex recovery may be different. This discrepancy in interpretation arises because the course of recovery for the more basic neurological functions, such as basic sensory functions, may have reached their asymptotic level prior to the time when the complete neuropsychological battery is generally administered or considered relevant. If less basic functions are used as external criteria for recovery's course, their recovery process is more likely to begin during the interval when neuropsychological assessments are relevant, thus the entire curvilinear process is visible to the investigator. This may explain why researchers using different measurements and different schedules of follow-up periods have found linear and curvilinear recovery courses.

## Age

An additional characteristic which has been reported to affect the rate of recovery is the age at which a person is injured (Long & Klein, 1990). Discrepancies between studies examining the effect of age upon recovery from head trauma appear to be related to the external criterion chosen as a measure of recovery as well as the age range and severity of injury of the subject population. In a study examining outcomes of head-injured children (three groups) and adults who had comparable derangement of anatomical structure and physiological responses, no difference was demonstrated. However, survival, and not recovery of function, was the outcome measure. Using neuropsychological, neurological, and school performance as external criteria of recovery, a comparison of recovery following closed head injury in children younger than 8 and those older than 9 found no significant differences among groups (Klonoff, Low, & Clark, 1977). A possible explanation for this lack of a significant difference is a narrow age range or a maturation effect.

In contrast to the previously mentioned research, studies using neuropsychological measures as external criteria of recovery have demonstrated consistent evidence that recovery from head trauma is poorer with increasing age (Bricolo, Turazzi, & Feriotti, 1980; Heiskanen & Sipponen, 1970; Oddy *et al.*, 1985; Overgaard, Christensen, Haase, Hein, Hvid-Hansen, Land, Pedersen, & Tweed, 1973; Reyes, Battacharyya, & Heller, 1981). Not only have significant declines in spatial and more complex integrative tasks been demonstrated with age, but data also suggest that this relationship is curvilinear (Long & Klein, 1990). The superior neuropsychological recovery of the young as compared to the aged may be attributed to the latter group's less flexible neural network (Miller, 1979), the lack of support systems, relying almost solely on a spouse (Oddy *et al.*, 1985), as well as an increased possibility of disease processes in the elderly population (i.e., Alzheimer's disease or strokes).

Bricolo and his colleagues (1980) followed 135 cases of brain-injured individuals who sustained a period of posttraumatic unconsciousness for a minimum of two weeks. Mortality increased steadily with age, from 16% of those under 20 years of age up to 78% of those over 60 years old. Conversely, the occurrences of satisfactory recoveries decreased with age from 43% of those under the age of 20 to 0% of those over the age of 60. The validity of these findings rests on the assumption that PTA connotes an equivalent measure of severity in the young and old. Russell and Smith (1961) noted the tendency for older subjects to have a longer PTA than younger subjects; however, this strengthens Bricolo and colleagues' age-differentiated findings. Furthermore, a review of the literature indicates that the morbidity rate of those individuals with severe head injuries (as demonstrated by a GCS of 8 or more) increases exponentially with age (Jennett and Teasdale, 1981).

Unfortunately, the effect that age has on recovery is not as clear-cut as it may initially appear. The basic problem in comparing young and old head-injured individuals is in the difficulty of finding instances in which age is the only differing variable. Another difficulty in many of these studies results from the fact that a large number of them use social and/or occupational readjustment as an assay of recovery (Miller, 1979). Employers may feel that there is a greater payoff when the employee who has sustained a head injury is younger due to the fact that they have more years of service once they have recovered. Another problem with comparing young and old individuals with head trauma is that a higher percentage of progressive as opposed to static pathology in the elderly may inflate the benefit that youth produces. Also, the young may not be using the damaged structures; thus, deficits will not become apparent until that part of the brain matures further. Whereas adults have attained the knowledge necessary to succeed in a competitive society, children are just commencing this process. Therefore, the two groups are affected by different stressors in the recovery process (Kriel, Krach, Bergland, & Panser, 1988). Despite the problems in analyzing the effect that age has upon recovery, clinical observations suggest that the young recover more quickly and show less long-term impairments than the old (Miller, 1984). Future research on the development of a recovery curve should consider age effects in order to substantiate this clinical impression.

An interaction between age and severity of injury has also been demonstrated with older subjects recovering more slowly and to a lesser degree than their younger counterparts with comparable lengths of PTA (Carlsson, Essen, & Lofgren, 1968). The effect which age may have on the recovery process may lower the highest level of recovery obtained as well as produce an overall slowing of recovery or extend the recovery process over a longer period of time. The expectations of the client and therapist should be lower when the client is over 50–60 years of age.

In order to investigate the validity of Long's clinically based model as well as advance the understanding of the process of recovery from head trauma and the factors that affect it, a retrospective, between-subjects design examined the performance of 163 individuals. The goal of this study was to examine two hypotheses derived from this review of the literature. First, it was hypothesized that the course of recovery is curvilinear as characterized by an initially rapid rate that gradually decelerates over time. Second, it was hypothesized that although the recovery course of all functions is curvilinear, more simple functions may appear linear because they have reached their asymptote of recovery prior to the interval during which neuropsychological assessments are administered.

## EXPERIMENTAL EVIDENCE

### Method

*Subjects*

In order to investigate the course of the recovery process as well as the contribution of various factors to the shape of this trajectory, Jones, Fahy, and Long (1989) retrospectively compiled data that were collected on head-injured patients who were referred for neuropsychological evaluation. Patients were referred by neurologists and neurosurgeons and underwent a comprehensive neuropsychological assessment which included the Wechsler Adult Intelligence Scale-Revised, the Halstead–Reitan Battery, the Wechsler Memory Scale, the Minnesota Multiphasic Personality Inventory, as well as other selected tests. Patients were excluded from the analysis based upon two criteria: (1) they were lacking information concerning severity of injury or (2) their severity of injury fell within the mildly impaired range based upon their PTA. The mildly impaired group was excluded because all of their PTAs were recorded as 1 whether the duration of unconsciousness lasted 2 or 23 hours. This method of recording is based upon the premise that individuals are not accurate enough, retrospectively, to assess PTA in spans less than one day. This resulted in a sample size of 163 individuals. This same subject sample was used for both experiments 1 and 2.

Table 15.3 lists the average age, years of education, and time since injury for these patients as a function of severity of injury (based upon PTA duration). The severity of injury demonstrated a slight trend in which a larger percentage of individuals with severities in the mild to moderate range were assessed within the first seven months (58% versus 42% in the severe to very severe range), whereas an equal percentage of individuals in each severity

TABLE 15.3. Mean Age, Education, and Time
since Injury as a Function of PTA

| PTA (group) | Mean age | Mean education | Mean time since injury (months) |
|---|---|---|---|
| Moderate ($n = 68$) | 32.375 | 11.875 | 6.917 |
| Severe ($n = 48$) | 30.158 | 12.658 | 6.342 |
| Very severe ($n = 47$) | 31.886 | 13.457 | 8.029 |

category were seen during the 13–18 month period. However, the assumption of homogeneity of variance was not significantly violated for the demographic variables across time. Heterogeneity of variance is a common problem with retrospective studies which can be partially addressed by using the appropriate statistical models.

## Experiment 1

The goal of this study entailed verifying the hypothesis that recovery from head trauma is a curvilinear process. This involved plotting the patient's time since injury against some external measure of recovery. The choice of the most appropriate measure for an external criterion of recovery was based upon the fact that one of the reasons for developing such a curve is to provide empirical support for the clinical model as well as provide the researcher with a model by which interventions can be evaluated. An overall index comes closer to mimicking the clinician's impression of recovery than an individual test and was, therefore, chosen as the external index of recovery. It was hypothesized that the relationship between the patient's time since injury and recovery, as measured by the Impairment Index, would be characterized by an initially rapid improvement followed by a gradual deceleration in the rate of recovery as the patient reaches his/her maximum outcome. This relationship would imply that time since injury would demonstrate a quadratic relationship with recovery.

### Procedure and Test Materials

Each patient's test performance was rated according to a modified version of the Halstead–Reitan Impairment Index. The Impairment Index is an overall measure of cortical integrity which has been highly accurate in discriminating between those with and without cerebral dysfunction (Reitan & Davison, 1974; Reitan & Wolfson, 1985). The modified version used in the assessment of these patients is based upon six measures of the Halstead–Reitan Battery (Finger Oscillation Test, Speech Sounds Perception Test, Seashore Rhythm Test, Tactual Performance Test-total time, Tactual Performance Test-memory, and Tactual Performance Test-location) and the Trails B Test. For each subject, the Impairment Index represented the percentage of these seven measures that fell within the impaired range of higher cortical functioning. This index describes behavior ranging from no impairment (0.0) to very severe impairment (1.0).

Trend analysis, a technique employing hierarchical regression analysis, allows the researcher to define the general shape of the curve by determining the greatest power to which the independent variable can be raised. The prediction of an individual's position in the recovery process based upon such a curve varies according to the degree of variance, becoming less reliable as the outer boundaries of the sample are reached. Trend analysis also enables the researcher to be able to examine simultaneously the general relevance of other factors, in addition to time since injury, which are thought to affect recovery. Relevant factors examined in this study include: severity of injury, as measured by the length of the individual's PTA, and age. Regression analysis is an appropriate technique for studies examining continuous independent variables (time and age) and employing a between-subjects design. This type of design does, however, introduce a larger amount of variance into the analysis.

*Results*

As was hypothesized, recovery from head trauma demonstrated a curvilinear relationship across time. The first step in the hierarchical regression analysis regressed the Impairment Index as an external measure of recovery ($M = .495$, $SD = .300$) on age, PTA duration, and time since injury (TSI). This resulted in a statistically significant linear relationship between the measure of recovery and the independent variables ($F = 8.44032$, $p = .000$). In the second step, the second-degree polynomial component ([time since injury]$^2$) was entered into the equation. The results of this step support a nonlinear trend by yielding a statistically significant, quadratic equation ($F = 7.725$, $p = .000$). In order to verify that the second-order function was the highest-order component which most accurately "fit" the relationship between time since injury and the Impairment Index, the TSI values were raised up to the fourth powers. Since these yielded nonsignificant equations, they were removed from the analysis. Finally, all possible interactions were entered. Table 15.4 presents a summary of the trend analysis and the significance attributed to the predictor variables entered at each step.

The beta weights for each of the predictor variables that compose the final regression equation (below) and the significance of each are listed in Table 15.5. Figure 15.2 represents the predicted curvilinear progression of recovery from head trauma across TSI. This curve was derived from points predicted by this equation using the Impairment Index (II) as a measure of overall recovery. The recovery of function prior to three months is not represented in this graph due to the lack of subjects tested during this time. Traditional neuropsychological batteries do not become sensitive to the behavioral changes until the patient has progressed through the acute phase of recovery (Figure 15.1). Moderately to severely injured patients enter the chronic phase later than mildly injured patients.

$$II = (.0371)TSI - (.0033)TSI2 + (.0019)PTA + (.0081)AGE + 0.1008$$

In order to investigate accurately the amount of variance that each of the independent variables (age, PTA (or severity of injury), time since injury, and time since injury squared) contributed to recovery, partial correlations were determined for each variable when entered last into the equation (Table 15.6). As suspected, each of these variables accounted for a significant amount of the variance of impairment. This attests to the significance of examining age, severity, and TSI when assessing the progress or predicting an individual's

TABLE 15.4.   Regression Analyses of the Impairment Index,
Trails A, and Trails B across Time since Injury

| Experiment | Dependent variable | Independent variables | $R^2$ | $\Delta R^2$ | $F$ |
|---|---|---|---|---|---|
| I | Impairment Index | 1. Age, PTA, and time since injury | .14 | .14*** | 8.44*** |
| | | 2. (Time)$^2$ | .17 | .03* | 7.73*** |
| II | Trails A (simple) | 1. Age, PTA, and time since injury | .05 | .05* | 2.63* |
| | | 2. (Time)$^2$ did not enter | | | |
| | Trails B (complex) | 1. Age, PTA, and time since injury | .13 | .13*** | 7.70*** |
| | | 2. (Time)$^2$ | .15 | .02* | 7.00*** |

$*p<.05$; $**p<.01$; $***p<.001$.

TABLE 15.5. Standardized Beta Weights for the Predictors
in the Recovery Curve Equation for Experiments I and II

| Experiment | Dependent variable | Independent variable | B | Beta | Sig T |
|---|---|---|---|---|---|
| I | Impairment Index | PTA | .002 | .189 | .011 |
| | | Age | .008 | .344 | .000 |
| | | Time since injury | .037 | .569 | .036 |
| | | (Time since injury)$^2$ | −.003 | −.594 | .028 |
| | | Constant | .101 | | .260 |
| II | Trails A | PTA | .092 | .127 | .100 |
| | | Age | .300 | .172 | .028 |
| | | Time since injury | −.224 | −.047 | .546 |
| | | Constant | 28.898 | | .000 |
| | Trails B | PTA | .161 | .091 | .219 |
| | | Age | 1.484 | .350 | .000 |
| | | Time since injury | 4.900 | .672 | .014 |
| | | (Time since injury)$^2$ | −.584 | −.563 | .038 |
| | | Constant | 23.548 | | .148 |

recovery from head trauma. Interestingly, age accounted for more of the variance than any of the other factors in the equation.

## Experiment 2

### Procedure and Test Materials

As mentioned previously, some studies in the literature suggest that recovery from head trauma is linear while others indicate that it is curvilinear. In the previous experiment, it was demonstrated that recovery (as measured by complex, integrative functions) is curvilinear, initially rapid and decelerating across time since injury. A hypothesis providing an explanation for the literature's discrepancies concerning the shape of the recovery curve postulates that when simple functions are used as external measures, they may be approaching their asymptotic level of recovery prior to the initial neuropsychological evaluation.

This hypothesis would suggest that the recovery of less complex functions following coma is initially very rapid, decelerating before more complex skills and possibly prior to the period during which a total neuropsychological evaluation is relevant. This is consistent with literature demonstrating that more complex skills recover more slowly than simple functions (Brooks et al., 1984; Mandelberg, 1975; van Zomeren & Deelman, 1978). During the period between the cessation of coma and the evaluation, patients must progress from a level at which they are incapable of completing these tasks to a performance approaching their final level of recovery. Miller (1984) suggests that if an overall, integrative measure of impairment is used to assess recovery, it is likely that the curvilinear component of recovery that exists for individual functions that compose this overall measure will be partially masked when these functions are averaged. Consistent with the proposed hypothesis, Miller's hypothesis would suggest that the rate of recovery of less

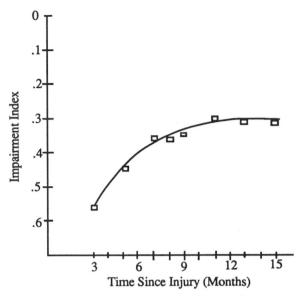

FIGURE 15.2. Recovery from head trauma as a function of time since injury.

complex functions would appear more rapid initially than more complex functions before decelerating.

In order to examine the relationship between task complexity and the shape of the recovery trajectory, two different parts of the Trail Making Test, Trails A ($M = 41.58$, $SD = 21.84$) and Trails B ($M = 102.15$, $SD = 53.98$), were selected as recovery measures. Both assessing perceptual-motor speed, Trails A and B contain a series of randomly placed circles filled with numbers from 1 to 25 which the subjects are instructed to connect consecutively. However, Trails B is a qualitatively more complex task than Trails A (Reitan, 1958). In addition to numbers, it contains circles filled with letters from A to Y. The complexity of the Trails B task is evidenced by the sequential "shifts" in attention which are required to alternate from alphabetical to numerical sequence. It was hypothesized that within the time during which complete neuropsychological assessments are relevant and, therefore, administered, Trails B would demonstrate a curvilinear recovery trajectory, whereas Trails A would appear linear due to more rapid recovery prior to the usual testing period.

TABLE 15.6. Percentage of Variance for Which Recovery's Predictor Variables Account

| Dependent variable | Age | PTA | Time since injury | (Time since injury)$^2$ |
|---|---|---|---|---|
| Impairment Index | 11.50*** | 3.50** | 2.38* | 2.62* |
| Trails A | 3.43** | 1.50 | 1.20 | 1.04 |
| Trails B | 11.90*** | 0.80 | 3.30** | 2.40* |

*$p<.05$; **$p<.01$; ***$p<.001$.

The analysis of the Trails A and B data supports the assumption that the discrepancy in the literature concerning the shape of the recovery curve is related to the complexity of the recovery measure. In order to test this assumption, a hierarchical regression analysis was performed on the Trails's tests using the same statistical format and subject sample as the analysis performed using the Impairment Index as the dependent variable. Thus, each patient's age and PTA duration were incorporated into the first step of the analysis along with their TSI value. $TSI^2$ was entered into the equation on the second step, followed by $TSI^3$ and $TSI^4$ on the third and fourth steps, respectively. Finally, all possible interactions were entered on the final step.

*Results*

As predicted, the regression analysis on Trails A did not reveal a curvilinear relationship as $TSI^2$ did not enter the equation. Although the resulting equation (below) only approached statistical significance ($F = 2.63, p = .05$), the shape of the curve suggests a linear relationship between Trails A and TSI during the time-since-injury interval assessed in this analysis (3–12 months). In contrast, the regression analysis of Trails B was statistically significant and revealed a curvilinear relationship between Trails B and time since injury ($F = 6.99, p = 0.000$, Figure 15.3). The steps involved in the trend analysis are presented in Table 15.4, and a summary of the beta weights of the final equation is displayed

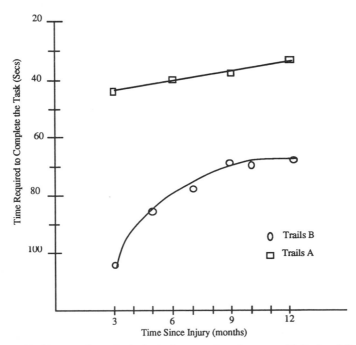

FIGURE 15.3. Significance of complexity in the interpretation of recovery: Trails A and Trails B.

in Table 15.5. In order to facilitate the interpretation of the contribution that each of the independent variables in this equation had on recovery, the percentage of variance for which each variable accounted is presented in Table 15.6. As in experiment 1, the independent variable which accounted for the largest amount of variance was age.

$$\text{Trails A} = 29 + (-.22)\text{TSI} + (.09)\text{PTA} + (.3)\text{AGE}$$
$$\text{Trails B} = 23.5 + (4.9)\text{TSI} - (.58)\text{TSI}^2 + (.16)\text{PTA} + (1.5)\text{AGE}$$

## DISCUSSION

Understanding the course of recovery in terms of overall functioning and individual skills has practical implications for both the clinician as well as the injured person and their family members. For the clinician and rehabilitative programs, having a clear conceptualization of the recovery of individual functions facilitates the most effective and cost-productive programs possible. By knowing the approximate rate of recovery of specific functions as well as the point at which recovery of specific skills begins, limited resources can be allocated to the relevant functions, at the pertinent times, and for the appropriate duration of time. An experimentally based, accurate recovery curve that can be visually presented to the patients and families would be beneficial to both clinicians and clients alike in terms of outcome. First, it would aid the family in seeing beyond the initial phases following injury as it assists in obtaining a general understanding of the recovery process. Second, it would aid the therapist–family team in setting realistic rehabilitative goals. A realistic strategy is imperative to maintaining the motivation that is necessary to maximize recovery through a period that is often extended and decreases motivation levels. Finally, it can be used as a measure against which the head-injured person's progress can be evaluated.

The results of the analysis using the Impairment Index as a measure of recovery suggest that the development of a general recovery curve is feasible. As was hypothesized, the curve depicts changes which are initially rapid and decelerate as the individual approaches his or her optimal level of recovery. These results are predicted by clinical (single case studies) and neuroanatomical literature; however, previous studies utilizing group data have failed to replicate this prediction with a more heterogeneous population. These findings are important because they empirically support the use of a single recovery curve that accounts for relevant individual factors (i.e., age, time since injury, severity, and complexity). Such a model of recovery promises to be beneficial both to the clinician in facilitating an understanding of the recovery process to patients and to the researcher as a guideline to evaluate the effects of different interventions. The data analyzed in this study suggest that the majority of recovery occurs within the first 12 months, a finding which, again, is consistent with the literature (see Table 15.2). It must be emphasized that the results of this analysis cannot be extrapolated to the mildly impaired population since they were not included in the analysis.

The analysis of the partial correlations of the independent variables from these experiments indicates that they provide valuable information concerning the personalization of an overall curvilinear recovery pattern to each individual's recovery. Age, time since injury, (time since injury)$^2$, and severity of injury all contributed significantly to the regression equation for recovery as a function of the Impairment Index. As expected, age (15–71 years old) and severity of injury (0–210 days) were negatively correlated with recovery, whereas time since injury (1–18 months) and (time since injury)$^2$ were positively correlated. Although it was hypothesized that all of these factors would significantly affect the course of recovery, it was not expected that age would account for a larger percentage of the variance than all other factors. These findings emphasize that recovery is a process unique to each individual and that the clinician needs to take these variables into consideration when predicting a person's recovery course or in evaluating the effectiveness of the intervention protocol. In addition, these findings accentuate the need for clinicians to employ age-corrected norms in evaluating the progress of their clients.

It was also postulated that the recovery literature's discrepancies concerning the shape of the recovery curve involve the complexity of the measure used as the external criteria of recovery. When complex functions are used, the majority of the recovery course occurs during the period in which complete neuropsychological batteries are relevant. In contrast, the majority of the more simple function's recovery may have occurred prior to the chronic phase of recovery during which neuropsychological assessment becomes relevant. If the researcher is examining the recovery of a function that has already reached an asymptotic level prior to assessment, it would appear linear during the time it was assessed. This means that the function must have reached this level rapidly and decelerated following the cessation of coma, because patients are obviously unable to perform these tasks while unconscious.

In support of this hypothesis, the results of the analysis comparing the curves of two levels of complexity of a task assessing perceptual-motor skills suggest that the less complex task (Trails A) appears to demonstrate a linear trend, whereas the more complex measure is represented by a significant quadratic relationship (Figure 15.3). However, patients must have reached this level of functioning prior to the assessment interval. Although knowing the course of recovery of a single function does not foster easy interpretation of the integrity of cortical functioning, information important to the planning of rehabilitative programs is obtained. That is, by knowing when the recovery process for various functions occurs, funding can be allocated during time intervals when recovery is most rapid.

The first experiment suggests that recovery, as depicted by an overall index most closely representing a clinician's prediction of a general recovery pattern, has a curvilinear course. This index is a composite of various functions which recover at different rates. The results of the second experiment in combination with Ommaya and Gennarelli's (1974) model may be used to explain why this pattern is not found by some researchers. Ommaya and Gennarelli demonstrate that functions vary in the rate of recovery as well as the point at which recovery begins. In order to further validate the hypothesis that all recovery is curvilinear, it is necessary for an investigation to utilize a prospective design to examine that recovery of a more basic task, such as Trails A, after patients regain consciousness.

An alternate interpretation may be that Trails A is not a sensitive measure of recovery. However, if this were the case, it is not likely that the linear relationship would have been significant ($p = .05$). The significance of the Trails's results should not be attributed to high variability as it was comparable to that of normal subjects and much lower than that of brain-damaged individuals in a study (Goul & Brown, 1970) norming the Trail Making

Tests on a sample of brain-damaged ($N = 93$) and normal individuals ($N = 106$) (Trails A: $SD = 21.8$ versus 39.3 and 17.3; Trails B: $SD = 54.0$ versus 76.7 and 46.2). Further prospective research using alternate measures of recovery is needed in order to rule out this possibility.

The major limitations of these studies originate from their retrospective design. First, retrospective research often limits a study to a between-subjects design since repeated evaluations were not available for most individuals. In a population in which heterogeneity is a perennial problem, this only serves to further augment the situation. Another limitation of a retrospective design specific to medical research is that patients who naturally seek assessment, particularly after a certain period of time following injury, represent a sample biased toward the more impaired range (Fordyce, Roueche, & Prigatano, 1983). Fortunately, this bias was relatively consistent over time in this study (i.e., similar percentages of patients at each level of severity, within each 3-month time period).

Another limitation of this study involves the population to which this recovery curve may be extrapolated. Due to a lack of representation of the mildly impaired individuals, the curve should not be used to predict this population's recovery. Future prospective research that can accurately record the length of their PTA should investigate their recovery curve. Finally, as with other retrospective studies involving head trauma patients, the sample did not include individuals who were seen immediately after their injury, due to the neuropsychological battery's inability to assess deficits during the acute phase. Persons who were approaching their premorbid level of functioning were most likely underrepresented in the sample because there is no longer a reason for them to seek a neuropsychological assessment.

Since the design of the study limited the time during which persons were actually assessed, clinicians must limit the use of the resulting equation for recovery within these bounds. Pedhazur (1982) emphasizes the dangers of extrapolating, or predicting performance outside of the range of the sample used in the study, on the basis of the regression equation. The fact that this phase of recovery is not observed by many researchers may be one reason why some studies do not find a curvilinear component to recovery. Possible measures which future prospective studies may utilize during the acute phase of recovery in order to obtain solid empirical data include the GCS or GOAT.

Outcome research is expensive and is often preceded by preliminary research in order to investigate the merit of its expense. Despite the limitations inherent in a retrospective design, the results appear to warrant the time and funding necessary for a tightly controlled, prospective, within-subjects, repeated-measures design in order to further investigate recovery, the factors which influence it, and its mechanisms. An alternate form of data analysis may be to treat the independent variables as code types and look for common patterns of recovery within the data, a method similar to that employed in the development of the Minnesota Multiphasic Personality Inventory. This may reveal information lost in the process of averaging heterogeneous group data. Future research should also investigate recovery as a function of other measures of overall impairment in order to assure that the Impairment Index is a true interval scale. This would ensure that a significant curvilinear trend was not due to the fact that the scale is "more compact" as time since injury increases. Other specific areas of interest include further research concerning other factors that may influence recovery, gathering data at the extreme time periods during the recovery process, and examining the issue of complexity with additional measures.

## CONCLUSION

This review began with the intent of answering a two-part question: despite the heterogeneity within the brain-injured population, can recovery be described by a single process, and, if so, is this process curvilinear? Both the review of the available neuro-anatomical and behavioral literature for factors that appear to affect the progression of recovery and the results of the current study support a model of recovery characterized by a single, orderly process, such as that proposed by Long and his colleagues. It is likely that the overall or general course of recovery is curvilinear, describing a process that is rapid at its onset and decelerates gradually as it approaches the maximum level of recovery.

The demand for more accurate predictors of outcome, and therefore a better under-standing of recovery, is increasing with the growing number of survivors of closed head trauma. The recovery curve, as based upon multiple regression of many variables which serve as predictors of outcome, promotes both of these demands. The recovery curve may also be employed as a measure against which deviations from the predicted course are used to evaluate the success of specific rehabilitative interventions for each patient.

In conclusion, there are three key components upon which additional models of recovery should focus in order to increase the knowledge and understanding of the recovery processes as well as the predictive outcome accuracy. First, recovery should be viewed as a multidimensional, yet orderly, process unique to each patient. Second, the model must be flexible enough to adjust to changes in the factors that have been demonstrated to influence recovery. Third, behavioral studies cannot ignore the neuroanatomical recovery with which the behavioral recovery is correlated.

## REFERENCES

Bond, M. R. (1975). Psychosocial outcome after severe head injury. *Ciba Foundation Symposium, 34,* 145–153.

Bond, M. R. (1983). Standardized methods of assessing and predicting outcome. In M. Rosenthal, E. Griffith, M. Bond, & J. Miller (Eds.), *Rehabilitation of the head injured adult* (pp. 97–113). Philadelphia: Davis.

Bond, M. R., & Brooks, D. N. (1976). Understanding the process of recovery as a basis for the investigation of rehabilitation for the brain injured. *Scandinavian Journal of Rehabilitation Medicine, 8,* 127–133.

Bricolo, A., Turazzi, S., & Feriotti, G. (1980). Prolonged posttraumatic unconsciousness: Therapeutic assets and liabilities. *Journal of Neurosurgery, 52,* 625–634.

Brooks, D. N. (1976). Wechsler Memory Scale performance and its relationship to brain damage after severe closed head injury. *Journal of Neurology, Neurosurgery, & Psychiatry, 39,* 593–601.

Brooks, D. N., & Aughton, M. E. (1979). Psychological consequences of blunt head injury. *International Rehabilitation Medicine, 1,* 160–165.

Brooks, D. N., Deelman, B. G., Van Zomeren, A.H., Van Dongen, H., Van Harskanp, F., & Aughton, M. E. (1984). Problems in measuring cognitive recovery after acute brain injury. *Journal of Clinical Neuropsychology, 6*(1), 71–85.

Brooks, D. N., Campsie, L., Symington, C., Beattie, A., & McKinlay, W. (1986). The five year outcome of severe blunt head injury: A relative's view. *Journal of Neurology, Neurosurgery, & Psychiatry, 49,* 764–770.

Brooks, D. N., Hosie, J., Bond, M. R., Jennett, B., & Aughton, M. E. (1986). Cognitive sequelae of severe head injury in relation to the Glasgow Outcome Scale. *Journal of Neurology, Neurosurgery, & Psychiatry, 49,* 549–553.

Butfield, E., & Zangwill, O. L. (1945). Re-education in aphasia: A review of 70 cases. *Journal of Neurology, Neurosurgery, & Psychiatry, 9,* 75–79.

Carlsson, C. A., Essen, C., & Lofgren, J. (1968). Factors affecting the clinical course of patients with severe head injuries. Part 1. Influence of biological factors. Part 2. Significance of posttraumatic coma. *Journal of Neurosurgery, 29*, 242–251.

Caveness, W. (1977). Epidemiologic studies of head injury. *Trauma, 18*(6), 61–66.

Dikmen, S., Reitan, R., & Temkin, N. R. (1983). Neuropsychological recovery in head injury. *Archives of Neurology, 40*, 333–338.

Dikmen, S., McLean, A., & Temkin, N. (1986). Neuropsychological and psychosocial consequences of minor head injury. *Journal of Neurology, Neurosurgery, & Psychiatry, 49*, 1227–1232.

Dikmen, S., Temkin, N., McLean, A., Wyler, A., & Machamer, J. (1987). Memory and head injury severity. *Journal of Neurology, Neurosurgery, & Psychiatry, 50*, 1613–1618.

Drudge, O., Williams, J. M., Gomes, F., & Kessler, M. (1984). Recovery from closed head injuries: Repeat testings with the Halstead–Reitan Neuropsychological Battery. *Journal of Clinical Psychology, 40*, 259–265.

Eichelberger, M. R., Mangubat, A., Sacco, W. S., Bowman, L. M., & Lowenstein, A. D. (1988). Comparative outcomes of children and adults suffering blunt trauma. *The Journal of Trauma, 28*(4), 430–434.

Fordyce, D. J., Roueche, J. R., & Prigatano, G. (1983). Enhanced emotional reactions in chronic head trauma patients. *Journal of Neurology, Neurosurgery, & Psychiatry, 46*, 620–624.

Fromm-Auch, D., & Yeudall, L. T. (1983). Normative data for the Halstead–Reitan neuropsychological tests. *Journal of Clinical Neuropsychology, 3*, 33–42.

Gensemer, I. B., Smith, J. L., Walker, J. C., McMurry, F., Indeck, M., & Brotman, S. (1989). Psychological consequences of blunt head trauma and relation to other indices of severity of injury. *Annals of Emergency Medicine, 18*(1), 9–12.

Gordon, V. L. (1989). Recovery from a head injury: A family process. *Pediatric Nursing, 15*(2), 131–133.

Goul, W. R., & Brown, M. (1970). Effects of age and intelligence on Trail Making Test performance and validity. *Perceptual & Motor Skills, 30*, 319–326.

Gulbrandsen, G. B. (1983). Neuropsychological sequelae of light head injuries in older children 6 months after trauma. *Journal of Clinical Neuropsychology, 6*, 257–268.

Head, H. (1926). *Aphasia and kindred disorders of speech*. London: Cambridge University Press.

Heiskanen, O., & Sipponen, P. (1970). Prognosis of severe brain injury. *Acta Neurologica Scandinavica, 46*, 343–348.

Jennett, B. (1976). Assessment of the severity of head injury. *Journal of Neurology, Neurosurgery, & Psychiatry, 39*, 647–655.

Jennett, B., & Bond, N. (1975). Assessment of outcome after severe brain damage. A practical scale. *Lancet, 1*, 480–484.

Jennett, B., & Teasdale, G. (1981). *Management of head injuries*. Philadelphia: Davis.

Jennett, B., Snoek, J., Bond, N., & Brooks, D. N. (1981). Long term neuropsychological outcome of closed head injury. *Journal of Neurology, Neurosurgery, & Psychiatry, 44*, 285–293.

Jones, C. L., Fahy, J., & Long, C. J. (1989, May). *Recovery from head trauma: A linear or curvilinear process?* Paper presented at the 6th Mid-South Conference on Human Neuropsychology, Head trauma: Acute care to recovery, Memphis, TN.

Klonoff, H., Low, M. D., & Clark, C. (1977). Head injuries in children: A prospective five year follow-up. *Journal of Neurology, Neurosurgery, & Psychiatry, 40*, 1211–1219.

Kolb, B. (1989). Brain development, plasticity, and behavior. *American Psychologist, 44*(9), 1203–1212.

Kriel, R. L., Krach, L. E., Bergland, M. M., & Panser, L. A. (1988). Severe adolescent head injury: Implications for transition into adult life. *Pediatric Neurology, 4*, 337–341.

Letcher, F., Corrao, P. G., & Ommaya, A. K. (1973). Head injury in the chimpanzee: Part II. Spontaneous and evoked epidural potentials as indices of injury severity. *Journal of Neurosurgery, 39*, 167–177.

Levin, H. S., Grossman, R. G., Rose, J. E., & Teasdale, G. (1979). long-term neuropsychological outcome of closed head injury. *Journal of Neurosurgery, 50*, 417–422.

Lezak, M. D., & Gray, D. K. (1984). Sampling problems and nonparametric solutions in clinical neuropsychological research. *Journal of Clinical Neuropsychology, 6*, 101–109.

Long, C., & Gouvier, W. (1981). *Cognitive sequelae following closed head trauma*. Paper presented at the Southeast Psychological Association meeting, Atlanta, GA.

Long, C. J., & Gouvier, W. D. (1982). Neuropsychological assessment of outcome following closed head injury. In R. N. Malatesha and L. C. Hartlage (Eds.), *Neuropsychology and cognition* (pp. 116–128). The Hague: Nijhoff.

Long, C. J., & Klein, K. (1990). Decision strategies in neuropsychology III: Determination of age effects on neuropsychological performance. *Archives of Clinical Neuropsychology*, *5*(4), 335–345.

Long, C. J., Gouvier, W. D., & Cole, J. C. (1984). A model of recovery for the total rehabilitation of individuals with head trauma. *Journal of Rehabilitation*, *50*(1), 39–45.

MacKenzie, E. J., Siegel, J. H., Shapiro, S., Moody, M., & Smith, R. T. (1988). Functional recovery and medical costs of trauma: An analysis by type and severity of injury. *The Journal of Trauma*, *28*(3), 281–297.

Mandelberg, I. A. (1975). Cognitive recovery after severe head injury, 2: Wechsler Adult Intelligence Scale during post-traumatic amnesia. *Journal of Neurology, Neurosurgery, & Psychiatry*, *38*, 1127–1132.

Mandelberg, I. A. (1976). Cognitive recovery after severe head injury. 3. WAIS verbal and performance IQs as a function of post-traumatic amnesia duration and time from injury. *Journal of Neurology, Neurosurgery, & Psychiatry*, *39*, 1001–1007.

Miller, E. (1979). The long term consequences of head injury: A discussion of the evidence with special reference to the preparation of legal reports. *British Journal of Social & Clinical Psychology*, *18*, 87–98.

Miller, E. (1984). *Recovery and management of neuropsychological impairments*. New York: Wiley.

Najenson, T., Sazbon, L., Fiselzon, J., Becker, E., & Schechter, I. (1978). Recovery of communicative functions after prolonged traumatic coma. *Scandinavian Journal of Rehabilitation Medicine*, *10*, 15–21.

Newcombe, F., Marshall, J. C., Carrivick, P. J., & Hiorns, R. W. (1975). Recovery curves in acquired dyslexia. *Journal of Neurological Sciences*, *24*, 127–133.

Oddy, M., & Humphrey, M. (1980). Social recovery during the year following severe head trauma. *Journal of Neurology, Neurosurgery, & Psychiatry*, *43*, 798–802.

Oddy, M., Coughlan, T., Tyerman, A., & Jenkins, D. (1985). Social adjustment after closed head injury: A further follow-up seven years after injury. *Journal of Neurology, Neurosurgery, & Psychiatry*, *48*, 564–568.

Ommaya, A. K. (1963). Head injuries: Aspects and problems. *Medical Annals of the District of Columbia*, *32*, 18–23.

Ommaya, A. K. (1968). The mechanical properties of tissues of the nervous system. *Journal of Biochemistry*, *2*, 1–12.

Ommaya, A. K. (1973). Computerized axial tomography: The EMI-Scanner, a new device for direct examination of the brain in vivo. *Surgical Neurology*, *1*, 217–222.

Ommaya, A. K., & Gennarelli, T. A. (1974). Correlation of experimental and clinical observations on blunt head injuries. *Brain*, *97*, 633–654.

Ommaya, A. K., & Jirsch, A. E. (1971). Tolerance of cerebral concussion from head impact and whiplash in primates. *Journal of Biomechanisms*, *4*, 13–22.

Overgaard, J., Christensen, S., Hasse, J., Hein, O., Hvid-Hansen, O., Land, A. M., Pedersen, K. K., & Tweed, W. A. (1973). Prognosis after head injury based on early clinical examination. *Lancet*, *2*, 631–635.

Pal, J., Brown, R., & Fleiszer, D. (1989). The value of the Glasgow Coma Scale and injury severity score: Predicting outcome in multiple trauma patients with head injury. *The Journal of Trauma*, *29*(6), 746–748.

Parker, S. A., & Serrats, A. F. (1976). Memory recovery after traumatic coma. *Acta Neurochirurgica*, *34*, 71–77.

Pedhazur, E. J. (1982). Trend analysis: Linear and curvilinear regression. In E. J. Pedhazur (Ed.), *Multiple regression in behavioral research, explanation and prediction* (pp. 396–435). New York: Holt, Rinehart & Winston.

Prigatano, G., Fordyce, D. J., Zeiner, H., Roueche, J. R., Pepping, M., & Wood, B. C. (1984). Neuropsychological rehabilitation after closed head injury in young adults. *Journal of Neurology, Neurosurgery, & Psychiatry*, *47*, 505–513.

Reitan, R. M. (1958). Validity of the Trail Making Test as an indicator of organic brain damage. *Perceptual & Motor Skills*, *8*, 271–276.

Reitan, R. M., & Davison, L. A. (1974). *Clinical neuropsychology: Current status and applications*. New York: Wiley.

Reitan, R. M., & Wolfson, D. (1985). *The Halstead–Reitan Neuropsychological Test Battery: Theory and clinical interpretation*. Tucson: Neuropsychology Press.

Reyes, R. L., Battacharyya, A. K., & Heller, D. (1981). Traumatic head injury: Restlessness and agitation as prognosticators of physical and psychological improvement in patients. *Archives of Physiological Medical Rehabilitation*, *62*, 20–23.

Rocca, B., Martin, C., Viviand, X., Bidet, P., Saint-Gilles, H., & Chevalier, A. (1989). Comparison of four severity scores in patients with head trauma. *The Journal of Trauma*, *29*(3), 299–305.

Russell, W. R., & Smith, R. (1961). PTA in closed head injury. *Archives of Neurology*, *5*, 4–17.

Teasdale, G., & Jennett, B. (1974). Assessment of coma and impaired consciousness. A practical study. *Lancet*, *2*, 81–84.

Thomsen, I. V. (1984). Late outcome of severe blunt head trauma: A 10–15 year second follow-up. *Journal of Neurology, Neurosurgery, & Psychiatry*, *47*, 260–268.

van Zomeren, A. H., & Deelman, B. G. (1978). Long-term recovery of visual reaction time after closed head injury. *Journal of Neurology, Neurosurgery, & Psychiatry*, *41*, 452–457.

Von Wowern, F. (1966). Posttraumatic amnesia and confusion as an index of severity in head injury. *Acta Neurologica Scandinavica*, *12*, 373–378.

Waechter, E., Phillips, J., & Holaday, B. (1985). Neuromuscular system. In E. Waechter & B. Holaday (Eds.), *Nursing care of children* (10th ed.) (pp. 1069–1079). Philadelphia: Lippincott.

Winogron, H. W., Knights, R. M., & Bawden, H. N. (1984). Neuropsychological deficits following head injury in children. *Journal of Clinical Neuropsychology*, *6*(3), 269–286.

# 16

# Neuropsychological Assessment of Traumatic Brain Injury in the Intensive Care and Acute Care Environment

## J. MICHAEL WILLIAMS

Most clinical neuropsychological evaluations of traumatic brain injury (TBI) are performed at least three months after the onset of injury. Although the neuropsychologist may assess a brain-injured patient early in recovery to establish severity or localization of injury, most evaluations of head trauma patients are used to establish functional ability levels and to plan for discharge placement and a rehabilitation program (Prigatano, Fordyce, Zeiner, Roueche, Pepping, & Wood, 1984). While currently few clinicians regularly practice in the trauma center, the use of neuropsychological assessment in the acute care environment represents a potentially new setting for neuropsychologists to monitor cognitive function. Early neuropsychological evaluation can also provide a valuable clinical service for the treatment and management of TBI.

In the context of the Intensive Care Unit or trauma center, most neuropsychological test batteries are cumbersome to administer, difficult for patients to complete, and so arcane and specific to neuropsychological diagnosis that they poorly assess cognitive functioning of patients with traumatic injuries. In order to provide an appropriate service, neuropsychologists have modified their techniques and, in some instances, have invented their own assessment battery for this atypical setting. These new testing procedures represent a reasonable expansion and growth in neuropsychological assessment technology. Novel

J. MICHAEL WILLIAMS • Neuropsychology Laboratory, Hahnemann University, Philadelphia, Pennsylvania 19102.

*HANDBOOK OF HEAD TRAUMA: Acute Care to Recovery*, edited by Charles J. Long and Leslie K. Ross. Plenum Press, New York, 1992.

approaches toward neuropsychological assessment not only include the traumatically brain injured (Prigatano *et al.*, 1984), but also encompass the dementia-related illnesses (Poon, 1986) and pediatric neuropsychology (Hynd & Obrzut, 1981). In each of these areas, there is strong motivation to create the new techniques which will enable clinicians to accurately and appropriately assess their patients.

The focus of this chapter will be the elaboration and development of assessment techniques for use in the acute-care TBI environment. There has been considerable research done in this setting (e.g., Levin, Benton, & Grossman, 1982) and new assessment techniques have been developed for these studies. This chapter begins with a summary of the research on the different clinical methods used to examine the cognitive abilities of trauma patients in the earliest phase of recovery. After reviewing this literature, a comprehensive clinical and research protocol for the assessment of head trauma patients, developed at Hahnemann University Hospital, will be presented.

## NEUROPATHOLOGY OF TBI IN RELATION TO EARLY COGNITIVE STATUS

Two major injuries occur when the cerebrum rapidly decelerates within the skull: shear injury and contusion. As the brain moves rapidly from back to front or side to side, axonal processes, support tissue, and the vascular systems are strained and damaged. The vascular damage produces hemorrhages and ischemia, whereas the axonal trauma produces direct neurological impairment. These factors are concentrated in the medial, interhemispheric areas of the cerebrum. Medial areas are subject to the greatest rotational forces during the rapid deceleration of the brain within the skull. Contusion occurs when the brain strikes the interior skull surfaces or other constraining structures, such as the falx. Contusion primarily injures cortical systems but can contribute to swelling, vascular insufficiency, and hemorrhage (Vogel, 1979; Gurdjian & Webster, 1958).

Rapid acceleration/deceleration, movement of the brain within the skull, shear injury, and contusion may all contribute to the formation of vascular trauma and hematoma. Hematomas are clear indicators of severe injury and develop in three basic forms: intracerebral, epidural, and subdural. The two factors which determine the relative severity of hematoma are the location of the mass of blood and the magnitude of displacement of the hematoma. In general, the most severe forms are the intracerebral and epidural. Intracerebral hematomas cause severe injury because of their location within the parenchyma of the brain. Their toxic and mass effects tend to injure subcortical structures and life-support systems in the brain stem. Significant intracerebral hematomas are almost always devastating and have been clinically identified as strongly predictive of mortality (Kerr, Kay, & Lassman, 1971).

Small parenchymal hemorrhages are also common in closed head injury and contribute to the swelling associated with severe injuries. They are most likely caused by the shearing forces of acceleration/deceleration. Most of these hemorrhages are small enough that they fall below the resolution of computer tomography scanning. Their full extent is often discovered at autopsy (Strich, 1961; Lewis, 1976).

If the patient survives the initial insult, both significant parenchymal and intracerebral hematomas have been clinically observed to produce generalized effects on brain function. These effects include coma, disorientation, agitation, and generalized cognitive decline.

Epidural and subdural hematomas vary greatly in their manifestations. Some are large and associated with considerable mass effect and neurological deficit; others are small and associated with virtually no brain injury. Most are treated surgically by evacuation. Clinically, they tend to have lateralizing neurological deficits which are attributable to pressure exerted on surrounding tissue and the toxic effect of blood. In general, epidural hematomas tend to form a mass of clotted blood and have prominent mass effects. Subdural hematomas usually consist of a smaller amount of blood layered over the cortex, with less mass effect. Of course, these descriptions are generalizations. Many subdural hematomas, for example, may consist of a large, layered mass of clotted blood. Neuropsychologists should carefully note the extent and location of hematoma. Their presence is generally predictive of worse cognitive outcome (Williams, Gomes, Drudge, & Kessler, 1984).

Another source of damage in traumatic injury is the general metabolic disturbances involving the control of virtually every biochemical process in the brain. These prominently include the metabolism of glucose and oxygen but also include the unique brain processes of neurotransmitter and axonal transport metabolism (Vogel, 1979). These latter processes are unique to the brain and their disruption produces widespread brain dysfunction.

The behavioral result of severe metabolic disturbance is an acute confusional state. Confusional states and delirium are common among patients with TBI, especially in the early stages of recovery (Plum & Posner, 1982). Delirium in such cases is usually short-lived and presumably resolves as metabolic processes recover. The determination and description of delirium from traumatic cerebral pathology is compromised by the presence of general sepsis, drug or alcohol intoxication, and medication effects. The most common situation which results in assessment difficulties and misinterpretation is when the patient presents at admission with delirium caused by alcohol or drug intoxication. Many intoxicated patients are delirious because of the drug agent and not because of cerebral trauma. Likewise, medication used for pain management or sedation may produce delirium in the early phases of recovery. The delirium produced by factors extraneous to the injury itself results in confusion and uncertainty in the measurement of coma, posttraumatic cognitive recovery, and in the prediction of outcome based on these factors. Since patients who are delirious will recover quickly, any predictions of outcome based upon assessment during the delirious state will be invalid.

These neuropathological changes are the major factors which produce the neurological impairment associated with TBI. Virtually none of these sources of injury are localizable to one area of the brain in a majority of cases or are typical of all injuries. Each case of TBI will have a unique cluster of these factors which can affect virtually any brain location.

Clinically, the end result of hematoma, swelling, and other pathology is functional impairment of the brain and neurological symptoms, encompassing the full breadth of neurological syndromes. Of course, the most prominent of these is coma. Among trauma patients, coma usually represents the result of injury to the brain stem and reticular activating system. Because of shearing forces and the dynamics of brain swelling, the brain stem is at differential risk of injury. Coma may also be exacerbated by metabolic disturbance, severe cortical damage, and other aspects of the injury. Other neurological symptoms which result from the pathological processes described here are cranial nerve syndromes, hemiparesis, acute aphasia, and seizure disorder. These symptoms suggest injury to localized brain areas and have been used as predictors of outcome.

## ASSESSMENT TOOLS FOR THE ACUTE-CARE TRAUMA CENTER

The overriding purpose of clinical assessment in the trauma center is to document cognitive function over the course of time for patients who usually begin at the lowest levels of cognitive ability and may recover to at least the average range. This unique situation requires measures which can be repeated and tests which allow assessment at the lowest levels of cognitive function. The following is a concise description of the instruments currently available at each stage of injury and recovery (Figure 16.1).

The assessment of coma level occurs at the earliest and most severe levels and represents a very simple, direct measure of cognitive function. Essentially, the examiner attempts to measure the general degree to which the cerebral cortex may be active. The unconsciousness referred to in the concept of coma is derived from the responsiveness of the cerebral cortex to various types of simple stimuli, such as pain and simple verbal command. Among all coma scales, responsiveness is scaled according to the following basic hierarchy: (1) unresponsiveness to any stimuli; (2) responsiveness only to pain; (3) responsiveness to verbal command; and (4) unconstrained, spontaneous responsiveness to verbal stimuli.

The role of cortical control at each stage of increasing responsiveness includes the construct of coma, and all coma scales reflect this hierarchy. They vary in the details of scaling the modalities of responsiveness. Some scales score only this general hierarchy (e.g., Grady Coma Scale; Cooper, Moody, Clark, Kirkpatrick, Maravilla, Gould, & Drane, 1979); other scales separately measure responsiveness in different modalities, such as eye opening, motor responses, and verbal responses (e.g., Glasgow Coma Scale [GCS]; Teasdale & Jennett, 1974) (Table 16.1). The GCS has a long history of research and clinical

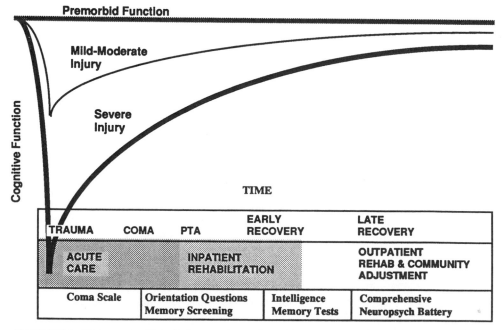

FIGURE 16.1. The general pattern of injury recovery and cognitive assessment instruments appropriate for each stage.

TABLE 16.1. The Two Major Types of Coma Scaling

Grady Coma Scale
 0 = Alert, oriented, may have posttraumatic amnesia
 1 = Lethargic, uncooperative, but does not lapse into sleep if left undisturbed
 2 = Stuporous; sleeps if undisturbed but is arousable
 3 = Deep stupor; moves purposefully only to deep pain
 4 = Decerebrate or decorticate; nonpurposeful response to deep pain; dilated pupils
 5 = Flaccid; does not respond to stimuli with any movements

Glasgow Coma Scale
 *Eye Opening*
   4—Volitional and purposeful eye opening
   3—Opens eyes to verbal command
   2—Opens eyes only to pain
   1—No eye opening

 *Motor Responses*
   6—Obeys verbal commands
   5—Localizes pain
   4—Flexion withdrawal
   3—Flexion decorticate regidity
   2—Extension decerebrate rigidity
   1—No motor responses

 *Verbal Responses*
   5—Patient is oriented and converses
   4—Patient is disoriented and converses
   3—Patient produces incorrect and inappropriate words
   2—Patient produces incomprehensible sounds
   1—No verbal responses

application. A minor drawback of the scale is that it is more difficult to use than a scale which does not separately scale modalities. Furthermore, there is a tendency among clinicians to only use the total score without attention to the behavior which went into the individual ratings that contributed to the overall score (Eisenberg & Weiner, 1987). This results in some misinterpretation of the total scale score. For example, some patients will have eye opening responses to verbal command and pain but no motor responses. The GCS total score will reflect a higher level of responsiveness than is probably the case if the subject made motor responses instead of eye opening. Another problem in interpretation results from the practice of paralyzing and immobilizing agitated patients with drug agents. Sometimes treatment programs will continue to document the coma score although the patient has been artificially rendered completely unresponsive. The coma rating in this situation has a completely different meaning than coma scores which are derived from cerebral impairment produced by the injury alone.

Aside from these minor inconsistencies, the GCS and others are likely valid measures of overall cerebral responsiveness and correspond to the construct of coma understood by most investigators. The few studies which have examined the interrelationship of coma scales have discovered them to be highly correlated (Cooper *et al.*, 1979).

## THE ASSESSMENT OF EARLY RECOVERY

Since cognitive functioning undergoes much change during recovery from traumatic injury, the nature and goals of patient assessment should also evolve and adapt to these changes exhibited by the patient. Trauma patients may have virtually any neuropsychological deficit as they recover from injury. Usually there are a variety of deficits, or impairments of attention and memory, resulting in generalized impairment of other abilities. Many focal deficits are masked by generalized impairment in the early stages. As a general rule of thumb, moderate to severe head injuries result in generalized and some discrete cognitive disability which resolves to a pattern of discrete, localized impairment. It is often not until substantial recovery has occurred that some discrete impairment, such as language disorder, is clearly noticeable and measurable. These deficits will persist through recovery of other abilities and become the permanent cognitive sequelae of the injury.

During the very early stages, both coma assessment and early cognitive assessment measure the generalized influence of severe injury. This is manifested as disorientation and memory disorder. Although the memory consolidation system may be completely intact, the generalized effects of the trauma produce confusion and severe attention deficits. These are commonly manifested as poor remembering.

The inability to remember new experiences is the common endpoint for all the deleterious influences on brain function which are associated with the injury. For this reason, assessment of cognitive status in the early recovery period usually focuses on memory function. Probably the most common strategy to assess alertness and general functional level is the use of informal orientation questions. Nurses, physicians, technicians, and others persistently ask orientation questions and base their prediction of outcome, treatment strategies, and general sense of recovery on the responses to these simple questions. This is documented in the medical chart by the familiar "AO × 3." Less consistently is inquiry made concerning memory for ongoing experiences. Therefore, conclusions regarding memory abilities based on informal orientation questions are far less reliable than formalized questionnaires of orientation and ongoing memory.

More formalized assessment measures include the Galveston Orientation and Amnesia Test (GOAT) and the mental status examination of orientation (e.g., Mattis, 1976). These brief questionnaires usually assess personal, place, and time orientation. As a rule of thumb, memory loss for basic personal information indicates a confusional state. Disorientation to place and time, with intact personal orientation, usually indicates memory disorder.

In the intensive care environment, orientation questionnaires and memory screening tests are often administered repeatedly. Although this violates psychometric principles which predict contamination of repeated scores by practice effects, failure or success on items is probably not associated with greater probability of success on future items. The points in recovery at which the patient becomes oriented are extremely important to assess and document because they are the benchmarks for treatment interventions and predictions about future outcomes.

After the trauma patient recovers to the point of orientation and intact memory for ongoing experiences, and the patient can focus and sustain attention, cognitive function can be assessed using conventional neuropsychological tests. However, the testable point in recovery usually coincides with the ability to attend and remember ongoing experiences. Since the early study of trauma, this approximate point in time was identified as the end of posttraumatic amnesia (PTA). The interval between time of injury and the time at which the patient retains ongoing experiences represents a salient feature or benchmark of recovery. It is considered to be predictive of later cognitive outcome (Bond & Brooks, 1976; Carlsson, Svardsudd, & Welin, 1987; Dikmen, McLean & Temkin, 1986b). If patients attain this level of function in a reasonable time, usually considered two weeks after injury, then the outcome will be good. If patients attain it after many weeks, then the outcome will be poor.

Of course, many trauma patients never become oriented and progress beyond the state of PTA.

As the patient attains middle to late recovery (Figure 16.1), there are two appropriate levels of neuropsychological assessment. Usually patients at this point in their recovery are intact enough to participate in an abbreviated intellectual assessment, such as an abbreviated intelligence scale and memory tests (Table 16.2). This assessment must be tailored to the patient's apparent level of attention and cooperation. On many occasions, it is impossible to examine a patient even using the tests suggested as an abbreviated battery.

The final level of examination includes the administration of a complete conventional neuropsychological test battery, or a screening of certain cognitive skills which appear intact, and then subsequent detailed testing of more impaired functions. Since traumatic injury can result in damage to any part of the brain, the examination must cover the full breadth of cognitive skills. As before, the extent of assessment is always governed by the patient's ability to sustain attention and cooperation.

## INJURY SEVERITY MEASURES AS OUTCOME PREDICTORS

Previous investigations of closed head injury outcome prediction have used a variety of measures of initial trauma severity and outcome. These measures include: abnormal neurological status (e.g., pupil abnormalities, cranial nerve palsy, and acute hemiparesis), duration of PTA, presence of hematoma, and severity and duration of coma. Methods of assessing outcome have ranged from simple mortality rates to cognitive and overall disability scales.

A variety of early neurological symptoms were found predictive of outcome in many studies (Gensemer, McMurray, Walker, Monasky, & Brotman, 1988; Jennett, Teasdale, Braakman, Minderhoud, & Knill-Jones, 1976; Levin & Grossman, 1978; Levin, Grossman, Rose, & Teasdale, 1979; Levin, Grossman, Sarwar, & Meyers, 1981; Rimel, Giordani, Barth, & Jane, 1982; Uzzell, Dolinskas, & Langfitt, 1988; Varney, 1988; Wilson, Wiedmann, Hadley, Condon, Teasdale, & Brooks, 1988). These studies revealed that the presence of abnormal neurological status, such as cranial nerve palsy, pupil abnormalities, and acute hemiparesis, was predictive of duration of unconsciousness, disorientation, and cognitive outcome. Pupillary abnormalities (e.g., fixed and nonreactive or dilated pupils) indicated poor prognosis in virtually all of the studies.

A number of studies have shown a relationship between duration of PTA and cognitive and psychosocial outcomes (Bond & Brooks, 1976; Carlsson et al., 1987; Dikmen,

TABLE 16.2.   Abbreviated Neuropsychological Evaluation[a]

General intelligence: Satz–Mogel WAIS, Quick Test, Slosson Intelligence Test
Memory: Memory Assessment Scales, Wechsler Memory Scale, LNNB Memory Subscale
Sensory screening: Sensory Perceptual Exam from the Halstead–Reitan Neuropsychological Battery
Motor function: Tapping Test, Motor Subscale of LNNB, selected subtests from LNNB
Aphasia/language screening: Aphasia Screening Test, selected items from Boston Diagnostic Aphasia Examination, selected items from LNNB
Academic skills: Wide Range Achievement Test

[a]LNNB: Luria–Nebraska Neuropsychological Battery; WAIS: Wechsler Adult Intelligence Scale.

McLean, & Temkin, 1986b; Mandleberg, 1976; McKinlay, Brooks, Bond, Matinage, & Marshall, 1981; Oddy, Humphrey, & Uttley, 1978; Uzzell *et al.*, 1988). A brief summary of these studies suggests that PTA best predicts cognitive function soon after the injury. As the patient recovers over the span of one year or more, cognitive function is less well predicted by PTA (Dikmen, McLean, & Temkin, 1986a; Mandleberg, 1976). Presumably factors such as premorbid status and rehabilitation experiences begin to play a greater role in prediction of outcome.

The next group of predictors involve signs of pathology and illness rather than direct indicators of neurological function. These include the presence of skull fracture, hematoma, and increased intracranial pressure. Skull fracture has been found unrelated to outcome in most studies (Levin *et al.*, 1979). However, Servadei, Ciucci, Pagano, Rebucci, Ariano, and Piazza (1988) did find that skull fracture predicted outcome only in cases of mild traumatic injury. These investigators theorized that the skull fractures predicted outcome because they were often associated with hematoma. Patients having a fracture and a hematoma had a worse outcome in comparison to the other cases of mild injury. In addition, both increased intracranial pressure and presence of hematoma have been consistently related to poorer outcome (Becker, Miller, & Greenberg, 1982; Fleichser, Payne, & Tindall, 1976; Vapalahti & Troupp, 1971).

The final and most studied area of outcome predictors involves using the assessments of impaired consciousness or coma. In general, studies examining coma level and duration have found strong, consistent relationships between level of impaired consciousness and most other outcome measures (Dikmen *et al.*, 1986b; Dikmen, Temkin, McLean, Wyler, & Machamer, 1987; Gensemer *et al.*, 1988; Klonoff, Costa, & Snow, 1986; Klove & Cleeland, 1972; Levin *et al.*, 1979, 1981; Lezak, 1979, 1987; Lundholm, Jepsen, & Thornval, 1975; Rimel *et al.*, 1982; Williams *et al.*, 1984). Furthermore, these studies found coma level to be the best predictor of outcome when compared to the previously mentioned severity measures. Indeed, many of these severity measures may be redundant with coma level in their prediction of outcome. For example, the mass effects of hematoma may compress the cranial nerves and brain stem thereby producing pupillary abnormalities and a severe coma. Therefore, coma probably represents a common end state for many of these traumatic sequelae. It emerges as the most reliable predictor because it represents a summary of much of the stress the brain has experienced.

## PREMORBID INDICES AS OUTCOME PREDICTORS

Although premorbid factors are often discussed in the prediction of intellectual and psychosocial outcome, this relationship has been largely neglected by researchers. For example, levels of premorbid intellectual skills, such as reading level, should be strong predictors of the same skills measured after the injury. A patient with poor reading skills before the injury should attain this level or lower after recovery. Likewise, it is assumed that premorbid vocational status should predict postinjury vocational status. Patients who are employable after recovering from TBI will tend to work in similar jobs as those they had before the injury. Numerous other examples can be cited of the prominent role that premorbid factors should have in outcome prediction. They will also play a major role in conceptualizing the treatment and outcome of rehabilitation programs (Prigatano *et al.*, 1984).

Many such examples and arguments appear in the literature on TBI, yet few studies have empirically examined these hypothesized relationships between premorbid indices and outcome following TBI. The probable reason for the paucity of research in this area is that methodologies have not been developed to directly assess premorbid function. Attempts at developing a scientifically valid methodology for estimating premorbid intelligence in cases of traumatic injury have been unsuccessful. If the patient had somehow received neuropsychological tests preceding the injury, then premorbid abilities could be factored into the patient's postinjury pattern of intellectual findings. Of course, no one is ever assessed premorbidly; thus, clinicians have been led to informally construct a premorbid characterization of the patient derived from family interviews and the medical and psychosocial history.

Although understudied, there have been some investigations which included premorbid measures, such as demographic variables (e.g., age, level of education, and gender), giving some suggestion of their predictive power. Age is shown to be predictive, whereas gender is not found to be predictive of outcome (Becker *et al.*, 1982; Jennett *et al.*, 1976; Jennett & Bond, 1975). Older subjects generally have greater mortality. The relationship of age and gender to outcome is probably constrained by the low variance of these variables among traumatically brain-injured patients. There is a strong bias for young adult males to be represented among these patients (Carlsson *et al.*, 1987). Using multivariate regression techniques and an estimate of premorbid cognitive function based on education and occupation, Williams *et al.* (1984) found that coma level and estimates of premorbid IQ were the most important variables in predicting cognitive outcome measured using the Wechsler Adult Intelligence Scale and Halstead–Reitan Neuropsychological Battery three to six months postinjury.

## THE HAHNEMANN TRAUMA ASSESSMENT PROTOCOL

The intention of the Hahnemann protocol was to design a clinical tracking battery and a set of procedures for assessing cognitive function at every stage in the early recovery from TBI. This mission resulted in two overall design requirements of the protocol. First, the protocol must be clinical in nature. This resulted in the inclusion of procedures which do not exist in a protocol designed only for research. The most significant are the procedures used to communicate neuropsychological test findings to other staff members in the trauma center. This entailed developing a new format for presenting neuropsychological data regarding which parts of the assessment to present to the staff members. Second, clinical procedures must also fit comfortably within the confines of the setting in which they are applied. In the trauma center, for example, one cannot administer long batteries of cognitive tests. Too many features of the setting mitigate against this: patients are in pain and distractible, and testing is often interrupted by medical tests and procedures.

Furthermore, the requirement that the protocol must assess the lowest levels of ability resulted in the creation of new reporting formats and new assessment instruments. Although a few instruments exist to assess low levels of ability, none have been integrated into an efficient clinical tracking system. This required the development of some new instruments as well as the reshaping of some already in use.

## The Summary Form

The foundation of the system is the Neuropsychological Laboratory Trauma Summary Form (Figure 16.2). This format was developed to communicate cognitive change over time in a format that was concise and understandable. The summary sheet consists of four major sections, each corresponding to the major phases of recovery. These focus on the assessment of coma, orientation, basic memory abilities, and comprehensive cognitive/memory assessment. The usual model for communicating test results to referral sources or others is the venerable neuropsychological report, a traditional narrative format which is a poor model for presenting information to an acute care team. Most team members do not have time to read such reports. Even those who have the time report that the language is so unfamiliar that they do not derive any benefit from reading it. The trauma center has such unique requirements for communication systems that traditional narrative reports have poor clinical utility.

## Coma

This protocol utilizes the GCS as the primary coma assessment instrument. The scale is used by all members of the trauma team and these assessments are summarized by the neuropsychology group and reported in the neuropsychology trauma report. The coma ratings are most often taken from critical care flow sheets or progress notes in the medical chart. It is rare for neuropsychology team members to assess coma for the most impaired patients. The administration of painful stimuli to assess coma is only done by nursing and medical staff. The neuropsychology team only monitors the values determined by these other team members. The response to verbal command for eye opening and motor function is commonly assessed by the neuropsychologist. At this level of coma assessment, the neuropsychologist probably assesses coma more often and reliably than other trauma staff. Once the patient is essentially responsive to verbal command and opens the eyes to command, the other trauma team members will only administer the coma scale sporadically and usually for the purpose of discovering some downward course in the patient's progress of recovery. After the patient recovers to the point of response to language, the acute care team is much less interested in coma as a measure of injury severity or recovery.

## Orientation

The patient's coma level is monitored daily until the patient can respond to orientation questions. At that point, the patient is administered the Hahnemann Orientation and Memory Examination (HOME; Appendix A). This instrument combines orientation questions with specific procedures for measuring retrograde and anterograde amnesia. It is based on many suggestions for orientation questionnaires. In particular, it was strongly influenced by the GOAT, and the GOAT score can actually be derived from the HOME. However, the HOME represents a significant improvement over the item content and scaling of other available instruments. The development of the HOME included a significant item expansion, clarification of interviewing methods for assessing retrograde and anterograde amnesia, improvement of item scaling, and inclusion of a new well-designed screening test of memory.

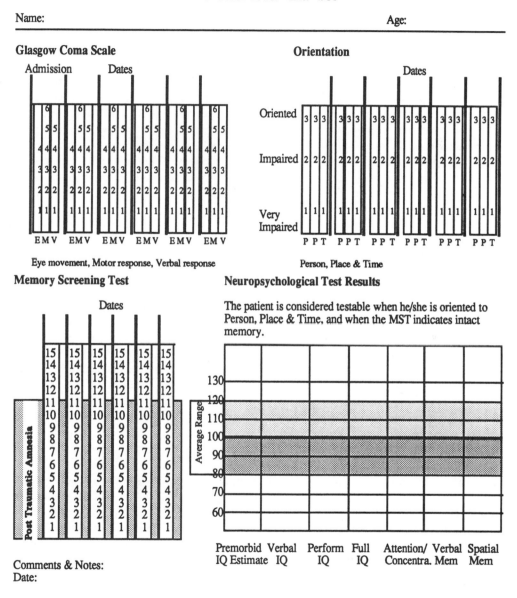

FIGURE 16.2. The Hahnemann Neuropsychology Laboratory Trauma Summary Form.

The HOME is organized into five major sections: (1) personal orientation; (2) place orientation; (3) time orientation; (4) retrograde/anterograde memory questions; (5) memory screening test. The personal orientation section consists of questions concerning well-learned personal information, such as the patient's name, address, phone number, occupation, and marital status. This is an expansion over previous questionnaires. The scaling of items was derived from administering the items to approximately 100 trauma patients. The scoring weights were derived from an analysis of the most commonly passed and missed questions of disoriented patients. Items which were most often passed were given the lowest weights, and remaining items were scaled upward based on their worst scale values and frequency of passed responses. For example, correct report of the name was discovered to be much easier than report of the current phone number. Therefore, a patient who reports only the name does not receive as many points for personal orientation as one who can report the phone number. This scaling procedure was also used with the place and time orientation questions. For example, the patient does not receive as many points for reporting the year as he/she receives for reporting the current day. Time and place orientation is assessed using conventional questions.

The HOME also includes questions for assessing anterograde and retrograde amnesia. The interview format for assessing memory for personal experiences is clearly the only way to measure retrograde and anterograde amnesia. Since the circumstances of traumatic injury preclude any systematic control of information presented to the patient, each patient's experience is therefore unique. The patient's simple description is the only way to assess knowledge for circumstances surrounding the accident.

The HOME includes suggestions for eliciting this information. Essentially, the examiner attempts to elicit a spontaneous description of events from the patient. The examiner should ask a variety of questions in order to elicit as much information as possible. Of course, many factors influence the reliability of this information. These include distractibility from pain, alcohol, drug, or medication intoxication, and stories told to the patient by family members while the patient is in the intensive care unit.

The magnitude of memory loss for events before the onset of trauma attributable to brain injury represents the degree of retrograde amnesia (RA). The event which is recalled correctly from the injury point back in time can be used as a reference point for the measurement of duration of RA. It is important to note the degree of memory loss for the interval in addition to the interval duration. Most previous studies have focused only on the duration. However, it is important to note the degree of memory loss during the interval. This will allow for comparison of density of anterograde amnesia and may highlight the deleterious effects of high alcohol levels and so forth which may have affected recall. It is unfortunate that the assessment of memory for these experiences must rely on such informal interview processes. The ratings and conclusion which result from these interview reports are strongly influenced and confounded by many factors outside the control of the examiner.

The final element of the HOME is the Memory Screening Test (Figure 16.3). The screening test consists of 15 cards in a booklet. Six pictures are printed on each card. The examiner shows a card and points to one of the six figures and instructs the patient: "Try to remember that I pointed to this figure. I will show this card to you again later and ask you to tell me which of these I pointed to before." The examiner then shows the 15 cards, one at a time, and points to one of the six figures on each card. After 15 cards are shown, the examiner then returns to the first card and says, "Which one of these did I point to before?" The patient then points out or names the figure which was indicated before. The score is

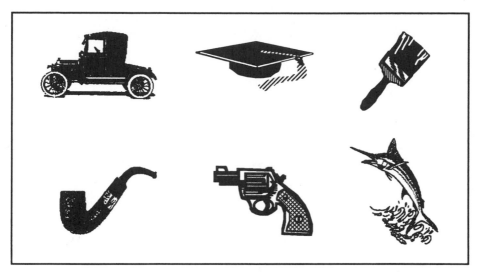

FIGURE 16.3. A representative item from the Memory Screening Test.

simply the number correct for the 15 trials. This score is recorded on the HOME summary table as a screening measure of anterograde memory ability. The score on this test in combination with the interview questions of current events constitutes the anterograde memory score. These two procedures also allow for the measurement of the construct of PTA duration.

After the examiner prompts the patient with open-ended questions and then follows with specific, follow-up questions designed to elicit details, the examiner makes an informal judgment of the degree and duration of retrograde amnesia and anterograde amnesia. These durations are summarized on the table at the top of the HOME. Likewise, the scores for personal, time, and place orientation are recorded. The values for general levels of impairment on this table were derived from analysis of the first 100 trauma patients administered the HOME. These values are still in the process of evaluation, and the results which emerge from further studies of the HOME may adjust them further.

## Neuropsychological Examination

The final step in the Hahnemann tracking system is to administer an abbreviated neuropsychological evaluation. This consists of the WAIS-R, Memory Assessment Scales (MAS), Sensory Perceptual Exam, motor tests, and other specialized tests (e.g., aphasia testing) suggested by the patient's unique deficits. The neuropsychological evaluation is designed to comprehensively screen cognitive abilities using a battery of tests which can be pragmatically used with most of the trauma patients at this stage of recovery. Of course, some patients are so impaired that they may only receive the HOME before discharge. Many such patients will receive neuropsychological evaluation later in recovery. A prominent feature of the acute-care setting these days is that trauma patients do not stay in the hospital for an extended period. As soon as they are medically stabilized, they are discharged to the rehabilitation setting or home.

The neuropsychological testing results are reported on the fourth major section of the trauma report (Figure 16.2). The summary table compiles the basic quotient measures for major constructs assessed by the WAIS-R and MAS. This table provides a concise presentation of neuropsychological test results in a format which can be viewed and comprehended quickly by trauma team members. This communication role of the trauma summary cannot be understated. It is difficult enough to have the usual referral sources pay attention to neuropsychological testing reports. The trauma center environment magnifies these difficulties tenfold. The trauma summary form is one method to present test findings in a graphic that can be apprehended at a glance.

Although all trauma patients receive these basic tracking tests, each patient has a unique pattern of deficits which are assessed using specialized tests. These deficits include visuospatial neglect, aphasia, frontal lobe syndrome, and lateralized motor and sensory findings. They vary with the extent of localized lesions derived from hematomas, cortical contusions, and other pathology. These unique deficits are assessed using conventional procedures, and these findings are reported in progress notes, team meetings, and consultation reports.

## Premorbid Abilities

Premorbid intellectual abilities are estimated using two major procedures. The first relies on the regression formula devised by Wilson, Rosenbaum, and Brown (1978). This formula utilizes the demographic variables of education, occupation, race, and gender to predict IQ. The second procedure is use of the ratings from the premorbid form of the Cognitive Behavior Rating Scales (CBRS; Williams, 1987). This scale requests family members to rate the patient on a wide array of everyday cognitive skill areas and manifestations of cognitive problems. The CBRS also requests family members to note the patient's history of schooling. This includes school grades, special class placement, and any history of problems in schooling. All of this information is considered, and a clinical prediction of premorbid intelligence is recorded on the summary form (Figure 16.2).

Although there is controversy surrounding the estimation of premorbid intellectual abilities, these estimates are often informally made in the trauma center and are used to conceptualize extent of injury and make clinical decisions. Because of the strong need to compare current abilities to premorbid status, trauma team members will make this comparison although estimating cognitive loss is uncertain and the psychologist disapproves. It is far preferable for the team to be guided by an estimate derived from the best of actuarial and clinical prediction methods derived from neuropsychology.

## Consultation Reports

The text which accompanies the neuropsychology summary chart consists of progress notes in the medical record, notes on the summary form itself, and formal consultation reports. In the trauma center, it is paramount to report findings quickly. Otherwise they will go unnoticed and have no bearing on the patient's care. Placement happens fast in the trauma center. If the neuropsychologist does not act quickly, then the pace of events will render the assessment useless. To a great extent, this simple feature of the trauma center environment has motivated many of the protocol design features used at Hahnemann.

As a result, the text descriptions which appear in the medical chart are also concise and use simple expository language. Obtuse or arcane psychological terminology is avoided. Conclusions and recommendations focus on the immediate decision-making which confronts the team. Such timely assessment of cognitive abilities can have great bearing on the patient's treatment and rehabilitation course. Most trauma team members understand and appreciate clear statements of the patient's cognitive abilities. Conventional neuropsychological reports which use unfamiliar terminology and do not focus on communication with the team will be ignored or neglected.

## PRELIMINARY RESULTS

At present, 176 patients have been followed on the Hahnemann protocol (Table 16.3). As can be seen, a majority of the trauma patients were young adult males who sustained their injuries in automobile accidents. This is consistent with most previous studies of trauma. The majority of the patients were admitted in a state of coma. Almost all of the patients were at least disoriented to time when first administered the HOME. In general, the sample conformed to the demographics and severity status of other samples studied from trauma centers (e.g., Becker *et al.*, 1982). However, the sample was distinct from groups collected from rehabilitation programs. The present sample included more patients who were mildly injured and recovered relatively quickly. Such patients are not usually referred to rehabilitation programs.

In general, the patients with severe injuries and low coma levels on the GCS became alert and at least oriented to place after 23 days. Of course, there was a group of patients who never recovered from coma and maintained either a persistent vegetative or an agitated, disoriented state. Five patients expired in the trauma center. However, patients with these poor outcomes were in the minority. Virtually all the patients at least emerged from coma.

Patients who eventually became oriented and recovered memory function emerged from coma very quickly. The average duration from injury to orientation was 9 days

TABLE 16.3. Characteristics of Preliminary Sample (*n* = 176)[a]

| Variable | Mean | SD | Min | Max | Measurement |
|---|---|---|---|---|---|
| Age | 36.11 | 14.58 | 14 | 80 | Years |
| Education | 12.47 | 2.59 | 4 | 21 | Years |
| Admit coma | 11.12 | 4.65 | 3 | 15 | Glasgow Coma Scale |
| Highest coma | 14.62 | 1.25 | 9 | 15 | Glasgow Coma Scale |
| Person orientation | 21.44 | 2.78 | 8 | 22 | HOME |
| Place orientation | 21.25 | 6.02 | 0 | 24 | HOME |
| Time orientation | 23.65 | 10.39 | 0 | 32 | HOME |
| Posttraumatic amnesia duration | 4.25 | 7.44 | 0 | 32 | HOME and GOAT |
| GOAT | 79.41 | 24.95 | 5 | 100 | |
| Memory Screening Test | 12.55 | 3.21 | 3 | 15 | Number correct |
| Glasgow Outcome Scale | 4.83 | 0.44 | 3 | 5 | Category Scale (1 to 6) |

Injury type: MVA 65%; falls 25%; other 10%
Gender: Males 76%
Presence of—hematoma: 12%; skull fracture: 18%; hemiparesis: 8%; pupillary abnormality: 14%

[a]HOME: Hahnemann Orientation and Memory Examination; GOAT: Galveston Orientation and Amnesia Test.

($SD$ = 13 days). The correlation between coma level (lowest GCS) and coma duration was statistically significant but low to moderate (Figure 16.4). The correlation between coma level and time until the patient was oriented was also low ($r$ = .43). Patients who persisted in coma for at least 15 days had a much poorer outcome, and some never attained orientation or basically intact memory function.

Measures of orientation derived from the HOME all demonstrated consistent inter-correlations in the moderate range. Contrary to most clinical lore and other studies of disorientation, this suggests that the areas assessed under disorientation are theoretically distinct. Most clinicians and researchers tend to integrate orientation to person, place, and time as one theoretical construct. The pattern observed here suggests that they are somewhat independent. Recovery of orientation also follows a characteristic pattern which suggests some independence. In general, patients who can be asked orientation questions are not disoriented to person unless they are delirious or premorbidly demented. The next area most resistant is orientation to place. Most patients who recovered to the point of being able to respond to the HOME correctly reported the city and state. They had greater

|  | Lowest GCS | Coma Duration | Hematoma | Skull Fracture | Pupil Abnormality | Hemiparesis | Person Orientation | Place Orientation | Time Orientation | GOAT Total Score | Memory Screening Test | PTA Duration | Retrograde Amnesia | Glasgow Outcome Scale |
|---|---|---|---|---|---|---|---|---|---|---|---|---|---|---|
| Lowest GCS |  |  |  |  |  |  |  |  |  |  |  |  |  |  |
| Coma Duration | .51 |  |  |  |  |  |  |  |  |  |  |  |  |  |
| Hematoma | .49 | .44 |  |  |  |  |  |  |  |  |  |  |  |  |
| Skull Fracture |  |  | .27 |  |  |  |  |  |  |  |  |  |  |  |
| Pupil Abnormality | .38 |  |  |  |  |  |  |  |  |  |  |  |  |  |
| Hemiparesis |  |  | .34 |  |  |  |  |  |  |  |  |  |  |  |
| Person Orientation | .28 |  |  |  |  |  |  |  |  |  |  |  |  |  |
| Place Orientation |  |  | .28 |  |  |  | .37 |  |  |  |  |  |  |  |
| Time Orientation | .26 |  |  |  |  |  | .40 | .56 |  |  |  |  |  |  |
| GOAT Total Score | .29 |  |  |  |  |  | .28 | .45 | .72 |  |  |  |  |  |
| Memory Screening Test | .28 | .37 |  |  |  |  | .39 | .44 | .47 | .42 |  |  |  |  |
| PTA Duration | .43 | .35 |  |  |  |  |  |  |  | .41 | .34 | .34 |  |  |
| Retrograde Amnesia | .44 |  |  |  | .35 |  |  |  |  | .34 |  |  |  |  |
| Glasgow Outcome Scale | .36 | .49 | .70 | .46 |  |  |  |  |  | .45 | .47 |  | .49 |  |

FIGURE 16.4. Statistically significant correlations between selected measures are presented. Coma level shows low but consistent correlations with virtually every other severity and outcome measure. Measures of memory ability and orientation to person, place, and time also show strong intercorrelations.

difficulty with the name of the hospital. All patients who were disoriented had difficulty reporting the time. They had greatest difficulty reporting the day of the week and the month. It was much easier to report the current year.

These findings suggest that responses to disorientation questionnaires are strongly influenced by anterograde memory processes, and there are a subset of items under each orientation heading which embody the construct of memory disorder. Such questions as "What is the current date?" or "What is the name of this hospital?" require the patient to have ongoing memory consolidation ability. There are another set of items which assess remote memory such as the patient's name or address. Many of these items can be scaled according to the recency of information exposure and the sensitivity of the item to anterograde amnesia. Items which request more remote knowledge are rarely failed; those items which request recent information are often failed. The concept of disorientation therefore rests on the commonly observed and studied phenomena associated with anterograde amnesia (Russell & Nathan, 1946). Amnesic patients cannot retain information presented recently but can recall remote knowledge consolidated in the past. A more theoretically consistent division of orientation items might therefore be to separately score person, place, and time items which request information which is recently acquired versus items which request remote information. Future analyses of the HOME will explore these notions and develop alternate scoring systems in order to best separate the constructs of disorientation, memory disorder, and delirium.


## SUMMARY

This chapter presented a model tracking system for measuring, documenting, and communicating cognitive status to members of the hospital team who treat cases of TBI in the acute care environment. Cognitive assessment in this environment is essential in order to monitor recovery, assess the influence of treatment, predict outcomes, and place patients in the best possible discharge settings. The model system proposed here relies strongly on abbreviated assessment instruments and alternative, concise, and efficient methods to present cognitive status information to the trauma team. The team will only use information from the neuropsychologist if it is presented in a timely fashion and in a format the team members can understand at a glance.

Preliminary findings concerning patient cognitive status, predictions of outcome, and utility of the tracking system are presented after approximately one year of data collection. In general, it was discovered that patients who sustained the more severe coma levels at admission had longer coma durations and worse cognitive outcomes. However, a subset of cases were characterized by severe initial comas but a quick recovery rate. These patients also had better overall outcomes than others of comparable severity.

The tracking battery and procedures performed well as a clinical system. Patients benefitted from an efficient monitoring of cognitive function. However, there are still some impediments to the use of cognitive data in decision-making in the trauma center. In general, only if a decision concerning a patient absolutely requires information about cognitive status do team members consult the neuropsychologist's report. Although the procedures described here increased the team members' understanding of the cognitive data, considerable attention must still be given to education of team members and enhancement of the use of cognitive data in the everyday management of trauma patients.

APPENDIX A

## *Hahnemann Orientation and Memory Examination (HOME)*

**J. Michael Williams, PhD & Sandra Koffler, PhD**

Name: _____ Date: _____ Date of Injury: _____

Age: _____ Education: _____ Occupation: _____

**Instructions:** Ask the patient each of the following questions. If the patient cannot respond, or responds incorrectly, then suggest three multiple choice alternatives. Circle point values on the right which correspond to the patient's performance. Sum these point values for each major section. The GOAT summary score is computed by subtracting the total "GOAT Fail" error points from 100.

| | Very Impaired | | Impaired | | Normal Limits |
|---|---|---|---|---|---|
| Personal Orientation | 0-5 | 6-11 | 12-17 | 18-20 | 21-22 |
| Place Orientation | 0-5 | 6-11 | 12-17 | 18-23 | 24 |
| Time Orientation | 0-6 | 7-13 | 14-17 | 18-23 | 24-32 |
| Anterograde Amnesia | 0-5 | 6-11 | 12-17 | 18-23 | 24 |
| GOAT | 0-33 | 34-65 | 66-70 | 71-75 | 76-100 |
| Memory Screen (Imm) | 1-3 | 4-5 | 6-8 | 9-10 | 11-15 |
| Memory Screen (24hrs) | 1-2 | 3-4 | 5-6 | 7-8 | 9-15 |

Duration of Retrograde Amnesia: _____   Duration of Anterograde Amnesia: _____

ILLNESS

*Personal Orientation:*

|   |   | Pass | Mult Choice Pass | Fail | GOAT Fail Points |
|---|---|---|---|---|---|
| 1. | What is your name? | 2 | 1 | 0 | 2 |
| 2. | What is your age? | 2 | 1 | 0 | |
| 3. | Where were you born? | 4 | 2 | 0 | |
| 4. | What is your date of birth? | 2 | 1 | 0 | 4 |
| 5. | What is your address? | 4 | 2 | 0 | 4 |
| 6. | What is your telephone number? | 4 | 2 | 0 | |
| 7. | Are you married? | 2 | 1 | 0 | |
| 8. | What is your occupation? | 2 | 1 | 0 | |

*Personal Orientation Subtotal:*

*Orientation to Place:*

|   |   | Pass | Mult Choice Pass | Fail | GOAT Fail Points |
|---|---|---|---|---|---|
| 9. | What state are we in? | 4 | 2 | 0 | |
| 10. | What city (town) are we in? | 6 | 3 | 0 | 5 |
| 11. | Where are you right now? | 6 | 3 | 0 | 5 |
| 12. | What is the name of this hospital? | 8 | 4 | 0 | |

*Place Orientation Subtotal:*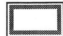

*Orientation to Time:*

**13. What is the year?**

GOAT score is computed by adding 10 for each year off, with a max of 30          **4    2    0** _____

**14. What is the month?**

GOAT score is computed by adding 5 for each month off, with a max of 15          **6    3    0** _____

**15. What *day* of the month is it?**

Give 4 pts. if the response is within 5 days of the correct day, or if the patient chooses the correct choice among multiple          **8    4    0** _____
choices. GOAT score is computed by adding 1 for each day off, with max of 5

**16. What day of the week is it?**

GOAT score is computed by adding 1 for each day off, with max of 7          **6    3    0** _____

**17. Without looking at your watch, tell me what time it is?**

Give 8 pts. for a response which is within one hour of the correct time. Give 4 pts if the response is within 2 hrs of the correct          **8    4    0** _____
time, or if the patient chooses correctly from multiple choices. Compute GOAT score by adding 1 for each 1/2 hour off, max of 5.

*Time Orientation Subtotal:*  ▢

**18. *Anterograde Amnesia:***

Prompt the patient to freely describe his/her accident, illness, the hospital setting, and events which have happened since admission. You may use prompts such as: **Why are you in the hospital now? Tell me what you know about your illness or injury. Tell me what you remember of the accident (or surgery, or other illness)? Describe a typical day in the hospital. Describe some things that have happened to you in the hospital.** Record the salient parts of the patient's response. Ask for details, such as what the patient had at the most recent meal, names of doctors, nurses etc. Give 6 points if the subject is correct and describes events in detail, and 3 points if the subject is correct but omits details.

**6    3    0**

**19. On what day were you admitted to the hospital?**          **6    3    0** _____

Award 6 pts if the patient is absolutely correct. Award 3 pts if the patient is within one day of the correct answer, or chooses correctly from multiple choices. If a patient reports that someone else has told him/her the day and thereby correctly reports the day, then this indicates intact memory and the patient receives 6 pts. GOAT is computed by adding 5 for an incorrect response

**20. How did you get here?**          **6    3    0** _____

Record the patient's response. Give 6 points if the subject is correct and describes events in detail, and 3 points if the subject is correct but omits details. If a patient reports that someone else has told him/her the manner of transport to the hospital and thereby correctly reports this information, then this indicates intact memory and the patient receives 6 pts. GOAT is computed by adding 5 for being unable to describe mode of transport to the hospital.

**21. Describe the first event you recalled after the accident (or illness). 6    3    0** _____

Record the salient parts of the patient's response. Ask for details concerning this event, such as whether the patient was with companions, date and time. Note the duration of Anterograde Amnesia. Give 6 points if the subject is correct and describes events in detail, and 3 points if the subject is correct but omits details. GOAT is computed by adding 10 for essentially being *unable* to make a response. Add 5 points to the GOAT if the subject makes a roughly accurate response but cannot give details.

*Anterograde Amnesia Subtotal:*  ▢

*Retrograde Amnesia*

**22. Tell me the last event you recall before the accident (or onset of illness).**

Record the patient's response. Note the duration of retrograde amnesia. This is the interval between the injury          _____
and the last event recalled. The GOAT score is computed by adding 5 points for an inaccurate response.

**23. Describe this event in detail. What was the date or time of the event?**

**Who was with you? Where were you?**

Record the salient features of the patient's response. Note the duration of retrograde amnesia. This is the interval between the injury and the last event recalled. The GOAT score is computed by adding 5 points for inability to report details of the event.

100 - (GOAT Fail Points) =                    (GOAT Score)

APPENDIX B: THE HAHNEMANN ORIENTATION AND MEMORY
EXAMINATION (HOME) AND A SAMPLE CONSULTATION REPORT

## Consultation Request

HAHNEMANN UNIVERSITY

| Date of request 7/18/90 | Desire consultation with Neuropsychology | |
|---|---|---|
| Requesting physician Dr. D. | Diagnosis Traumatic Brain Injury | Name Plate Area |
| REASON FOR CONSULTATION | Evaluation of cognitive abilities | |

| Physician or service | Was notified on | AT | BY AM PM | At Extension | Direct Office | Other |
|---|---|---|---|---|---|---|
| | | | | | | |

TL is a 23-year-old SWF involved in a MVA on 5/16/89. She was unconscious at the scene of the accident and was intubated. Upon admission, she was disoriented X3, combative, and was moving all extremities. Her admission Glasgow Coma Score was judged to be a 6. CT of the head on 5/16 revealed a left frontal contusion, which was largely resolved by 5/18. The patient is S/P splenectomy, has fractured ribs and a fractured right scapula. The patient's disorientation and agitation was resolved by 5/23, when she was noted to be alert, oriented, and able to remember ongoing events. She had a remarkably accelerated recovery of cognitive abilities relative to the initial severity of the injury and coma.

TL is a flight attendant who is currently between jobs. She was an above average student in high school and attended two years of college. She was given the *Wechsler Adult Intelligence Scale—Revised*, the *Memory Assessment Scales*, the *Wide Range Achievement Test*, and her mother completed the premorbid assessment form of the *Cognitive Behavior Rating Scales*. The following are findings from testing on 5/25/89.

*Findings:* Cognitive and memory testing indicate that she is currently functioning

### Neuropsychological Test Results

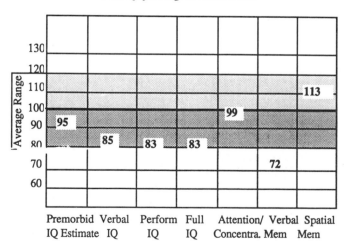

generally in the low average range. She has relative strengths in attention and concentration. Her academic skills and general fund of information are relatively poor. Her verbal and performance IQ scores are in the low average range (see figure on page 290). The results of the achievement test indicate that her current reading, spelling, and arithmetic abilities are approximately at the sixth grade level. These abilities are probably mildly diminished from premorbid levels. This drop in ability is probably a result of fatigue and the general effects of the trauma and hospitalization.

She performed in the mildly impaired range on test of verbal memory and delayed recall. Her visuospatial memory was average to above average. This relative difference in verbal versus visuospatial memory is most likely the persistent result of left hemisphere injury. It is recommended that she be reevaluated before returning to work.

## REFERENCES

Becker, D. P., Miller, J. D., & Greenberg, R. P. (1982). Prognosis after head injury. In J. R. Youmans (Ed.), *Neurological surgery*. Philadelphia: Saunders.

Bond, M. R., & Brooks, D. N. (1976). Understanding the process of recovery as a basis for the investigation of rehabilitation for the brain injured. *Scandinavian Journal of Rehabilitation Medicine*, 8, 127–133.

Carlsson, G. S., Svardsudd, K., & Welin, L. (1987). Long-term effects of head injuries sustained during life in three male populations. *Journal of Neurosurgery*, 67, 197–205.

Cooper, P. R., Moody, S., Clark, W. K., Kirkpatrick, J., Maravilla, K., Gould, A. L., & Drane, W. (1979). Dexamethasone and severe head injury. *Journal of Neurosurgery*, 51, 307–316.

Dikmen, S., McLean, A., & Temkin, N. R. (1986a). Neuropsychological and psychosocial consequences of minor head injury. *Journal of Neurology, Neurosurgery, & Psychiatry*, 49, 1227–1232.

Dikmen, S., McLean, A., & Temkin, N. R. (1986b). Neuropsychologic outcome at one-month postinjury. *Archives of Physical Medicine & Rehabilitation*, 67, 507–513.

Dikmen, S., Temkin, N., McLean, A., Wyler, A., & Machamer, J. (1987). Memory and head injury severity. *Journal of Neurology, Neurosurgery & Psychiatry*, 50, 1613–1618.

Eisenberg, H. M., & Weiner, R. L. (1987). Input variables: How information from the acute injury can be used to characterize groups of patients for studies of outcome. In H. S. Levin, J. Grafman, & H. M. Eisenberg (Eds.), *Neurobehavioral consequences of closed head injury*. New York: Oxford University Press.

Fleichser, A. S., Payne, N. S., & Tindall, G. T. (1976). Continuous monitoring of intracranial pressure in severe closed head injury without mass lesions. *Surgical Neurology*, 6, 31–34.

Gensemer, I. B., McMurry, F. G., Walker, J. C., Monasky, M., & Brotman, S. J. (1988). Behavioral consequences of trauma. *The Journal of Trauma*, 28, 44–49.

Gurdjian, E. S., & Webster, J. E. (1958). *Head injuries, mechanisms, diagnosis and management*. Boston: Little, Brown.

Hynd, G. W., & Obrzut, J. E. (1981). *Neuropsychological assessment and the school-age child: Issues and procedures*. New York: Grune & Stratton.

Jennett, B., & Bond, M. (1975). Assessment of outcome after severe brain damage. *Lancet*, 1, 480–487.

Jennett, B., Teasdale, G., Braakman, R., Minderhoud, J., & Knill-Jones, R. (1976). Predicting outcome in individual patients after severe head injury. *Lancet*, 1, 1031–1034.

Kerr, T. A., Kay, W. K., & Lassman, L. P. (1971). Characteristics of patients, type of accident, and mortality in a consecutive series of head injuries admitted to a neurosurgical unit. *British Journal of the Society of Medicine*, 25, 179–185.

Klonoff, P. S., Costa, L .D., & Snow, W. G. (1986). Predictors and indicators of quality of life in patients with closed head injury. *Journal of Clinical & Experimental Neuropsychology*, 8, 469–485.

Klove, H. W., & Cleeland, C. S. (1972). The relationship of neuropsychological impairment to other indices of severity and head injury. *Scandinavian Journal of Rehabilitation Medicine*, 4, 55–60.

Levin, H. S., & Grossman, R. G. (1978). Behavioral sequelae of closed head injury. *Archives of Neurology*, 35, 720–727.

Levin, H. S., Grossman, R. G., Rose, J. E., & Teasdale, G. (1979). Long-term neuropsychological outcome of closed head injury. *Journal of Neurosurgery*, *50*, 412–422.

Levin, H. S., Grossman, R. G., Sarwar, M., & Meyers, C. A. (1981). Linguistic recovery after closed head injury. *Brain & Cognition*, *12*, 360–374.

Levin, H. S., Benton, A. L., & Grossman, R. G. (1982). *Neurobehavioral consequences of closed head injury*. New York: Oxford University Press.

Lewis, A. J. (1976). *Mechanisms of neurological disease*. Boston: Little, Brown.

Lezak, M. (1979). Recovery of memory and learning functions following traumatic brain injury. *Cortex*, *15*, 63–72.

Lezak, M. (1987). Relationship between personality disorders, social disturbances and physical disability following traumatic brain injury. *Journal of Head Trauma Rehabilitation*, *2*, 57–69.

Lundholm, J., Jepsen, B. N., & Thornval, G. (1975). The late neurological, psychological, and social aspects of severe traumatic coma. *Scandinavian Journal of Rehabilitation Medicine*, *7*, 97–100.

McKinlay, W. W., Brooks, D. N., Bond, M. R., Matinage, D. P., & Marshall, M. M. (1981). The short-term outcome of severe blunt head injury as reported by relatives of the injured persons. *Journal of Neurology, Neurosurgery, & Psychiatry*, *44*, 527–533.

Mandleberg, I. A. (1976). Cognitive recovery after severe head injury. 3. Wechsler Adult Intelligence Scale Verbal and Performance IQ's as a function of post traumatic amnesia duration and time from injury. *Journal of Neurology, Neurosurgery, & Psychiatry*, *39*, 1001–1007.

Mattis, S. (1976). Mental status examination for organic mental syndrome in the elderly patient. In L. Bellak & T. Karasu (Eds.), *Geriatric psychiatry. A handbook for psychiatrists and primary care physicians*. New York: Grune & Stratton.

Oddy, M., Humphrey, M., & Uttley, D. (1978). Subjective impairment and social recovery after closed head injury. *Journal of Neurology, Neurosurgery, & Psychiatry*, *41*, 611–616.

Plum, F., & Posner, J. B. (1982). *The diagnosis of stupor and coma*. Philadelphia: Davis.

Poon, L. (1986). *Clinical memory assessment of older adults*. Washington, DC: American Psychological Association.

Prigatano, G. P., Fordyce, D. J., Zeiner, H. K., Roueche, J. R., Pepping, M., & Wood, B. C. (1984). Neuropsychological rehabilitation after closed head injury in young adults. *Journal of Neurology, Neurosurgery, & Psychiatry*, *47*, 505–513.

Rimel, R. W., Giordani, B., Barth, J. T., & Jane, J. (1982). Moderate head injury: Completing the clinical spectrum of brain trauma. *Neurosurgery*, *11*, 344–351.

Russell, W. R., & Nathan, P. W. (1946). Traumatic amnesia. *Brain*, *69*, 280–300.

Strich, S. J. (1961). Shearing of nerve fibers as a cause of brain damage due to head injury: A pathological study of twenty cases. *Lancet*, *2*, 443–448.

Teasdale, G., & Jennett, B. (1974). Assessment of coma and impaired consciousness. A practical scale. *Lancet*, *2*, 81–84.

Uzzell, B. P., Dolinskas, C. A., & Langfitt, T. W. (1988). Visual field defects in relation to head injury severity. *Archives of Neurology*, *45*, 420–424.

Vapalahti, M., & Troupp, H. (1971). Prognosis for patients with severe brain injuries. *British Medical Journal*, *3*, 404–407.

Varney, N. R. (1988). Prognostic significance of anosmia in patients with closed head injury. *Journal of Clinical & Experimental Neuropsychology*, *10*, 250–254.

Vogel, F. S. (1979). Pathology of trauma of the nervous system. In G. L. Odom (Ed.), *Central nervous system trauma research status report* (pp. 114–122). Bethesda: NINCDS, National Institutes of Health.

Williams, J. M. (1987). *The Cognitive Behavior Rating Scales*. Odessa, FL: Psychological Assessment Resources.

Williams, J. M. (1990). *The Memory Assessment Scales*. Odessa, FL: Psychological Assessment Resources.

Williams, J. M., Gomes, F., Drudge, O. W., & Kessler, M. (1984). The prediction of outcome from closed head injury by early assessment of trauma severity. *Journal of Neurosurgery*, *61*, 581–585.

Wilson, J. T. L., Wiedmann, K. D., Hadley, D. M., Condon, B., Teasdale, G., & Brooks, D. N. (1988). Early and late magnetic resonance imaging and neuropsychological outcome after head injury, *Journal of Neurology, Neurosurgery & Psychiatry*, *51*, 391–396.

Wilson, R. S., Rosenbaum, G., & Brown, G. (1978). An index of premorbid intelligence. *Journal of Consulting & Clinical Psychology*, *46*, 1554–1555.

# 17

# Traumatic Brain Injury

## Outcome and Predictors of Outcome

DONALD A. TAYLOR

### SCOPE OF THE PROBLEM

Traumatic brain injury (TBI) affects over 400,000 people each year in the United States (Kalsbeck, McLaurin *et al.*, 1980). Mortality following severe TBI varies between 30% and 60% (Bartkowski & Lovely, 1986). One multicenter study of TBI in an adult population identified 51% mortality with 36% having good recovery or moderate disability and 13% having severe disability or being in a vegetative state (Jennett, Teasdale *et al.*, 1987). In children and adolescents, there was a 33% mortality, 51% of the patients had a good outcome or moderate disability and 16% were severely disabled or were in a vegetative state (Berger, Pitts, & Lovely, 1985). The Medical College of Virginia, demonstrating the value of intensive management, found 30% mortality with 60% good outcome/moderate disability, 8% severe disability, and 2% persistent vegetative state (Becker, Miller *et al.*, 1977). A study of pediatric head injury from the same institution reported 24% mortality, 68% good outcome/moderate disability, 6% severe disability, and 2% persistent vegetative state (Ward & Alberico, 1987). Thus, although good outcome or moderate disability varies widely depending on age and level of care, the incidence of severe disability/vegetative state is relatively constant despite age or type of care. Approximately 40,000 patients will have poor outcome annually with 32,000 being severely disabled and 8000 remaining in a vegetative state.

DONALD A. TAYLOR • Cumberland Hospital, New Kent, Virginia 23124.

*HANDBOOK OF HEAD TRAUMA: Acute Care to Recovery*, edited by Charles J. Long and Leslie K. Ross. Plenum Press, New York, 1992.

## DEFINITION OF CONCEPTS

A significant problem in assessment of outcome in TBI is an imprecision in the definition of concepts, specifically *coma* and *vegetative state*. The correct use of terms and appropriate definition of terms is essential before one can evaluate prognosis in TBI.

*Coma* refers to a state of unarousable psychologic unresponsiveness in which the patient lies with eyes closed. These patients show no recognizable response to external stimulus or the expression of inner needs (Medical Research Council, Brain Injuries Committee, 1941). Unfortunately, a number of terms to grade degree of or severity of coma have emerged, confusing the definition of coma as noted above. For example, *semicoma* refers to the patient who can be aroused (through noxious stimulation) to a state of nonspecific movement or stirring.

This type of imprecision in terminology led to the creation of more objective coma grading systems, such as the Glasgow Coma Score (Jennett & Teasdale, 1977). Thus, a numerical score can be used to quantify severity of consciousness alteration and correlate severity of injury with outcome. However, the meaning of the term *coma* is lost as only the lowest Glasgow Coma Score possible refers to a state of no recognizable response to external stimulus or inner need. Therefore, based on the Glasgow Coma Score, many TBI patients are not classified as being in coma (by strict definition), but are rather in a state of less than normal arousability when certain stimuli are applied.

Similar problems exist with the use of the term *vegetative state*. This term refers to return of wakefulness with apparent total lack of cognitive function. Operationally, sleep–wake cycles exist and eyes open spontaneously in response to verbal stimuli. The patient spontaneously maintains blood pressure and respiratory control. There are no discrete localizing motor responses, and receptive and expressive language are absent (Levy, Knill-Jones, & Plum, 1978; Plum & Posner, 1980). The term *vegetative state* underscores the significant discrepancy between preserved vegetative (autonomic) functions and severe cognitive disability (Plum & Posner, 1980). Unfortunately, the term *persistent vegetative state* is frequently confused with, or substituted for, the term *vegetative state* implying prognosis when sufficient clinical data to establish prognosis are not available. This desire to avoid the prognostic implication of the term *vegetative* has led to use of a variety of other terms—*coma vigil, apallic syndrome, neocortical death*.

## RECENT DEVELOPMENTS IN TBI

In the last 20 years tremendous advances have been made in the neurosurgical management and intensive care of severe TBI. Recognition of enlarging intracranial mass lesions (clots) by clinical course and subsequent surgical evacuation of the clot(s) has been known to improve outcome since before the era of modern medicine. The development of special neuroimaging procedures, such as computed tomography of the brain, and their immediate availability in the emergency room setting has led to early identification of operable clots even before deteriorating clinical course revealed their presence. These neuroimaging modalities also allowed better identification of brain swelling (edema) and elucidation of edema and increased pressure inside the head as a major source of mortality and morbidity. Perhaps the greatest single advance in the management of severe TBI has been the development of intracranial pressure monitoring. Secondary injury to the brain may result from increased intracranial pressure and resultant reduction in blood flow to the brain. In many cases the outcome can be improved by medical or surgical reduction of the increased intracranial pressure, thus improving blood flow to the brain. Thus, the development of neuroimaging procedures was a significant help to the neurosurgeon managing a patient with severe TBI.

Despite these advancements in management, the mortality and morbidity following severe TBI remain significant (Jennett et al., 1987; Berger et al., 1985). Furthermore, a large number of severe TBI victims (47% to 72%) do not have injury requiring surgical treatment (Bowers & Marshall, 1980; Levati et al., 1982). These patients may have relatively long duration of coma, and recovery is often incomplete. Prolonged survival of patients in persistent coma or vegetative state has led to increasing concerns regarding: (1) cost of care, (2) cost/benefit ratio, and (3) hardship on the family who has a relative in a state of "living death."

Clearly, a better understanding of the pathology and pathophysiology of severe TBI is necessary both *in vivo* and *in vitro*. Three relatively recent developments have set the stage for modern investigation into management and prognosis of coma following severe TBI by allowing identification of more homogeneous subgroups of coma patients. They are:

1. Improved understanding of the pathology and pathophysiology of TBI
2. Improved brain imaging techniques
3. Improved clinical neurophysiology monitors

## Pathophysiology

Pathological analyses of severe TBI have often been incomplete or difficult because of the secondary damage to the brain by hypoxia and ischemia. Evaluation during life has previously been hampered by relatively crude neuroimaging technique and the relatively gross application of clinical neurophysiology tests such as the routine electroencephalogram (EEG). The long-held hypothesis that prolonged coma in the absence of obvious gross intracranial lesion was due to brain-stem injury was based as much on conjecture as on actual data obtained from coma patients.

The demonstration of a unique constellation of pathological findings (e.g., diffuse axonal injury) following pure acceleration–deceleration injury has allowed better understanding of the clinical course following severe TBI by emphasizing the presence of widespread white matter injury (Adams, Graham et al., 1982). In the past, the existence of diffuse axonal injury following TBI has been a controversial issue because of secondary changes in the brain that may occur due to hypoxia–ischemia. However, the development of an animal model for pure acceleration–deceleration injury which delineated a unique pathology of diffuse axonal injury in primates led to the clear recognition of these pathological findings in humans and the separation of diffuse axonal injury from secondary effects of hypoxia–ischemia (Gennarelli, Thibault, Adams et al., 1982). Failure to awaken from coma may be primarily due to malfunction of ascending cortical arousal systems due to diffuse axonal injury (i.e., primary brain-stem malfunction and/or failure of transmission through ascending fiber tracts due to diffuse axonal injury).

Diffuse axonal injury represents an identifiable syndrome clinically and pathologically. Patients with pure diffuse axonal injury are comatose from impact and do not have surgical intracranial mass lesions. The gross and microscopic pathology of diffuse axonal injury may not be identified by computerized tomography (unless as nonspecific "atrophy"). Diffuse axonal injury is the neuropathophysiological injury responsible for most cases of prolonged coma following TBI.

Improved understanding of neuropathophysiology of TBI allows better understanding of the etiology of coma and underscores the continuum of injury and clinical state. Thus, diffuse axonal injury may be responsible for coma with good recovery and coma leading to persistent vegetative state. Differences in outcome may be related to the degree and not the kind of pathological damage. Focal areas of cerebral contusion and general hypoxic–ischemic injury may further complicate the clinical course and also significantly affect outcome.

## Neuroimaging Techniques

Improved computerized tomography resolution has allowed better identification of the petechial hemorrhages associated with diffuse axonal injury which are typically seen in the corpus callosum and dorsal brain stem. The importance of these findings may not be in the direct identification of injury caused by the relatively small hemorrhage, but the indirect identification of diffuse axonal injury which is inferred by their presence. The use of MRI scanning may allow more direct identification of white matter injury (Han, Kaufman et al., 1984).

## Clinical Neurophysiology Monitors

The EEG is a well-known measure of ongoing cortical electrical activity (actually allowing visualization of summated excitatory and inhibitory postsynaptic potentials). In coma there may be slowing of the EEG background and improvement in EEG background may parallel clinical improvement (Mizrani & Kellaway, 1984).

Evoked potential analysis, however, allows a more direct and oftentimes more valuable analysis of central nervous system stimulation through visual, auditory, and somatosensory modalities. In particular, the somatosensory evoked potential allows assessment of conduction in somatosensory pathways from spinal cord to medulla to thalamus and to cortex. Newer techniques will allow direct evaluation of corticospinal motor pathways by direct stimulation of motor cortex. Both somatosensory and motor evoked potentials provide a direct measure of conduction through major fiber tracts and, thus, a direct evaluation of diffuse axonal injury. Absence of the somatosensory evoked potential N20 response (thalamus–cortex) is a reliable predictor of persistence in vegetative state in adults (Hume, Cant, & Shaw, 1981) and children (Frank, Furgiuele, & Etheridge, 1985).

## PREDICTORS OF OUTCOME

Many types of information have been reported that allow prediction of outcome following severe TBI. These include: (1) extent of injury; (2) age; (3) prehospital care; (4) neurological examination (Glasgow Coma Score, etc.); (5) intracranial pressure; (6) cellular injury markers; and (7) clinical neurophysiology examinations.

## Extent of Injury

Extent of injury influences outcome whether the injury is due to the primary traumatic event or due to secondary injury. However, it is usually the injuries that are secondary to the primary traumatic event which are most likely to be managed in the posttraumatic medical setting. Of these secondary impairments, the most sinister is hypoxic–ischemic injury. Hypoxic–ischemic injury may be due to multiple trauma involving heart and lungs or may be due to increased intracranial pressure. Increased intracranial pressure may lead to decreased perfusion pressure of the brain which results in hypoxic–ischemic injury. Increased intracranial pressure may also lead to various herniation syndromes, wherein mechanical forces produce brain injury directly or indirectly by compromise of blood supply. Infection (meningitis) associated with traumatic cerebrospinal fluid leak may also be a cause of secondary injury. All types of secondary injury may adversely influence outcome following severe TBI.

## Age

Young age may influence outcome almost independent of level of coma. Outcome data on 85 children (ages 4 months to 18 years) collected between 1975 and 1977 using the Glasgow Outcome Scale revealed that 77% of patients with score of 3 or 4 and 100% of patients with score of 5–8 made good recovery. These patients progressed to good recovery of moderate disability as scored by the Glasgow Outcome Scale (Bruce et al., 1979). Similar trends for good recovery in younger patients have been noted in other published series (Ward & Alberico, 1987; Narayan, Greenberg et al., 1981).

## Prehospital Care

Analysis of prehospital care has provided interesting results in severe TBI outcome prediction. Lokkeberg and Grime (1984) found that time to intubation (control of airway) had a positive correlation with outcome, while mode of transport and time of transport (up to 4 hours) did not correlate with outcome. Thus, airway control (and reduction of hypoxemia) improves outcome, while rapid transport is not so valuable without control of airway and support of blood pressure. Their study also supported the premise that increasing severity of injury has negative impact on outcome while younger age has more positive influence on outcome.

## Neurological Examination

The neurological examination has proven to be a very valuable outcome predictor in severe TBI. The Glasgow Coma Score is an abbreviated, stylized, reproducible, and quantifiable neurological examination which has been found very suitable for assessment of level of consciousness following TBI (Teasdale & Jennett, 1974). It is remarkable that such a relatively simple evaluation scale has proven to be such a reliable predictor to outcome. The reliability of the Glasgow Coma Score in predicting outcome may be enhanced by combination with clinical data such as patient age, pupil reaction, and eye movements (oculocephalic responses) (Jennett, Teasdale, Braakman, et al., 1979; Choi, Ward, & Becker, 1983).

The most widely used and accepted measurement of outcome following severe TBI is the Glasgow Outcome Scale (Jennett & Bond, 1975). The Glasgow Outcome Scale uses five gross outcome categories: (1) death, (2) persistent vegetative state, (3) severe disability (conscious but disabled), (4) moderate disability (disabled but independent), and (5) good recovery. Thus, the Glasgow Outcome Scale heavily emphasizes functional independence with respect to motility, transportation, and social life. Emotional and cognitive dysfunction, however, may be a source of extreme disability even in a patient with a relatively good Glasgow Outcome Scale level. When the Glasgow Coma Score is used to *predict* outcome, the Glasgow Outcome Scale is the usual *measurement* of outcome.

Recovery following severe TBI is variable, and rarely does the patient return to the premorbid level of functioning. Thus, a patient with no meaningful environmental interaction one month after injury may then begin to rapidly improve or may remain at a clinical plateau for a period of time before improvement occurs. Assignment of outcome, therefore, must take into account both functional level and *time from injury*. Some patients will advance to their highest functional level 6 months after injury as measured by the Glasgow Outcome Scale, while others may continue to have meaningful recovery months or years after injury (Jennett & Bond, 1975; Jennett, Teasdale, Braakman *et al.*, 1976; Jennett *et al.*, 1979; Mahoney, D'Souza, & Freeman, 1981).

In addition, significant meaningful improvement may occur with attendant improvement in quality of life even in patients who remain within a specific Glasgow Outcome Scale level. Alternative measures of outcome may be more appropriate than the Glasgow Outcome Scale in patients with moderate or severe disability. Severe disability and, thus, bad outcome from one point of view, may be reasonable quality of life with meaningful interaction from another perspective.

Several studies using the Glasgow Outcome Scale have cited that most patients reach their best level of recovery within 3 to 6 months of injury (Lange-Crossach, Riebel, & Grumme, 1981; Jennett *et al.*, 1976). Other studies have reported significant improvement in functional level beyond 6 months and extending into years following the injury (Mahoney *et al.*, 1981). Therefore, time from injury is a significant, but variable, factor in outcome assessment following severe TBI. There is definite need to better discriminate between patients who demonstrate early improvement versus patients who improve later in order to allow for better use of relatively limited resources for rehabilitation care.

## Intracranial Pressure

Intracranial pressure monitoring has not only allowed improvement in the intensive care of TBI, but the pattern of intracranial pressure may assist in outcome prediction. Narayan *et al.* (1981) reported the correlation between intracranial pressure and outcome (see Table 1).

## Cellular Injury Markers

Cerebrospinal fluid cellular injury markers such as creatinine kinase or myelin basic protein and blood creatinine kinase have been reported to correlate with outcome in TBI. In these cases they are primarily indicators of extent of brain injury. In certain select situations these markers may have special value in assisting with outcome prediction. In general,

TABLE 17.1. Intracranial Pressure as It Relates to Outcome (%)

| Intracranial pressure course (ICP) | Number of patients | Outcome (%) | | |
|---|---|---|---|---|
| | | Good outcome/ moderate disability | Severe disability/ vegetative | Dead |
| Normal throughout | 74 | 80 | 4 | 16 |
| Elevated ICP | 59 | 36 | 13 | 51 |
| High, then normal | 6 | 50 | 17 | 33 |
| Normal, then high | 44 | 39 | 16 | 45 |
| High throughout | 9 | 11 | 0 | 89 |

however, they do not significantly improve outcome prediction over that given by the Glasgow Coma Score.

## Clinical Neurophysiology

Recently, increasing interest has been directed toward the use of clinical neurology testing (EEG and evoked potentials) in predicting outcome.

### EEG

From the earliest days of clinical neurophysiology, the EEG has been known to correlate with alteration of consciousness (Berger, 1931; Gibbs, Davis, & Lennox, 1935). Animal models on EEG changes due to concussion demonstrate an immediate EEG amplitude suppression (at the time of concussion) that is followed by a relatively short period of background slowing before return to normal (Williams & Denny-Brown, 1941). The generalized slowing of the human EEG following head trauma correlates well with depressed level of consciousness.

Regardless of the EEG pattern correlating significantly with level of consciousness, the development of a simple, reproducible "coma score" based on clinical examination that correlated with outcome minimized, at first, the need for clinical neurophysiological studies in head-injured individuals (Jennett & Bond, 1975; Jennett *et al.*, 1976). Furthermore, as the field of neurotraumatology emerged as an area of specialty, several factors probably contributed to the failure of the routine EEG to be widely used to monitor the patient with TBI. These included:

1. Development of the Glasgow Coma Score
2. Correlation of Glasgow Coma Score with outcome
3. ICU environment hostile to prolonged routine EEG
4. Manpower needs to run technically satisfactory EEG in ICU
5. Costs associated with #4
6. The magnitude of data produced with hours of routine EEG recording
7. Patient technical problems including:
   a. Head bandages
   b. Scalp edema

   c. Other monitoring devices on the head
   d. Muscle artifact
8. Neurosurgeons often don't read EEGs
9. Neurologists often not interested in TBI
10. Development of neuroimaging—especially computerized tomography

In particular, the development of computerized tomography highlighted the weakness of the EEG in identifying or localizing focal surgical lesions—thus making the EEG of considerably less value to the neurosurgeon involved in acute management of the TBI patient.

Although there are significant correlations between distinct EEG patterns seen following TBI and outcome, these patterns are no better predictors of outcome than the Glasgow Coma Score (Bricolo, 1976; Chatrian, White, & Daly, 1963; Synek, 1988).

Recently, because of an increase in the number of TBI survivors with severe disability or persistent coma, there has been a renewed interest in EEG measurements. The traditional EEG has been enhanced through the use of computer-assisted Fourier transform analysis of the EEG along with better display techniques (Compressed Spectral Array [CSA]) that allow the compression of large amounts of EEG information into brief, readable, "eye-appealing" packets. Using these techniques, several authors have shown that slow, monotonous CSA has unfavorable outcome, while return of or persistence of alpha and theta frequencies in the CSA may indicate a good or a better outcome than if the alpha and theta frequencies remained absent (Bricolo, Turazzi, Faccioli, Odorizzi, Sciarretta, & Erculiani, 1978; Cant & Shaw, 1984). Although it was hoped that the technological improvements of the EEG would lead to a more accurate and reliable predictor of outcome, these techniques are at best as good in predicting outcome following TBI as a clinical exam that is quantified according to the Glasgow Coma Score.

## Sensory Evoked Potential

Sensory evoked potential evaluation has been shown to be useful in TBI outcome prediction whether studied as a single modality or as several modalities in combination. Several factors have contributed to the clinical utility of this methodology:

1. Sensory evoked potential data can be elicited when the clinical exam may be limited by medication (muscle paralyzing agents or barbiturates).
2. The short-latency sensory evoked potentials are minimally, if at all, affected by medications (barbiturates).
3. Quantitative data (interpeak latencies and central conduction times) as well as qualitative data can be determined.
4. Given the current understanding of the neuropathology of TBI, especially diffuse axonal injury, measurement of conduction through neuronal pathways is appealingly straightforward.

## Brain-stem Auditory Evoked Potential

Brain-stem auditory evoked potential is quite stable and resistant to the effect of medications such as the barbiturates. Loss of the latter components of the brain-stem auditory evoked potential bilaterally or absence of the brain-stem auditory evoked potential correlates well with brain death (Kaga, Nagai, & Takamori, 1985). Papanicolaou, Loving, Eisenbert, Raz, and Contreras (1986) found prolonged wave V latency-distinguished patients in the vegetative or dead categories Glasgow Outcome Scale from higher outcome categories.

Kaga and colleagues (1985) were able to show that analysis of the middle and long latency components to auditory stimulus coupled with the brain-stem auditory evoked potential increased confidence in predicting survival from coma. Normal brain-stem auditory evoked potential, middle and long latency components predicted survival in 100% of cases while normal brain-stem auditory evoked potential and middle latency components predicted survival in 91%.

Karnaze and colleagues (1985) in a preliminary study of 45 patients with TBI combined clinical indices of injury with auditory and brain-stem evoked potentials to create a 40-point Neurophysiological Coma Scale (see Table 2).

Of 45 patients studied, 39 had an initial score of 8 or less (severe injury) while 6 had a score of 9 to 11 (moderate injury). Scores of 20 or more predicted favorable outcome: 31 of 39 patients with scores of 20 or above had favorable outcome. All 6 patients with scores of less than 20 had unfavorable outcome. The Neurophysiology Coma Scale was found to have predictive accuracy of 82% compared to the Glasgow Coma Score with 71% accuracy. Moreover, there were no falsely pessimistic predictions with the Neurophysiology Coma Scale (Karnaze, Wincr, & Marshall, 1985).

## Visual Evoked Potentials

Anderson et al. used graded flash visual evoked potentials as a predictor of outcome in their series of 39 TBI patients (Anderson, Bundlie, & Rockswold, 1984). They found flash visual evoked potentials to be poorly tolerated by patients not deeply in coma or paralyzed. They successfully recorded flash visual evoked potentials in 12 of 39 patients—all of whom had normal ERGs. They determined that flash visual evoked potentials were a good indicator of unfavorable outcome, but not of favorable outcome (Anderson et al., 1984).

Gupta et al. (1986) studied monocular pattern-shift visual evoked potentials in 33 patients who had been comatose from several hours to several days. Evaluations were performed 6 to 24 months after head injury. Cognitive ability was based on a scale modified for the Rancho Los Amigos Scale. Patients who were moderately or severely impaired were

TABLE 17.2.   Neurophysiological Coma Scale

|                                        | Possible points | Range |
|----------------------------------------|-----------------|-------|
| Age                                    | 5               | 2–5   |
| Glasgow Coma Score                     | 15              | 3–15  |
| Pupillary reactions                    | 5               | 0–5   |
| Oculocephalic reflex                   | 5               | 1–5   |
| Brain-stem auditory evoked potentials  | 5               | 1–5   |
| Auditory evoked potentials             | 5               | 1–5   |
|                                        | 40              | 8–40  |

TABLE 17.3.   Pattern-Shift Visual Evoked Potentials
and Cognitive Functioning (Gupta *et al.*, 1986)

| Cognitive impairment | $N$ | $N$ (% abnormal pattern-shift visual evoked potential) |
|---|---|---|
| Mild | 9 | 1 (11%) |
| Moderate | 18 | 7 (39%) |
| Severe | 6 | 3 (50%) |

more likely to have abnormal pattern-shift visual evoked potentials compared to the mildly cognitively impaired group (see Table 17.3).

*Somatosensory Evoked Potentials*

Somatosensory evoked potentials have been found to be reliable predictors of favorable or unfavorable outcome in victims of TBI (Walser, Emre, & Janzer, 1984; Goldie, Chiappa, Young, & Brooks, 1981; Hume & Cant, 1981; Anderson *et al.*, 1984; Rumpl *et al.*, 1983; Lutschg *et al.*, 1983). In all cases absence of all components of somatosensory evoked potentials or absence of components past the P15 response suggested unfavorable outcome. In addition, prolongation of the central conduction time was noted to correlate with outcome.

*Multimodality Evoked Potentials*

Multimodality evoked potentials provide the most accurate and reliable prediction of outcome of all the clinical neurophysiological monitors. In all articles reviewed, the authors use grading systems for evoked potential data based on number of identifiable waveforms, absolute latencies, interpeak latencies, amplitude, or some combination of these.

Greenberg and associates (1977) were among the first to apply multimodality evoked potentials to outcome predictions in TBI. In 1977 they analyzed multimodality evoked potentials in 51 comatose patients with severe TBI and graded them on a scale of I (best) to IV (worst). By the 3rd day from injury, somatosensory evoked potentials significantly correlated with outcome; and, by the 14th day, both somatosensory evoked potentials and brain-stem auditory evoked potentials had predictive value. Of the patients who had grade I or II multimodality evoked potentials by day 3, 80% became responsive by day 30 (Greenberg *et al.*, 1977).

In 1981, Narayan *et al.* reported the results of a prospective study of 133 severely head-injured patients admitted to the Medical College of Virginia from May 1976 to September 1979. They evaluated a combination of clinical data including age, Glasgow Coma Score, pupillary response, presence of surgical mass lesions, extraocular mobility, and motor posturing as well as computerized tomography, intracranial pressure data, and multi-modality evoked potentials (Narayan *et al.*, 1981). They used the linear logistic regression model to apply these data singly or in combination to outcome prediction in individual patients. Using the Glasgow Outcome Scale they predicted categorization of patients into two groups: (1) good recovery/moderate disability and (2) severe disability/vegetative/dead.

They found multimodality evoked potential data alone represented the most accurate single prognostic indicator with 91% correct predictions (25% at the over 90% confidence level). As in other studies, they reported no falsely pessimistic predictions based as multimodality evoked potentials alone. Moreover, they found that the combination of multimodality evoked potential data *and* clinical examination data gave 89% prognostic accuracy with 64% over the 90% confidence level and only 4% falsely pessimistic errors.

Clearly, clinical neurophysiological monitors are valuable, if not essential, in the care of the severe TBI patient. Early in the course of neurointensive care, EEG and evoked potential data allow gross monitoring of cortical activity and objective assessment of conduction along certain neural pathways. Serial assessment of these data allows localization of injury, better monitoring of treatment variables, and better outcome prediction. The combination of multimodality evoked potential data and clinical data currently provide the best combination of prognostic accuracy, reliability, and confidence. Emergence of new clinical neurophysiological techniques (such as motor evoked potentials) will no doubt further contribute to the quality of care of head injury victims.

## SUMMARY

Of these predictors of outcome, the Glasgow Coma Score remains the benchmark for prediction when using the Glasgow Outcome Scale to measure outcome. Clinical neurophysiology offers great potential for the future in this area. Evoked potential measurement directly assesses conduction through neuronal pathways and may be uniquely valuable in assessing the extent of diffuse axonal injury.

The spectrum of neurological disability following severe TBI is a continuum with coma, vegetative state, and severe disability being levels of function and not prognostic categories per se. Persistent coma or persistent vegetative state are statements of prognosis indicating no chance for advancement in functional level or state. Therefore, these terms should only be used when every reasonable attempt has been made to identify more meaningful functional level over a period of months to years. Many predictors of outcome have been presented, but none are clearly better than the Glasgow Coma Score. Certain clinical neurophysiology monitors such as the sensory evoked potentials may improve reliability of outcome prediction and ultimately be valuable in defining the persistent vegetative state.

## REFERENCES

Adams, J. H., Graham, D. I., *et al*. (1982). Diffuse axonal injury due to non-missile head injury in humans: An analysis of 45 cases. *Annals of Neurology, 12,* 557–563.

Anderson, D., Bundlie, S., & Rockswold, G. (1984). Multimodality evoked potentials in closed head trauma. *Archives of Neurology, 41,* 369–379.

Bartkowski, H. M., & Lovely, M. P. (1986). Prognosis in coma and the persistent vegetative state. *Journal of Head Trauma Rehabilitation, 1,* 1–5.

Becker, D. P., Miller, J. D., *et al.* (1977). The outcome from severe head injury with early diagnosis and intensive management. *Journal of Neurosurgery, 47,* 491–502.

Berger, H. (1931). Uber das elektrnkephalogrqmar des menschen III, Mitteilung. *Archiv fuer Psychiatrie und Nervenkrankheiten, 94,* 16–60.

Berger, M. S., Pitts, L. H., & Lovely, M. (1985). Outcome from severe head injury in children and adolescents. *Journal of Neurosurgery, 62,* 194–199.

Bowers, S. A., & Marshall, L. F. (1980). Outcome in 200 consecutive cases of severe head injury treated in San Diego County: A prospective analysis. *Neurosurgery, 6,* 237–242.

Bricolo, A. (1976). Electroencephalography in neurotraumatology. *Clinical Electroencephalography, 7,* 184–197.

Bricolo, A., Turazzi, S., Faccioli, F., Odorizzi, F., Sciarretta, G., & Erculiani, P. (1978). Clinical application of compressed spectral array in long term EEG monitoring of comatose patients. *Electroencephalography & Clinical Neurophysiology, 45,* 211–25.

Bruce, D. A., *et al.* (1979). Pathophysiology, treatment and outcome following severe head injury in children. *Child's Brain, 5,* 174–191.

Cant, B. R., & Shaw, N. A. (1984). Monitoring by compressed special array in prolonged coma. *Neurology, 34,* 35–39.

Chatrian, G. E., White, L. E., & Daly, D. (1963). Electroencephalographic patterns resembling those of sleep in certain comatose states after head injury. *Electroencephalography & Clinical Neurophysiology, 15,* 272–280.

Choi, S. C., Ward, J. D., & Becker, D. P. (1983). Chart for outcome prediction in severe head injury. *Journal of Neurosurgery, 59,* 294–297.

Facco, E., *et al.* (1985). Is the auditory brain-stem response (ABR) effective in the assessment of post-traumatic coma? *Electroencephalography & Clinical Neurophysiology, 62,* 332–337.

Frank, L. M., Furgiuele, T. L., & Etheridge, J. E. (1985). Prediction of chronic vegetative state in children using evoked potentials. *Neurology, 35,* 931–934.

Gennarelli, T. A., *et al.* (1982). Influence of the type of intracranial lesion on outcome from severe head injury. *Journal of Neurosurgery, 56,* 26–32.

Gennarelli, T. A., Thibault, L. E., Adams, J. H., *et al.* (1982). Diffuse axonal injury and traumatic coma in the primate. *Annals of Neurology, 12,* 564–574.

Gibbs, F. A., Davis, H., & Lennox, W. G. (1935). The electroencephalogram in epilepsy and in conditions of impaired consciousness. *Archives of Neurology & Psychiatry, 34,* 1133–1148.

Goldie, W., Chiappa, K., Young, R., & Brooks, E. (1981). Brain-stem auditory and short-latency somatosensory evoked responses in brain death. *Neurology, 31,* 248–256.

Greenberg, R. P., & Ducker, T. B. (1982). Evoked potentials in the clinical neurosciences. *Journal of Neurosurgery, 56,* 1–18.

Greenberg, R., *et al.* (1977). Evaluation of brain function in severe human head trauma with multimodality evoked potentials, part 1: Evoked brain-injury potentials, methods, & analysis. *Journal of Neurosurgery, 47,* 150–162.

Greenberg, R., *et al.* (1977). Evaluation of brain function in severe human head trauma with multimodality evoked potentials, part 2: Localization of brain dysfunction and correlations with post-traumatic neurological conditions. *Journal of Neurosurgery, 47,* 163–177.

Greenberg, R. P., Newlon, P. G., *et al.* (1981). Prognostic implications of early multimodality evoked potentials in severely head-injured patients. *Journal of Neurosurgery, 55,* 227–236.

Gupta, N. K., *et al.* (1986). Visual evoked response in head trauma: Pattern-shift stimulus. *Neurology, 36,* 578–581.

Hall, K., Cope, N., & Rappaport, M. (1985). Glasgow Outcome Scale and Disability Rating Scale: Comparative usefulness in following recovery in traumatic head injury. *Archives of Physical Medicine & Rehabilitation, 66,* 35–37.

Han, J. S., Kaufman, B., *et al.* (1984). Head trauma evaluated by magnetic resonance and computed tomography: A comparison. *Radiology, 150,* 71–77.

Hume, A. L., & Cant, B. R. (1981). Central somatosensory condition after head injury. *Annals of Neurology, 10,* 411–419.

Hume, A. L., Cant, M. P., & Shaw, M. A. (1979). Central somatosensory conduction time in comatose patients. *Annals of Neurology, 5,* 379–384.

Jennett, W. B., & Plum, F. (1972). The persistent vegetative state: A syndrome in search of a name. *Lancet, 1,* 734–737.

Jennett, B., & Bond, M. (1975). Assessment of outcome after severe brain damage. A practical scale. *Lancet, 1,* 480–484.

Jennett, B., & Teasdale, G. (1977). Aspects of coma after severe head injury. *Lancet, 1,* 878–881.

Jennett, B., Teasdale, G., Braakman, R., *et al.* (1976). Predicting outcome in individual patients after severe head injury. *Lancet, 1,* 1031–1034.

Jennett, B., Teasdale, G., Braakman, R., *et al.* (1979). Prognosis of patients with severe head injury. *Neurosurgery, 4,* 283–289.

Jennett, B., Teasdale, G., *et al.* (1987). Prognosis of patients with severe head injury. *Neurosurgery, 40,* 291–298.

Kaga, K., Nagai, T., & Takamori, A. (1985). Auditory short, middle and long latency responses in acutely comatose patients. *Laryngoscope, 95,* 321–325.

Kalsbeck, W. D., McLaurin, R. I., *et al.* (1980). The national head and spinal cord injury survey: Major findings. *Journal of Neurosurgery, 53*(Suppl.), 19–31.

Karnaze, D., et al (1982). Localizing and prognostic value of auditory evoked responses in coma after closed head injury. *Neurology, 32,* 299–302.

Karnaze, D., Winer, J., & Marshall, L. (1985). Auditory evoked potentials in coma after closed head injury: A clinical-neurophysiological coma scale for predicting outcome. *Neurology, 35,* 1122–11265.

Kindsay, K. W., *et al.* (1981). Evoked potentials in severe head injury—Analysis and relation to outcome. *Journal of Neurology, Neurosurgery & Psychiatry, 44,* 796–802.

Lange-Cossach, W., Riebel, W., & Grumme, T. (1981). Possibilities and limitation of rehabilitation after traumatic apallic syndrome in children and adolescents. *Neuropediatrics, 12,* 338–365.

Levati, A., *et al.* (1982). Prognosis of severe head injuries. *Journal of Neurosurgery, 57,* 779–783.

Levy, D. E., Knill-Jones, R. P., & Plum, F. (1978). The vegetative state and its prognosis following non-traumatic coma. *Annals of the New York Academy of Sciences, 315,* 293–306.

Lokkeberg, A. R., & Grime, R. M. (1984). Assessing the influence of non-treatment variables in a study of outcome from severe head injury. *Journal of Neurosurgery, 61,* 254–262.

Lutschg, J., et al (1983). Brain-stem auditory evoked potentials and early somatosensory evoked potentials in neurointensively treated comatose children. *American Journal of Disabled Children, 137,* 421–426.

Mahoney, W. J., D'Souza, B. J., & Freeman, J. M. (1981). Surprising good outcome of prolonged coma after severe head injury. *Annals of Neurology, 10,* 286.

Mizrani, E. M., & Kellaway, P. (1984). Censoral concussion in children: Assessment of injury by electroencephalography. *Pediatrics, 73,* 419–425.

Narayan, R., Greenberg, R., *et al.* (1981). Improved confidence of outcome prediction in severe head injury: A comparative analysis of the clinical examination, multimodality evoked potentials, CT scanning and intracranial pressure. *Journal of Neurosurgery, 54,* 751–762.

Newlon, P. G., & Greenberg, R. P. (1984). Evoked potentials in severe head injury. *The Journal of Trauma, 24,* 61–66.

Newlon, P. G., Greenberg, R. P., *et al.* (1982). The dynamics of neuronal dysfunction and recovery following severe head injury assessed with serial multimodality evoked potentials. *Journal of Neurosurgery, 57,* 168–177.

Papanicolaou, A., *et al.* (1984). Evoked potential correlates of post-trauma amnesia after closed head injury. *Neurosurgery, 14,* 676–678.

Papanicolaou, A., Loving, D., Eisenbert, H., Raz, N., & Contreras, F. (1986). Auditory brain stem evoked responses in comatose head-injured patients. *Neurosurgery, 18,* 173–175.

Pfurtscheller, G., *et al.* (1985). Clinical relevance of long-latency SEPs and VEPs during coma and emergence from coma. *Electroencephalography & Clinical Neurophysiology, 62,* 88–98.

Plum, F., & Posner, J. B.(1980). *The diagnosis of stupor and coma* (3rd ed.). Philadelphia: Davis.

Rosenberg, C., Wogensen, K., & Starr, A. (1984). Auditory brain-stem and middle and long-latency evoked potentials and coma. *Archives of Neurology, 41,* 835–838.

Rosenblum, W. I., et al (1981). Midbrain lesions: Frequent and significant prognostic feature in closed head injury. *Neurosurgery, 9,* 613–620.

Rumpl, E., Prugger, M., *et al.* (1983). Central somatosensory conduction time and short latency somatosensory evoked potentials in post-traumatic coma. *Electroencephalography & Clinical Neurophysiology, 56,* 583–596.

Scherg, M., Cramon, D., & Elton, M. (1984). Brain-stem auditory evoked potentials in post-comatose patients after severe closed head trauma. *Journal of Neurology, 231,* 1–5.

Shaw, N. A., & Cant, B. R. (1984). The effect of experimental concussion on somatosensory evoked potentials. *Australian Journal of Experimental Biology & Medical Science*, *62*, 361–371.

Stablein, D. N., *et al*. (1980). Statistical methods for determining prognosis in severe head injury. *Neurosurgery*, *6*, 243–248.

Stone, J. L., Ghaly, R. F., & Hughes, J. R. (1988). Electroencephalography in acute head injury. *Journal of Clinical Neurophysiology*, *5*, 125–133.

Stone, J. L., Ghaly, R. F., & Hughes, J. R. (1988). Evoked potentials in head injury and states of increased intracranial pressure. *Journal of Clinical Neurophysiology*, *5*, 135–160.

Synek, V. M. (1988). Prognostically important EEG coma patterns in diffuse anoxic and traumatic encephalopathies in adults. *Journal of Clinical Neurophysiology*, *5*, 161–174.

Teasdale, G., & Jennett, B. (1974). Assessment of coma and impaired consciousness. A practical scale. *Lancet*, *2*, 81–84.

Walser, H., Emre, M., & Janzer, R. (1986). Somatosensory evoked potentials in comatose patients: Correlation with outcome and neuropathological findings. *Journal of Neurology*, *233*, 34–40.

Ward, J. D., & Alberico, A. M. (1987). Pediatric head injury. *Brain Injury*, *1*, 21–25.

Williams, D., & Denny-Brown, D. (1941). Cerebral electrical changes in experimental concussion. *Brain*, *64*, 223–238.

# V

# Individual Therapy and Family Issues in Rehabilitation

# 18

# Group Psychotherapy with Brain-Damaged Adults and Their Families

WARREN T. JACKSON and WILLIAM DREW GOUVIER

In the past, cognitive and behavioral sequelae of neurological insult were thought to contraindicate psychotherapeutic intervention with brain-damaged adults. Recently, however, the cultivation of awareness of deficits, self-appraisal techniques, and adaptive skills have become important objectives for postacute rehabilitation of such patients. Meeting these objectives can be a critical obstacle to successful community reentry. In this context, psychotherapy is becoming a viable therapeutic tool (Rosenthal, 1989).

Psychotherapy is a broad and multiply defined concept. Many schools of thought have proposed theories of psychopathology and how it should be therapeutically addressed (Patterson, 1986). In order to advance the status of the field with respect to working with the brain-damaged, interventions for the brain-damaged should be operationalized in terms of their outcome in three areas: (1) adaptive behavioral functioning, (2) cognitive functioning, and (3) psychosocial adjustment to disability. The mode of psychotherapeutic treatment must be research-based, and its outcome must be evaluated. Unfortunately, little work has been done to empirically validate psychotherapy with brain-damaged adults. The purpose of this chapter is to summarize the work that has been done in this area, and to present a framework for application of group psychotherapy principles to brain-damaged adults and their families. A number of specific group formats that have appeared in the recent literature are described. In an effort to provide information useful to practitioners working in different settings, both inpatient and outpatient therapeutic settings are explored. Also included is a presentation of the structure currently used at the Louisiana State University Psychological Services Center for concurrent outpatient group psychotherapy of brain-damaged individuals and their families.

---

WARREN T. JACKSON and WILLIAM DREW GOUVIER • Department of Psychology, Louisiana State University, Baton Rouge, Louisiana 70803-5501.

*HANDBOOK OF HEAD TRAUMA: Acute Care to Recovery*, edited by Charles J. Long and Leslie K. Ross. Plenum Press, New York, 1992.

## THE CLINICAL RELEVANCE OF GROUP PSYCHOTHERAPY

The advantages of psychotherapy in a group context are well documented for general psychiatric populations (Vinogradov & Yalom, 1989; Yalom, 1985), disabled and/or neurologically impaired persons (Crawford & McIvor, 1985; Salhoot, 1984), and for elderly nursing home patients (Gugel & Eisdorfer, 1985). In addition, a number of studies have compared the treatment outcome of group psychotherapy to that of individual psycho- therapy. In a recent review of 32 studies comparing individual versus group treatment of interpersonal problems, Toseland and Siporin (1986) documented no significant difference in 24 of the studies (75%). The other 8 studies reported that group psychotherapy was more effective than individual psychotherapy. Thus, with its general clinical efficacy established, group psychotherapy might be applied to a brain-damaged population with expected results at least equal to those of individual treatment.

Carberry and Burd (1983) were among the first to identify the specific clinical benefits of group treatment of brain-injured patients:

1. The group format provides additional support and decreased isolation, as well as a source of group identification and belongingness.
2. A secure environment is created that allows a freeing-up of the patient's defenses in order to begin the process of overcoming denial of disabilities and resistance to growth.
3. The group format provides an opportunity to model, practice, and refine behavior (e.g., job interviews, asking for a date, making telephone calls, planning a trip, asserting oneself, modifying aggressive responses, etc.).
4. The group provides an opportunity for reality testing of how one is perceived by others. There are many opportunities for constructive corrective feedback (e.g., "you are not listening," etc.) as well as more positive feedback (e.g., "you really expressed that clearly," etc.).
5. The group format facilitates group members gaining a realistic picture of strengths and weaknesses. Often there is either a denial of problems or the opposite—a feeling that "everything is wrong with me." The group interaction pushes through rigid stances and encourages a more flexible mode of thinking and self-appraisal.
6. The group format provides a spirit of competition, caring, and concern that helps the person get outside of himself/herself, overcome egocentricity, and adopt a more humane stance.
7. The group format sets up expectations, by brain-damaged patients, for brain- damaged patients, which pushes toward more competent and independent function- ing. Group members have a real sense from their own experience as to when someone is avoiding, manipulating, or exaggerating symptoms. This can be used in a confrontive and yet supportive manner and seems best when done by the group members themselves.

The clinical efficacy of group psychotherapy is complemented by its efficiency. Group treatment is both an efficient use of therapeutic resources, and a cost-effective setting for meeting the needs of patients. More patients can be treated when time, space, psychological and/or social work personnel, and other resources are limited. In the context of postacute inpatient rehabilitation, when large numbers of patients must be seen by a limited staff of psychosocial treatment team members, the patient-to-staff ratio is often too high to allow for much individual contact. Thus, group meetings allow for important psychotherapy to be conducted. In an outpatient setting, the same considerations apply. Patient and family member groups can be held concurrently in different meeting rooms of the same clinic. This format simplifies scheduling for both the clients and the clinic, and reduces the demand for space that might otherwise occur with individual sessions.

## PSYCHOTHERAPY AFTER BRAIN DAMAGE

The cognitive and behavioral sequelae of brain injury are many, and their full description is beyond the focus of this chapter. The psychosocial and personality disturbances common after brain injury, however, are particularly pertinent to a discussion of group psychotherapy. These psychosocial sequelae involve personality changes, emotional reactions to injury, and premorbid characterological styles (Prigatano, 1986a). Such symptomatology is amenable to clinical intervention. Psychotherapy can substantially reduce patients' discomfort and improve their psychological adjustment (Cicerone, 1989).

In his review of research on personality disturbances following brain injury, Prigatano (1986a) proposed four broad classes of maladaptive functioning: (1) anxiety and the catastrophic reaction; (2) denial of illness, or anosognosia; (3) paranoia and psychomotor agitation; and (4) depression, social withdrawal, and amotivational states. Each of these classes of behavior will be outlined below without detailed reference to neuroanatomical correlates. Rather, the treatment of these symptom classifications within a group psychotherapeutic setting is emphasized.

Patients confronted with a sense of loss secondary to traumatic brain injury often experience a catastrophic reaction characterized by, but not limited to, anxiety, irritability, mistrust of others, hopelessness, helplessness, anger, and phobic behavior. These patients have a strong need to discharge this anxiety, and they frequently do so inappropriately. The group psychotherapy environment is especially well suited to the cathartic ventilation of these emotions (Vinogradov & Yalom, 1989). The patients can share their inner despair and anxiety in a group without fear of rejection. In addition, they can receive feedback about the social appropriateness of their cathartic content and the mode of expression used. This feedback is guided by the therapist, and supplemented by the group members. The intensity of the catastrophic reaction can be greatly attenuated as the patient begins to replace the belief that he or she is unacceptable and unlovable, with a sense of self-acceptance fostered in the group.

Denial of illness, or anosognosia, is a particular issue of significance with head-injured patients, and is often a major focus of psychotherapeutic intervention (Cicerone, 1989). Often, when brain-damaged patients fail to recognize the nature and severity of their limitations, rehabilitative treatment outcome and subsequent community reintegration is disrupted. Fortunately, group psychotherapy seems to have a robust effect in addressing denial issues. Cicerone (1989) outlined three interventions that can be applied in a group setting. The first intervention involves the process of accurate self-appraisal. Here, the patient with denial of deficits may be asked, "How sure are you that you can do that? What would it mean if you're unable to do what you think you can?" (p. 109). The second type of intervention is more directive and behaviorally oriented. In this scenario, an anosognostic patient might be confronted with, "You're still making more mistakes than you said. I think you have to slow down and correct your errors ... or you could change your goal. Which do you want to do?" (p. 109). The third intervention, simply, is a combination of the previous two. Each of these interventions is very effective in a group setting because the therapist can use peer feedback to enhance the discrepancy between reality and the denying patient's perception of it.

The third class of maladaptive behavioral functioning apparent after brain injury is comprised of paranoid thinking and psychomotor agitation. Often during the postacute phase of rehabilitation, patients are easily confused and they show signs of paranoid ideation. They may also be disoriented, restless, agitated, and even combative. This complex of behaviors can be modified in the group setting. In this case, modeling appears to be critical therapeutic variable. The paranoid and/or agitated patient often grows more manageable when surrounded by peers who are displaying calm and compliant behavior. Of course, extremely combative or explosive patients may not be appropriate for group psychotherapy without an adjunct pharmacological intervention, but doubtless, even agitated patients can sometimes benefit from the opportunity to learn how their behavior is perceived by others. Often, these patients have little insight as to the social effects of their behavior. The group environment can help patients develop such insight. In addition, the paranoid ideation experienced by these patients can be effectively addressed in a group. The consensual reality of the group is usually more persuasive than the individual reality of a lone staff member.

Depression and social withdrawal make up the final class of psychosocial disruption secondary to brain insult. These affective problems are of special concern to the rehabilitation treatment team because they often result in a weak commitment to work hard in rehabilitation therapies. In addition, family members struggle a great deal with patients who are unwilling to develop higher levels of independent functioning. Depressive symptomatology includes feelings of worthlessness, helplessness, guilt, and a loss of interest in other people (Prigatano, 1986a). These features differ from those experienced in a normal catastrophic reaction in that they persist in the face of positive reinforcement from the environment (e.g., improved functional ability or increased social acceptance) that would typically lessen sadness over loss of function. Thus, group work should attempt to change the patients' cognitions about self and foster interest in activities designed to promote self-esteem. Social withdrawal is often both a result of depression and a source of its continuance. Feelings of helplessness and worthlessness, coupled with repeated failures in coping with the environment, lead many brain-damaged patients to withdraw from their contact with others. This reaction tends to perpetuate itself as the resultant isolation confirms feelings of worthlessness. Social isolation, however, does not always occur in the context of depression. Patients are reinforced for seeking the least aversive environment, where minimal demands are placed on their impaired ability. Although this withdrawal behavior may be adaptive in the shortrun, it is ultimately to the detriment of their continuing rehabilitation. Psychotherapy in a group setting is especially suited to addressing isolation issues because it places withdrawn patients in a controlled social environment in which they can cope more easily. In a group, the therapist can attenuate the potential for social failure, creating a sense of social efficacy. In addition, feedback from the therapist and other group members helps withdrawn patients to form more realistic cognitions about the way they are perceived by others.

As outlined above, individuals who have suffered a brain injury often show certain patterns of psychosocial and personality disturbance that can greatly interfere with the rehabilitation process. The role of treatment, particularly in the case of psychotherapy, is to (1) facilitate the rehabilitative efforts of the therapeutic staff, (2) maximize the recovery potential of the patient, and (3) assist the family in adjusting to the reality of living with a characterologically altered brain-injured patient (Lezak, 1978). Prigatano (1986b) outlined the goals of psychotherapy after brain injury as follows:

1. Provide a modeling component that helps patients understand what has happened to them.
2. Help patients deal with the meaning of the brain injury in their lives.
3. Help patients achieve a sense of self-acceptance and forgiveness of others.
4. Help patients make realistic commitments to work and personal relationships.
5. Improve patients' social competency across situations.
6. Provide specific behavioral strategies for deficit compensation.
7. Instill a sense of realistic hope. (p. 71)

Prigatano also sets out a number of guidelines that he has found useful in providing the most effective group psychotherapy to brain-damaged adults.

1. Do not make it too easy for the patient to begin psychotherapy or a rehabilitation program.
2. Decide what constellation of individual and group psychotherapy sessions will be necessary.
3. Plan what topics you are going to introduce in a given therapy session.
4. Separate cognitive problems from emotional and motivational problems in therapy sessions, at least in the beginning.
5. In the group setting, provide a model of personality difficulties and teach patients how to cope with them.
6. Reinforce awareness of deficits in self and others.
7. Help each patient recognize how his or her personal background contributes to the rehabilitation progress.
8. Point out the power of the group to reduce the sense of personal discomfort and to enhance a sense of belonging.
9. Obtain permission to give honest feedback (both painful and pleasant) within the context of the group setting.
10. Filter information and feedback to the patient in doses the patient can handle so that he or she can begin modifying socially incompetent behavior.
11. Do not be afraid of using humor and analogies to get your point across, but do not lessen the seriousness of the business at hand.
12. Be clear about the problems that need to be worked on, and periodically publicly review progress in writing.
13. Constantly remind yourself and the patient of the following:
    a. that you will strive to be honest and face the truth about his or her strengths and weaknesses;
    b. that you do not have all the answers but are committed to helping the patient change where possible; and

   c. that there are no miracles in rehabilitation or psychotherapy—only hard work.
14. Remind the patient that the pot of gold at the end of the rainbow is not necessarily happiness. The goal is to be independent, to be able to take care of one's needs and to be productive. (pp. 71–74)

Prigatano and his associates have contributed much to the application of group psychotherapeutic intervention to the brain-damaged population. As work in this area has developed, a growing awareness of the unique needs of the families of brain-damaged individuals has also begun to emerge. It is to this topic that attention will now be turned.

## IMPORTANCE OF FAMILY GROUP TREATMENT

Family distress following brain injury has become a growing concern of rehabilitation professionals in recent years. In fact, the treatment of family reactions to head injury, stroke, and other neurological disorders is becoming an integral part of holistic rehabilitative efforts. A growing literature has begun to document family problems arising from the brain-damaged patient's dependency, cognitive deficits, and impaired adjustment to disability (Lezak, 1988). Additionally, the moral and psychological problems that confront family caregivers are being examined (Callahan, 1988; Lezak, 1978).

Empirical research has begun to unravel the relationship between brain-damaged adults, their family members, and rehabilitation outcome. The role of the family has been established as a critical variable in stroke rehabilitation. One group of researchers used the McMaster Family Assessment Device (FAD) and clinical data from 60 stroke patients to predict outcome at six months and one year intervals poststroke (Evans, Bishop, Matlock, Stranahan, Halar, & Noonan, 1987). Results indicated that family functioning was a better predictor of hospital stay than baseline ratings of typical predictors of stroke outcome, such as demographic variables. As measured by the FAD, problem-solving scores, family communication skills, and patient self-care ability predicted patient adjustment. In addition, ratings of behavior control (e.g., the family's pattern of coping with difficult situations) and affective responsiveness of the family (e.g., ability to respond with appropriate quality and quantity of emotion) predicted stroke-related rehospitalization during the poststroke interval. In a related study, Evans, Bishop, Matlock, Stranahan, Smith, and Halar (1987) used the FAD to determine the relationship between family function and poststroke treatment adherence. The caregivers of 60 stroke patients were assessed five months after patient discharge from a stroke care unit. Better functioning families were found to score consistently high on items related to treatment adherence. Once again, family problem solving, communication, and affective involvement were significant predictors.

Families that are functioning well in the domains outlined above should not automatically be assumed to be providing the best care possible for the rehabilitating patient (Callahan, 1988). In fact, family denial of deficits and/or differences in perception of the degree and types of changes may limit long-term progress in rehabilitation. Hendryx (1989) compared the differences in perceived relative importance of cognitive, emotional, and physical changes between a group of head-injured adults and their families. The comparison indicated that family members tended to rate the patients' emotional changes as most severe, whereas the brain- damaged patients rated their cognitive changes as more extreme than their changes in emotion. Degree of physical change was rated the most consistently between groups. These differences in perception about the extent of cognitive and emotional changes may stem from the family's denial and/or lack of awareness of the sequelae of brain damage (Hendryx, 1989), although they may also relate to anosognostic changes in the patient. Family members readily observe the patient's outward display of frustrations, yet they may not relate the source of frustration to the patient's cognitive deficits. Thus, it is often easier for the family to note emotional difficulties as the primary result of head injury, rather than to come to terms with the implications of permanent cognitive impairment. In situations such as this, educational and psychotherapeutic interventions may be indicated.

In order for successful intervention to take place with the families of the brain-injured, it is important to recognize the specific cognitive and behavioral deficits affecting family functioning. Rosenthal and Geckler (1986) identified eight primary deficits likely to disrupt normal family functioning. Most of these deficit areas have been described with some detail in above sections concerning psychosocial sequelae of brain injury; thus, a brief outline of the areas will suffice here. The deficit areas that affect family functioning are as follows: (1) presence of cognitive deficits, especially in the areas of attention and concentration, complex information processing, memory and new learning, and problem solving; (2) disorders of communication, including aphasia, dysarthria, and apraxia; (3) emotional regression that includes heightened dependency, constant attention-seeking, inappropriate affect, and temper tantrums; (4) frontal lobe behavior, encompassing such behaviors as aspontaneity, lethargy, flat affect, irritability, loss of initiative, amotivation, disinhibition, and impaired abstraction ability; (5) social withdrawal, as a function of lowered self-esteem and other negative self-perceptions that lead to isolation; (6) inappropriate social behavior, including verbal and motoric perseveration, pathological laughter, and inappropriate sexual behavior; (7) depression, often observed in the form of decreased activity level, negative self-statements, negative affect, reports of feeling worthless and hopeless, suicidal ideation, and vegetative indicators such as social withdrawal, sleep disturbance, and loss of appetite; and finally (8) inability to resume premorbid role in the family, which is often associated with feelings of anxiety, grief, anger, and guilt among various family members. Later sections on inpatient and outpatient group psychotherapy with family members of brain-damaged adults will address modes of intervention specific to these problem areas that affect family functioning.

Having enumerated the specific problems of brain-damaged adults that directly affect their families, attention will now be turned to the stages of family adaptation to the disabled individual. Lezak (1986) presented an insightful conceptualization of six different reaction patterns, or stages, displayed by families as they develop an understanding and acceptance of the psychosocial sequelae of brain injury (Table 18.1). Lezak was quick to point out that her model allows for idiographic experience of the stages at different rates of progression and with varying degrees of linearity. In addition, the stages tend to overlap, and individuals can progress forward and backwards among them. The primary function of her model, then, is to provide a conceptual framework within which family members can work through the various emotions associated with the traumatic brain injury. A description of Lezak's stage model follows.

Stage one begins during hospitalization and lasts up to three months after discharge.

TABLE 18.1.   Stages in the Evolution of Family Reactions[a]

| Stage | Time since discharge (months) | Perception of patient | Expectation | Family reaction |
|---|---|---|---|---|
| I | 0–1 to 3 | Mildly difficult | Full recovery in one year | Relief |
| II | 1–3 to 6–9 | Uncooperative, unmotivated, and self-centered | Full recovery if try harder | Anxiety |
| III | 6–9 to 9–24 | Irresponsible, self-centered, and irritable | Independent if given proper help | Depression, guilt, and defeat |
| IV | 9 and up | Difficult, childlike, dependent | Little or no change | Depression, "trapped" |
| V | 15 and up | Difficult, childlike, dependent | Little or no change | Mourning |
| VI | 18 to 24 and up | Difficult, childlike, dependent | Little or no change | Detached |

[a]Adapted from Lezak (1986).

During this time family members typically perceive the brain-damaged individual as moderately difficult to manage. This is attributed to environmental factors or patient variables such as fatigability and weakness due to inactivity. Family members often expect full recovery by approximately one year's time. Stage one is generally a time of relative happiness for the family. Members are relieved that the patient has finally come home from the hospital and expectations for a return to "normal" run high.

As the family's optimism and energy from stage one diminish, stage two begins and continues until nine months postdischarge. Now, family members often become anxious as the brain-damaged person's deficits and emotionally disturbing behaviors persist. The patient begins to be perceived as uncooperative, unmotivated, and self-centered. Family members may become bewildered by the changes in the personality of the patient. During this stage, the expectation for full recovery is maintained, contingent on the increased desire and effort of the patient to improve.

Stage three develops out of a worsening stage two. This stage lasts up to two years after patient discharge, but may continue indefinitely. The tendency at this stage is for family members to perceive the unimproved patient as irresponsible, self-centered, irritable, and lazy. The family members believe that improvements can be made if they can find the "right" way to help the patient overcome deficits. This belief often results in feelings of discouragement, guilt, depression, and fears of "going crazy," as attempts to motivate the patient repeatedly fail.

Like stage three, the fourth stage can continue indefinitely. Stage four is characterized by the developing perception that the brain-damaged family member is now a different person than before: more childlike and difficult to manage. This realization is usually agonizing for the family, and feelings of depression, despair, and burden are typical. At this point, the family begins to acknowledge that the brain-damaged individual has reached close to maximum recovery, and little or no additional change is expected.

Such a marked change in the way the family perceives the patient can lead to the mourning reaction characteristic of stage five. This stage usually occurs some time after 15 months postdischarge, yet unlike stages three and four, stage five is typically time-limited. The patient is still perceived as a difficult childlike dependent with little hope for improvement. Unlike stage four, however, grief feelings rather than depression dominate this time period as family members give up hope that the premorbid personality will return.

Stage six often follows a successful resolution of stages four and five. During this stage, role adjustment and reorganization are signs of healthy functioning. Family members are still engaged with the brain-damaged patient on a physical and financial level, yet they are able to establish a sense of emotional detachment that allows them to rebuild a meaningful life and avoid social isolation. By the time families reach stage six, much of the emotional pain associated with the compromised member is resolved. Once again, specific interventions appropriate for each stage will be outlined below in the section on outpatient group psychotherapy with families.

Lezak's stage model presents a useful and believable portrayal of the psychosocial difficulties experienced by the patient's family after traumatic brain damage, and even when families fail to follow the model's stages precisely, the model still offers a framework within which much teaching can be conducted, and family members have a schema within which to understand their own experiences. As noted previously, the quality of family functioning is highly correlated with rehabilitation outcome. Therefore, it follows that one important component of treating the brain-damaged adult is providing psychological services for the family members. Salhoot (1984) proposed that group treatment strategies are especially effective in meeting the needs of families. Several direct benefits of group psychotherapy with families were presented by Power and Dell Orto (1980). First, the group format facilitates the transfer of information about brain damage from professional staff and between members of different families. Through the group process, the family gains a sense of competence, and the understanding that their feelings are shared by others. Second, the group environment is an excellent place for family members to reorganize patterns of relating to one another. Exposure to the communication problems experienced by other families and their subsequent methods of coping aids in the normalization of intrafamilial relating. Third, contact with other families engaged in the coping process acts to renew awareness of internal family strength and mobilize resources. Fourth, the group format enables family members to identify their own needs that are often ignored as they attend to the patient's needs. Group members provide support for guiltless recognition of such needs.

In summary, brain-injured persons suffer multiple cognitive, behavioral, and psychosocial difficulties. These problem areas directly affect the psychological well-being of the family, which in turn has a reciprocal effect on the patient's rehabilitation outcome. The primary conclusion that can be drawn from an understanding of the relationship between the brain-damaged adult and the family is that successful psychotherapeutic treatment of the brain-injured patient *must* include concurrent treatment of the family. The first part of this chapter has presented the basis for this conclusion and argued for the treatment of both patient and family in a group setting. The rest of the chapter will present the most current methods of applying group psychotherapy in both inpatient and outpatient settings.

## INPATIENT GROUP PSYCHOTHERAPY

The framework for inpatient group psychotherapy with brain-damaged adults and their families is somewhat different from that of the group treatment format usually encountered in a psychiatric environment. Rather than participating in group on a psychiatric ward,

brain-damaged patients receive psychotherapy on a rehabilitation unit. Inpatient rehabilitation psychotherapy groups are usually limited to weekly or biweekly meetings due to time
constraints imposed by the multidisciplinary treatment team. These groups are open to a
steady flow of new admissions and discharged patients. Usually, a single therapist runs the
groups due to staff demands. In addition, the time frames of these groups range from several
weeks to a few months, making it difficult for the group to pursue many issues in depth
unless group sessions are offered at least several times a week. A discussion of inpatient
group psychotherapy with brain-damaged adults is presented next, followed by recommendations for treatment of their families.

## The Brain-Damaged Patient

Vinogradov and Yalom (1989) remind the group therapist working with special
populations that when working under time constraints, the goals must be specific, attain-
able, and tailored to the capacity and potential of the group members. General goals suited
to an inpatient population such as "restoration of function" and "preparation for discharge"
must be more specifically operationalized.

Because of the heterogeneity of brain-damaged patients in rehabilitation, two or three
different groups may be established. One group might focus on issues concerning adjustment to ability. This group is most suitable for the higher functioning patients on the unit,
and it can be referred to as a "class" in order to more easily involve some patients who
might be somewhat resistant to psychological services. Another group ("class") might
address the needs of lower functioning patients who are confused and disoriented.
Reorientation and basic cognitive retraining is the emphasis in this group. Finally, ad hoc
groups can be formed as needed for intermediate level patients or special subpopulations
(e.g., young adults, women, veterans, etc.). Accurate assessment of cognitive, behavioral,
and psychosocial functioning is important for appropriate group placement of patients.

As noted in the introduction, little research has been published that attempts to
document specific group formats and to empirically validate psychotherapeutic outcome.
Recently, however, more work has begun in this area. Several current applications of group
psychotherapy to brain-damaged inpatients follow.

### Reality Orientation

Corrigan, Arnett, Houck, and Jackson (1985) developed an orientation group to
improve attention deficits, confusion, and anterograde amnesia in brain-injured patients.
Seven specific behavioral objectives were used to measure (1) orientation, (2) attention, (3)
immediate retention, (4) episodic recall, and (5) use of memory aids. For example,
objective one states, "Patient is oriented to the day, date, and year 80% of the time over a
2-week period (time orientation aids such as calendars and clocks may be used)" (p. 627).
Ratings of the patients' daily performance in each of the objective domains (interrater
reliability of 0.875) were aggregated to obtain a weekly summary score. The researchers
found that the weekly aggregate score is a good index of recovery during posttraumatic
amnesia, with high correspondence to qualitative changes in patient progress.

Corrigan and colleagues deserve credit for establishing and implementing such
specific objectives in its orientation group. As the authors point out, however, the limited

data do not indicate that this form of group intervention alone resolves disorientation, confusion, and anterograde amnesia, but there is no reason to believe that such programs interfere in any way with recovery, either. Nonetheless, definitive conclusions concerning the effectiveness of an orientation group await controlled outcome studies.

## Cognitive Retraining

Leer (1986) reported the development of a cognitive retraining activity group for brain-damaged patients. The purpose was to enhance orientation, cognition, and social skills. The group was led by two therapists who met with five to seven patients three times a week for 45 minutes. During the group, the patients performed specific tasks with individualized objectives that were carefully planned beforehand by the therapists. After the group sessions, each patient's observed level of functioning was recorded on an observation sheet using a weighted hierarchy numerical scoring system that assessed a number of cognitive and social areas. Leer's findings indicate that most patients made significant gains by participating in the cognitive retraining group.

Leer's conclusion may be somewhat premature due to the fact that there is no mention of comparison to control in his report. In addition, the assessment methodology is rather subjective. The design of the group itself, however, appears quite promising. Such a cognitive retraining activity group certainly may see an increased acceptance into the mainstream of inpatient rehabilitation, especially if it can offer something significantly distinct from occupational and recreational therapy.

## Coping Skills

In order to aid brain-damaged adults in their emotional adjustment to their disability and improve their social skills, Leer and Sonday (1986) developed a Client Coping Skills Group. According to this design, a psychologist and a social worker met one to two times weekly with a group of five to seven patients. The group was structured so that specific information relevant to its composition could be covered, but it was flexible enough to allow members to share personal experiences and concerns as needed. After each session, a number of emotional and social areas were assessed using an observation protocol similar to that described above (Leer, 1986). The authors reported that clinically observable gains were documented in most group members.

The Client Coping Skills Group and the cognitive retraining activities group described previously exemplify the use of different groups to meet the diverse needs of a hetero-geneous rehabilitation population. In addition, the number of patients can be kept to an optimal number when two, or even three different groups are offered on a unit. As noted above, however, the therapeutic efficacy of these groups lacks empirical validation by controlled outcome, and more objective assessment techniques are needed.

## The Prigatano Model

The Prigatano neuropsychological rehabilitation group (1986b) has developed a detailed approach to group psychotherapy with brain-damaged inpatients. The group has a comprehensive topical structure that is conducted according to the goals and guidelines presented in an earlier section of this chapter. Although little empirical analysis is available on outcome, the 24 topics appear to address most psychological needs germane to this population.

The topics used by Prigatano's rehabilitation team is as follows: Topic 1, orientation to group psychotherapy; Topic 2, evaluation of patients' emotional reaction to their brain injury (c.g., each patient is asked: "What have been your emotional reactions to your brain injury?"); Topic 3, evaluation of patients' perception of family reactions to their brain injury (e.g., the question is asked: "What do your relatives see as your emotional reaction to your brain injury?"); Topic 4, personality change (e.g., "How has your personality changed since your brain injury?"); Topic 5, family perception of personality change (e.g., "How do your relatives see your personality at the present time? Do they think there has been any change? What is their evidence for this?"); Topic 6, differences between patient and family perspective (e.g., "If relatives could change anything in your emotional reaction or your personality following the injury, what would they change and why?"); Topic 7, evaluation of patients' objective assessment of their problems (e.g., "If you could change your emotional reaction or personality following your brain injury, what would you change and why?"); Topic 8, nature of catastrophic reaction; Topic 9, general information about emotional and motivational problems following brain injury is presented in the form of lists, and patients are asked to determine which problems in the lists apply to them; Topic 10, patients get feedback from their peers on their problem lists; Topic 11, review of functional neuroanatomy is given, and the specific medical history of each patient is discussed in terms of the correlation between their neuropsychological deficits and their emotional and motivational disturbances; Topic 12, discussion of emotional reaction to specific neuro-psychological deficits; Topic 13, peer feedback about emotional functioning is given to each patient; Topic 14, patients again generate problem lists and receive peer feedback concerning the accuracy of their lists; Topic 15, body image after brain injury; Topic 16, self-confidence; Topic 17, paranoid ideation; Topic 18, denial of illness; Topic 19, sexual dysfunction; Topic 20, social isolation and withdrawal; Topic 21, problems in dealing with spouse and children; Topic 22, dealing with relatives other than spouse and children; Topic 23, emotions related to employment and unemployment; Topic 24, patients are presented with the psychiatric model of group psychotherapy to determine nature of advances made (Yalom, 1985). In other words, the group is conducted as if the treatment outcome goals are symptom relief and character change, rather than restoration of function and preparation for discharge.

The Prigatano model is an excellent application of many aspects of traditional group psychotherapy to patients recovering from brain injury. The content of the sessions, however, is only appropriate for higher functioning patients who may be many months postinjury. Thus, the Prigatano model may see its most appropriate application in a long-term inpatient rehabilitation facility.

*Videotaping*

The use of videotape as a feedback modality for social skills training and self-awareness development has gained recent popularity in group treatment settings. Helffen-stein and Wechsler (1982) reported significantly greater improvements in the (1) trait anxiety, (2) self-concept, and (3) social skills of a group of newly brain-injured patients who received several hours of videotaped feedback of their social interactions, compared to a control group who got no such feedback. Alexy, Foster, and Baker (1983) presented a description of their use of videotape feedback in group sessions with brain-damaged adults two to six months postinjury. In biweekly sessions, two or three therapists meet with three to eight patients in an activity room equipped with a videotape camera and a TV monitor. After initial welcome and introductions, one of the therapists describes the purpose of the group as follows:

> Many people who have had a head injury often experience some difficulty in observing themselves as they interact with others. This ability to observe one's self is called *self-awareness*. By videotaping patients as they interact with each other, they can play-back on the TV monitor what they did and decide for themselves what they liked and what they didn't like. With the help of the group and its leaders, patients can decide if there are things they wish to change in their interactions and relations with others. (p. 8)

The first half of the hour-long session is used to videotape group participants as they talk about common patient issues (e.g., rehabilitation progress, discharge plans, family issues, adjustment to disability), and display noticeable behaviors (e.g., stereotypies, laughing, fidgeting). In addition, there is a review of specific target behaviors that particular patients need to concentrate on during the session.

The second half of the group session is devoted to viewing the videotape recorded in the first half. The videotape is stopped at approximately two-minute intervals, and the patient who was highlighted is asked to critically evaluate his or her behavior. Next, other group members are asked to give feedback. When the entire videotape has been viewed in this manner, the remaining time is used to review each patient's progress with individual target behaviors. The behavioral goals that these authors have addressed in group include: (1) improvement of attention and concentration, (2) increased voice volume, (3) ability to monitor rate of speech, (4) increased relevance of speech, (5) reduced perseverative speech and stereotypies, (6) increased empathetic responses to peers, (7) decreased inappropriate laughter and regressive responses, and (8) improved posture.

In addition to presenting the way videotape feedback group is conducted, Alexy *et al.* (1983) suggested several methods for enhancing group effectiveness. These suggestions are summarized as follows:

1. Include patients who function at different levels.
2. Identify and focus on specific target behaviors.
3. Encourage each participant to identify target behaviors toward the beginning of each group.
4. Encourage patients to define their own target behaviors.
5. Encourage generalization of target behaviors [via] a dual approach: (a) encourage patients to practice their behaviors between sessions, and (b) encourage other staff, family, and friends to remind and reinforce patients for practicing their target behaviors.
6. Provide ample opportunity for patients to reflect on the audio-visual feedback.
7. Allow patients to establish direction of group process.
8. Model the behavior expected from patients. (pp. 9–10)

Using this psychotherapeutic technique, the authors report that the group sessions have facilitated the development of more adaptive social skills in most treated patients. This format is promising, but systematic outcome studies are needed to empirically validate this group treatment modality.

## The Family

Group psychotherapy with family members while the patient is still hospitalized differs greatly from outpatient techniques described below. Unrealistic expectations for patient recovery, denial of deficits, and emotional shock are only a few of the family variables that limit the effectiveness of inpatient group psychotherapy with family members. However, psychology staff can lay important groundwork for later intervention at this time.

The goals for inpatient group treatment of family members can be stated as follows: (1) to present information about brain damage and an orientation to the typical course of rehabilitative treatment, (2) to instill an awareness of the commonalities between different families, (3) to provide emotional support, and (4) to create an environment for catharsis. The family support group may be led by a psychologist and a case manager or social worker. Other members of the treatment team (e.g., physical, occupational, and speech therapists) may rotate into the group to provide information about discipline-specific topics. Typically, this group is divided into two parts: (1) an initial didactic component, and (2) a more traditional group format. In addition to its overt purpose, the didactic component also serves to break the ice among group members and establish a sense of common concern. After the didactic goal is satisfied, introductions are given around the table with brief patient histories. From then on, the group is completely unstructured, allowing family members to discuss perceived relevant issues. The entire group session need only last 45 minutes to an hour. Although it is usually the case that psychotherapeutic effect will be limited during inpatient work with the family, inroads can be made that will facilitate later treatment.

## OUTPATIENT GROUP PSYCHOTHERAPY

The format of group psychotherapy with brain-damaged adults and their families on an outpatient basis is distinct in several ways from inpatient treatment. Sessions are no longer conducted on the rehabilitation unit. Now, groups are held in a meeting room of the local mental health clinic or medical center. Often co-therapists are available to run weekly outpatient groups. The time frames of these groups now range from several weeks to several months, or even years, depending on the specific design. In addition, the tone of the groups is less formal than it was during inpatient treatment. Refreshments are usually served to help emphasize the supportive social aspects of the session. A discussion of outpatient group psychotherapy with brain-damaged adults will first be presented, then family treatment issues and techniques will be addressed.

## The Brain-Damaged Patient

Participation in outpatient group psychotherapy usually requires that the brain-damaged individual has made a moderately good cognitive and behavioral recovery. The patient does not have to be living independently or even functioning at a very high level, but he or she must have the capacity and potential to benefit from group content that focuses on issues of adjustment to disability with development and maintenance of appropriate psychosocial functioning. Three broad goals for group psychotherapy with the brain-injured are as follows: (1) reeducation, (2) resocialization, and (3) support.

As with the inpatient treatment literature, empirical studies are scant for outpatient populations. Current trends, however, have yielded some documentation of techniques and treatment outcome in this area of growing interest. Several recent applications of group psychotherapy to brain-damaged outpatients are presented below.

## Cognitive–Social Retraining

Carberry and Burd (1983) reported qualitative success in their cognitive and social retraining group. The group consisted of a maximum of eight patients and two co-therapists, meeting every week for 20 weeks. The format of the group was semiflexible, striking a balance between a structured topical emphasis and sensitivity to various affective concerns. Specific strategies and techniques used to develop social skills included (1) enhancing listening skills, (2) summarizing, (3) presentation of self to others, (4) storytelling technique, (5) empathy building tasks, (6) role playing, (7) counseling, and (8) humor. Although the authors have presented a creative and sensitive portrayal of the group psychotherapeutic process, very little hope currently exists for the reliable and valid measurement of social skills such as "empathy." It should be noted once again that treatment objectives must be very specific and well defined in order to document therapeutic effectiveness.

A recent paper by Hibbard, Grober, Gordon, and Aletta (1990) outlined a protocol for modifying traditional cognitive therapy techniques to address the problem of poststroke depression. Specific strategies for using cognitive therapy techniques with commonly observed sequelae such as anosognosia or denial were discussed, and the vital importance of providing adjunct services to the families of the patients was emphasized as well. Cicerone (1989) also offered a thoughtful paper on psychotherapy with brain-damaged patients, in which he encouraged therapists to separately examine contributions related to (1) neuropsychologically based personality changes, (2) emotional reactions to the injury, and (3) magnification or minimization of premorbid response styles. He asserted the goal of therapy is not to cure the damaged brain, but more realistically, to reduce discomfort and promote adjustment.

## Basic Social Skills

Social skills training offers a well-researched tool for treating deficiencies in social behavior in populations ranging from mentally retarded children to depressed adults. This problem-focused technique has been applied to the skill deficits among brain-damaged populations as well. A fine example of recent research in this area (Brotherton, Thomas, Wisotzek, & Milan, 1988) described the use of multiple baseline single case design in the treatment of four individuals who had survived severe traumatic brain injuries at least two years before. This straightforward program included components of instruction/education, modeling, behavioral rehearsal, video feedback (cf. Alexy et al., 1983; Helffenstein &

Wechsler, 1982), and social reinforcement. One-year follow-up data were collected in order to examine the longevity of treatment outcomes. The authors concluded that their program worked better in altering simple motoric behavior (e.g., posture, self-stimulation) than more complex verbal–social behavior.

### Coping and Problem-Solving Skills

Interventions targeting these skills areas attempt to enhance a patient's behavioral repertoire by training different ways to think and behave in stressful situations. Rose (1989) outlined several characteristics believed to be important in running a coping skills group with brain-damaged patients. Suggestions included encouraging peer tutoring to foster skills acquisition, evaluating treatment outcome empirically, and promoting generalization of treatment effects to novel situations. Foxx, Martella, and Marchand-Martella (1989) described their efforts to provide problem-solving training to three brain-damaged adults. Using a set of programmatic techniques to facilitate acquisition and retention of the problem-solving repertoire, the authors targeted areas such as community transportation, correct self-administration and monitoring of medications, basic assertiveness, and emergency awareness. Their program report stated that the intervention led to relatively prompt acquisition of new behaviors that lasted at least up to the six month follow-up, and also seemed to generalize to settings other than those used in training.

## The Family

Lezak (1978) proposed that the characterological alterations seen among brain-damaged patients, along with subsequent changes in family dynamics, put the family unit under a great deal of stress for which family members are typically unprepared. She recommended counseling family members to set realistic expectations, learn behavior management principles, be alert to their own needs, and to feel unselfish about meeting those needs. According to the author, family preparedness to cope with a brain-damaged member is a factor that can affect the recovery process, and that family members need to be prepared to deal with their own psychosocial problems related to the injury of their loved one (Lezak, 1986, 1988).

The need to establish clearer expectancies for recovery is evident in research that examines the concordance of complaints from patients and their families. Typically there is more disagreement about what problems persist after head injury than agreement. Agreement tends to relate to physical limitations rather than cognitive or emotional limitations (Gouvier, Uddo-Crane, & Brown, 1988; Hendryx, 1989).

The importance of cohesive family functioning in recovery from brain injury cannot be overemphasized. Evans, Bishop, Matlock, Stranahan, Halar *et al.* (1987) have reported evidence that rehospitalization following stroke is predicted by measures of family control and emotional closeness, and patient adjustment is predicted by family communication and  problem-solving skills. Further evidence suggests that patients from more functional families are more likely to comply with their treatment regimes than patients from dysfunctional families (Evans, Bishop, Matlock, Stranahan, Smith *et al.*, 1987). Freidland and McColl (1987) reported that measures of social support predict psychosocial symptomatology among brain-damaged patients, accounting for about 15% of the variance.

While not perfect prediction, the authors argued that an "especially strong protective effect was produced by community social support" (p. 475).

While family cohesion and social support may help promote recovery from brain injury, the effort to provide an optimal environment for recovery may be more that a family can sustain without doing irreparable damage to the family structure. Callahan (1988) made the observation that our society offers little moral recognition for the families who take care of their brain-injured, and thus, this activity offers no real extrinsic rewards. He points out that the conflict arises when a family is subjected to what appears to be a justifiable moral claim to care for a loved one, but it becomes a claim they cannot endure. Conversely, the ability to meet an endurable claim ought not be a factor in establishing the justifiability of a claim. Unless these considerations are acknowledged, the end result may be the dissolution of a family unit, typically leaving one family member burdened with all responsibilities. Other family members are left "burned out" from their previous efforts, disinclined to contribute any more to the patient's care.

Our efforts at Louisiana State University have begun to address the needs common to many metropolitan and rural areas of the country: the needs of patients and their families that continue long after most formal rehabilitation efforts have drawn to a close. Once rehabilitation is "over," many patients and their families have continued need for support, education, and guidance. Often, this follow-up care can extend for a period of years, addressing new problems that arise as patients attempt to reenter the mainstream of society.

To address these needs, we have developed a 12-week program of weekly group sessions designed for patients and their families. Separate groups for patients and their families are conducted in order to minimize the scheduling, caretaking, and transportation difficulties that would arise with groups held at different times. The program is designed so that complementary topics are addressed in each group, and the specific content is tailored to the needs of the groups' members. For example, one topic is motivation. In the patient group, the emphasis is on how to "get themselves moving," and in the family group, the emphasis is on how they can create conditions that maximize the likelihood of the patient being motivated to work hard in continuing rehabilitation. Some of the other topic areas include the following: management of thoughts, emotions, and behavior; interviewing skills; accessing community resources, and accepting limitations without yielding to them. We are currently collecting data at Louisiana State University, in order to determine the effectiveness of this group program. Waiting-list control group data are also being collected.

## CONCLUSION

It is encouraging to note that there is now a sufficient literature on group therapy with the brain-injured to allow the present review to be written. Ten, or even five years ago, there would not have been enough work in this area to review. This chapter has examined a number of points raised over the past few years, including the applicability of psycho-therapy in treating psychological changes following brain injury. Many lists and task hierarchies have been presented uncritically with the goal of offering group therapists a sampling of current techniques in the area. These are not intended to be viewed as absolute facts or rigid guidelines until such claims are supported by research data. Much of what has been presented here represents the untested speculations of practitioners. However, it is from these speculations that testable hypotheses can be derived. It is our hope that in updating this review five years hence, a much greater proportion of empirical studies will be available.

## REFERENCES

Alexy, W. D., Foster, M., & Baker, A. (1983). Audio-visual feedback: An exercise in self-awareness for the head injured patient. *Cognitive Rehabilitation, 1*(6), 8–10.

Brotherton, F. A., Thomas, L. L., Wisotzek, I. E., & Milan, M. A. (1988). Social skills training in the rehabilitation of patients with traumatic closed head injury. *Archives of Physical Medicine & Rehabilitation, 69*, 827–832.

Callahan, D. (1988). Families as caregivers: The limits of morality. *Archives of Physical Medicine & Rehabilitation, 69*, 323–328.

Carberry, H., & Burd, B. (1983). Social aspects of cognitive retraining in an outpatient group setting for head trauma patients. *Cognitive Rehabilitation, 1*(6), 5–7.

Cicerone, K. D. (1989). Psychotherapeutic interventions with traumatically brain-injured patients. *Rehabilitation Psychology, 34*(2), 105–114.

Corrigan, J. D., Arnett, J. A., Houck, L. J., Jackson, R. D. (1985). Reality orientation for brain injured patients: Group treatment and monitoring of recovery. *Archives of Physical Medicine & Rehabilitation, 66*, 626–630.

Crawford, J. D., & McIvor, G. P. (1985). Group psychotherapy: Benefits in multiple sclerosis. *Archives of Physical Medicine & Rehabilitation, 66*, 810–813.

Evans, R. L., Bishop, D. S., Matlock, A.-L., Stranahan, S., Halar, E. M., & Noonan, W. C. (1987). Prestroke family interaction as a predictor of stroke outcome. *Archives of Physical Medicine & Rehabilitation, 68*, 508–512.

Evans, R. L., Bishop, D. S., Matlock, A.-L., Stranahan, S., Smith, G. G., & Halar, E. M. (1987). Family interaction and treatment adherence after stroke. *Archives of Physical Medicine & Rehabilitation, 68*, 513–517.

Foxx, R. M., Martella, R. C., & Marchand-Martella, N. E. (1989). The acquisition, maintenance, and generalization of problem-solving skills by closed head-injured adults. *Behavior Therapy, 20*, 61–76.

Freidland, J., & McColl, M. A. (1987). Social support and psychosocial dysfunction after stroke: Buffering effects in a community sample. *Archives of Physical Medicine & Rehabilitation, 68*(8), 475–480.

Gouvier, W. D., Uddo-Crane, M., & Brown, L. M. (1988). Baserates of post-concussional symptoms. *Archives of Clinical Neuropsychology, 3*, 273–278.

Gugel, R. N., & Eisdorfer, S. (1985). The role of therapeutic group programs in a nursing home. *Rehabilitation Psychology, 30*(2), 83–92.

Helffenstein, D., & Wechsler, F. (1982). The use of Interpersonal Process Recall (IPR) in the remediation of interpersonal and communication skill deficits in the newly brain injured. *Clinical Neuropsychology, 4*, 139–143.

Hendryx, P. M. (1989). Psychosocial changes perceived by closed-head-injured adults and their families. *Archives of Physical Medicine & Rehabilitation, 70*, 526–530.

Hibbard, M. R., Grober, S. E., Gordon, W. A., & Aletta, E. G. (1990). Modification of cognitive psychotherapy for the treatment of post-stroke depression. *The Behavior Therapist, 13*(1), 15–17.

Leer, W.B. (1986). Brain injured activity group for cognitive retraining in a rehabilitation setting [Abstract, Proceedings of the 5th Annual Meeting of the National Academy of Neuropsychologists]. *Archives of Clinical Neuropsychology, 1*(1), 55.

Leer, W. B., & Sonday, W. E. (1986). Brain injured client coping skills group in a rehabilitation setting [Abstract, Proceedings of the 6th Annual Meeting of the National Academy of Neuropsychologists]. *Archives of Clinical Neuropsychology, 1*(3), 277.

Lezak, M. D. (1978). Living with the characterologically altered brain-injured patient. *Journal of Clinical Psychiatry, 39*(7), 592–598.

Lezak, M. D. (1986). Psychological implications of traumatic brain damage for the patient's family. *Rehabilitation Psychology*, *31*(4), 241–250.

Lezak, M. D. (1988). Brain damage is a family affair. *Journal of Clinical & Experimental Neuropsychology*, *10*(1), 111–123.

Patterson, C. H. (1986). *Theories of counseling and psychotherapy* (4th ed.). New York: Harper & Row.

Power, P. W., & Dell Orto, A. E. (1980). Approaches to family intervention. In P. W. Power & A. E. Dell Orto (Eds.), *Role of the family in the rehabilitation of the physically disabled*. Baltimore: University Park Press.

Prigatano, G. P. (1986a). Personality and psychosocial consequences of brain injury. In G. P. Prigatano, D. J. Fordyce, H. K. Zeiner, J. R. Roeche, M. Pepping, & B. C. Wood (Eds.), *Neuropsychological rehabilitation after brain injury* (pp. 29–50). Baltimore: Johns Hopkins University Press.

Prigatano, G. P. (1986b). Psychotherapy after brain injury. In G.P. Prigatano, D. J. Fordyce, H. K. Zeiner, J. R. Roeche, M. Pepping, & B. C. Wood (Eds.), *Neuropsychological rehabilitation after brain injury* (pp. 67–95). Baltimore: Johns Hopkins University Press.

Rose, S. D. (1989). Coping skill training in groups. *International Journal of Group Psychotherapy*, *39*(1), 59–78.

Rosenthal, M. (1989). Response to "Psychotherapeutic interventions with traumatically brain-injured patients." *Rehabilitation Psychology*, *34*(2), 115–116.

Rosenthal, M., & Geckler, C. (1986). Family therapy issues in neuropsychology. In D. Wedding, A. M. Horton, Jr., & J. Webster (Eds.), *The neuropsychology handbook: Behavioral and clinical perspectives* (pp. 325–344). Berlin: Springer.

Salhoot, J. T. (1984). Group therapy and rehabilitation. In D. W. Krueger (Ed.), *Rehabilitation psychology: A comprehensive textbook* (pp. 61–68). Rockville, MD: Aspen Systems.

Toseland, R. W., & Siporin, M. (1986). When to recommend group treatment: A review of the clinical and research literature. *International Journal of Group Psychotherapy*, *32*, 171–201.

Vinogradov, S., & Yalom, I. D. (1989). *Concise guide to group psychotherapy*. Washington, DC: American Psychiatric Press.

Yalom, I. D. (1985). *The theory and practice of group psychotherapy* (3rd ed.). New York: Basic Books.

# 19

# Family Involvement in Cognitive Recovery following Traumatic Brain Injury

THOMAS A. NOVACK, THOMAS F. BERGQUIST, and GERALD BENNETT

Prior to addressing the specifics of cognitive recovery strategies to be used by the family, issues related to involvement of family members in a rehabilitation program need to be discussed. A great deal is at stake for the family of a head-injured person. The impact of head injury on family members has been addressed in multiple publications documenting the potentially devastating effect on family health and stability. Rosenbaum and Najenson (1976), in an Israeli population, found that wives of head-injured individuals were more likely to be depressed and less likely to have a stable support network than the wives of persons with paraplegia or uninjured males. Kozloff (1987) was able to document decreasing social support for head-injured persons and their families as the time since injury increases. Finally, multiple studies coming from Glasgow, Scotland (Livingston, Brooks, & Bond, 1985; Livingston, 1987; Brooks, Campsie, Symington, Beattie, & McKinlay, 1987) indicate the extreme burden placed on family members by head-injured individuals even up to seven years postinjury.

The cognitive and behavioral problems experienced by head-injured individuals leave the family perplexed as to how to cope, and, as a result, dissolution of the family network is not uncommon following head injury. A sense of loss of control seems to permeate many of the comments of family members of head-injured individuals (as well as the head-injured

THOMAS A. NOVACK, THOMAS F. BERGQUIST, and GERALD BENNETT • Spain Rehabilitation Center, Department of Rehab Medicine, University of Alabama at Birmingham School of Medicine, Birmingham, Alabama 35294.

*HANDBOOK OF HEAD TRAUMA: Acute Care to Recovery*, edited by Charles J. Long and Leslie K. Ross. Plenum Press, New York, 1992.

persons themselves); they simply do not know what to do to improve the situation and feel that what they *are* doing is not effective. Unfortunately, in the United States, services for individuals several years postinjury are hard to find and expensive. Consequently, over the long run, families are often isolated in terms of professional contact, and the problems associated with head injury often make it difficult to establish a firm social network or consistent support from the extended family. The situation is not one that will be remedied by any specific treatment program; severe head injury results in permanent changes in brain functioning which will have (in the majority of cases) an impact on everyday life even with the best of rehabilitation programs. A better conception of the problem is to consider how families might be aided in coping with the situation more effectively. Some solutions are quite obvious, such as family counseling, attending local support groups sponsored by the National Head Injury Foundation, and increased social outreach. However, endeavors in these areas are often not made until a significant problem exists, and by that time it is often difficult to relieve the stress. From a prevention standpoint, it may be easier to intervene with family members earlier during the recovery process (even while the head-injured person is still hospitalized) to provide the family with a framework for their interactions with the head-injured person.

What has been lacking thus far for the families in many situations is the definition of a specific role in the rehabilitation program. Many family members fall into old, familiar roles (such as being parent to a young child) which may not be appropriate for dealing with a head-injured person. However, this is what is familiar and therefore what will be attempted initially. What is required is a new definition of roles for family members: family members have to be provided with information and training which allows them to impact the recovery process, literally a rationale for how to interact with a head-injured person.

## AREAS OF CONFLICT WITH FAMILY MEMBERS

At present, family members generally have an undefined role at rehabilitation centers. Staff members may view family members as a hindrance to treatment. In fact, there are problems associated with having family members present at a rehabilitation center. First, families tend to get in the way due to their physical presence and frequent questions. Staff may perceive that the rehabilitation program is like a well-oiled machine in which the family represents grit in the wheels. The presence of family members is considered a diversion away from the actual tasks of the rehabilitation team. Second, staff often develop performance jitters in the presence of family members. Understandably, it is difficult to perform when a family member is closely observing staff work with a patient. Such observation implies potentially negative evaluation of staff performance. As a result, it is not uncommon for staff to ask family members to leave the room or therapy area when they are working with a patient. Third, staff regard having to talk with family members and deal with their emotional distress as a diversion of professional time from the patient and, therefore, begin to resent questions and comments from the family. Fourth, rehabilitation staff often become tired of having to repeat information for family members. Family members in a rehabilitation center commonly do not fully process information the first time they hear it and the necessity of repetition is well known. This can become very tedious and leads to unfounded concerns that the family may be in the midst of denial or intellectually subnormal. Fifth, there is a common concern among rehabilitation professionals that if families are invited to participate in patient care, they will literally "camp out" at the rehabilitation center and at the bedside of the injured family member. Once the family is in that position, it is very difficult to ask them to leave. The possibility of a confrontation with the family frightens staff. This issue is especially troublesome when families have been staying around the clock with an injured relative on a neurosurgical unit. Finally, families may express opinions which are perceived by staff as being unrealistic given the status of the patient. Romano (1974) provided several examples of denial by family members, for instance, believing that the injured person will awake from a coma as if from sleep. In a rehabilitation center the denial may take more subtle forms, such as believing that following several weeks of rehabilitation the person will be totally recovered, or that reflexive movements represent intentional, functional abilities, or that some medication or inter-personal conflict with a therapist is standing in the way of the injured person's progress in multiple areas. Many staff members seem to regard it as an inherent part of working in the rehabilitation setting to challenge unrealistic attitudes of family members. Such challenging may turn into confrontation between staff and family with potentially destructive conse-quences. Once family members perceive staff members as disagreeing with them about the recovery potential of the patient, the credibility of that staff member in the family's eyes may diminish greatly, which undermines future communication.

## UNDERSTANDING FAMILY MEMBERS

Instead of minimizing family involvement in a rehabilitation program, it would be better to try to understand the emotional status of family members and how they perceive the rehabilitation situation to help increase the effectiveness of family involvement. At the Spain Rehabilitation Center, 36 primary caretakers (22 mothers, 3 fathers, 7 wives, 3 husbands, 1 cousin) of injured patients were followed during the acute rehabilitation phase to determine levels of anxiety, depression, and the ability to objectively evaluate level of disability. Family members were able to rate level of disability using the Disability Rating Scale accurately in comparison to a professional familiar with the effects of head injury (Tables 19.1 and 19.2). Based on the results of the Beck Depression Scale, relatively few (4/36) family members were clinically depressed on patient admission, which fell to two depressed family members by discharge. Thus, depression was not a significant factor for family members. On the other hand, anxiety (as measured by the State–Trait Anxiety Scale) was a significant problem, with 12 family members (33% of the sample) being in the clinically anxious range at the time of patient admission, which had dropped to 3 anxious individuals by the time of discharge. Thus, many family members were anxious at the time of admission but much improved by discharge. The level of anxiety of family members

TABLE 19.1.   Family versus Professional
in Rating Disability at Admission

|  | Mean | SD | Range | Correlation (w/professional) |
|---|---|---|---|---|
| Family | 12.4 | 6.2 | 4–23 | .97 |
| Professional | 13.5 | 6.5 | 5–25 |  |

TABLE 19.2.   Family versus Professional
in Rating Disability at Discharge

|  | Mean | *SD* | Range | Correlation (w/professional) |
|---|---|---|---|---|
| Family | 7.2 | 5.8 | 1–26 | .94 |
| Professional | 7.1 | 5.5 | 3–23 |  |

cannot be explained by the disability level of the head-injured person: correlations between scores on the State–Trait Anxiety Scale and disability level were uniformly nonsignificant (Tables 19.3 and 19.4). Thus, no matter how impaired the patient was on admission, family members were still quite anxious. Obviously, there is not a simple relationship between disability level and the family's emotional distress; other factors are necessary to understand the anxiety level. Although objective evidence is lacking, it is reasonable to assume that part of the problem for family members is that they perceive the situation as being unpredictable, which generates anxiety. Even for the milder injuries, the ultimate outcome is difficult to predict at the time of acute rehabilitation and that uncertainty generates anxiety among family members. Also contributing to the anxiety may be the fact that while a person is in acute rehabilitation, the role of the family is left undefined, which leaves members wondering what they should be doing to promote recovery. There may also be an assumption that what they have been doing is not that helpful. Therefore, defining a role for family members at the time of acute rehabilitation and thereafter may be helpful in diminishing some of the anxiety they experience.

Despite the problems associated with having family members present on a regular basis at a rehabilitation center, defining a role for family members and thus having them participate in the rehabilitation process should be perceived as a necessity rather than something that is simply desirable. Since there is no appreciable correlation between family anxiety and the level of disability of the head-injured person, it follows that the family anxiety cannot be addressed simply by treating, and thus improving, the head-injured person. The anxiety has to be addressed in other ways, sometimes in a subtle fashion. Families are often sensitive to being treated as patients themselves on the assumption that such treatment will draw attention away from the injured person, where the treatment is most needed. Therefore, formal family therapy often is difficult to achieve in an acute rehabilitation setting. A more subtle approach, but still effective, is to define a specific role for the family and thus direct the expenditure of their energy and attention on constructive tasks.

TABLE 19.3.   Correlations
for Admission Variables

|  | Disability level | Depression |
|---|---|---|
| Depression | .25 | — |
| Anxiety | −.12 | .41 |

TABLE 19.4. Correlations
for Discharge Variables

|            | Disability level | Depression |
|------------|------------------|------------|
| Depression | −.10             | —          |
| Anxiety    | −.14             | .58        |

Those who work with families in rehabilitation settings are aware that, for the most part, family members want to help. However, they need clear direction as to how to help. Most have never had experience with rehabilitation and therefore should not be expected to understand the rationale for rehabilitation and how it is accomplished. Also, it is well known from learning theorists (but not often applied) that learning is best accomplished by observation followed by performance under supervision and, finally, independent performance. Such training cannot take place with family members on a single day; it needs to be spread out over time. Thus, the typical approach of training families on the day of discharge from a rehabilitation center is simply inadequate. In this situation staff is almost ensuring that the family will not be able to carry out activities at home and therefore jeopardizing generalization of progress seen at the rehabilitation center. In any new endeavor, such as family member participation in a rehabilitation program, it is important to create a feeling of self-efficacy in which the person believes that what he/she is doing is valid and will have impact. Literally, the family members should feel that they can make a difference in the injured person's recovery. Otherwise, tasks recommended by the therapists are viewed as inconsequential and intrusive. Development of such self-efficacy occurs over time with multiple contacts between the family member, the injured person, and therapists, with the family member being able to perceive the impact of various procedures on the head-injured person.

Involving the family in the rehabilitation program also emphasizes that professional time with the patient is actually limited, which is not often acknowledged. For instance, appointments for physical therapy and cognitive remediation may occupy several hours of a patient's day at the rehabilitation center, but little attention is given to evening hours when time is often spent with the family. Looked at objectively, it is obvious that head-injured individuals (even in an inpatient setting) spend more time with their families than with specific therapists. It is a waste for patients not to use the time with the family in a therapeutic fashion. Another seldom acknowledged fact is that family members may understand the problem better than the professionals. Professionals are adept at expounding about the effects of head injury but overlook the important fact that the head injury happened to a particular person with whom they are not in the least familiar. To the extent that family members are more familiar with the head-injured person, they are more likely to have an impact in training and should be able to gauge particular moods and responses much more effectively than staff members. Professionals are not good at giving credit where credit is due with regard to the family: professionals know about head injury but not the injured person. Finally, involvement of the family in the rehabilitation program increases the chances of generalization of progress to the home setting, which is the ultimate goal of inpatient rehabilitation. If family members can demonstrate understanding of the principles of rehabilitation, specific application of procedures, and build a sense of self-efficacy concerning those interventions, there is a much greater likelihood that the family will actually carry through with some of those interventions at home.

Given that it is desirable that family members be involved in a rehabilitation program during acute rehabilitation and thereafter, the question remains as to how the family is to be involved and at what level. While role definition for families can realistically emphasize involvement in any area in the rehabilitation program, the focus of this chapter is on family participation in cognitive remediation efforts. Sohlberg and Mateer (1989) differentiate process-specific cognitive rehabilitation (which emphasizes work in specific deficit areas using a theoretical, repetitive, and hierarchical approach) and generalized stimulation (which emphasizes stimulation in multiple areas without the theoretical background or hierarchical approach). It would be presumptuous to think that families could become experts in process-specific rehabilitation following a relatively brief interaction with professionals. On the other hand, the provision of generalized stimulation is well within the capability of most families and represents a principle which is relatively easy to understand: the more the person is asked to think and to react to the environment the more likely they will progress in terms of their cognitive skills. Sohlberg and Mateer (1989) accurately note that there is no indication based on objective data that generalized stimulation results in significant improvement in cognitive functioning. The evidence simply does not exist at this point, although it would be premature to totally neglect the potential impact of such stimulation. From a logical standpoint, it is better to provide some organized stimulation than no stimulation at all. In a home setting this distinction may have tremendous impact on how family members interact with a head-injured person. On the one hand, with a conception of generalized stimulation, family members will interact with a head-injured person and provide an assortment of tasks. Without that rationale, however, the head-injured person could encounter a day full of passive activities, such as watching television for many hours. It should also not be overlooked that part of the reason for involving families in a generalized stimulation program is to focus the attention and energies of family members and thus diminish the level of anxiety experienced by primary caretakers. Thus, such training for families may not only benefit the head-injured person but may also help the family. The concern over whether generalized stimulation actually expedites recovery of cognitive functions in a laboratory situation should not be overlooked, but neither should that concern be used as a means of belittling the efforts of family members.

## FAMILY INVOLVEMENT IN COGNITIVE REMEDIATION DURING ACUTE REHABILITATION

What families need to learn about cognitive remediation in order to engage in a generalized stimulation program usually can be attained by attending appointments with therapists in a rehabilitation setting. The importance of consistency in presentation, repetition, and structure needs to be emphasized and demonstrated for the family. Techniques of simplifying material when necessary for the head-injured person and prompting to obtain responses are also very important. It is a common and understandable tendency for family members to provide answers when head-injured individuals are struggling rather than provide cues so the head-injured person can eventually derive the answer. The need for reward also needs to be discussed directly. Families often overlook the fact that even with simple responses reinforcement is very important, even if it is just a short, positive comment. Families seem to overlook the potential beneficial impact of such simple interventions. Finally, the importance of purpose should be stressed with families. The head-injured person needs to be given some idea of why he or she is engaging in certain tasks, particularly if the tasks are mundane. The more realistic the task can be in the sense of duplicating life skills, the more the head-injured person will likely be motivated to perform the task. An explanation of what is to be gained by engaging in a task and how to rate performance is necessary.

Family involvement in cognitive recovery should not be limited to those head-injured individuals who are fully responsive and cooperative. Families can be helpful in cases where the head-injured person is still in coma or extremely agitated. For instance, coma stimulation procedures can be taught to family members who can then employ such procedures at times when therapists are not available, such as in the evening. In fact, families may be more effective at this than therapists. It is reasonable to assume that someone in the midst of coma or in a transitional stage to consciousness will respond more readily to a familiar voice and face than to an unknown person. The family can also be important in providing information about the injured person's likes and dislikes in such areas as music. With this information the treatment staff can then stimulate the patient with desired music. In dealing with the agitated head-injured person the family's presence can also be extremely helpful. A familiar person being present is often important in minimizing the anxiety and disorientation which may serve as the basis for agitation. Family members can be taught procedures for orienting the injured person, redirection when that person becomes fixated, and how to employ behavioral management when the injured person becomes restless/agitated. By having family members work with the staff in this fashion, episodes of agitation by the injured person will be minimized in duration and frequency. At the Spain Rehabilitation Center, arrangements are made with family members, if possible, for someone to be with the agitated patient 24 hours a day initially, which is then tapered over several days as the patient improves. Initially, it is very important to have family members available in the evening hours when time is less structured for the injured person, since those are the times when episodes of restlessness/agitation are more often going to occur.

With proper direction family members can supplement the work of professional staff regarding cognitive recovery. In the area of orientation, for example, the family can provide photos and scrapbook materials to prompt the injured person's recall of events from prior to the injury. The family can also provide social updates on friends and the circumstances of the accident. Such information is often not available to treatment staff and may promote orientation to a greater extent than professional interventions. Family members can also be of help by obtaining local newspapers and ensuring that the injured person monitors daily news broadcasts to help with knowledge of current events. While these suggestions seem logical and, if asked, most family members could generate these ideas themselves, family members will not initiate these procedures unless directed by staff. In many respects a medical setting is intimidating to most people and there is a general feeling that one must wait until told to do something for fear of interfering with the rehabilitation program. Therefore, staff should not be bashful about directing family members by providing suggestions for activities, while also listening for ideas generated by the family.

Family members can also provide unique experiences with regard to memory functioning. For instance, families are aware of plans for upcoming holidays and for events which occurred at previous holidays. They can also help the injured person keep track of visitors and upcoming, family-related events (such as weddings, births, graduations, etc.). With direction, the family can then be taught how to evaluate the head-injured person's recall of such information over time and provide prompting when necessary. To the extent that such information is of interest to the head-injured person, effort will be expended in trying to recall the information as compared to the random word lists often presented in formal cognitive remediation.

Families can provide unique interventions with regard to improvement of spatial skills. Simply exploring the rehabilitation center with the injured person and expecting the injured person to recall directions is helpful. Fairly simple (but often overlooked) activities such as board games, Ping-Pong, or billiards (the ubiquitous games of rehabilitation centers) can be helpful in developing spatial skills. The latter tasks not only fit into development of spatial skills but also focus on recreational skills. Unfortunately, recreation is often considered a tertiary concern at a rehabilitation center, even though it may have a tremendous impact on the head-injured person's mood and willingness to participate in therapies. Obviously, if a task is considered recreational in that it is fun, challenging but obtainable, and interesting, it is more likely to be accomplished by the head-injured person. Therefore, recreational tasks should not be overlooked in a rehabilitation program, including even the simplest of games. Television viewing can also be done in a responsible fashion; if not to excess. Asking the head-injured person to keep track of events during a TV show and asking what is to happen next in a story line or sporting event alters television viewing from a passive activity to a more active endeavor. Trips outside the hospital should not be overlooked as an important component to treatment. If properly directed, family members can make such out-trips an educational venture.

Finally, families can be of real benefit in a rehabilitation center in working on reasoning skills. Everyday activities can be used as projects in sequencing, such as placing pictures in the family album or writing a letter. Family members providing problems related to time (hours, days, months, season, years) is also helpful in terms of reasoning and orientation. Although a question such as "How old will you be in 1995?" may seem simple on the surface, it actually requires several sequential steps to derive a correct answer. Exercises in convergent and divergent thinking can also be incorporated in everyday conversations and tasks. Asking the head-injured person for advice as to how to deal with a particular problem at home incorporates reasoning, as do simple verbal guessing games where sequential clues are offered.

Despite the problems that may occur at times with having families present in a rehabilitation center on a regular basis, the potential benefits of family involvement in the overall rehabilitation process (and specifically cognitive recovery as discussed here) cannot be overlooked. It needs to be emphasized that family involvement in this case does not negate professional responsibility; the involvement of family members is to supplement, not replace, professional activities. Total responsibility for cognitive recovery (or any other aspect of rehabilitation) cannot be placed solely in the hands of the family. Overall, rehabilitation facilities tend to err in the opposite direction, that is, not giving families enough guidance for participation in the program. The need for direction also needs to be emphasized since family members will often not initiate activities that they feel will be helpful for fear of somehow interfering with the rehabilitation program. Clear communication between therapists and families is obviously required: therapists should never assume that family members understand a concept or can apply a procedure unless it has been specifically discussed and, if necessary, demonstrated by the family.

## GENERALIZED STIMULATION IN THE HOME SETTING

Family members, most often parents, are ultimately responsible for head-injured individuals who are unable to return immediately to independent living at the time of discharge from a rehabilitation program. Family members are often understandably anxious at having the head-injured person come home due to perceived changes in personality, cognition, and physical ability. They are unsure as to what to do to expedite further recovery, which again evolves into a question concerning roles. What role is a family member to assume when a head-injured person comes home? To answer this question one must consider the type of environment that is presumed desirable for head-injured individuals. There is general agreement that an unstimulating, passive environment is not desirable. Thus, the daily routine of watching ten hours of television while resting on a sofa would not be advocated. Family members, therefore, need to understand how they can generate a more active, stimulating environment in the home. Unfortunately, often due to brain injury, head-injured persons are unable to generate such an environment themselves. Once again, professional staff are needed to direct family members as to their involvement in the recovery program. In addition to the obvious impact on activity level, a home stimulation program also carries with it more subtle effects on the family and head-injured individuals. For instance, a home program establishes expectations for the patient and the family by defining the roles each is to fulfill. The communication to the injured person is that he or she is expected to be active and continue to recover, while the family is told through the program that they are expected to continue working with the head-injured person and not tolerate passivity. Such a program also helps families feel useful, rather than waiting for recovery to take place in a magical fashion. A home program is by definition future oriented and helps family members and head-injured individuals maintain perspective regarding continued recovery. Finally, such a program helps the family to define a hierarchy of stimulation for the head-injured person. A home stimulation program not only avoids excessive passivity, it also helps avoid overstimulation by directing families as to what tasks might be challenging to the head-injured person at particular points throughout recovery. Thus, it helps avoid the situation in which the family actually expects too much of the head-injured person, rather than too little.

Fortunately, ideas for a home-based generalized stimulation program can be obtained from multiple sources, such as the Basic Thinking Skills series (Harnadek, 1977) and the Thinking Skills Workbook (Carter, Caruso, & Languirand, 1984), which describe tasks in areas such as attention, concentration, memory, and reasoning. Craine and Gudeman (1981) provide an extensive list of activities with designation as to relative difficulty, area of cognitive function addressed, and modality of presentation. Ideas with regard to language functioning and verbal reasoning can be obtained from Holloran and Bressler (1983), and Novack, Bergquist, Bennett, and Hartley (1987) provide some ideas specifically focusing on home stimulation for head-injured individuals (Appendix A). Finally, a recently published manual, Head Injury: A Home Based Cognitive Rehabilitation Program (1989), may be helpful in generating ideas for activities as well as dealing with behavioral problems exhibited by the head-injured persons. These materials can be used in conjunction with established procedures at the rehabilitation center in providing a home stimulation program for use by the family of a head-injured individual. Although the focus is on general stimulation, it is helpful to pick out some tasks in particular deficit areas. It is important to designate levels at which the task be performed with ease initially so that family and the injured person do not become frustrated.

In addition to developing stimulation activities, it is also beneficial to utilize existing stimulation activities, such as games. Games are excellent sources of generalized stimulation in that they often require some degree of reasoning, involve extended attention, and are interesting. Everyone, family members and head-injured individuals alike, has experience with games and can return to those games with relatively little prompting. The cognitive skills required vary across games. For instance, bingo requires relatively little reasoning skill, whereas checkers is more demanding in this respect. Chess, on the other hand, is even more complex than checkers. Therefore, it is possible for the professional to select games which would be suitable for the head-injured individual at virtually any stage of recovery. Novack *et al*. (1987) have provided a listing of popular games (Appendix B) and a breakdown of what areas of cognitive functioning are involved in those games.

It is helpful to provide families with some idea of how to progress with a task, rather than just providing them with the task alone. Novack *et al*. (1987) provide different stages for each task presented, with later stages being more complex than earlier stages. In the area of attention and concentration, for instance, there are several tasks listed, including the shell game (modeled after the old carnival game). Under the shell game there are four different stages, each one more complex than the last. At the easiest stage there are two clear containers with a single marble, so the trainee can actually see the marble while it is being moved about. At the next stage two identical opaque containers are used so the trainee can no longer see the marble. Slow increase in the amount of time spent moving the containers is also recommended at stage two. At stage three, three or more opaque containers are used, whereas at stage four, three or more opaque containers and two or more distinctly colored marbles are used. Therefore, the trainee must attend to different stimuli simultaneously. Setting up the task in this way allows some measure of success as the trainee progresses from one stage to the next. This may increase motivation to continue with the program, both for the family and the injured individual.

When a head-injured person is discharged from the Spain Rehabilitation Center, the family is provided with a list of home stimulation activities. One person (usually whoever has most often attended therapy sessions) is designated as the leader of the home stimulation program. Of the entire activity list, particular tasks are circled as being particularly appropriate for the injured person, and an arrow is placed next to one of several stages as the suggested beginning point for the family. Each of the tasks is discussed and questions are answered, including demonstrations if confusion is evident. Games which would be appropriate for a particular head-injured person are endorsed by an asterisk among a listing of games, and particular games are discussed. For the most part, families are familiar with the games listed and often indicate that such games are in the home. As a means of allaying fears about expense, family members are always advised that there is no expectation that they buy the games or any materials to complete the cognitive program. However, if friends or other family members have particular games or materials in their homes it would be appropriate to borrow those materials for a period of time. Families are also advised that it is unnecessary to attempt each task or game every day, rather the aim is to stimulate the injured person on a daily basis using a variety of tasks. It is important for the family leader to establish a daily schedule of activities, including time for exercise, cognitive stimulation, household responsibilities (if possible), trips out of the home (visiting friends, grocery shopping, going to the library), and rest periods. Cognitive stimulation is likely accomplished best in a nondistracting area that can be used repetitively. Approximately one week after discharge from the rehabilitation center the family leader is contacted to find out if there have been any problems since discharge and to address questions concerning the cognitive program. At scheduled follow-up appointments the stimulation program is discussed and alterations recommended.

The use of television and video games always needs to be addressed with families at the time of discharge since these are such prevalent activities in our culture. Watching television as a reinforcement or as a means of relaxation at periods throughout the day is appropriate and can be made part of the variation in activities. As already noted, it is possible to make watching television a cognitive task in itself with another person prompting the head-injured individual to recall information and focus on future developments in a television show. What has to be avoided if at all possible is the head-injured individual watching many hours of television daily. Video games can be viewed in much the same way as watching television; as a form of relaxation and reinforcement. Video games can be very helpful, but too much time spent in such activity is detrimental. Fortunately, many of the video games today require more than just response speed and fine motor control; careful examination of the available games indicates that reasoning and memory functioning are required for successful performance. Therefore, family members should be encouraged to make use of the video games available with the qualification that playing time should be interrupted by other activities on a regular basis.

Use of computers in the home setting is also being addressed with family members with increasing frequency. Personal computers are appearing in more homes and therefore are available to more head-injured individuals. Selection of appropriate computer software for head-injured individuals is extremely difficult. Unfortunately, much of the software designed for head-injured individuals and used in cognitive remediation settings is too sophisticated for the average family member and also prohibitively expensive. An alternative source of software is an educational supply store, but the materials (understandably) will often focus solely on academic skills and are presented in a juvenile format. Finally, it may be worth visiting the local public library where software may be available on loan. Due to the large number of computer programs which are available today, it is very difficult to make specific recommendations regarding the needs of head-injured individuals in terms of software. In fact, entire books have been published (Apple Computer Resources in Special Education and Rehabilitation, 1987) focusing on available software for this type of application.

The effectiveness of a home stimulation program is open to speculation. It is difficult to imagine a research project with adequate controls which would establish, in an experimental sense, whether such intervention results in significant cognitive gains. As is often the case in rehabilitation, one is left recommending procedures which are logical for recovery, but for which there is no objective proof of effectiveness. At a subjective level, the experience at the Spain Rehabilitation Center suggests that the home stimulation program is very effective in focusing the attention of family members on maintaining a stimulating and active lifestyle for the head-injured person. While virtually every family member interviewed reports that the home stimulation program activities have been used at least periodically, the most avid reports relate to the use of games with the head-injured individual. The reason for the more extensive use of games is fairly simple: games are fun for the head-injured person and the family member and therefore there is no arm twisting involved. Families may also use the home stimulation activities as a springboard to develop their own activities which may actually be more functional for the head-injured person. If the impact of a home stimulation program provided by professionals is only indirect, such as in helping the family generate their own ideas about activities, professional time is still well spent.

## SUMMARY

If dealt with in an understanding manner, family members can expedite recovery from head injury. In order for rehabilitation professionals to adequately utilize the resources of the family, these professionals must overcome some well-established prejudices against having family members actively participating in a rehabilitation program. Establishing a well-defined role for family members will help to focus their attention and efforts while diminishing anxiety over the lack of role definition. If the rehabilitation program can be viewed as a cooperative effort between the head-injured person, his or her family, and the rehabilitation professionals, the prospects for recovery are increased. In many respects the head-injured person and his or her family are the primary players, while the rehabilitation professionals assume a supporting role and are on stage for only a few minutes of the entire play. It is only logical that rehabilitation professionals should attempt to use all the resources available to promote the patient's recovery including the ability of the family to provide generalized stimulation at the rehabilitation center and at home. Although the effectiveness of the family interventions described in this chapter have not been established in an objective sense, it is difficult to imagine treating a head-injured individual and his family in any other fashion.

## APPENDIX A: EXAMPLES OF HOME STIMULATION ACTIVITIES

Note: To progress to the next stage in any task the trainee should master the easier stage by completing the task successfully at least three times. Further practice is not harmful.

### Attention and Concentration

*Task 1—Shell Game*

This is a variation of the old carnival game in which the person must identify which of several containers holds the object.

Stage I—Materials: Two clear glasses and a marble. Directions: Turn the glasses upside down, placing the marble underneath one with the trainee watching. Ask the trainee to point to the glass containing the marble. Once this has been accomplished move the glasses and ask the trainee to indicate once again. Repeat several times.

Stage II—Materials: Two identical opaque containers and a marble. Directions: Same as Stage I. At this stage the trainee can no longer see the marble in the container. On repetitions, slowly increase the amount of time spent moving the containers.

Stage III—Materials: Three or more opaque containers and one marble. Directions: Same as previous stages.

Stage IV—Materials: Three or more opaque containers and two or more distinctly colored marbles. Directions: Place all marbles under separate containers with the trainee watching. Ask the trainee to identify where each colored marble may be found. Move the containers about and ask again. Repeat several times, increasing the time spent moving the containers.

## Task 2—Cancellation Tasks

Given an array of items, the trainee is expected to select out specified items and "cancel" them.

Stage I—Materials: An 8 × 11 sheet of white paper with the letters K B L Z B O Y across the middle in large print. Directions: Ask the trainee to mark out all the B letters. This could be done with shapes (square, triangle, circle, hexagon, etc.) or numbers. Repeat several times with different sequences and search letters (or shapes or numbers).

Stage II—Materials: An 8×11 sheet with two rows of letters (or shapes or numbers). Directions: Same as Stage I. Repeat with variations in the material.

Stage III—Materials: An 8 × 11 sheet of paper with three or more rows of letters (or shapes or numbers). Directions: Same as Stage II.

Stage IV—Materials: An 8 × 11 sheet with several rows of upper and lower case letters. Directions: Tell the trainee to mark out a single letter, both upper and lower case. Repeat with varied material.

Stage V—Materials: An 8×11 sheet with several rows of upper and lower case letters (or numbers or shapes) in which particular patterns are embedded (for example: the letters I N Q or the number sequence 2 8 7). Directions: Ask the trainee to cancel the sequence whenever encountered. Repeat with varied material.

Stage VI—Materials: An 8 × 11 sheet with several rows of letters in which three-letter words are imbedded (for example: I P H O G Q Z). Spacing must be equal throughout. Directions: Ask the trainee to find the words.

## Task 3—Time Sense

Being aware of the passage of time is a subtle, but complex form of attention. Materials for all stages: Stopwatch and score pad.

Stage I—Directions: Give stopwatch to trainee and instruct to start watch when told and stop it at ten seconds. With the watch in full view of the trainee tell trainee to start watch. Repeat with variations in time up to one minute. When trainee can stop watch within one to two seconds of goal consistently, move on to Stage II.

Stage II—Directions: After trainee has started watch announce the time to stop, between 8 and 60 seconds with the trainee able to see the watch at all times. Repeat with variations in time span. Once consistently accurate, move on to Stage III.

Stage III—Directions: The trainee should not be allowed to see the stopwatch. The trainee is asked to tell the trainer when 10 seconds have passed since the stopwatch was started. Counting out loud should be encouraged at first. Repeat with variations in the time span up to two minutes. With increasing time, a wider span of error should be anticipated. For every 10 seconds of time span, 1.5 seconds' variation should be allowed. Thus, for 30 seconds as the goal, a response by the trainee between 25.5 and 34.5 seconds would be acceptable.

Stage IV—Directions: Same as for Stage III except that the trainer is to fill in the time with conversation, questions, etc. The trainee must try to keep track of the passing seconds despite these distractions. A larger range of error is acceptable: 2 seconds for every 10 seconds of time span. So for 30 seconds as a goal, a response between 24 and 36 seconds is acceptable.

*Task 4—Number Sequences*

To successfully complete number sequences, the trainee must actively attend to the pattern and anticipate the next response.

Stage I—Directions: Ask the trainee to say or write the numbers 1 to 10 in sequence. If either of these is difficult, present the 10 numbers written on individual squares of paper and ask the trainee to order the numbers by sight. Repeat several times, increasing the number span if the trainee succeeds. The trainer could also use the alphabet, days, and months for sequencing in this manner.

Stage II—Directions: Ask the trainee to sequence numbers by odd, even, or 10s (count by odd numbers, count by even numbers, count by 10s). Begin by providing the initial four digits in the sequence, either written or spoken, for the trainee. Repeat several times, altering the directions (odd versus even) and the starting point. When consistent success is evident, go on to Stage III.

Stage III—Directions: Provide the trainee with the first four digits of a sequence in which a set number is added or subtracted each time (for example: 3—7—11—15). Instruct the trainee as to the steps to be taken (for example: add 4 each time). Repeat with variations.

Stage IV—Directions: Same as Stage III except that the trainer does not specify the operation to be employed (for example: don't tell the trainee to add 4 each time). This requires that the trainee figure out what has to be done.

Stage V—Materials: Scratch paper for trainee. Directions:
Same as Stage IV except that operations can now include multiplication. At this stage the trainer might also employ other sequences, particularly the alphabet (for example: call out every third letter of the alphabet).

Stage VI—Materials: Scratch paper. Directions: Ask for sequences in reverse order (for example: count backwards from 20, name the alphabet backwards, name the months backwards). Counting backwards by three or some other variation would also be suitable.

*Task 5—Careful Listening*

Stage I—Directions: Ask trainee to raise hand when a particular letter is said (for example: P) and then say aloud letters in a random fashion. Remind trainee to raise hand if designated letter is missed. Say designated letter frequently (averaging 1 out of every 5 letters) with variation.

Stage II—Directions: Same as Stage I except trainee is asked to raise hand to two letters (for example: D and X).

Stage III—Materials: Dictionary. Directions: Instruct trainee to raise hand when a particular letter appears in a word. Then read aloud words randomly from the dictionary.

Stage IV—Materials: Magazine articles. Directions: Instruct trainee to raise hand when particular words are read aloud (the word can be common, such as "the," or appear infrequently in the article). Read articles aloud.

## Motor Speed

The goal is to increase the trainee's rate of motor response and general coordination, particularly with the hands.

### Task 1—Finger Tapping

Materials for all Stages: Preferably a typewriter or home computer with a keyboard.

Stage I—Directions: Ask the trainee to tap a single key on the board as rapidly as possible for 10 seconds with one finger on the preferred hand. Score is the number of letters typed. Allow 20 seconds of rest and repeat. Do this five times. If a typewriter is not available, have the trainee tap the table with one finger and count the taps. Repeat this cycle with several individual fingers on both hands.

Stage II—Directions: Have the trainee tap two keys with two fingers on the same hand, alternating between the keys, for 10 seconds. Allow a rest period and repeat. Change fingers and/or hands after five trials.

Stage III—Directions: Have the trainee alternate between tapping two keys, one with a finger from the left hand, the other with a finger on the right hand. Repeat as instructed in Stages I and II.

Stage IV—Directions: Using four fingers of the right hand, have the trainee press four keys in sequence for 30 seconds. Repeat several items, then try the left hand. Introduce variations in the sequence.

### Task 2—Nuts and Bolts

Materials for all Stages: 100 nuts and 100 matching bolts approximately one inch long. Three empty shoe boxes. If nuts and bolts are not available, any two small items could be used (for example: buttons, paper clips, coins).

Stage I—Directions: Place the nuts in one box and place an empty box approximately 12 inches away. Using the right hand, ask the trainee to place nuts one at a time into the empty box. After some practice assess speed by allowing 30 seconds to transfer. Score is how many nuts are transferred in that time. When one hand tires, switch to the other hand.

Stage II—Directions: Place all the nuts in one box. Arrange two empty boxes on each side of the full box, about 12 inches away. Ask the trainee to place individual nuts in empty boxes, alternating between the two. If the trainee stops alternating, provide a reminder. Assess speed as in Stage I. When one hand tires, switch to the other hand.

Stage III—Directions: Place three boxes in a row with full box in middle, as in Stage

II. Ask trainee to transfer nuts one at a time using both hands simultaneously. The left hand is to fill the box on the left, the right hand the box on the right. Time and score as in Stages I and II.

Stage IV—Directions: Arrange boxes as in Stage III. Place both nuts and bolts in center box. Using the left hand, the trainee is to place the nuts in the box on the left, and with the right hand place the bolts in the box on the right. Correct errors when they occur. Encourage the use of both hands simultaneously and look for approximately equal numbers of items in each box. Periodically switch the task: right hand for nuts, left hand for bolts. Time for 60 seconds.

Stage V—Directions: Place nuts in one box and bolts in the others. Instruct the trainee to pick up a bolt with one hand and a nut with the other and screw the nut on the bolt a few turns (just enough so they do not come apart). The completed assembly is to be placed in the remaining empty box. Allow practice and then time for 60 seconds. As performance improves increase the time allotted to two minutes, then three, etc.

### Constructional–Spatial

The ability to function in two- or three-dimensional space is extremely important to our daily functioning and is often impaired by brain injury.

#### Task 1—Centering

Materials for all Stages: Pencil and unlined paper.

Stage I—Directions: Draw a straight line on the paper and ask the trainee to mark each end of the line with a pencil mark. Correct any errors. Then ask the trainee to mark the center of the line. Provide feedback and repeat, varying the length of lines.

Stage II—Directions: Draw a straight line on the paper and ask the trainee to divide it into thirds. Provide feedback and repeat. Vary the length of the line, number of divisions (for example, fourths, fifths) and the orientation of the line (vertical, diagonal, horizontal).

Stage III—Directions: Draw an enclosed figure (for example: circle or square) and ask the trainee to place a dot in the center of the figure. Repeat with varying figures of different sizes.

Stage IV—Directions: Draw a square and ask the trainee to divide the square into four equal portions using intersecting lines. Then ask the trainee to place a dot at the center of each of the smaller squares. Repeat with varying size squares. As performance improves, make the division more demanding. For instance, ask for six or nine square created by intersecting lines.

#### Task 2—Right-Left Orientation

Stage I—Directions: Have the trainee identify body parts on the right and left. For instance, ask him/her to touch the right ear. Provide guidance if necessary.

Stage II—Materials: A front view drawing or picture of a person (such as from a magazine), including both arms and legs. Directions: Holding the picture in front of the trainee, ask the trainee to point out the pictured person's right and left features (which are opposite to the trainee's right and left). If there is some confusion, reverse the drawing so that the pictured person's right and left correspond to the trainee's. If necessary, keep reversing in this fashion.

Stage III—Directions: Ask the trainee to identify right and left body parts on the trainer with the trainer sitting next to the trainee and facing the same direction.

Stage IV—Directions: Ask the trainee to identify right and left body parts on the trainer with the trainer sitting and facing the trainee.

Stage V—Directions: Ask the trainee to touch body parts in a specific manner. For instance, ask the trainee to touch his/her left ear with the right hand or the right leg with the left heel.

### Task 3—Connecting the Dots

Materials for all Stages: Two pieces of paper with multiple nine-dot squares on each (see below).

```
.   .   .

.   .   .

.   .   .
```

Stage I—Directions: The trainer draws a line connecting two of the dots in one square. Using another sheet, the trainee duplicates the line on a nine-dot square. Repeat several times using a new square each time.

Stage II—Directions: The trainer connects two dots and then a third in a continuous line. The trainee duplicates this. Repeat several times using a new square each time. When performance is accurate on three consecutive trials, connect four dots. Do not let the lines cross. Ask the trainee to duplicate. As performance allows, keep connecting more dots but without crossing lines. Initially, allow the trainee to see the standard as it is drawn. As this is mastered, the trainee can be presented with complete designs.

Stage III—Directions: Connect at least four dots and cross lines. Ask the trainee to duplicate. As performance warrants, the trainer may increase the number of dots connected. To add complexity, the number of dots in the square can be increased.

### Task 4—Locating Squares

Materials: For Stages I to V a sheet of paper with multiple $3 \times 3$ square matrixes (like a tic-tac-toe grid) marked horizontally with letters and vertically with numbers will be required.

Stage I—Directions: Ask the trainee to point to the squares under the letter B and then to the squares in row 2. Do this for other columns and rows.

Stage II—Directions: Ask the trainee to point to the intersection of row 2 and column B. Encourage the use of a finger for pointing as a means of structuring the task. Do the same thing for other columns and rows.

Stage III—Directions: Point to a square and ask the trainee to provide the row number and column letter (for example: row 1, column C).

Stage IV—Directions: Give the trainee a row number and column letter and ask him/her to place an "X" in the proper square. Stage V—Directions: Play tic-tac-toe with the trainee providing only coordinates which the trainee must fill in (for example: "I select 3B").

Stage VI—Materials: Increase the number of squares by adding new rows and columns to the grid labeling each by number or letter. Directions: Continue to ask the trainee to locate squares given coordinates.

Stage VII—Materials: A 10x10 grid labeled as above. Directions: Each player locates "ships" on the grid out of sight of the other. For instance, one ship could be several squares positioned in a row, column, or diagonally. The size and number of ships can be varied. Each player is then to take turns in trying to guess the location of the other person's ships given three guesses per turn. If a player provides the coordinates of an opponent's ships, the opponent indicates this by saying "hit." When all squares comprising a particular ship are guessed, the ship is considered sunk. The player who sinks all his/her opponent's ships wins. This game can be made more complex by adding more rows and columns.

Stage VIII—Materials: Television listing for one day. Directions: An everyday task involving visual search is reading a television schedule. The trainee must first locate the time on the listing and then look for the program and channel. Provide a listing of a time and channel and ask what program will be aired (for example: "What will come on Channel 4 at 8:00 pm?"). The trainer can make a list of such questions and let the trainee work alone.

### Task 5—Drawing Figures

Materials for all Stages: Colored pencils and unlined paper.

Stage I—Directions: With the trainee watching, the trainer draws a shape beginning with the most simple, such as a horizontal or vertical line, circle, square, or triangle. Given a different colored pencil, the trainee is to trace the edge of the figure. Repeat several times varying the figure. As performance allows, the figure may become more complex, such as a hexagon, octagon, etc.

Stage II—Directions: Have the trainee shadow trace figures. For best results the original page with figures to be traced should be taped to the table with a clean sheet of paper taped over the top.

Stage III—Directions: Provide dotted outlines of figures on a clean sheet with the expectation that the trainee fill in the figures. The more dots provided, the easier the task. For greatest complexity, a dot at each corner of the figure is all that should be provided.

Stage IV—Directions: Ask the trainee to copy figures on a clean sheet, matching the standard in terms of size and orientation. Once geometric shapes are mastered, move on to drawing of objects, such as a house, automobile, tree, etc.

Stage V—Directions: The trainee should draw geometric figures to command, that is, without a standard from which to copy. Once geometric shapes are mastered, the drawing of objects to command can be attempted.

### Task 6—Puzzles

Stage I—Materials: Two- to four-piece flat puzzles (can be made by cutting a page from a magazine in several pieces). Directions: Initially show the completed puzzle to the trainee and dismantle in his/her presence. Have the trainee assemble, with guidance if necessary. If the trainee is performing well, present him/her with the dismantled pieces, never having seen the completed puzzle.

Stage II—Materials: Flat puzzles with varying numbers of pieces, up to 100. Directions: Allow the trainee to assemble the puzzle. If the puzzle comes with a picture of the completed product, allow this to be used for guidance.

Stage III—Materials: Building blocks of varying sizes. Directions: The trainer builds two-dimensional constructions (for example, towers, walls) which the trainee is asked to duplicate with the trainer's standard in full view. Repeat with varying constructions.

Stage IV—Materials: Same as Stage III. Directions: The trainer uses blocks to make three-dimensional constructions (for example: a pyramid, a "house"). With this standard in view the trainee is to duplicate. Repeat with increasing complexity in the construction. For instance, the construction need not be symmetrical.

## Task 7—Mazes

Materials: Paper and pencil mazes of varying complexity which may be purchased at an educational supply store or some newsstands.

Directions: Have the trainee attempt the mazes, beginning with the simplest. Initially it may be necessary for the trainer to draw an exit line and the trainee trace the line. As performance warrants, go on to more complex mazes.

## Task 8—Map Location

Stage I—Materials: Hand-drawn map of the neighborhood. Directions: With the trainee's pen at "home" on the map, give directions which the trainee will follow with the pen. For instance, tell the trainee to go east and turn right on a particular street. Repeat with trainee starting at home and vary directions.

Stage II—Materials: A map as in Stage I with stores and other important locations included. Colored pencils. Directions: Direct the trainee to get from home to important locations using different colored pencils for each location. On outside excursions, ask the trainee to direct the way. It may be helpful to take the map.

Stage III—Materials: City map. Directions: Point out two locations on the map and have the trainee determine the shortest route between the two.

Stage IV—Materials: Road atlas of the United States. Directions: Ask trainee to designate a route between points in two cities, including interstate highways and city streets.

## Language Skills

The following tasks are intended for persons who are able to communicate through language at a basic level by comprehending, speaking, reading, or writing.

## Task 1—Word Search

Stage I—Materials: Write four letters with a three-letter word inserted (example: PDOG). Directions: Ask the trainee to underline the word. Generate as many letter sequences with inserted words as possible.

Stage II—Materials: Write four letters with a three-letter word inserted in reverse (example: XTAC). Directions: Ask the trainee to underline the word. Generate as many sequences as possible to provide practice.

Stage III—Materials: A four by four (4x4) block of letters with a word inserted on each row. Example:

```
T   A   G   H
P   A   N   D
X   W   H   Y
P   I   N   A
```

Directions: Ask the trainee to underline each word.

Stage IV—Materials: Four by four (4 × 4) block as in Stage III but with words presented vertically. Directions: Ask trainee to circle words.

Stage V—Materials: Four by four (4 × 4) letter block as in Stage III but with words reversed in each row. Directions: Ask trainee to underline words.

Stage VI—Materials: Four by four (4 × 4) letter block as in Stage III with words presented in any format: rows, columns, or reversed. Directions: Ask trainee to circle words.

Stage VII—Directions: Increase the complexity of the task by adding rows and columns of letters and presenting longer words.

### Task 2—Crossword Puzzles

Crossword puzzles of varying difficulty are available through newsstands and educational supply stores. It may be appropriate to begin with simpler puzzles intended for children and work up to more complex puzzles.

### Task 3—Hangman

Materials: Paper and pencil.

Stage I—Directions: The trainer thinks of a word and draws spaces corresponding to the number of letters (example: _____). A scaffold with noose is also drawn. The person is then given chances to guess letters in the word. If a letter in the word is guessed, that space is filled in. If the letter is not in the word, then a body part (for example, head, trunk, arm) is added to the figure on the scaffold. The challenge is to guess the word before the man on the scaffold is complete and thus "hung." Provide a definition of the word being sought and write down letters guessed within sight of the trainee.

Stage II—Directions: Same as above except a definition of the word is not provided. Write down letters guessed by the person. This prevents duplication of guesses.

Stage III—Directions: Same as above but do not provide definitions and do not write down guesses.

### Task 4—Fill in the Blank

Materials: Paper and pencil.

Stage I—Directions: A sentence is provided with a space for a missing word. The sentence with the missing word is accompanied by a picture to which the sentence refers. (Example: Picture of a red ball with the sentence "The color of the _____ is red.").

Stage II—Directions: No picture is provided but the missing word is easily determined in the context of the sentence. (Example: "The color of grass is _____ .")

Stage III—Directions: Sentences are provided with multiple blanks which can be filled by more than one word. (Example: "_____ , _____ , and _____ are some of the animals that can be seen at the zoo.")

## Reasoning/Problem Solving

### Task 1—Locating Information in the Newspaper

Materials: Local newspaper.

Stage I—Directions: Ask the trainee about information from the front page, such as headlines, the date, and name of the paper.

Stage II—Directions: Ask the trainee to locate sections of the paper, such as sports, business, and classified ads.

Stage III—Directions: Ask for specific information without indicating the section in which it can be found. For instance, ask for the score of baseball games (or any seasonal sport), movies showing in town, and weather information (low temperature, high temperature, etc.).

Stage IV—Directions: Ask for specific information involving a decision. For instance, the trainer is interested in buying a car, such as a small foreign car, for a given price and ask the trainee to provide a list of cars for sale that meet the criteria.

### Task 2—Ordering Numbers

Materials: Small pieces of paper with a number written on each.

Stage I—Directions: Give the trainee three numbers and ask him/her to arrange in order from lowest to highest.

Stage II—Directions: Start with three numbers to be arranged and then hand the trainee other numbers, one at a time, to be inserted in the sequence.

Stage III—Directions: Given three numbers, ask the trainee what the numbers have in common (for instance, odd or even, multiples of each other, or another common number).

### Task 3—Problem Situations

Materials: Paper and pencil.

Stage I—Directions: Provide a written list of steps involved in a simple task, such as brushing teeth. For example:

Brush teeth.

Take out toothpaste and toothbrush.

Ask the trainee which comes first, second, etc.

Stage II—Directions: Ask the trainee how to go about more complex tasks, such as scrambling eggs or changing a tire on a car. Ask for details about what is done. If an important step is left out, ask the trainee where it should go.

Stage III—Directions: Present problem situations in which decisions are required and no clear sequence of behavior is evident. For instance, ask the trainee how he/she would respond to running out of gas in the car, finding that he/she had no money while standing at the cash register of a store, losing his/her wallet, being lost in a new city, being improperly dressed at a formal party.

### Task 4—Reasoning from General to Specific

Materials: Paper and pencil.

Stage I—Directions: Given a general heading (such as tools, animals, plants, countries, occupations, foods, sports), ask the trainee to generate as many items in that area as possible. If the trainee is stumped, hints are permissible. For instance, in generating the names of animals, the trainer could advise the trainee to think of the zoo or the farm. For foods you could suggest thinking of the grocery store.

Stage II—Directions: Same as Stage I except the possible responses to the general heading are more limited. For instance, asking which sports involve running, use of balls, water contact, use of a racquet, more or less than five players, or physical contact between players. This involves a decision process in which the trainee must rule out inappropriate items.

Stage III—Directions: Tell the trainee that you bought something at the grocery store and that he/she must figure out what it is by asking questions. Encourage the trainee to ask very general questions at first (for example: "Is it a vegetable?" or "Is it a meat?") rather than very specific questions (such as: "Is it a cucumber?"). Once more, general questions are answered, more specific questions can be asked. Initially, allow as many questions as necessary. After the trainee has guessed correctly on a few items, start to limit the number of questions allowed the trainee, starting with 30, down to 20, then to 15.

### Task 5—Categorization

Stage I—Materials: A list of 30 items each belonging to one of three categories (for example: food, furniture, clothing). Directions: Ask the trainee to sort the items according to category. If the trainee is unable to determine the categories, they may be provided.

Stage II—Materials: A list of 30 items all from the same general category but which can be subdivided (for example: a list of food items than can be divided into meats, vegetables, and dairy products). Directions: Ask the trainee to sort the items into three categories but do not specify the categories.

Stage III—Materials: A listing of paired items that have something in common (for example: chair–couch, steak–pork, book–newspaper). Directions: Ask the trainee what each pair of items have in common. Ask for more than one answer if possible (for example: a book and a newspaper are both written and both are made of paper).

### Task 6—Budgeting

Materials: Make up a budget with entries for each month in the following areas: rent, food, electricity, car.

Stage I—Directions: Ask the trainee during which month a particular expenditure (such as electricity) was highest (or lowest).

Stage II—Directions: Ask for yearly totals of expenditures in all areas. Alter the amounts spent in each category and add other categories (for example: entertainment, clothing).

Stage III—Directions: Ask the trainee to determine how much money would be required each month to live within the budget. Break this down further into weekly income and finally hourly wage. Include consideration of taxes at a rate of 10 percent.

## Task 7—Sequencing Comics

Materials: Sunday or daily comic composed of several pictures (panels) in sequence.

Stage I—Directions: Cut entire comic strip from the paper and then cut strip into two pieces, leaving panels intact. Ask the trainee to put the two pieces in proper sequence from left to right. Trainee is not to see the comic strip before cutting. Ask the trainee to explain the story line after the two pieces are placed together.

Stage II—Directions: Same as Stage I but comic strip is cut into three pieces.
Stage III—Directions: Same as Stage II but comic strip is cut into four or more pieces.

## Task 8—Coding

Materials for Stages I to III: A coding key as follows:
$0 = *$;  $1 = @$;  $2 = \$$;  $3 = ($;  $4 = )$;  $5 = \%$;  $6 = '.$;  $7 = +$; $8 = !$; $9 = ?$

Stage I—Directions: Write symbols corresponding to numbers and ask trainee to identify each number based on the key.

Stage II—Directions: Write a sequence of symbols corresponding to familiar numbers, such as the trainee's phone number, age, or zip code.

Stage III—Directions: Write a sequence of symbols corresponding to random numbers of varying length which the trainee must then decipher.

Materials for Stages IV to VIII: A = Q; B = W; C = E; D = R; E = T; F = Y; G = U; M = I; I = O; J = P; K = A; L = S; M = D; N = F; O = G; P = H; Q = J; R = K; S = L; T = Z; U = X; V = C; W = V; X = B; Y = N; Z = M.

Stage IV—Directions: Write letters and have trainee identify letter intended based on the key.

Stage V—Directions: Write a sequence of letters which, when deciphered by the trainee, will spell familiar words, such as names and places.

Stage VI—Directions: Write a sequence of letters which, when deciphered by the trainee, will spell random words of varying length.

Stage VII—Directions: Write a sequence of letters with spaces between words which, when deciphered by the trainee, will result in full sentences.

Stage VIII—Directions: Ask the trainee to transcribe full sentences into code.

## Memory/Orientation

### Task 1—Recall of Pictures and Places

Materials: Two decks of playing cards.
Stage I—Directions: Place two different cards from the same deck face up on a table and allow trainee to view for five seconds, then turn cards face down. Ask trainee to point

to the proper card as it is named. Increase number of cards to a maximum of five as trainee progresses.

Stage II—Directions: Select identical cards from each of two decks to form two pair (for example: two king of spades, two nine of diamonds). Place cards face up in front of trainee for five seconds and then turn over. Ask trainee to match cards. If match is not successful turn cards back over in place. Keep repeating until trainee gets correct pairings. Remove correctly paired cards from the table.

Stage III—Directions: Increase number of pairings to three with a challenge to trainee to minimize the number of turns before the table is empty of cards. Remember to remove cards when correctly paired. Keep increasing number of pairings to a maximum of 15 pairs as trainee progresses. Increase time to view cards face up by five seconds for each additional pairing. (For example: six pairs is allotted 30 seconds' viewing time.)

Stage IV—Directions: Select five cards in sequence (for example: three, four, five, six, seven of clubs) and place in random order face up in front of trainee, then turn face down after five seconds. Ask trainee to turn cards over in sequence. Turn card back over if incorrect choice is made.

Stage V—Directions: Increase the number of cards in the sequence, allowing one more second of viewing time for each card added, to a maximum of eight.

### Task 2—News Events

Stage I—Directions: Pick out one major news event that the trainee is to recall on request during the day. Provide cuing as needed.

Stage II—Directions: Trainee is to watch a national news broadcast on television and write down (or verbalize with trainer writing) the major news events as each is presented. Recall later in the day is expected with cuing provided by written notes.

Stage III—Directions: Same as Stage II except that a written listing of major events is to be done after the news broadcast is complete.

Stage IV—Directions: Trainee is to derive a list of major news events from the front page of the local paper with a short summary of the facts. Recall later in the day is expected.

### Task 3—Orientation to Time

Stage I—Directions: Provide the trainee with a large calendar in a central, permanent location. Check the calendar with the trainee at the same time each day. Cross off days that have passed. Write important events on the calendar.

Stage II—Directions: Ask the trainee for the month, day, year, and day of week just prior to checking the calendar.

Stage III—Directions: Ask the trainee to provide the date of a day removed in time. For instance, ask what the date will be tomorrow, next week, 10 days ago, etc. Ask the number of weeks or months until, or since, important dates, such as Christmas, birthdays, etc.

### APPENDIX B: POPULAR GAMES SUITABLE FOR COGNITIVE STIMULATION

Below is an alphabetical list of games that are commercially available which could be used in a cognitive stimulation program. This list is by no means comprehensive. The manufacturer of the game is provided after each entry (unless the game is available through several manufacturers) along with a listing by number of the cognitive skills required. The number coding of cognitive skills is as follows:

1. Perceptual accuracy—All games require perceptual (usually visual) accuracy to some extent but some focus on accuracy as a goal.
2. Spatial organization—Games requiring, as a basic focus, organization of material in two or three dimensions.
3. Perceptual-motor functioning—Basically this entails fine motor functioning or motor speed when it represents a primary component of the game.
4. Verbal skills—Games addressing the generation of words or other verbal material.
5. Arithmetic skills—Games in which basic arithmetic plays a central role, including the handling of money.
6. Convergent problem-solving—The emphasis here is on piecing together solutions in a step-wise fashion, an essential component to effective strategy.
7. Divergent problem-solving—Flexibility in approach is the hallmark. In other words, diverging from step-by-step solutions to generate new strategies.
8. Sequencing—This is often a component of convergent and divergent problem-solving but, in some cases, is a goal in itself.
9. Memory—All games require ongoing monitoring and recall as part of the game process but some games focus on memory itself; that is, the ability to retrieve information from long-term storage.

The complexity of the games varies a great deal and is very difficult to rate in a consistent fashion. However, even complex games can be made more simple by altering rules, such as by removing special cards and liberalizing time constraints. For instance, the game Uno (International) can be simplified by removing all special cards, such as Draw Four and Reverse.

Aggravation (Lakeside)—6
Backgammon—2,5,6
Bargain Hunter (Milton Bradley)—5,6
Battleship (Milton Bradley)—2,6
Bed Bugs (Milton Bradley)—3
Bingo—2
Boggle (Parker Brothers)—4,7
Checkers—2,6
Chess—2,6,7
Clue (Parker Brothers)—6
Connect Four (Milton Bradley)—2,6
Conquest of the Empire (Milton Bradley)—1,6
Dominoes—1,2
Erector Sets—2,3,6
Etch-A-Sketch (Ohio Art)—2,3
Foursight (Lakeside)—2,7
Gridlock (Ideal)—1,2,6
Lego—1,2,3
Life (Milton Bradley)—5,6

Lincoln Logs (Playskool)—1,2,3
Lite-Brite (Hasbro)—1,2,3
Lotto (Edu-Cards)
Farm Lotto—1,6
Go-Together Lotto—1,6
Object Lotto—1
Zoo Lotto—1,6
The World About Us Lotto—1,6
Luck Plus (International)—1,5
Mastermind (Pressman)—2,6
Memory (Milton Bradley)
Animal Families—2,9
Fronts & Backs—2,9
Original—2,9
Step by Step—6,8
Mling (Suntex)—6,7,8
Models, plastic replica—1,2,3,8
Monopoly—5,6
Mystery Mansion—6
Othello—2,6
Paint-by-Numbers—1,2,3
Parcheesi (Selchow & Righter)—6
Password (Milton Bradley)—4,6,9
Pay Day (Parker Brothers)—5,6
Pente (Parker Brothers)—2,6
Perquacky (Lakeside)—4,7,9
Picture Tri-Ominoes (Pressman)—1
Pic Up Stik (Steven)—3
Racko (Milton Bradley)—8
Rage (International)—6,8
Risk (Parker Brothers)—2,6,7
Sabotage (Lakeside)—6,7
Scotland Yard (Milton Bradley)—2,6,8
Scrabble—2,4,7,9
Smath (Pressman)—2,5,6
Sorry (Parker Brothers)—6
Think & Jump (Pressman)—2,6
Toss Across (Ideal)—3
Tri-Ominoes (Pressman)—1
Tripoley—1,8
Uno (International)—1,8
Verbatim (Lakeside)—4,7,9
Whodunit (Selchow & Righter)—6
Word War (Whitman)—4,6,7,9
Word Yahtzee (Milton Bradley)—4,7,9
Yahtzee (Milton Bradley)—5,6

# REFERENCES

*Apple computer resources in special education and rehabilitation*. (1987). Allen, TX: DLM Teaching Resources.

Brooks, N., Campsie, L., Symington, C., Beattie, A., & McKinlay, W. (1987). The effects of severe head injury on patient and relative within seven years of injury. *Journal of Head Trauma Rehabilitation*, 2, 1–13.

Carter, L. T., Caruso, J. L., & Languirand, M.A. (1984). *The thinking skills workbook*. Springfield, IL: Thomas.

Craine, J. F., & Gudeman, H. E. (1981). *The rehabilitation of brain functions*. Springfield, IL: Thomas.

Harnadek, A. (1977). *Basic thinking skills*. Pacific Grove, CA: Midwest Publishing.

*Head injury: A home based cognitive rehabilitation program*. (1989). Houston: HDI Publishers.

Holloran, S. M., & Bressler, E. J. (1983). *Cognitive reorganization: A stimulus handbook*. Oregon: C.C. Publications.

Kozloff, R. (1987). Networks of social support and the outcome from severe head injury. *Journal of Head Trauma Rehabilitation*, 2, 14–23.

Livingston, M. G. (1987). Head injury: The relative's response. *Brain Injury*, 1, 8–14.

Livingston, M. G., Brooks, D. N., & Bond, M. R. (1985). Patient outcome in the year following severe head injury and relative's psychiatric and social functioning. *Journal of Neurology*, 48, 876–881.

Novack, T. A., Bergquist, T. F., Bennett, G., & Hartley, D. (1987). Cognitive stimulation in the home environment. In J.M. Williams & C. J. Long (Eds.). *The rehabilitation of cognitive disabilities* (pp. 149–169). New York: Plenum Press.

Romano, M. D. (1974). Family response to traumatic head injury. *Scandinavian Journal of Rehabilitation*, 6, 1–4.

Rosenbaum, M., & Najenson, T. (1976). Changes in life patterns and symptoms of low mood as reported by wives of severely brain-injured soldiers. *Journal of Consulting Clinical Psychology*, 44, 881–888.

Sohlberg, M.M., & Mateer, C.A. (1989). *Introduction to cognitive rehabilitation: Theory and practice*. New York: Guilford Press.

# 20

# Closed Head Injury and Family Structure

## Factors Contributing to Dysfunctional Dynamics

BOBBY G. GREER, MARY ANNE KNACK,
and ROB ROBERTS

Considerable attention has been given in the literature to the impact of closed head injury on the family (Brooks, 1984; Brown & McCormick, 1988). Stressors, as well as other factors, contributing to posttrauma family adjustment have been delineated (Braciszeski, 1987). This chapter will review this other work and will propose another perspective from which to view family restructuring after closed head injury.

The family with a handicapped member is, by definition, severely stressed (Bubolz & Whiren, 1984). There is a limited supply of physical and psychic energy in a family system necessary to maintain the system and when energy of both types is being used to deal with a handicapped member, who may never be able to contribute much to the system, that system can easily become overwhelmed. The stresses inherent in the family of the victim of traumatic brain injury (TBI) are often compounded by outside forces such as inflation, unemployment, unsafe housing and myriads of other social conditions.

TBI in a family member brings about many stressors for the family. First, there is the impact of the trauma on the family member involved. There is the constant threat of death during the acute care stage. Second, the family must adjust to the long-term aftereffects

BOBBY G. GREER and ROB ROBERTS • College of Education, Memphis State University, Memphis, Tennessee 38152.     MARY ANNE KNACK • Department of Counseling and Personnel Services, Memphis State University, Memphis, Tennessee 38152.

*HANDBOOK OF HEAD TRAUMA: Acute Care to Recovery*, edited by Charles J. Long and Leslie K. Ross. Plenum Press, New York, 1992.

of TBI on the functioning of the involved family member. For example, it has been found that families experience less difficulty accepting the motor and memory dysfunctions resulting from brain injury than accepting the personality changes which are often the sequelae of TBI (Thomasen, 1974; Brooks & Aughton, 1979).

According to Panting and Merry (1972), 60% of relatives of head-injured patients required tranquilizers or sleeping pills as a direct result of the stress of the brain injury on the family. Kozloff (1987) stated, "professional and family support diminishes as money and medical indications for therapy decrease" (p. 20). Oddy, Humphrey, and Uttley (1978) concluded that stress did not diminish with time for the families of head-injured individuals. Brooks, Capsie, Symington, Beattie, and McKinlay (1987) claim that even after seven years, levels of stress are still high, especially in cases of brain injury where posttraumatic amnesia lasted over 14 days. Another very real stressor is the financial burden of the medical care costs of TBI. In addition, as reported by Jacobs (1985), the indirect costs of TBI, including lost wages and loss of educational opportunities, have been reported by such families to be a definite drain on family resources.

Families develop coping mechanisms to deal with such stressors. Braciszeski (1987) lists a number of both constructive and destructive mechanisms utilized by families. These coping mechanisms include shock, denial, hope, and protectiveness. In the postacute care phase, shock is not normally present. Denial, however, is very prevalent (Braciszeski, 1987; Brown & McCormick, 1988; Kahoe, Kundu, & Hollingsworth, 1988). Denial can take many forms, from total denial (client is temporarily sick or asleep) to more subtle forms (client's deficits are temporary and his/her memory, etc. will return). Romano (1974) reports that the denial seen in TBI families is unlike any other due to its tenacious, long-term nature. In a study of 13 families followed for up to four years postinjury, Romano stated that none of the families moved beyond the denial stage. In fact, she reports that in individuals who do display moving beyond the denial stage, pressures from other family members force these individuals to return to the denial stage, or risk alienation from the other members who perceive them as traitors.

In addition to the above stressors directly related to the impact of TBI on the family, there are indications in the literature that many social dysfunctions often exist in such families prior to injury (Braciszeski, 1987; Kaplan, 1988; Jones, 1990). In one such study, alcohol and drug abuse, marital and/or interpersonal problems, disruptive or acting out behaviors were found to exist in more than 38% of the cases (Braciszeski, 1987). In addition, Jones (1989) reports that in families with a TBI member the incidence of abusive drinking premorbidly was 40 to 51%. Therefore, it is most likely that non-injury-related dysfunctions occur in a significant proportion of TBI families.

Family intervention efforts following closed head injury have tended to focus on educating about TBI, training family members to assist and to stimulate cognitive rehabilitation, or addressing the emotional issues for the individual brought about by TBI. For education, Kahoe *et al.* (1988) point out the initial need of most families for "understanding the cognitive and emotional state of the patient" (p. 207). This acquaints family members with the typical problems they may encounter in a cognitive, didactic manner. These authors also caution that the family should not be overwhelmed with too much information at this point. An example of the family as cognitive retrainers is to be found in the chapter in this book by Novack, Bergquist and Bennett. Braciszeski (1987) presents a currently used framework for working through the socioemotional issues involved in TBI families. This approach focuses more on the emotional status of the other family member than on the needs of the injured members. It is with this approach that the grief, guilt, and despair of the noninjured members of the family are dealt with in a therapeutic manner (Kahoe *et al.*, 1988).

## FAMILY DYSFUNCTION AND TBI

The remainder of this chapter will focus on intervention with TBI families through the family systems approach. A unique perspective to be used here is that many of the affected families were dysfunctional prior to the occurrence of the closed head injury and, therefore, such dysfunctions compound any therapeutic interventions involving the family. For example, if the affected family member was injured while in an intoxicated state, there is likely to be some resentment and blaming of the "victim." In many cases, the intoxication was not an isolated incident, but rather a recurrent pattern of behavior. The feelings of the family regarding this form of acting out behavior then become an integral part of the intervention process.

Family systems theory has developed in this century partly as a result of observations by clinicians that individuals who made good progress in treatment often regressed when returned to the family (Bateson, 1959; Haley, 1959; Jackson, 1961; Jackson & Weakland, 1959). An awareness developed that the family, just like other systems, could not be treated in a piecemeal fashion. In a reciprocal manner, effective treatment for the individual usually required dealing with the larger family system, or the existing forces would once again exert their pressure on the changed individual, so the family would again reach homeostasis.

Just as individuals have a developmental cycle, families have a similar cycle over time that helps negotiate the tasks required for that phase in the living process. The order of the particular life cycles is arbitrary as the family continues to expand, contract, or realign over and over with each generation. Each stage has its own set of tasks necessary to successfully prepare for the following stage (Carter & McGoldrick, 1989).

The first developmental stage consists of launching the young adult from the parental home. The tasks necessary for this stage are the acceptance by the young person of emotional and financial responsibility for self. This involves differentiation from the family of origin, development of a meaningful peer network, and establishment of vocational and financial independence.

The second stage focuses on the newly married couple and the establishment of a new family system, to which each individual brings elements of both families of origin, but blended in a way to produce commitment to a new family system. Included in this stage is the realignment of relationships with extended families and friends to include the spouse.

The third stage involves young children in the new family system. Necessary to accepting new members into this family system is realignment of the existing couple's relationship to make room for children. This includes negotiating the child rearing, financial, and household tasks. More adjustment is needed among the extended family to include parenting and grandparenting roles.

The fourth stage involves families with adolescent children. Necessary to this stage is the loosening up, or increased flexibility, of family boundaries to encourage and accommodate increasing independence of the adolescent children and adjustment to the aging of the grandparents. At this stage, typically there is a review and possible rededication to midlife marital and career issues.

In the fifth stage, the young adult is launched from the home. In this stage the boundaries of the family are most permeable. Children leave, they marry and bring new members into the family, they have their own children, and often death begins removing members from the system. The principal tasks of this stage are the renegotiation of the marital dyad, learning to interact with grown children as adult to adult instead of parent to child, establishing relationships with in-laws and grandchildren, and dealing with aging and death of elderly parents.

The sixth stage focuses on families in later life who need to accept and adjust to the shift of generational roles and influence. Included in this is adapting to declining physical vigor; death of a spouse, siblings, and other peers; developing meaningful roles in the family; supporting the younger generation and preparation for their own death by a life review and attempt at integration (Carter & McGoldrick, 1989).

Satir (1973) refers to "troubled" families rather than dysfunctional families. By this, Satir refers to families who do not seem to have developed the skills and abilities to resolve long-standing problems. She describes the "hopelessness, helplessness, the loneliness" (p. 12) in these families where members have never learned to be friends with each other, to support each other, or to trust each other. One of the biggest problems in these families is the lack of resources to encourage the growth of individual members, even infants and young children. Frequently, the adults in such troubled families were, themselves, raised in an environment that was similarly deficient in encouraging growth and development of the individual members, such that significant deficits have been present over several generations.

Minuchin (1974) distinguishes between stuck families, or families with "growing pains," and pathological families. He indicates that stuck families are those who are having trouble negotiating a life-cycle change while pathological families are those "who in the face of stress increase the rigidity of their transactional patterns and boundaries, and avoid or resist any exploration of alternatives" (p. 61). This implies that the pathological family may need much more extensive therapy, than does the "stuck" family, to achieve a satisfactory adjustment to the stress of a head-injured family member.

It can be seen from the above description of stages of family evolution that the effects of a traumatic brain injury on a family member will depend to a large extent on the stage of family development at the time of injury. For example, since a large proportion of TBI are males, ages 18 to 35 (Brown & McCormick, 1988), it is easy to see how such an injury could delay, sometimes permanently, the launching of the young adult from the home, the establishment of a new family, or the integration of new children into the existing family system. In fact, depending on the severity of the concomitant disabilities, the TBI member might reassume a child's role in the family system, or be made to assume such a role by other family members. Such a family may have the continual care of such an individual, attenuating the family developmental cycle.

The combination of previous dysfunctions in the TBI family, the stresses brought about by the injury's consequences, as well as the accompanying attenuation of the family development cycle further compounds the family's situation, often to the breaking point. Frequently, more dysfunctions will develop in the family in the form of other health problems, behavior problems in other family members, marital strife, chemical abuse, emotional problems, or a variety of other life style manifestations of stress.

It is critical that the family therapist trying to address the problems of the TBI family, understand the other dysfunctions, or "troubles," which often already exist in these families. This includes an understanding of preexisting problems, family life- cycle stages and stresses, the unique stressors brought about by the head trauma, and preexisting family attitudes toward health problems, which can impact the adjustment and functioning of the family system.

Often a family genogram elicits attitudes toward illness as well as dysfunctional patterns that can be modified or used as a beginning point for instilling some hope, some interrelatedness, and some sense of empowerment in order for the family to learn to have confidence in their ability to resolve problems (McGoldrick & Gerson, 1989). If a family is only familiar with dealing with acute and/or terminal illness, they may not have the knowledge or expectations that produce the best possible outcome for the injured individual as well as the rest of the family. This may be partly the reason for the persistent nature of denial observed by Romano (1974). If such families had only experienced acute illnesses, then the persistent expectation that the individual will "wake up and be normal again" has some experiential validity. A typical example is a mother who has observed relatives caring for family members with terminal cancer. It is a painful, emotional, and physically draining experience, but there is a definite ending point. With a TBI individual, however, the injured family member often outlives the primary caretaker. A woman or man devoting the majority of his or her energy to caring for an adult child who is brain injured may eventually feel depressed, stressed, isolated, and guilty for resenting their situation. Through their intense attentiveness to the injured individual, such caretakers may actually perpetuate and increase the dependency of the head-injured survivor. In the literature on dysfunctional families, this pathological attentiveness is referred to as enabling or co-dependence. This phenomenon has two adverse effects. First, the injured individual's full potential is not realized and, second, the caretaker neglects his or her own needs and those of other family members to care for the injured charge (Wegscheider, 1981).

TBI begins with an acute onset where the extent of the injury is unknown and, in fact, whether the individual will survive from the trauma is uncertain for a time. This acute, life-threatening phase has its own peculiar kind of stresses and requires a readjustment of the family structure, roles, and affective coping; all of which must be accomplished over a very compressed time span. It requires rapid mobilization of crisis management skills and some families are better equipped than others to deal with rapid change and the intense strain of this stage (Roland, 1989). Frequently the family member or members who adapt well to this stage will not function well later in the chronic phase. Typically, with TBI, after the initial stabilization and rehabilitation phase, the biological course stabilizes and the individual is characterized by some clear-cut deficits or residual functional limitations. For the family focused on total recovery, it may be extremely difficult to accept the permanence of the member's decreased level of functioning, not just the physical or organic limitations, but the personality changes as well. The family member who adjusted to the preinjury emotionally stable young adult often has a difficult time readjusting to the postinjury emotional lability, irritability, or the childlike qualities on a long-term basis (Brooks, 1984; Lezak, 1986).

Brooks and Aughton (1979) studied 89 closed head injury cases where the stressors on the family were investigated. All the major objective burdens the families reported were related to mental and emotional changes, such as irritability, slowness, tiredness, tension/anxiety, impatience, depression, anger, personality change, memory disturbance, and complaining. The least burdensome changes reported were in the areas of physical change, sensory change, or another mixed group of unrelated changes such as trouble with the law and expressing suicidal thoughts. Further analysis showed that "physical disabilities appear completely unimportant as predictors of stress within the family, except in the specific case of urinary incontinence" (p. 164). The most critical predictors of stress in the family are, in descending order, childish behavior, loss of interest, change in sex life, depression, and tension/anxiety.

## IMPLICATIONS FOR LONG-TERM FAMILY INTERVENTION

In order to maximize the long term adjustment of families of individuals who sustain TBI, education, support, and family therapy are critical. Often, the piecemeal approach to treatment leaves strategic gaps in these areas with the bulk of therapeutic resources being focused on assessing and rehabilitating the injured individual. The above review of available literature on the adjustment of families to TBI indicates "head injury causes serious personality change, serious emotional disability and often childish, demanding and irritable and aggressive behavior" (Brooks, 1984, p. 144). Such changes place a serious burden, that appears to be chronic, on the family (Brooks *et al.*, 1987). With suitable and supportive treatment, many families could be assisted in the process of caring for their head-injured family member. An ideal treatment team approach would involve rehabilitation counselors and family therapists as a follow-up to inpatient treatment for the family, in addition to continuing therapeutic services for the injured family member.

### Education

Family members need continued education all through the rehabilitation of their family member (DePompei & Zarski, 1989; DePompei, Zarski, & Hall, 1988; Oddy *et al.*, 1978). In the early stages following the trauma, they need to be educated in a general way about the nature of head injury and the recovery process. Though they often are not ready to accept the extent of their family member's impairment, they need to hear in an objective fashion the range of outcome possibilities. This helps prepare them for the time when they will be more able to be realistic about the recovery potential of their loved one. Specific information should be given to family members in limited amounts, allowing them time to process the full meaning of such information. Too often, near the time of discharge from inpatient care, the family is giving a "crash course on TBI" as it relates to their family member. Such families are ill-prepared to absorb the totality of such information, let alone process it. Both patient and family will often need to be informed numerous times before they can absorb the full measure of their circumstance. An important consideration is to tailor the amount of information and the quality of the information to fit the demographics of the patient and his/her family. Such "demographics" would include educational level, sophistication regarding medical information, and the emotional and financial resources of the family. Often such information is best learned in groups with other families who are dealing with similar circumstances.

It is very important that all family members be involved in educational sessions. It is imperative that the whole family know what to expect in dealing with their impaired family member. Often when information is passed through the family piecemeal, it becomes very distorted over time, much like in the old game of "gossip." Providing the family with information in a clear and consistent manner will avoid much confusion within the family. Often information sessions need to be scheduled especially for the convenience of the family. It is worth some trouble on the part of the therapist to be able to make sure that all family members are included in the counseling and planning involved in these sessions. Family members should be encouraged to bring up their own concerns about the situation so they can be addressed by the professionals. Time spent in these sessions usually helps tremendously in the process of accepting and adapting to the new family system that has emerged as the result of adjusting to the head injury and concomitant changes in structure and function of its members.

## Support

As time goes on, families begin to get past the crisis stage and are becoming ready for more focused support and assistance. At this stage more specific information about any communications impairment and its possible consequences should be examined, including how these deficits will be manifested in the home. Counseling sessions are often helpful in assisting families in developing coping behaviors and structure to minimize problems of reorganizing the family to accommodate the brain-injured individual. The counseling experience also is helpful at identifying those families who may need more intensive work to make a satisfactory adjustment. Family support groups often help to break the isolation of families and provide a level of support over time that professionals are not able to provide.

Many families have reported that relatives and friends were very helpful and supportive at the time of the injury but, in the chronic stages, they seemed to tire of hearing of the problems involved and were available very little, if at all. Wives of head-injured men have reported tensions between themselves and their husband's family (Kozloff, 1987; Rosenbaum & Najenson, 1976). Given the dissatisfaction that is frequently reported by the wives of head-injured men, it can be assumed that parents might be afraid of the burden left to them if their sons' wives should leave their husbands. Support groups, such as those offered through the National Head Injury Foundation and the Head Trauma Support Project, may be able to assist families in a reorganizational structure which will not bring undue hardship on any one family member.

Day-care centers and sheltered workshops can be critical support systems for family members as well as providing input and meaning for the injured individual. These settings would be logical places for group therapy to take place. Prigatano and Klonoff (1988) stated that group feedback to patients can be invaluable, as patients may accept suggestions and criticisms from peers more readily than from therapists: "Group therapy can also be valuable in helping less aware patients become more sensitive to their negative social impact on others" (p. 53). Needless to say, these individuals may also be able to accept suggestions from their groups quicker than they would from their families. Brooks (1984) says that brain-injured persons often have no idea or comprehension of the extent of their own behavior changes from premorbid levels, even if they were lonely, had lost contact with old friends, and had troublesome relationships with their families.

Particular attention should be given to the special burden borne by the women in families with TBI members, whether in the role of wife, mother, or, in some cases, oldest sister. Societal and personal expectations often leave women the largest share of the burden for caring for difficult and demanding family members. Buck and Hohman (1981) found that the spouses of male spinal cord injured bore an undue amount of stress relative to other family members. With changing societal and personal expectations, it can no longer be assumed that women will always be available for the caretaker role. When women "continue to play the role of server and unpaid worker" (McGoldrick, 1989, p. 62) while also working outside the home, stresses can quickly build to the breaking point. If the goal of family counseling and therapy is to maximize the satisfaction of *all* family members, it is no longer reasonable to expect women to assume the major burden of care for the TBI family member (Enns, 1988). Kozloff stated the following:

> It is the woman in the role of mother or wife who ultimately becomes the head-injured man's sole source of task-oriented and emotional support. It is she who alters her life, gives up her job, friends, and social life to care for her head-injured son or husband. She must reconcile her obligations to care for her husband or son with her other responsibilities and in doing so often puts her own health, marriage, and the rest of her family at risk. (p. 21)

Rosenbaum and Najenson (1976) compared the wives of paraplegics and the wives of brain-injured men one year after injury. The wives of brain-injured men reported more depression, more irritability, more physical complaints, and more insomnia than the wives of paraplegics. They also tended to experience a crisis at about a year after injury when the reality of the permanent nature of their husband's condition really sank in. The wives of the brain-injured men reported their husbands were more self-oriented and had more childlike dependency than the paraplegic husbands, even though the paraplegic husbands exhibited more of these tendencies than normal husbands. Their study also reported severe sexual difficulties for the wives of head-injured men that seemed to stem from the problems with interpersonal sensitivity and intimacy; the wives revealing a tendency to dislike any physical contact with their husbands. The sexual difficulties in paraplegic couples seemed more related to the spinal cord injury. The social isolation of the brain-injured wives was more extreme than for the paraplegic wives. This apparently was related to the better social sensitivity and awareness of the paraplegic husbands and the insensitive behavior of the brain-injured husbands.

Lezak (1978) discusses the myriad of problems facing the spouses of brain-injured patients. The social problems of spouses of head injury survivors are enormous. They are not divorced or widowed, and yet they do not have partners and are not eligible to get one. Mourning is not allowed as the mate is still alive though often in such altered form that the spouse no longer considers the relationship a marriage. Severe social and personal restrictions often prevent a person from divorcing an injured and changed spouse. When there were severe problems to begin with, the injury frequently prolongs an already unhappy situation. The spouse has no legitimate outlet for sexual and affectional needs to be met, though in many cases the injured partner is not capable of providing for those needs. Rosenbaum and Najenson (1976) conclude that while support and nurturing for the wives of head-injured men would certainly be of assistance, a more productive approach would be to train "the disabled man to acquire the appropriate interpersonal skills needed to make him once again a source of positive reinforcement to his wife" (p. 888).

Prigatano and Klonoff (1988) discuss the major ingredients to psychological health. Building on Freudian theory, they state that the ability to work and to love are essential ingredients that enable a person to learn "to behave in his or her own best self-interest"

(p. 48). While neuropsychological testing can often effectively evaluate a person's ability to work, the ability to love is often more subtle and more complex. The major ingredients of love are passion, intimacy, and commitment (Sternberg, 1986), and while passion is often present in head-injured individuals, it often is too disinhibited and unchecked. This type of passion may result in inappropriate behavior that seriously interferes with the ability to be intimate. Prigatano and Klonoff observe "it is difficult for a healthy spouse to have a sense of intimacy with a partner who behaves more like a child than an adult" (p. 51). Often spouses of these patients have said it is like having an extra child on their hands than any kind of a partner or helpmate.

## Therapy

Families who are not able to move to some workable level of reorganization often need more intensive and extensive professional help. The extent of the need for family therapy will depend on many of the factors discussed in the present chapter, i.e., amount of premorbid dysfunction, the community and financial resources, the preinjury role of the injured family member, as well as the history of the family's ability to cope with prior illnesses and/or disabilities. Some families become stuck in their own grief over the loss of the person with whom they had developed a deep and meaningful relationship. Such family members will need assistance in order to move on with their lives and to accept the head-injured member as a family loved one. With such support and assistance, such families often achieve the reorganization necessary for the maintenance of homeostasis and fulfillment of the family's function, i.e., the enhancement of growth in each member.

While therapy and family counseling cannot spare the family members or the patient the pain of the losses and adjustments associated with traumatic head injury, mental health professionals who understand how head injury disrupts families can help them cope with the grief, frustration, and reorganization necessary for full family functioning. It is critical that family members and the injured member be told that the problem behaviors and the family's reaction to them are natural, given their situation. This will help relieve "the patient and family of many of the self-doubts, guilts, and fears for their sanity that tend to pile up" (Lezak, 1986, p. 249) as they realize the extent and lasting nature of their loss. It is also important for professionals to help the family understand they move back and forth between stages of acceptance of their reality, and that is the necessary process of adjusting to their changed circumstances. Martin (1988) says "adaptation is clearly not a static, one-time event, but rather is a very complex, fluid process that may fluctuate over time" (p. 469).

Family members often develop dysfunctional responses to their injured family member. These responses can include blaming the patient for his/her impulsiveness and poor social and cognitive skills, taking over responsibility for areas that would be better handled by the patient, using rigid power and authority to maintain position, avoiding any responsibility for any of the problems in the family, denying the severity of the deficits and trying to "get back to normal" when it is impossible to reestablish premorbid functioning, and controlling the activities unnecessarily for their family member rather than letting them choose (DePompei et al., 1988).

There are many intervention strategies to offset these dysfunctional patterns and frequently need to be employed periodically in the adjustment process. The first is education which is dealt with in more detail above. The second is developing family awareness of their own reactions to the changed behavior of their family member and learning techniques to deal with those behaviors. This can be done by practicing "active listening" techniques to learn to really hear the injured family member. Often education concerning nonverbal communication, and videotaping family interactions can be beneficial. Rehearsing and role-playing more positive or supportive reactions to problem behavior may also be very helpful. For example, a parent who is irritated and annoyed by tangential speech can learn to interrupt with a restatement of the individual's opening comment to get them back on target again. It is best to let the family members discover and rehearse what is natural to them, but often they may be inspired by some suggestions by the therapist. These sessions also give the counselor an excellent chance to model appropriate behavior and responses to the head-injured individual. Reframing in more positive terms the behavior of the head-injured survivor is also helpful for family functioning. For example, if a mother can understand that her adult child's rocking behavior is a reaction to stress or fatigue, she will be less likely to be defensive and irritated by it. A stressed wife may believe her injured husband's clumsy attempts to do laundry are a way of annoying her. If she can see that it is his attempt to be helpful and responsible, she may very well be able to help structure the task so he will be successful with it.

Periodic reviews are needed to assess the progress of the communication and cooperation of the family and how therapy can continue to improve that goal. A frank discussion of what is working and what is not working is important. DePompei *et al.* (1988) caution that family members need to understand "they are learning ways to interact with their head-injured survivor, and that they are not being trained to assume the role and responsibilities of the treating professionals" (p. 21).

Family members also need to hear how important it is for them to take care of themselves first or they will not be able to continue giving the patient good care (Lezak, 1978). Often family members can be motivated to take better care of themselves if they are convinced it will help their family member. They cannot hear this too many times in the process of adjusting to the reality of living with a head-injured family member. Rest, leisure, hobbies, and "adequate opportunities for a change of pace and respite from the responsibilities of patient care" (p. 595) are necessary for the continued mental and physical health of caretakers.

Family caretakers also need encouragement to rely on their own judgment in conflicts with the injured family member or any other family member. Only the caretaker knows the actuality of being responsible for the injured family member and the truth of his/her own limits. When other family members get an opportunity to periodically take full responsibility for the patient for a period of time, they often back off and cease giving so much free advice and opinions.

At times, it becomes necessary to make other living arrangements for the injured family member. On these occasions, it is important to help the responsible family members process their situation, and their feelings about it, so they can become reasonably comfortable with the decision. One instance when placement outside of the home may be appropriate is when the physical and emotional safety of minor children are involved. Often with counseling, caretakers can learn to manage belligerent family members, but when these have proven to be unworkable there may be no other recourse. When a caretaker knows the decision was made with concern for all involved and with consideration of all possible solutions, he/she is usually able to accept the reality with some peace.

## CONCLUSION

The needs of head-injured patients and their families are not being met with existing rehabilitation services which focus mainly on the physical handicaps in the patient (Brooks, 1984). The recent changes in services which focus more on counseling, therapy, and advocacy for the patient in addition to physical rehabilitation will, in the long run, be more efficient because of the reduction in the burdens on the families of these individuals. Families will be less likely to sacrifice the overall goal of the families in the interests of the injured member, leading to better rehabilitation prospects and increased family stability. As Prigatano and Klonoff (1988) stated, "perhaps effective psychotherapy cures very little but does manage problems much better" (p. 52).

A brief look at the ramifications of family functioning, in the face of TBI in one of its members, shows that even the healthiest and most highly functioning of families premorbidly need an array of services above the typical individual cognitive, physical, and vocational rehabilitation services. All families need help processing the vast changes that ensue in their family systems and the helping professional must have a good working knowledge of family systems as well as of brain injury rehabilitation. These families will invariably need support, counseling, and education. Families who were not at a relatively healthy level of functioning premorbidly, may also benefit from extensive therapy to try to achieve a better level of functioning. While this requires a major investment in time and resources, the payoff of functioning, stable families able to provide support and assistance for their loved ones is well worth the investment.

## REFERENCES

Bateson, G. (1959). Cultural problems posed by a study of schizophrenic processes. In A. Auerback (Ed.), *Schizophrenia: An integrated approach*. New York: Ronald Press.

Braciszeski, T. L. (1987, May). *Family system issues associated with closed head injuries*. Paper presented at the 8th Annual Children's Center Conference, Detroit, MI.

Brooks, D. N., & Aughton, M. E. (1979). Psychological consequences of blunt head injury. *International Rehabilitation Medicine*, *1*, 160–165.

Brooks, N.(1984). Head injury and the family. In N. Brooks (Ed.), *Closed head injury: Psychological, social and family consequences*. London: Oxford University Press.

Brooks, N., Capsie, L., Symington, C., Beattie, A., & McKinlay, W. (1987). The effects of head injury on patient and relative within seven years of injury. *Journal of Head Trauma Rehabilitation*, *2*(3), 1–13.

Brown, B.W., & McCormick, T. (1988). Family coping following traumatic head injury: An exploratory analysis with recommendations for treatment. *Family Relations*, *37*(1), 12–16.

Bubolz, M. M., & Whiren, A. P. (1984). The family of the handicapped: An ecological model for policy and practice. *Family Relations*, *33*, 5–12.

Buck, F. M., & Hohman, G.(1981). Personality, behavior, values and family relations of children of fathers with spinal cord injury. *Archives of Physical Medicine*, *68*, 432–438.

Carter, B. C., & McGoldrick, M. (1989). The changing family life cycle: A framework for family therapy. In B. Carter & M. McGoldrick (Eds.), *The changing family life cycle: A framework for family therapy*. Boston: Allyn & Bacon.

DePompei, R., & Zarski, J. J. (1989). Families, head injury, and cognitive-communicative impairments: Issues for family counseling. *Topics in Language Disorders*, *9*(2), 78–79.

DePompei, R., Zarski, J. J., & Hall, D. E. (1988). Cognitive communication impairments: A family-focused viewpoint. *Journal of Head Trauma Rehabilitation*, *3*(2), 13–22.

Enns, C. Z. (1988). Dilemmas of power and equality in marital and family counseling: A feminist perspective. *Journal of Counseling and Development*, *67*, 52–55.

Haley, J. (1959). The family of the schizophrenic. *Journal of Nervous & Mental Disease*, *129*, 357–374.

Jackson, D. D. (1961). Family therapy in the family of the schizophrenic. In M. Stern (Ed.), *Contemporary psychotherapies*. Glencoe, IL: The Free Press.

Jackson, D. D., & Weakland, J. H. (1959). Schizophrenic symptoms and family interaction. *Archives of General Psychiatry*, *1*, 616–621.

Jacobs, H. I. (1985). *The family as a therapeutic agent: Long term rehabilitation of the head injured patient*. Unpublished manuscript, National Institute for Handicapped Research.

Jones, G. A. (1989). Alcohol abuse and traumatic brain injury. *Alcohol Health & Research World*, *13*(2), 104–109.

Kahoe, J. L., Kundu, M. M., & Hollingsworth, D. K. (1988). Impact of brain injury on the family and the role of the rehabilitation counselor in the postacute rehabilitation setting. *Rehabilitation Education*, *2*(3/4), 205–212.

Kaplan, S. P. (1988). Adaptations following serious brain injury: An assessment after one year. *Journal of Applied Rehabilitation Counseling*, *19*(3), 3–8.

Kozloff, R. (1987). Networks of social support and the outcome from severe head injury. *Journal of Head Trauma Rehabilitation*, *2*(3), 14–23.

Lezak, M. D. (1978). Living with characterologically altered brain injured patient. *Journal of Clinical Psychiatry*, *39*, 592–598.

Lezak, M. D. (1986). Psychological implications of traumatic brain damage for the patient's family. *Rehabilitation Psychology*, *31*(4), 241–250.

McGoldrick, M. (1989). Women and the family life cycle. In B. Carter & M. McGoldrick (Eds.), *The changing family life cycle*. Boston: Allyn & Bacon.

McGoldrick, M., & Gerson, R. (1989). Genograms and the family life cycle. In B. Carter & M. McGoldrick (Eds.), *The changing family life cycle: A framework for family therapy*. Boston: Allyn & Bacon.

Martin, D. A. (1988). Children and adolescents with traumatic brain injury: Impact on the family. *Journal of Learning Disabilities*, *21*(8), 464–470.

Minuchin, S. (1974). *Families and family therapy*. Cambridge, MA: Harvard University Press.

Oddy, M., Humphrey, M., & Uttley, D. (1978). Stresses upon the relatives of head-injured patients. *British Journal of Psychiatry*, *133*, 507–513.

Panting, A., & Merry, P. (1972). The long-term rehabilitation of severe head injuries with particular reference to the need for social and medical support for the patient's family. *Rehabilitation*, *38*, 33–37.

Prigatano, G. P., & Klonoff, P. S. (1988). Psychotherapy and neuropsychological assessment after brain injury. *Journal of Head Trauma Rehabilitation*, *3*(1), 45–56.

Roland, J. (1989). Chronic illness and the family life cycle. In B. Carter & M. McGoldrick (Eds.), *The changing family life cycle: A framework for family therapy*. Boston: Allyn & Bacon.

Romano, M.D. (1974). Family response to traumatic head injury. *Scandinavian Journal of Rehabilitation Medicine*, *6*, 1–4.

Rosenbaum, M., & Najenson, T. (1976). Changes in life patterns and symptoms of low moods as reported by wives of severely brain-injured soldiers. *Journal of Consulting & Clinical Psychology*, *44*(6), 881–888.

Satir, V. (1973). *Peoplemaking*. Palo Alto, CA: Science & Behavior Books.

Sternberg, R. J. (1986). A triangular theory of love. *Psychological Review*, *93*, 119–135.

Thomasen, I.V. (1974). The patient with severe head injury and his family—a follow-up of 50 families. *Scandinavian Journal of Rehabilitation Medicine*, *8*, 180–183.

Wegscheider, S. (1981). *Another chance: Hope and health for the alcoholic family*. Palo Alto, CA: Science & Behavior Books.

# VI

# Vocational Evaluation and Job-Oriented Rehabilitation

# 21

# Vocational Evaluation and Planning

## ROB ROBERTS

The individual with traumatic brain injury (TBI) is perhaps the most challenging client in terms of designing an appropriate, useful, and meaningful vocational evaluation. A primary reason for this difficulty is the change in cognitive, behavioral, and physical functioning that may take place as a result of a head injury (Musante, 1983). In addition, the occupational, social, and familial aspects of the person's life that are affected require the evaluator to be conscious of making recommendations that have long-term implications.

In order to address the vocational impact of TBI, this chapter will focus upon the vocational evaluation process, the testing instruments that are particularly useful in assessing persons with TBI, and program planning as it relates to reentry into the community. First, vocational evaluation is distinguished from neuropsychological evaluation in terms of process and outcomes of the evaluation. Second, the tools used in evaluation that appear the most appropriate for assessing adults with TBI are outlined. Finally, vocational planning for entry or reentry into the community is discussed based on the results of the evaluation and the placement strategies available to the rehabilitation counselor.

## THE VOCATIONAL EVALUATION PROCESS

Vocational evaluation may be defined according to the client population served and the setting in which the evaluation occurs (Pruitt, 1986). The staff of a vocational evaluation unit who work primarily with adults with mental retardation, for example, may define the purpose, instruments used, and outcomes differently from a unit that works with disadvantaged or physically handicapped populations. For purposes of this chapter, Power (1984) defines vocational assessment as a "comprehensive, intradisciplinary process of evaluating an individual's physical, mental, and emotional abilities, limitations, and tolerance in order

---

ROB ROBERTS • College of Education, Memphis State University, Memphis, Tennessee 38152.

*HANDBOOK OF HEAD TRAUMA: Acute Care to Recovery*, edited by Charles J. Long and Leslie K. Ross. Plenum Press, New York, 1992.

to identify an optimal outcome for the disabled or handicapped person" (p. xiv). Comprehensive refers to the fact that the evaluator incorporates medical, psychological, social, vocational, educational, cultural, and economic data within the total evaluation process (Pruitt, 1986). Intradisciplinary refers to the broad base of knowledge garnered from various disciplines called upon to interpret and synthesize test results.

Selection of the instruments to be administered is not arbitrary; it involves developing and writing a plan to structure the evaluation (CCWAVES, 1987). Perhaps the most unique aspect of vocational evaluation as practiced in the public sector is the individual's participation in the evaluation process, where the client, as consumer and participant, is expected to be involved in the planning and implementation of services (McAlees, 1990). Upon completion of testing, test data are interpreted and synthesized to assist the individual to understand work-related strengths and deficits, identify occupations consistent with the individual's interests and aptitudes, and decide upon the objectives necessary to achieve a specific vocational goal. Thus, vocational evaluation attempts to predict whether or not the person will be able to work as well as what type of work a person will be able to do (Power, 1984). Making these predictions requires a dynamic and interactive process that is client centered throughout.

Vocational evaluation usually occurs when it is determined by the referring person or agency that additional assessment is needed. Individuals with a disabling condition who apply to the state vocational rehabilitation agency (VR) receive an initial interview and screening by a rehabilitation counselor to determine eligibility. In the case of head injury, the individual usually applies for VR services between one and two years postinjury. Generally, the potential client decides to apply for services when he or she has experienced difficulty after returning to a former employment and/or the client and family decide that assistance is needed to identify and prepare for an alternate occupation. For persons with mild or moderate TBI, the need for VR services becomes evident when problems occur after return to work or return to a former occupation becomes difficult if not improbable (Corthell & Tooman, 1985; Musante, 1983). There is also evidence that even individuals who have experienced a minor concussion may experience cognitive or behavioral problems in social and work settings (Long & Novack, 1986; Wood, Novack, & Long, 1984).

In addition to the public sector rehabilitation programs, there are private rehabilitation facilities that specialize in comprehensive programs of therapy and treatment including evaluation and community placement. Since many private rehabilitation facilities specializing in head trauma offer comprehensive services, the individual and family may not always select public VR services. The southeast region, for example, includes the Atlanta Rehabilitation Institute, Lakeshore, Rebound, and Roosevelt Warm Springs. However, the average stay in acute care facilities is 90 to 120 days at an average cost of $575 per week (National Head Injury Foundation, 1988) and individuals without adequate medical insurance benefits to cover long-term treatment may look to the public rehabilitation sector for evaluation and job placement services.

Various factors impact upon the capacity of the adult with TBI to return to his or her former work (Kenig, Morse, Flaherty, Guzik, & Minassian, 1986). The individual's level of premorbid functioning, nature and severity of the injury, and age at onset influence the amount of recovery and postinjury adjustment and, ultimately, the client's vocational options. Typically, the vocational options that follow rehabilitation services fall along a continuum and include a highly structured day activity program, sheltered workshop, volunteer work, part time employment in a former or related occupation, or return to full time employment (with or without support) in the community. Along with attempting to maximize the individual's vocational potential are the programs and services needed to increase independent living. It is the task of the vocational evaluator to predict the client's potential, the services needed to eliminate or minimize attitudinal and physical barriers, and determine the capacity that the interests of the client are best served.

It becomes obvious that, to accurately predict the client's potential, the vocational evaluator must be able to integrate prior diagnostic information including medical and neuropsychological assessments with what is known about the client from the vocational assessment. The focus is on identifying the current and potential levels of vocational functioning and matching as broad a range of occupational alternatives as possible. In fact, the National Rehabilitation Association (1987) points out that vocational assessment of individuals with TBI should involve an analysis of abilities that are more global or generic as opposed to job specific, thereby focusing upon the individual's residual skills to increase work options.

Traditionally, the objective of neuropsychological assessment has differed substantively from that of vocational evaluation. For example, Kolb and Whishaw (1985) identify the goals of neuropsychological assessment as:

> . . . (a) diagnosis and localization of the presence of cortical damage or dysfunction, (b) facilitation of patient care as well as rehabilitation, (c) identification of unusual brain organization that may occur in left handers or in people with childhood brain injury, (d) localization of lesions, and (e) evaluation of deficits and outcome related to pharmacological treatment. (p. 672)

However, recent evidence in the literature suggests that the trend in neuropsychology is toward development of comprehensive test batteries designed to evaluate a range of neurologically mediated, higher cognitive functioning (Lewis & Sinnett, 1987). Much of the test data gathered in the neuropsychological examination center upon cognitive functioning (e.g., receptive and expressive language, attention and memory, sensory and perceptual functioning), whereas the vocational evaluation is apt to be more diverse in terms of the behaviors assessed (e.g., interest, aptitude). Also, vocational evaluation is more likely to be future work oriented in that the evaluator attempts to determine (a) whether or not the person can fulfill a vocational role and at what level, (b) the impact of disabilities upon the person's return to work, (c) if there are behaviors or emotional problems that may interfere with the person's ability to maintain work, (d) motivation toward work and/or rehabilitation, (e) any additional medical or physical limitations, (f) if the expressed job interests are realistic, and (g) the capacity for the person to benefit from a skills training program. In contrast, the goal of neuropsychological assessment is diagnosis aimed at understanding and changing behavior, with equal importance and attention placed upon the comprehensive assessment (Kolb & Whishaw, 1985).

## EVALUATION OF THE TBI REFERRAL

At the outset, there are several factors which should be considered prior to evaluation of persons with TBI (Corthell & Tooman, 1985). First is the individual's ability to participate in the evaluation process. Even a cursory review of the literature suggests that the range of impairments resulting from head injury and the capacity of the individual to return to a preinjury level of functioning are dependent upon the type of injury and course of recovery (Ben-Yishay, 1986; Long, Gouvier, & Cole, 1984; Musante, 1983). Therefore, the amount of residual functioning will play an important role in accurately assessing and predicting client behavior in other settings. Ben-Yishay (1986) has generated questions to be answered following head injury that may serve as a guide for the evaluator in analyzing the client's current vocational status and involve the ability to, or capability for:

1. Initiate and sustain mental acts to engage in purposive behaviors
2. Pay attention and concentrate
3. Muscular coordination, physical agility, and manual dexterity
4. Execute simple and complex perceptual–motor, visual, and visual–motor–spatial acts involved in all of the "practical" activities of everyday life
5. Memory functions (i.e., the ability to recall relevant information from past experiences, learn and to assimilate new information, and apply what has been learned appropriately, in specific situations)
6. Reasoning abilities (i.e., the various types of thinking, the capacity to form and exercise "good judgment," and the ability to engage in effective problem-solving activities in a manner fitting the particular circumstances of life)
7. Social communication skills, the various social and behavioral "repertoires," and the capacity to maintain previously established intimate relationships and/or personal friendships
8. Ego strength (i.e., how effectively can he/she absorb the tragedy of the head injury, how resilient is he/she emotionally, and to what extent can he/she bounce back with determination to overcome)
9. Malleability (i.e., what is his/her capacity to open up, to become influenced by and to respond to people's coaxing, encouragement, demands, and inspirations while undergoing rehabilitation)

Second, the evaluator should consider the purpose or reason(s) for conducting the evaluation. The questions which the referral source will want answered influence the duration of the evaluation and the tests to be administered. In the former case, a short-term evaluation may fail to uncover potentially significant deficits with the result that the final recommendations may be inappropriate or irrelevant. In the latter case, the selection of testing instruments, based on a clearly defined rationale and consideration of the client's needs, increases the likelihood that the evaluation is comprehensive and thorough enough to answer the referring person's questions and provide accurate measures of abilities.

Third, the evaluator should begin to generate initial hypotheses about the individual's potential to return to work. Analysis of the functional limitations, behavior, retention of preinjury skills, potential for acquiring needed skills, medical and psychoneurological diagnostic information, and evaluator knowledge of community resources and employment opportunities (Corthell & Tooman, 1985) will assist the evaluator in planning for, and individualizing, the evaluation.

Finally, the evaluation and testing should be structured not only to identify client strengths and limitations, but to learn if the client retains any skills which may be transferrable to other work settings and determine adaptations that have been made, or are necessary, to compensate for decreased functions (Long et al., 1984). The client's stamina during the testing may be an indicator of how easily he or she will become fatigued, at least initially, if placed in a job. Another important area for concern during evaluation are client behaviors as they relate to seeking and maintaining work, functioning in the community, and entering into social situations and settings. Appropriate social and interpersonal behaviors appear to be a significant factor in maintaining a job for individuals with disabilities (Wright, 1980). Further, the evaluator should attempt to include a specified period of situational assessment in order to assess the client's work behaviors and patterns. Included in the situational assessment are observation and measurement of productivity, attendance, reaction to supervision and co-workers, on/off task behaviors, frustration tolerance, persistence, dependability, and approach to and organization of work. Thus, information gained from a situational assessment can be useful in identifying behaviors that may interfere with gaining part or full time work as well as providing measurement of specific work behaviors.

The type of instruments used in vocational evaluation are important to the amount of useful information gained from the evaluation. The sensitivity of instruments to individuals with impaired cognitive, emotional, behavioral, motor, and physical functioning should be investigated (Kundu, 1988; Vander Kolk & Stewart, 1988). In addition, the head-injured adult differs from other disabled populations by not responding to traditional methods of vocational evaluation (Musante, 1983). The individual with TBI who is unaccustomed to difficulty with understanding social nuances, being a dependent adult, or adapting to a set of rules may invalidate evaluation results. The individual's state of readiness for evaluation, attitude toward testing and the rehabilitation process, medication, family support, and level of adjustment to the brain injury also potentially influence the outcome of evaluation.

In the course of planning and structuring the vocational evaluation, it becomes evident that numerous factors may impact upon attempts to predict outcome in terms of independent living and occupational alternatives. Howard and Sbordone (undated) have outlined a series of statements that may be used to address outcome following head injury and thus give the evaluator a fair estimate of overall potential:

1. Preinjury predictors
   a. History of general achievement of life goals, skills and attitudes
   b. Previous social skills and relationships
   c. History of learning disability
   d. Level of intelligence
   e. History of academic achievement
   f. Substance abuse and criminal history
   g. Nature of general character and self-control (appropriate/adjusted)
   h. Nature of the family system
   i. Emotional and personality characteristics
   j. Age at time of injury
   k. Similarity of pre- and postinjury vocational skills
   l. Presence of previous and/or later brain injuries
   m. History of stress management skills
2. Medical/neurological predictors
   a. Glasgow Coma Scale rating at time of initial admission of 7 or higher

    b.  Duration of coma less than 6 hours and posttraumatic amnesia less than 24 hours

    c.  Rate of recovery of functions and time lapsed since date of injury

    d.  Location of the primary brain damage (localized versus diffuse)

    e.  Secondary sources of brain damage (e.g., bleeding, infection)

    f.  Posttraumatic seizure disorder

    g.  Presence of depressed skull fracture

    h.  Dependence on medications

    i.  Abnormal EEG patterns

3. Behavioral predictors

    a.  Self-awareness of errors and behavioral deficits

    b.  Motivation and goal orientation in rehabilitation tasks

    c.  Persistence in rehabilitation tasks and activities

    d.  Ability to ambulate freely in the environment

    e.  Judgment and reasoning skills

    f.  Mental flexibility and shifting of attention

    g.  Sensory–motor skills

    h.  Level of independence in self-care skills

    i.  Self-initiation of tasks and activities

    j.  Concern and empathy for others' feelings

    k.  Success–failure ratio in daily living

    l.  Level of activity and agitation

    m.  Degree of recent memory deficit

    n.  Severity of catastrophic reaction

    o.  Optimism and positive attitude

    p.  Effectiveness of communication skills

    q.  Effectiveness of planning skills

    r.  Speed of thinking

4. Environmental predictors

    a.  Presence of a "key" person in the family

    b.  Involvement of family in treatment

    c.  Family support and acceptance

    d.  Family realistic about patient's deficits and outcome

    e.  Organization of the treatment team—interdisciplinary team treatment

    f.  Presence of a "key person" on the staff

    g.  Appropriateness of team goals to expected long-term outcome

    h.  Individual treatment plan

    i.  Continuity and coordination of entire rehabilitation process

    j.  Structure, consistency, and repetition in daily activities

    k.  Success in environmental interactions

    l.  Financial and insurance resources

    m.  Rewards for successful progress

    n.  Support groups and resources for family and patient

5. Other areas

    a.  Driving

    b.  Sexual behavior

    c.   Personal hygiene
    d.   Bowel and bladder continence
    e.   Safety
    f.   Independent living

## TESTS USED IN VOCATIONAL EVALUATION

The techniques that are used in vocational evaluation include (a) behavioral observations, (b) interviews, (c) psychometric tests (e.g., interest, personality, aptitude, achievement), (d) work samples (i.e., simulations of actual work), and (e) situational assessment. There are various recognized procedures for conducting testing according to the evaluation setting and population served (Power, 1984). Whatever the particular method, the availability of published testing products appears to address the evaluator's need for obtaining adequate test data for basing vocational decisions and recommendations. The testing equipment discussed in this section has been selected for review based on the capacity to aid in observation of performance and, at the same time, provide a measure of vocationally relevant behaviors of adults with TBI. It should also be noted that the appearance here of a certain test is not meant as an endorsement but, based on the author's experience, is indicative of the belief that is of particular value in assessing persons with traumatic head injury. Also, the instruments described herein are by no means an exhaustive listing of the range of psychometric tests or work samples.

It is important to emphasize, at the outset, that the use of a single test or measurement to examine one or more facets of a person's behavior should be, in the author's opinion, avoided in vocational evaluation. It is the usual practice for the evaluator to administer more than one test to measure a particular behavior (e.g., interest, aptitude, achievement). In the case of work performance, several units of a particular work sample system are often administered to obtain an overall picture of work patterns, skills, and aptitudes. Of equal importance is the client's participation through joint client–evaluator development of the evaluation plan (Rehabilitation Act, 1973). Client participation involves sharing decisions about what tests are to be administered, interpretation of test results (how the results affect client goals and what the client knows about him- or herself), and agreement upon a final vocational goal and recommendations related to the individual's vocational objective. The basic tools used by the evaluator include psychometrics, work samples, and, if available, a situational assessment.

## PSYCHOMETRICS

### Interest Inventories

*Career Occupational Preference System (COPS)*

The COPS (R. Knapp & Knapp, 1981) is designed as a brief inventory to assist with career guidance and decision making. Career information is presented by relating the individual's interests to 14 occupational clusters, several of which are subdivided into professional and skilled levels. There are 168 items containing descriptive statements about tasks performed in various jobs. Examinees respond by indicating the degree of like or dislike for each item (e.g., "like very much"). Examples of occupational clusters are Professional Science, Skilled Technology, and Communication. The COPS inventory may be used in conjunction with the Career Ability Placement System (CAPS; Knapp & Knapp, 1976), and the Career Orientation Placement and Evaluation Survey (COPES; Knapp & Knapp, 1978) to coordinate interests with the individual's aptitudes and values. The self-interpretation profile and guide is useful for career exploration and decision making by leading the individual toward selecting training and educational programs that match high-interest areas. The adult with TBI who does not retain at least a sixth to eighth grade reading level may have difficulty in completing the inventory. Alternate testing methods such as reading each item aloud to the examinee or using a prerecorded cassette tape may be used.

### Wide Range Interest–Opinion Test (WRIOT)

The WRIOT (Jastak & Jastak, 1979) inventories work interests by presenting sets of pictures or drawings of work-related activities. It consists of 450 pictures arranged in 150 combinations of three. The examinee selects two activities from each set of three drawings according to one which he or she perceives is most liked and one which is least liked. Additional scores are obtained to provide the evaluator with an estimate of the examinee's attitudes toward risk, ambition, motivation to work at demonstrated skill level, and sex stereotype. The WRIOT provides a measure of interest (T-Scores) for 18 occupational clusters (e.g., Art, Mechanics, Office Work, Social Service, Athletics). According to the authors, the initial normative group consisted of adolescent and adult males and females representing all levels of education and various occupations. The tested group consisted of minorities, rehabilitation clients, and individuals from the general population (Jastak & Jastak, 1979). Scoring templates labeled by sex and norm tables according to sex and age group are provided. The WRIOT may be modified by assisting the examinee with marking items if physical or speech restrictions interfere with self-administration. Descriptions of each of the pictured activities are also available if the examinee has questions concerning a particular drawing.

### Aptitude

### Career Ability Placement Survey (CAPS)

The CAPS (L. Knapp & Knapp, 1981) consists of eight, five-minute ability tests including Mechanical Reasoning, Spatial Relations, Verbal Reasoning, Numerical Reasoning, Language Usage, Word Knowledge, Perceptual Speed and Accuracy, and Manual Speed and Dexterity. Norms for the 1981 version of the CAPS were based on a national sample of approximately 6000 students from five geographical areas including both rural and urban samples and minorities. The tests are self-scoring which is useful when testing large groups. Raw scores are converted to stanines with aptitude for each occupational grouping determined by totaling the stanine score that is associated with a particular occupational group. Thus, it is possible to not score well on one or two subtests and still demonstrate potential for success in several occupational work groups. Since the CAPS uses the same 14 occupational clusters as the COPS, interest and aptitude scores may be compared on the profile forms to determine which work groups contain similarly high cumulative scores.

## Detroit Tests of Learning Aptitude-Second Edition (DTLA-2)

The DTLA-2 (Hammill, 1985) was designed for use with individuals ages 6 through 17-11 (Hammill, 1985) and contains 11 subtests. Based on the original work of Baker and Leland (1967), the DTLA-2 evolved from the concepts that aptitude and intelligence are closely related, that aptitude tests are built to sample behaviors common to all people in a society, and that aptitudes are generally acquired incidentally; a reference to the intrinsic capacity for future learning. The DTLA-2 was standardized with a sample of over 1500 individuals residing in 30 states. Raw scores may be converted into standard scores, percentile ranks, and age equivalencies. The subtests, and what each purports to measure, are shown in Table 21.1.

## Woodcock–Johnson Psycho-Educational Battery-Revised (WJ-R)

The WJ-R (Woodcock & Johnson, 1989) is designed to measure cognitive abilities, scholastic aptitudes, and achievement (Woodcock & Mather, 1989). The revised test battery consists of tests of standard (1–7 and 22–26) and supplemental batteries (8–21 and 31–35) for cognitive ability and tests of achievement, respectively. Tests of cognitive ability measure long-term retrieval, short-term memory, processing speed, auditory and visual processing, comprehension-knowledge, and fluid reasoning factors. Tests of achievement measure curricular areas including reading, mathematics, written language, knowledge (e.g., science), and skills (e.g., applied problems) and has two forms (Form A and Form B) matched in content.

The WJ-R has sufficient age range and content to be useful for educational or clinical purposes and from preschool to geriatric age levels (Woodcock & Mather, 1989). Current uses of the WJ-R include diagnosis of deficits in cognitive abilities and achievement, identifying discrepancies in aptitude/achievement, intracognitive, and intra-achievement, program placement, planning, evaluation, student guidance, and research. The tests may also be modified for individuals with hearing, visual, and physical impairments.

TABLE 21.1. Detroit Tests of Learning Aptitude, Second Edition: Description of Subtests

| Subtest | Measures |
|---|---|
| Word Opposites | Vocabulary; knowledge of antonyms |
| Sentence Imitation | Rote sequential memory; grammar |
| Oral Directions | Listening comprehension, short-term memory, and attention |
| Word Sequences | Short-term verbal memory and attention |
| Story Construction | Storytelling ability |
| Design Reproduction | Attention, manual dexterity, short-term visual memory, spatial relations |
| Object Sequences | Attention and visual short-term memory |
| Symbolic Relations | Problem solving and visual reasoning |
| Conceptual Matching | Ability to see theoretical or practical relationships between objects |
| Word Fragments | The ability to form closure and recognize partially presented familiar words |
| Letter Sequences | Short-term visual memory and attention |

## Work Samples

*Valpar Work Sample System*

The Valpar Component Work Sample Series is comprised of 16 individual units designed to simulate jobs found within the labor market. Each component is related to a group of jobs that reflect worker characteristics similar to those measured by the work sample. The individual is rated according to the length of time taken to complete the work sample and the number of errors made. Time and error scores are then compared to the appropriate norm group to determine a percentile rating which, in turn, indicates the person's potential for success within a certain job family.

There are several features of the Valpar that make it suitable for testing performance levels of adults with TBI. First, the work samples coincide with the worker traits (i.e., aptitudes) associated with each job found in the Dictionary of Occupational Titles (DOT). Thus, if the client performs at least at the 50th percentile (average level) on a particular unit, it may be assumed that he or she meets the minimum aptitudes for comparable jobs. Second, separate tables for each of eight norm groups are available for comparison of the client's scores. By comparing the client's scores to these standardization samples, the evaluator may determine which normative group best represents the current level of performance. In addition, since the normative groups appear hierarchical in relation to levels of independent living and vocational functioning, the evaluator may also estimate whether or not the individual's performance is near that of persons with entry level skills for jobs represented by the particular work sample. A brief description of each norm group is given below; the individual work sample components, measures, relationship to work performed, worker requirements, and occupations are provided in Table 21.2.

1. *Institutional Retarded—Sheltered Living*: moderate to severely retarded (FSIQ = 15–60), age 16–40, males and females, little opportunity for eventual placement in community.
2. *Institutional Retarded—Independent/Community Living*: mild to moderate retardation (FSIQ range of 40–78), age 16–40, males and females, eventually placed in the community.
3. *General Population—Disadvantaged*: mentally handicapped, physically disabled, youthful offenders and farm workers, age 16–60, males and females.
4. *San Diego Employed Workers*: males and females, employed in the community for a minimum of six months, age 18–60, jobs included sorter, machine operator, assembler, carpenter, fork lift operator, cashier, electronics assembler, secretary.
5. *Air Force*: male and female service personnel, maintained Air Force position for a minimum of six months to 20 years, age 18–42.
6. *Deaf*: students from school for the deaf, ranged from severe and profound congenitally deaf, high to low communication skills, age 16–20, males and females.
7. *Skill Center*: unemployed, low-income persons, age 16–55, males and females.
8. *Methods, Time, Motion (MTM)*: the MTM standardization process analyzes an individual's performance in terms of the basic motions required to perform it (Valpar, 1987). On the MTM scale, scores near the 100% level signify performance comparable to persons with entry level skills for jobs requiring that type of activity rather than a performance level demonstrated by a particular group of individuals.

## Comprehensive Batteries

*Apticom Aptitude Test*

The Apticom Aptitude Test was developed to assess vocational aptitudes, occupational interests, and work-related math and language skills and is appropriate for use in schools, rehabilitation, industry, and job training programs (Harris, Dansky, & Gannaway, 1985; Harris, Dansky, Zimmerman, & Gannaway, 1985). It is computer assisted and contains a series of plastic-coated panels, a dexterity board, and an answer probe which the examinee uses to select answers. The probe is also used as part of two dexterity tests. The three batteries consist of 11 aptitude tests, two achievement tests, and an interest inventory. With the exception of the interest inventory, each test is timed by an internal clock and includes a practice section. The evaluator controls the testing by moving various toggle switches in the back of the Apticom unit to start and stop individual tests, administer the aptitude, interest, achievement, and dexterity tests, and print out scores and individual reports. Individual scores are then matched against the jobs contained in the computer's memory bank and those that match are printed out in the final report. The evaluator may also select, and compare scores to, normative samples based on eighth through twelfth grade and adult. A standard error of measurement may be added automatically to each score.

According to Harris, Dansky, Zimmerman, and Gannaway (1985), the constructs used with the Apticom Aptitude Test Battery were adopted from the *Dictionary of Occupational Titles* (U. S. Department of Labor, 1977), *Handbook for Analyzing Jobs of Labor* (U. S. Department of Labor, 1972), and the *Guide for Occupational Exploration* (U. S. Department of Labor, 1979), and correspond to the definitions found in the General Aptitude Tests Battery (GATB; U.S. Department of Labor, 1982). The aptitude portion of the Apticom was standardized on unemployed persons referred by state employment offices in Canada and the United States. The population sampled ranged in age from 16 to 60 years and was compri... ...ional level of the sample was 11.8 years and ...re briefly defined and listed below.

**TABLE 21.2.** Valpar Work Sample Components

| Component | Measures |
|---|---|
| 1. Small Tools (Mechanical) | Understanding of and ability to work with small tools |
| | Work in a very small space using fingers and hands |
| 2. Size Discrimination | Ability to perform work tasks requiring visual size discrimination |
| 3. Numerical Sorting | Ability to use numbers and numerical series |
| 4. Upper Extremity Range of Motion | Upper extremity range of motion include the shoulder, upper arm, forcarm, elbow, wrist, and hand. |
| | Related factors include neck and back fatigue, finger dexterity, and finger tactile sense |
| | Two separate scoring procedures enable evaluator to record client reaction to muscular stress positions |
| 5. Clerical Comprehension and Aptitude | Ability to perform a variety of basic clerical tasks |
| | Aptitude to learn basic clerical tasks |
| 6. Independent Problem Solving | Ability to perform work tasks requiring visual comparison and selection of abstract designs |
| | Basic independent problem-solving ability |
| 7. Multi-Level Sorting | Make decisions while performing work tasks requiring physical manipulation and visual discrimination of color, color–number, color–letter, and a combination of color–letter–number |
| 8. Simulated Assembly | Ability to work at an assembly task requiring repetitive manipulation |
| | Bilateral use of upper extremities |
| 9. Whole Body Range of Motion | Agility of person's gross body movements of trunk, arms, hands, legs, and fingers |
| | A second scoring procedure records the person's physical reactions to muscular stress |
| 10. Tri-Level Measurement | Ability to perform very simple to very precise inspection and measurement tasks |
| 11. Eye–Hand–Foot Coordination | Ability to use eyes, hands, and feet simultaneously and in coordinated manner |

| Work performed | Work requirements | Occupations |
|---|---|---|
| 1. Fabricating, inspecting, repairing | Eye–hand coordination | Automobile mechanic |
| | Manual/finger dex... | Brake... |
| | Spat... | |

TABLE 21.2. (*Continued*)

| Work performed | Work requirements | Occupations |
|---|---|---|
| 5. Clerical tasks | Plan | Typist |
| | Follow instructions | Correspondence clerk |
| | Work under supervision | Records custodian |
| | Complete tasks according to priorities | File clerk |
| | | Library assistant |
| | Communicate effectively | Audit clerk |
| | Concentrate for long periods of time | Desk clerk |
| | | Timekeeper |
| | Detect errors | Shipping clerk |
| | Speed/accuracy | Office helper |
| 6. Carry out prescribed actions in relation to information | Understand, follow orders | Diet clerk |
| | Spatial/form perception | Kitchen food checker |
| | Eye–hand coordination | Shipping clerk |
| | Finger/manual dexterity | Office helper |
| | Work with standards | Counter clerk |
| | Adapt to a routine | Mail clerk |
| | Attention to detail | Food assembler |
| | Avoid errors | Review records |
| | | Parts inspector |
| | | Counter attendant |
| 7. Manual skills, apply knowledge related to materials, tools, and crafts | Meet prescribed standards | Laboratory tester |
| | Dextrous use of hands, tools | Photographer |
| | Operate machines/equipment | Parking meter collector |
| | Use persuasive techniques | Sales agent |
| | Provide personal services | Hair stylist |
| | | Photoengraver |
| 8. Placing/removing materials | Motor coordination | Duplicating machine operator |
| | Physical stamina | Dry-cleaner helper |
| | Follow instructions | Farmhand |
| | Finger/hand dexterity | Conveyor loader |
| | Enjoy routine/repetitive work | Line assembler |
| | Sustained attention to machine | Conveyor operator |
| 9. Physical performance | Stooping | Manipulating |
| | Kneeling | Feeding-offbearing |
| | Crouching | Investigating |
| | Reaching | Driving–operating |
| | Handling, feeling, seeing | Set up/operate machine |
| 10. Apply body of knowledge related to tools, materials, and crafts | Learn/apply craft techniques | Machinist |
| | Use independent judgment | Machine setup |
| | Attain prescribed standards | Injector assembler |
| | Apply shop mathematics | Tester, motors |
| | Perceive small differences | Brake inspector |
| | Attain prescribed tolerances | Plumber |
| | Work with hands | Maintenance repairer |
| | Manual/finger dexterity | Drafting |
| | Eye–hand coordination | |
| 11. Start, stop, observe functioning of machines | Understand machines | Laundry worker |
| | Eye–hand–foot coordination | Shoe repairer |
| | Spatial discrimination | Equipment operator |
| | Manual dexterity | Drill press operator |
| | Enjoy working with machines | Sewing machine worker |
| | Follow instructions | Sheet metal worker |
| | Atention to detail | Tow-truck operater |
| | Visual acuity | Forklift operator |
| | Physical stamina | Conveyor line operator |

*Exploration* (GOE; U. S. Department of Labor, 1979) and are further defined in terms of skills and experience levels. For example, OAP 01 (Artistic) includes 01.01 (Literary Arts) and 01.08 (Modeling) and OAP 06 includes 06.01 (Production Technology) and 06.03 (Quality Control). Within each OAP category are the job titles which pertain to that particular occupational category (e.g., editor).

The third battery, Educational Skills Development, provides measures of mathematical and language development. The range of problems in Mathematical Development include tasks ranging from adding and subtracting two-digit numbers to modern algebra and calculus. Language Development includes measures of ability to recognize two- and three-syllable words, reading (up to college level), and grammar.

In administering the Apticom to adults with TBI, the evaluator should be prepared to exercise some caution in interpreting the test results. Because of the reading level inherent in many of the word and math problems, individuals functioning at the lower end of academic achievement will have difficulty completing certain sections of the aptitude and education batteries. In addition, individuals with physical impairments in the upper and lower extremities will have difficulty manipulating the probe and performing the dexterity tests. Examinees whose aptitude and educational scores do not match their occupational interests or who have physical or academic impairments, are not likely to obtain a listing of job titles. The advantage in using the Apticom is that the evaluator may manipulate the data entry in terms of selecting or not selecting certain report options or omitting an entire battery (e.g., Interest), thereby obtaining a listing of jobs and data that may be compared with other evaluation results. However, reports generated in this manner should be interpreted with some caution and a note of this made to the referring counselor.

### McCarron–Dial System (MDS)

The MDS is used to assess the educational and vocational potential of the neuropsychologically disabled (ND) including mental retardation, cerebral palsy, brain trauma, and learning disabilities (McCarron & Dial, 1986). The MDS is based on a neuropsychological model which incorporates the traditional views of brain function as well as the concepts of Luria.

The MDS identifies five neuropsychological factors as predictive of vocational competency for the ND population: verbal–cognitive, sensory, motor, emotional, and integration–coping (behavior). Although McCarron and Dial (1986) report that an orthogonal factor analysis of the predictor data suggests that the five factors are actually three, a clearer picture of the factors being measured and instruments used is provided if the five factors are retained. The primary methods used to gather data include (a) case history to identify critical incidents; (b) behavioral observations or the observation and recording of critical behaviors including distractions, problems in following directions, low frustration tolerance, reluctance to attempt difficult or unfamiliar tasks, poor self-concept, difficulties in organization, poor sense and use of time, perceptual deficits, neuromotor deficits, poor response to criticism, defensiveness, impulsivity, propensity for depression, immature attention seeking, memory deficits, poor adaptability, attention problems, anxiety, poor social perception, inadequate or inappropriate social behavior; (c) standardized testing (e.g., WAIS, BVMGT); and (d) integration of functional levels, strengths, and deficits from which programming goals and intervention strategies may be identified.

the rehabilitation counselor assists the client to understand his or her diagnostic information including the vocational evaluation and how these results relate to developing appropriate vocational goals and objectives. In planning services to meet the individual's vocational objective, the counselor also estimates the time frames when the objectives should be met, along with the appropriate service providers. When considering the decreased physical, cognitive, and behavioral characteristics of adults with TBI (Price, 1986), it becomes clear that client-directed vocational planning must emphasize long-term case management and services appropriate to maintaining successful job placement. Indeed, as Price (1986) states, there is an increased concern among vocational evaluators regarding the need for extended evaluations and ongoing, repeated evaluations that focus on changes that may occur over time. Similarly, in planning the rehabilitation program, counselors are concerned with the factors that impact upon the client's adjustment to, and progress in, training programs and work settings. To do this, the counselor should become familiar with the standard battery of instruments used in neurological assessment in order to better understand test results and how the results may impact upon counselor–client decisions for employment training and placement. There are several models described in the literature that emphasize various components of the job placement process with adults with TBI. The approaches generally recognized as most useful for the TBI population are described in the next section.

## APPROACHES TO JOB PLACEMENT

Fraser (1988) has developed and revised a set of guidelines for job placement based on severity level and defined according to the percent of Halstead–Reitan tests outside normal limits. A key issue in job placement is the pattern of interpersonal deficits related to TBI that impact upon the selection of a job placement approach. Thus, a linear model was discarded in favor of a decision tree for which the severity and type of neuropsychological, employment, and emotional/interpersonal variables formed the basis for choosing a placement strategy. Often, failure to establish and maintain appropriate interpersonal relationships on the job with supervisors and co-workers is a primary reason for loss of employment among individuals with disabilities. Therefore, understanding the nature of the disabling condition as well as client assets and deficits is useful in deciding upon the type of support or intensity of intervention needed in job placement. The decision tree model as developed by Fraser is shown in Figure 21.1.

Fawber and Wachter (1987) have modified the traditional approach to vocational rehabilitation to include cognitive retraining and psychosocial services, involving a psychologist familiar with brain–behavior relationships and the VR process. A second component in placement is the place and train approach used in supported employment, in which the client is placed following vocational evaluation and then trained at the job site. This model emphasizes the need to provide supportive services throughout placement and long-term following after placement. Treatment aspects of the model include addressing cognitive and emotional needs of the client, awareness of the implications of skill deficits, and development of behaviors appropriate to the work site. Specific techniques include (a) task-specific training for a position prior to placement, (b) structured failure to increase the client's awareness of his or her strengths and weaknesses, (c) videotaped feedback sessions,

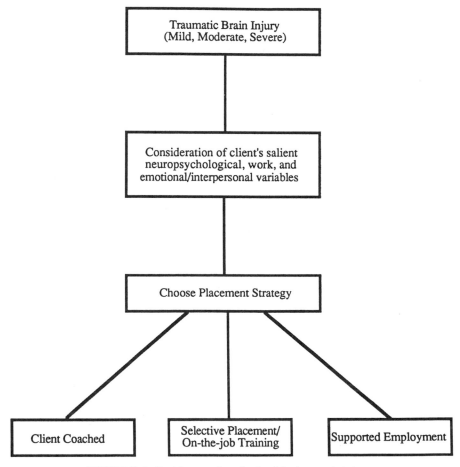

FIGURE 21.1. Decision tree for selecting job placement strategy.

(d) individualized and flexible training programs, (e) placement specialist or job coach, (f) employer education, (g) increasing job demands in small increments, and (h) increasing the client's skills toward competitive employment. Selectivity of job site, job analysis, placement site education and training, and family support relative to the client's cognitive, physical, and psychosocial strengths and deficits are also important considerations prior to placement.

Because the ability to generalize and maintain learning across settings is especially difficult for adults with TBI (Leland, Lewis, Hinman, & Carrillo, 1988), treatment and training programs need to focus on assisting the client to establish behavior changes beyond the rehabilitation setting. The particular strategy may differ but is generally identified as a functional approach (Cochran, undated; Herring,1988; Traphagan,1988). Leland *et al.* (1988) propose an integrated transdisciplinary team approach for retraining functional activities. Enhancing the generalization of skills involves (a) emphasizing the relevance of the skills to be learned, (b) incorporating important elements of the targeted environment into the learning setting (Ellis, 1965), (c) consistently reinforcing newly learned skills across persons and settings, and (d) teaching strategies for dealing with real world problems in real world settings (Kelly, 1982). The transdisciplinary team conducts an integrated evaluation and synthesizes assessment information from each discipline into a single plan that reflects realistic outcome goals, objectives, and treatment.

Another model which has been successful in placement efforts for adults with TBI is the supported work model (Wehman, Kreutzer, Wood, Morton, & Sherron, 1988). Supported employment merges behavior modification with physical medicine treatment for those with serious head injury (Wehman *et al.* 1988). Supported employment is defined in the *Federal Register* (1987) as follows:

> Paid employment in an integrated work setting for individuals who, because of their handicaps, need ongoing support to perform that work. Supported employment is limited to persons with severe handicaps for whom competitive employment has not traditionally occurred. It includes transitional employment for individuals with chronic mental illness.

It is perhaps obvious that the federal definition is limited since it does not address (a) the quality of the workplace, (b) level of wage or advancement, (c) the value or importance of the work performed, (d) access to public transportation, restaurants, or shops, and (e) whether or not the work is suited to the client. Therefore, O'Brien and Lyle (1987) have identified indicators of quality of life in considering supported employment options.

1. *Community presence*: sharing ordinary places that define community life such as car pools, breaks, and lunch.
2. *Choice*: experience of autonomy in everyday matters and in life-defining matters. The opportunity to choose from a selection of careers and programs.
3. *Competence*: opportunity to perform functional and meaningful activities with whatever level or type of assistance is required. Marketing individual capacity rather than disability to employers.
4. *Respect*: having a valued place among a network of people and valued roles in community life.
5. *Community participation*: experience of being part of a growing network of personal relationships that include close friends and a wide variety of people.

There are several models of supported employment that may be beneficial in assisting the adult with TBI to regain work experience and/or enter employment consistent with his or her abilities. The Supported Employment Training Project at the University of Kentucky (1989) provides a brief description of each model in a recently published training manual.

1. *Enclave*: a group of up to eight people with disabilities and a full-time supervisor who work in a community business. The supervisor and/or workers with disabilities may be employed by either the participating business or the supported employment program that facilitated the placement.
2. *Mobile Work Crew*: a group of eight people with disabilities and a full-time supervisor (employed by the supported employment program) who travel together to work sites in the community. They perform contract work for community businesses.
3. *Benchwork*: a group of up to eight people who work in a private business (typically

owned by the supported employment program) that produces goods on a subcontract basis or as a prime manufacturer. The business also employs an unspecified number of persons who do not have disabilities.

4. *Job Coach*: an individual with a disability is hired by a community business and receives one-to-one training support from a job coach. The job coach is employed by the supported employment program and initially provides full-time support. The job coach's intervention decreases as the worker's independence increases, although long-term follow-up is provided.

## STRATEGIES IN THE WORKPLACE

Strategies that may be used to increase the likelihood that placement will be successful are important to the rehabilitation specialist working with the adult with TBI. While head injury does not necessarily preclude employment, return to employment in a previously held job may be unrealistic because ability levels may no longer be sufficient to fulfill the job demands (Fraser, Dikman, McLean, Miller, & Temkin, 1988). Research suggests that there are various interventions available for working with the adult with TBI in the employment setting. For example, Vieceli (1986) discusses some basic strategies according to cognitive, executive, physical, psychosocial, and communication deficits, which are given in Table 21.4.

Cohen (1985) also describes training methods that are useful in working with individuals with severe brain damage. In addition to understanding the client's problems stemming from TBI, Cohen addresses several dimensions related to assessing TBI prior to training, including quality of work, work speed, level of assistance required, basic work skills, orientation to time, attitudes to work and colleagues, appearance, and vocational range. His specific model includes the strategies outlined in Table 21.5.

Research over the past six years indicates that treatment strategies have been designed not only for training (Lynch, 1984), but are oriented to the professional working with, and the employer who hires, adults with TBI (Dense, Deboskey, Burton, Cook, Lowe, McHenry, & Morin, 1987). Lynch (1984) describes various strategies of treatment involved in teaching a work task involving:

a. *Simplification*: reducing the requirements of a task to a level at which the patient can perform adequately; gradually increasing the complexity of the task as the patient masters each increment of difficulty.

b. *Amplification*: enhancement of a stimulus in order to ensure timely and accurate reception by the patient. Highlighting or emphasizing subtle cues (e.g., bright red tags in left page so patient will attend), louder auditory or more vivid visual inputs for arousal.

c. *Feedback*: provides regulatory information to individual at the time a task is performed. Should be continuous and immediate. Involves constructive criticism and words of encouragement, videotaping.

d. *Substitution*: substituting one intact system or behavioral ability for another. Using different set of muscles or different sequences of movements.

e. *Redundancy*: repetition for perceptual–motor skills training, memory retraining,

TABLE 21.4. Vocational Rehabilitation Strategies

| Category | Deficit | Strategies |
|----------|---------|------------|
| Cognitive | Memory impairment | Daily recording system |
| | | Job modification to "routinize" daily tasks |
| | | Educating the employer and co-workers about memory deficits, susceptibility to distractions, inability to perform simple tasks, lengthiness of training, retraining, or on-the-job training needed to learn and internalize a new routine, use of visual prompts and physical cues |
| | Attentional deficits | Short training periods |
| | | Concise and brief directions or checklists |
| | | Reinforcement |
| Executive | Disorganization | Organize task into blocks of related activites |
| | Poor work quality | Use of checklists to monitor quality |
| Physical | Motor impairment | Physical repositioning |
| | | Adapted work stations |
| | | Orthotic devices |
| | | Consult with physical or occupational therapist |
| | Sensory impairment | Quiet, uncluttered, well-lighted work environment |
| | Questionable safety | Moderate climate in work environment |
| | | Avoid placement around hazardous machinery |
| | | Monitor level of stress |
| Psychosocial | Inappropriate behavior | Consider simulated work environment or sheltered work setting to address problems initially |
| | | Self-monitoring strategies, videotaping |
| | | Supportive counseling |
| Communication | Speech/language deficits | Speech/language pathologists |
| | | Communication devices or techniques for nonverbal clients |

TABLE 21.5. Training Methods for Individuals with Severe TBI

| Problem/deficit | Intervention |
|-----------------|--------------|
| Skills/habits | Environmental design: use of special devices, eliminate distractions, reminders |
| | Practice and rehearsal |
| | Modeling reinforcement, feedback, and monitoring |
| Comprehension | Task analysis |
| | Information processing through alternate systems |
| Memory | Use of note pad, repetition of information |
| | Use of multiple, active and passive, verbal and written information systems |
| Awareness | Group discussions |
| Expectations | Problem-solving techniques, brainstorming, reality testing |
| Depression | Empathy, acceptance, encouraging a sense of hope |
| | Cognitive restructuring to change interpretation of reality |
| | Increasing rate and strength of reinforcing events in patient's life |
| Interpersonal | Instructions, modeling, and role play |
| Fatigue | Testing for best time interval for working |
| | Improving sleeping habits |
| | Elimination of drug intake |

speech or language therapy. Enhance development of more automatic performance of motor, cognitive, or speech skills.

f. *Family involvement in treatment and conferences.*
g. *Development of outcome measures and follow-up.*

Dense *et al.* (1987) have developed practitioner-oriented strategies for coping with the personal reactions to persons with brain injury that stem from the frustration, anger, or helplessness felt in working with severely disabled individuals. First, practitioners may need to resolve unrealistic expectations by becoming informed on the topic, studying the work of others, and identifying one's own unrealistic expectations. Second, reducing frustration may occur by reassessing the validity of our expectations, reexamining goals for client, identifying the most frustrating tasks to practitioner and client, identifying and discriminating behaviors that can be changed or modified from those that cannot, and designing and implementing behavior management strategies for behavior that can be changed. Third, interventions to manage anger may be implemented, including identifying unrealistic expectations, goals, tasks, and behaviors that are the greatest source of anger; using humor and covert, positive self-talk; using assertive not aggressive communication; and enlisting another person's help in problem solving. In addition to the above are feelings of helplessness and guilt for which the practitioner might design instruction, with which successful outcomes are most likely, consult a colleague for alternate ways to help, and learn from one's own mistakes.

## SUMMARY

Evaluation of, and planning, rehabilitation services with adults with TBI presents a unique opportunity for the vocational evaluator and rehabilitation counselor to develop and implement assessment and service delivery options. The vocational evaluator should be cognizant of testing instruments that are sensitive to the TBI population and provide information that is useful in assisting the client to make realistic vocational choices. A working knowledge of neuropsychological instruments is necessary for understanding cognitive deficits resulting from the injury and estimating residual skills. In decisions regarding selection of evaluation instruments, attention should be given to those that provide a measure of vocational strengths. Situational assessment may be used to evaluate actual work behaviors that could impact upon job seeking and job retention. Decisions pertaining to intervention, job training and placement are based on integration of the results of neurological assessment and the vocational evaluation.

The rehabilitation counselor is primarily responsible for planning rehabilitation services that incorporate assessment information needed to identify services consistent with the individual's abilities and vocational objectives. Placement decisions based on the client's residual skills may include sheltered employment, part- and full-time employment, or a combination of supported and community employment options. The literature suggests that various models and interventions are appropriate for training and job placement and may be successfully applied to modify or adjust for the cognitive, behavioral, and social deficits common to persons with mild and moderate head injury. Finally, there is increasing evidence in the literature to indicate that rehabilitation practitioners should be receiving specialized training in in-service education programs (Farish, 1988; McMahon, Shaw, & Mahaffey, 1988). In addition, students in rehabilitation education or counseling programs can receive the necessary knowledge and experience, to intervene more effectively and efficiently in treatment programs, by enrolling in introductory neuropsychology courses and requesting specialized practicum in head trauma facilities.

## REFERENCES

Alcazaren, E. (1988). Medical and rehabilitation aspects in traumatic brain injury. *Rehabilitation Education*, *2*(3/4), 165–170.

Baker, H., & Leland, B. (1967). *Detroit tests of learning aptitude: Examiner's handbook*. Indianapolis, IN: Bobbs-Merrill.

Ben-Yishay, Y. (1986). The role of clinical neuropsychology in the diagnosis and rehabilitation of the head injured person. *Head injury: Help, hope and information*. New York City: New York State Head Injury Association, Inc.

Cochran, W. (undated). *Rehabilitation of the traumatically head injured*. Hot Springs: University of Arkansas, Regional Rehabilitation Continuing Education Program.

Cohen, J. (1985). Vocational rehabilitation of the severely brain damaged patient: Stages and processes. *Journal of Applied Rehabilitation Counseling*, *16*(4), 25–30.

Commission on Certification of Work Adjustment and Vocational Evaluation Specialists (CCWAVES). (1987). *Standards and procedures manual for certification in vocational evaluation*. Arlington Heights, IL: Author.

Corthell, D., & Tooman, M. (1985). *Rehabilitation of traumatic brain injury (TBI)*. Menomonie: University of Wisconsin–Stout, Stout Vocational Rehabilitation Institute.

Dense, C., Deboskey, D., Burton, J., Cook, C., Lowe, L., McHenry, D., & Morin, K. (1987). *Teaching the head injured: What to expect*. Tampa, FL: Tampa General Rehabilitation Center.

Dunn, D. (1973). *Situational assessment: Models for the future*. Menomonie, WI: Materials Development Center.

Ellis, H. (1965). *The transfer of learning*. New York: Macmillan Co.

Farish, J. (1988). Emphasizing traumatic brain injury in rehabilitation counselor training programs. *Rehabilitation Education*, *2*(3/4), 237–244.

Fawber, H., & Wachter, J. (1987). Job placement as a treatment component of the vocational rehabilitation process. *Journal of Head Trauma Rehabilitation*, *2*(1), 27–33.

*Federal Register*. (1987, August). The state supported employment services program; final regulations, p. 30551. Washington, DC: U.S. Government Printing Office.

Fewell, S. (1989, March). Situational assessment in an integrated setting for survivors of traumatic head injury. *The issues papers: Fourth national forum on issues in vocational assessment*, St. Louis, MO.

Fraser, R. (1988). Refinement of a decision tree in traumatic brain injury job placement. *Rehabilitation Education*, *2*(3/4), 179–184.

Fraser, R., Dikman, S., McLean, A., Miller, B., & Temkin, N. (1988). Employability of head injury survivors: First year post-injury. *Rehabilitation Counseling Bulletin*, *31*(4), 276–288.

Hammill, D. (1985). *Detroit tests of learning aptitude—2*. Austin, TX: Pro-Ed.

Harris, J., Dansky, H., & Gannaway, T. (1985). *Apticom: System operation, administration, and scoring manual*. Philadelphia, PA: Vocational Research Institute, Jewish Employment and Vocational Service.

Harris, J., Dansky, H., Zimmerman, B., & Gannaway, T. (1985). *Apticom: System technical manual*. Philadelphia, PA: Vocational Research Institute, Jewish Employment and Vocational Service.

Herring, S. (1988). Cognitive and psychosocial complications following traumatic brain injury (TBI). *Rehabilitation Education*, *2*(3/4), 171–177.

Howard, M., & Sbordone, R. (undated). *Outcome from head injury*. Bradenton, FL: The Center at Manatee Springs.

Jastak, J., & Jastak, S. (1979). *Wide range interest–opinion test*. Wilmington, DE: Jastak Associates, Inc.

Kelly, J. (1982). *Social skills training*. Berlin: Springer.

Kenig, J., Morse, A., Flaherty, M., Guzik, J., & Minassian, R. (1986). Neuranatomical considerations in brain injury. In P. Morse (Ed.), *Brain injury: Cognitive and prevocational approaches to rehabilitation*. New York: The Tiresias Press.

Knapp, L., & Knapp, R. (1976). *Career ability placement survey (CAPS)*. San Diego: Educational and Industrial Testing Service (EdiTS).

Knapp, L., & Knapp, R. (1981). *Career ability placement survey (CAPS) manual*. San Diego: Educational and Industrial Testing Service (EdiTS).

Knapp, R., & Knapp, L. (1978). *Career orientation placement and evaluation survey (COPES)*. San Diego: Educational and Industrial Testing Service (EdiTS).

Knapp, R., & Knapp, L. (1981). *Career occupational preference system manual*. San Diego: Educational and Industrial Testing Service (EdiTS).

Kolb, B., & Whishaw, I. (1985). *Human neuropsychology*. San Francisco: Freeman.

Kundu, M. (1988). Guest editor's introduction. Approaches to traumatic brain injury. Special issue. *Rehabilitation Education*, 2(3/4), 159–162.

Leland, M., Lewis, F., Hinman, S., & Carrillo, R. (1988). Functional retraining of traumatically brain injured adults in a transdisciplinary environment. *Rehabilitation Education*, 31(4), 289–297.

Lewis, L., & Sinnett, R. (1987). An introduction to neuropsychological assessment. *Journal of Counseling & Development*, 66(2), 126–130.

Long, C., & Novack, T. (1986). Postconcussion symptoms after head trauma: Interpretation and treatment. *Southern Medical Journal*, 79(6), 728–732.

Long, C., Gouvier, W., & Cole, J. (1984). A model of recovery for the total rehabilitation of individuals with head trauma. *Journal of Rehabilitation*, 50(1), 39–45, 70.

Lynch, W. (1984). A rehabilitation program for brain-injured adults. In B. Edelstein & E. Couture (Eds.), *Behavioral assessment and rehabilitation of the traumatically brain-damaged*. New York: Plenum Press.

McAlees, D. (1990). New directions for rehabilitation facilities. *Vocational Evaluation & Work Adjustment Bulletin*, 23(1), 25–30.

McCarron, L., & Dial, J. (1986). *McCarron–Dial evaluation system: A systematic approach to vocational, educational, and neuropsychological assessment*. Dallas, TX: McCarron–Dial Systems.

McMahon, B., Shaw, L., & Mahaffey, D. (1988). Career opportunities and professional preparation in head injury rehabilitation. *Rehabilitation Counseling Bulletin*, 31(4), 344–354.

Musante, S. (1983). Issues relevant to the vocational evaluation of the traumatically head injured client. *Vocational Evaluation & Work Adjustment Bulletin*, 16(2), 45–49, 68.

National Head Injury Foundation. (1988, January). *The role of NHIF in rehabilitation and public policy*. Paper presented at the meeting of the Regional Traumatic Brain Injury Conference, Atlanta, GA.

National Rehabilitation Association. (1987). *The traumatically brain injured*. Washington, DC: Author, Institute on Rehabilitation Issues.

O'Brien, J., & Lyle, C. (1987). *Framework for accomplishment: A workshop for people developing better services*. Decator, GA: Responsive Systems Associates.

Power, P. (1984). *A guide to vocational assessment*. Austin, TX: Pro-Ed.

Price, P. (1986). Facilitating client-directed vocational planning in head injured adults. *Vocational Evaluation & Work Adjustment Bulletin*, 19(3), 117–119.

Pruitt, W. (1986). *Vocational evaluation*. Menomonie, WI: Walt Pruitt Associates.

Traphagan, J. (1988). *Community re-entry*. Southborough, MA: National Head Injury Foundation.

U.S. Department of Labor, Employment and Training Administration. (1977). *Dictionary of occupational titles* (4th ed.). Washington, DC: U.S. Government Printing Office.

U.S. Department of Labor, Employment and Training Administration. (1979). *Guide for occupational exploration*. Washington, DC: U.S. Government Printing Office.

U.S. Department of Labor, Employment and Training Administration. (1982). *Manual for the USES general aptitude test battery. Section 1: Administration and scoring (Forms A and B)*. Washington, DC: U.S. Government Printing Office.

U.S. Department of Labor, Manpower Administration. (1972). *Handbook for analyzing jobs*. Washington, DC: U.S. Government Printing Office.

Valpar International Corporation. (1987). *Evaluator's handbook: Instructions and normative data*. Tucson, AZ: Author.

Vander Kolk, C., & Stewart, W. (1988). Characteristics of and intervention for persons with minor traumatic head injury. *Rehabilitation Education*, 2(3/4), 213–219.

Vieceli, B. (1986). *A sampling of vocational rehabilitation strategies for the traumatically head injured client.* Southborough, MA: National Head Injury Foundation.

Wehman, P., Kreutzer, J., Wood, W., Morton, M., & Sherron, P. (1988). Supported work model for persons with traumatic brain injury: Toward job placement and retention. *Rehabilitation Counseling Bulletin, 31*(4), 298–312.

Wood, F., Novack, T., & Long, C. (1984). Post-concussion symptoms: Cognitive, emotional, and environmental aspects. *International Journal of Psychiatry in Medicine, 14*(4), 277–283.

Woodcock, R., & Johnson, M. (1989). *Woodcock–Johnson Psycho-Educational Battery-revised.* Allen, TX: DLM Teaching Resources.

Woodcock, R., & Mather, N. (1989). WJ-R tests of achievement: Examiner's manual. In R. W. Woodcock & M. B. Johnson (Eds.), *Woodcock–Johnson Psycho-Educational Battery-revised.* Allen, TX: DLM Teaching Resources.

Wright, G. (1980). *Total rehabilitation.* Boston: Little, Brown.

# 22

# Job-Oriented Rehabilitation

## MICHAEL McCUE

Severe head injury typically results in a number of physical, cognitive, and emotional limitations. Most commonly, problems such as impulsivity, the inability to learn effectively, remember new information, and control behavior, as well as a lack of self-awareness are found in persons who have sustained severe head injury. In addition, depending upon the nature and location of the injury, a myriad of other limitations may occur (e.g., hemiparesis, emotional lability and affective disturbances, perceptual difficulties, and language problems). Because of the broad nature and severity of problems associated with traumatic brain injury (TBI), vocational rehabilitation with this population is difficult (Ben-Yishay, Silver, Piasetsky, & Rattok, 1987; Brinkley, 1989; Brooks, McKinlay, Symington, Beattie, & Campsie, 1987; Kreutzer, Wehman, Morton, & Stonnington, 1988).

Studies which have attempted to address the vocational outcome of TBI have produced varied findings. Kay, Ezrachi, and Cavallo (1988) reviewed and reported on 37 studies which examined vocational outcome of persons with TBI. These studies spanned a 40-year period from 1945 to 1985. Of those studies reporting at least a one-year follow-up, employment rates ranged from 20% to 96%. Unfortunately, the lack of standardized methodology prevents drawing conclusions from this pool of literature. Design difficulties include variability in the range of head injury severity among samples, the lack of a uniform criterion for "return to work," the lack of verification of work performance status, and the absence of reliable and standardized follow-up periods (Ben-Yishay *et al.*, 1987).

Despite the divergent findings reported, it appears that severely head-injured persons demonstrate a poor likelihood of becoming employed, and an even poorer prognosis for successfully returning to their previous jobs (Brinkley, 1989; Brooks *et al.*, 1987; Fraser, Dikmen, McLean, Miller, & Temkin, 1988; Oddy, Coughlan, Tyerman, & Jenkins, 1985). Of those who do return to work, a majority continue to report difficulties related to their head injuries that jeopardize job maintenance (Fraser *et al.*, 1988).

---

MICHAEL McCUE • Behavioral Neuropsychology Associates, Pittsburgh, Pennsylvania 15222.

*HANDBOOK OF HEAD TRAUMA: Acute Care to Recovery*, edited by Charles J. Long and Leslie K. Ross. Plenum Press, New York, 1992.

## CRITICAL FACTORS INFLUENCING SUCCESSFUL RETURN TO WORK

Before beginning a discussion of recommended service components for vocational rehabilitation of TBI, several internal and external factors influential in successful job-oriented rehabilitation are worth noting. Given the breadth of potential presentations of TBI in individuals, internal factors which mediate successful outcome can be quite varied, though a few seem to stand out as very important. One key factor is accurate appraisal of strengths and functional limitations, or insight. Related to this is the ability to see how deficits might impact work performance and the ability to self-monitor performance accuracy and rate. Self-awareness is also required for the individual to actively deal with workplace performance problems, including accepting accommodations and modifications in work approaches or demands.

Prigatano (1989) reports that unawareness of deficit is the factor most responsible for vocational failure in persons who have sustained TBI. The unawareness syndrome is difficult to treat. The problem of inaccurate self-appraisal should be approached from an educational and experiential perspective, with a realization that noticeable change may take a long time. Individuals should be provided with accurate, straightforward information about their functional strengths and weaknesses, as these relate to their everyday and work experiences. Group feedback and videotape playback and discussion may be somewhat effective in providing this feedback. Individuals should also have the opportunity to experience the natural consequences of their behavior as a means of shaping their accurate appraisal of their skills and limitations. These persons may have to fail at a job, or jobs, before the level of awareness of their abilities becomes more consistent with their actual functional capacities.

A second key internal factor is adequate behavioral control. Impulsivity, inappropriate verbalizations, poor social skills, and perseverative behaviors, even if relatively subtle, can have a detrimental effect on successful workplace integration. Positive response to behavioral treatment approaches is likely to enhance employability. Critical to the development of effective behavior management programming is the identification of a unique and meaningful set of reinforcers for each individual (Killiam, Diambra & Fry, 1990).

While it is well established that substance abuse is a significant risk factor for TBI (Field, 1976), difficulties associated with substance abuse also seriously jeopardize vocational outcome post-TBI. Wehman and Goodall (1990) recommend comprehensive screening for, and treatment of, current substance abuse prior to involvement in job-oriented rehabilitation.

Physical communication and mobility impairments, which may be associated with TBI, may present significant vocational handicaps in this population. Persons who present with "visible" communication and/or mobility handicaps are unlikely to benefit from the development of job options which circumvent these problems. The types of vocational positions relied upon as options with non-brain-damaged, physically handicapped individuals often require intact cognitive skills and are, therefore, often inappropriate for the TBI survivor. Thus, the presence of language communication and mobility problems may compound the cognitive and behavioral problems associated with TBI and make vocational integration more difficult.

Finally, affective disturbances, depression in particular, influence employability. This is compounded in persons who demonstrate "adynamia" or difficulty in mobilizing energy to initiate and complete a task or engage in an activity. Adynamia is thought to be a biological condition of underarousal which undermines involvement in rehabilitation efforts. In persons with this presentation, efforts must be made to energize the individual toward active participation in rehabilitation. Ben-Yishay and his colleagues have developed group treatment interventions that have been shown to be effective in confronting adynamia (Ben-Yishay, Diller, & Rattok, 1978).

External factors, or environmental influences, also impact the individual's potential to successfully return to work. Flexibility on the part of the employer to allow for modified scheduling, gradual immersion into the work responsibilities, and support from supervisors and staff are critical. Sometimes this flexibility and support is available from the onset, while in other cases, support and modifications may have to be advocated for and negotiated by the client and rehabilitation staff. Regardless, this flexibility and potential for support is absolutely essential to the reintegration of workers who have sustained TBI.

Another external factor includes the availability of resources for providing support on the job (perhaps for a brief period of tooling up or developing accommodation strategies) and in the living environment, because disruption outside of the workplace can have devastating effects on the individual's abilities at work.

A third important factor is family involvement. It is not sufficient to obtain the passive support of the family for the return to work. The family must be actively involved in the process. Assisting in the job search, designing accommodations and modifications, and trouble-shooting or problem solving are examples of ways in which families can be proactively involved in resumption of the worker role by TBI survivors.

The factors listed above are those that seem to influence the employability of many of the individuals who have sustained TBI. However, for each individual, a unique set of factors is likely to determine employability and treatment approaches. Individualized, functionally oriented assessment is required to determine the factors which may influence each person's successful rehabilitation in the workplace.

## PROGRAMMATIC RECOMMENDATIONS
## FOR JOB-ORIENTED REHABILITATION

Without specialized, comprehensive, long-term services targeted to vocational rehabilitation, successful reintegration into the workplace is unlikely. The remainder of this chapter will present programmatic recommendations for comprehensive job-oriented rehabilitation with persons who have sustained TBI. Information will be presented on assessment for vocational rehabilitation, vocational rehabilitation planning, pre-vocational treatment strategies, and employment options, including supported work. In the process of job-oriented rehabilitation, these strategies do not exist along a linear continuum. Rather, the ideal process is one where assessment and treatment are ultimately carried out in the work environment, through one or more employment options. Figure 22.1 illustrates the process of job-oriented rehabilitation. The following is a description of the various components in the vocational rehabilitation of TBI.

## ASSESSMENT FOR VOCATIONAL REHABILITATION

Central to the task of providing rehabilitation services to an individual with TBI is obtaining a clear understanding of how the disability impairs or impedes vocational and

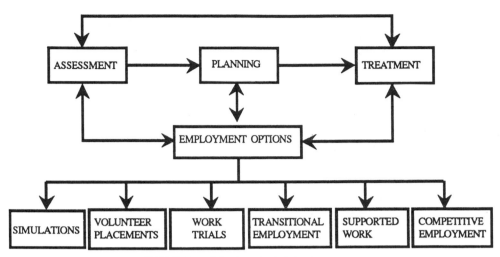

FIGURE 22.1. Job-oriented rehabilitation process.

independent living functioning. Unlike physical disabilities, the cognitive manifestations of disability are not easily quantified and the impact of specific cognitive deficits is difficult to ascertain. Obtaining functionally useful information in the vocational rehabilitation process is optimally done by observing individuals in their natural environment. However, the feasibility of doing this early in the rehabilitation process is quite limited. Often, it is very difficult to identify a vocational objective or evaluate the client in the natural environment during early phases of rehabilitation with clients with severe disabilities. Given both the nature and severity of deficits associated with TBI, assessment for vocational rehabilitation is more realistically defined as a process of ongoing information gathering using all methods and findings toward the objective of identifying functional capabilities. Further, this assessment should involve predictions about how these capabilities will be manifested in the independent living, work, or training environments.

Traditional approaches to assessment of this population (e.g., neuropsychological assessment) are effective in identifying the broad range of deficits which may result from a TBI. However, these approaches may not be effective in detailing how these deficits might interact with task and environmental demands to impact the individual's functioning in real life situations (Cicerone & Tupper, 1990). In fact, results of psychological assessment procedures can be quite misrepresentative of an individual's actual functional level (Naugle & Chelune, 1990). Therefore, a combination of assessment approaches which target real life functioning is required for vocational rehabilitation purposes, including clinical interviews, neuropsychological assessment, functional behavioral assessment, and vocational evaluation. Detailed job analysis to identify the specific environmental demands, which the person will encounter at work, is also critical. The overall purpose of the evaluation is to document the specific cognitive, behavioral, physical, and emotional deficits which present as obstacles to meeting everyday functioning and work demands. A highly individualized rehabilitation approach for each client may then be developed.

## Vocational Interviewing

The initial vocational rehabilitation contact with the client is typically in the form of a clinical interview. A history is taken which includes information on the nature of the brain injury, the client's perception of his/her deficits, medical history, educational and vocational background, social and family history, support systems, and previous rehabilitation experiences. Interviews with significant others in the client's environment, preferably a family member, should also be performed. This is to validate details relating to the client's injury and premorbid history, and to obtain an observer's perspective of the client's current functional abilities. It may be necessary to interview a number of individuals to assure the collection of all pertinent information. Interviewing the client's previous employer or supervisor will also provide critical information regarding premorbid vocational competencies, demands that will face the client upon return to work, and the potential for support, flexibility, and/or modifications in the client's position upon return.

Careful review of medical and rehabilitation records should also be undertaken to obtain information such as medication and medical complications (e.g., seizures, persistent headaches, sensory and motor impairment). These factors may have important safety ramifications for work. Review of previous rehabilitation approaches which were either successful or unsuccessful may also provide clues about which approaches will be effective in the work setting.

Clinical vocational interviewing and record review provides an initial working knowledge of the client and a basis for gathering functional information. Despite concerns regarding the validity of client self-appraisal and self-report, the initial source of information about what a client can or cannot do should always be that individual's description. Subsequent information gathered in the rehabilitation process can be used to build upon that initial data base, and validate that information, if necessary.

## Neuropsychological Assessment

A comprehensive battery of psychological and neuropsychological tests should be administered to rehabilitation clients as they approach vocational integration (or reintegration) to address cognitive, perceptual, language, motor, and behavioral characteristics. However, in using neuropsychological assessment to identify functional and vocation abilities, one must examine the validity of this application of these assessment approaches. There is evidence that a significant relationship exists between results of neuropsychological assessment and vocational functioning in neuropsychiatrically disabled individuals (Dennerll, Rodin, Gonzalez, Schwartz, & Lin, 1966; DeTurk, 1975; Dikmen & Morgan, 1980; Heaton, Chelune, & Lehman, 1978; Mackworth, Mackworth, & Cope, 1982; Morris, Ryan, & Peterson, 1982; Newnan, Heaton, & Lehman, 1978; Schwartz, Dennerll, & Lin, 1968).

With respect to planning, neuropsychological assessment may yield information on such topics as identification of a rehabilitation goal, delineation of remedial or rehabilitative strategies that are required and the degree to which these are required for a particular objective, compensatory and/or accommodation strategies which might be used in overcoming deficits, identification of areas in need of skill development (e.g., social skills), therapeutic or counseling needs, and specific vocational training or placement needs.

Clinical hypotheses or predictions about real world competencies posed on the basis of neuropsychological tests require knowledge and expertise in three areas:

1. A clear, clinical knowledge of the skills and abilities that are being measured. In this case, behaviors to be measured are those which might be associated with TBI. For example, in order to make predictions about how difficulties in executive functioning would interfere with vocational performance, one would have to have a thorough appreciation for the types, degree, and intensity of disorders of executive functioning.
2. Technical expertise in the test procedures. Such expertise includes an appreciation for the range of behaviors required for adaptive or intact performance, and strong interpretive skills for addressing difficulties or performance failures.
3. An understanding of, and appreciation for, the demands of the situation or environment one is attempting to make predictions about. The performance on standardized tests must be related to the demands of the environment for it to be functionally relevant. For example, knowledge that, among other competencies, a clerical/receptionist job required a significant degree of auditory attention, moderately complex verbal comprehension and expression, and fine bimanual coordination, would be essential in making a prediction about whether or not an individual could perform on that job.

Psychologists and neuropsychologists are well trained and experienced in points 1 and 2 above. However, in order to generate sound hypotheses for vocational rehabilitation from psychological and neuropsychological tests, the psychologist or neuropsychologist must develop knowledge and expertise in evaluating the demands of the vocational environment. Without a clear sense of the outcome environment one tries to predict, test scores are of limited use in contributing to our understanding of how an individual will function in work or other aspects of everyday living.

In summary, while acknowledging that most psychological and neuropsychological tests were not developed to predict behavior in the natural environment, and extensive validation does not exist for this purpose, there is increasing evidence to suggest that standardized measurement of cognitive and behavioral skills on psychological and neuropsychological tests are well correlated with performance in the daily living and work environments. Furthermore, the ability to make such predictions about real world behavior is enhanced when test data are combined with specific knowledge about the environment and the demands which exist within that environment. Finally, when inferences are made about functional abilities from psychological tests, because of the lack of established validity for this purpose, further testing of such inferences, or working hypotheses, is required throughout the vocational rehabilitation process. This continued testing of clinical hypotheses can be accomplished through functional assessment.

## Functional Assessment

Functional assessment may be defined as the analysis and measurement of specific behaviors which occur in real environments and are relevant to life or vocational goals (Halpern & Fuhrer, 1984). Functional assessment always involves an interaction between the purposeful or "goal-directed" behavior and environmental conditions such as people, rules, physical barriers, or schedules. Because the demands placed upon a person differ from one environment to another and from one occupation to another, functional assessment must always be an individualized process.

The ideal mechanism for valid study of real world behavior is to directly observe individuals confronted by demands in their natural environment. In order to measure cognitive behavior in the natural environment, some method of quantifying and qualifying the behavior is required. While several functional assessment measures exist (e.g., Functional Assessment Inventory, Crewe & Athelstan, 1984; Rehabilitation Indicators, Diller, Fordyce, Jacobs, Brown, Gordon, Simmens, Orazem, & Barrett, 1983), these approaches do not adequately address the measurement of cognitive and problem-solving skills. A primary limitation of functional assessment instruments has been the restricted range of activities they address (Haffey & Johnston, 1990; Indices, 1979). In order to plan interventions to overcome limitations associated with TBI, procedures must address the functional impact of cognitive disabilities. The Pre-Vocational Checklist developed at the NYU Center for Head Trauma and Stroke (Silver, Ezrachi, Kay, Rattok, Piasetsky, & Ben-Yishay, 1988) holds promise as a valid and reliable measure of complex cognitive behaviors in the vocational environment. This checklist provides for detailed behavioral analysis of a wide range of cognitive, language, problem-solving, and work responses in a work evaluation environment. The checklist also may be applied in a number of settings in which cognitive demands are placed upon the client. These settings range from more restrictive environments, such as the psychological testing or the clinical treatment setting, to naturalistic observation in the client's work or living environment.

Functional assessment should span the entire rehabilitation process. Initial assessment should be conducted within the clinical or rehabilitation setting, in conjunction with other forms of assessment and early treatment. Subsequent assessments can be performed in a variety of vocational environments such as in volunteer placements or work trials. Ultimately, assessment will be conducted in the actual workplace. Functional assessment data can be gathered throughout the entire process, using direct behavioral observation. Such observation may be facilitated by the use of rating scales such as the Prevocational Checklist (Silver *et al.*, 1988)

Active involvement of the client throughout the assessment process improves the validity and reliability of the information gathered and enhances the client's understanding of and investment in the rehabilitation process. Client involvement in gathering functional assessment information is also seen as a therapeutic approach to gaining more accurate self-appraisal and insight into strengths and limitations because it is not a clinical process; rather, it is the observation and recording of behavior that occurs in real environments in response to real life demands.

## Vocational Assessment

All clients should have access to a variety of techniques for exploring their vocational strengths, weaknesses, interests, and aptitudes. While a preliminary vocational assessment, using paper and pencil vocational interest and aptitude tests, may be used to identify directions for vocational counseling, the purpose of such assessment should not be to definitively identify a vocational option. With persons with severe cognitive limitations, these tests are often of limited use. Vocational interest and preference tests may be used to preliminarily narrow down the field of vocational choices with each client and identify directions which might be explored in more detail by the client and vocational counselor.

Vocational evaluation in a workshop setting may also be used to obtain information on aptitudes and work behaviors, and assessment of the client's cognitive and behavioral responses to worklike demands. Vocational evaluation programs which specialize in TBI should be utilized because behaviors associated with TBI (e.g., inattention, impulsivity) often interfere with participation in more traditional, work-sample vocational evaluation approaches.

## VOCATIONAL REHABILITATION PLANNING

In order to identify and access the appropriate rehabilitation interventions prior to, and during employment, a rehabilitation plan which is problem-oriented should be developed. A comprehensive functional assessment should identify all problem or deficit areas. A plan for ameliorating each of the areas of deficit should also be specified. This specification should include what is to be done, when, for how long, and by whom. It should also specify the target behavior or criterion which indicates resolution of the problem. There should be a one-to-one correspondence between each functional limitation and a strategy or set of strategies for addressing the obstacle. Such a system promotes treatment focus upon the specific functional manifestations of a disability and the unique presentations of each individual rather than treating "head injury" generically. Planning should actively involve the client.

In planning job-oriented interventions, four classes of rehabilitation strategies might be applied. These include:

1. The initial inclination in rehabilitation is to attempt to *remediate or fix* the area of deficit. In this case, through the application of direct treatment approaches, the individual learns new skills to overcome the area of deficit. Cognitive rehabilitation of a memory deficit is one approach that illustrates the "fix" approach. Another example might be self-relaxation techniques learned by an individual to cope with anxiety triggered by specific aspects of the workplace.
2. A second strategy might be to *compensate* for an area of deficit. This approach is based upon the client using internal assets to overcome or compensate for an area of deficit. For example, a client might use strong "hands-on" learning abilities to learn new tasks when memory or verbal material is problematic.
3. Third, an individual may *accommodate* for an area of deficit. Accommodations are based on the use of external or environmental aids or modifications to overcome an area of deficit. Accommodations may be environmental modifications, such as adjusting schedules or rules, alterations in the physical environment, the use of prosthetic devices (calculators, notebooks, schedules), or the use of strategies (note-taking procedures, scheduling, mnemonic devices).
4. A final strategy would be *avoiding or circumventing the area of deficit*. For example if a client presents with a deficit in interpersonal skills, one might choose occupations in which work is not contingent upon interaction with other individuals.

For example, in developing a rehabilitation plan with an individual who experiences difficulties paying attention to auditory information, strategies might include a combination of compensatory (information presented in writing when possible, to capitalize upon strengths in written language skills), accommodation (information always presented in the supervisor's office where distractions are minimal), rehabilitation (client will be trained to attend to a particular type of auditory cue for brief time periods), and circumvention (vocational placements in nondistracting, quiet environments will be sought).

Typically, a number of functional limitations are identified and a plan for each limitation is specified. While this type of job-oriented rehabilitation planning requires a great deal of information, knowledge about the client, and time, such a procedure assures that obstacles to the attainment of client goals will be individually addressed in the rehabilitation planning process.

## PREVOCATIONAL TREATMENT STRATEGIES

Once a rehabilitation plan has been developed, a number of strategies will have been identified for addressing obstacles to employment and independent living. While these are almost all initiated during the prevocational stages of the rehabilitation process, such treatments may also be applied later in the rehabilitation process, in the natural environment. Within the context of job-oriented rehabilitation for TBI, the following strategies are recommended: direct treatment approaches (including cognitive and behavioral rehabilitation); accommodations, modifications and compensatory strategies; career counseling and vocational exploration; and job development and placement.

### Direct Approaches

Several "direct treatment" approaches may be required in implementing a viable vocationally oriented rehabilitation program for TBI survivors. These may be group and individually administered treatments and should address the functional/behavioral problems that impact the individual in the vocational environment, or in the living environment which would interfere with the ability to maintain employment. A variety of intervention methodologies may be applied using a direct treatment approach to job-oriented rehabilitation. These include such techniques as memory, attention, perceptual, impulse control, social skills, and problem-solving training. Individualized behavioral therapeutic techniques should also be applied if indicated. The focus in all of these approaches is developing basic competencies required for entry into the vocational environment.

Individual treatments such as cognitive remediation (e.g., memory or attention training) should be designed and tested prevocationally and implemented as "in vivo" strategies in the workplace. This requires that cognitive rehabilitation work done be oriented to community-based application. For example, memory strategies should focus on relevant learning requirements which will face the client and should utilize strategies which can be implemented outside of the clinical or rehabilitation setting. Behavioral management and treatment strategies should be similarly applied. Such treatments are described in detail in other chapters of this book and will not be elaborated upon here. When it is not feasible to implement strategies "in vivo," generalization of effects to each client's real life experiences should be stressed.

## Accommodations, Modifications, and Compensatory Strategies

In many cases it may not be feasible, appropriate, or cost effective to attempt to directly treat an area of deficit, particularly when the deficit may be ameliorated through modifications in the work demands or environment, or through the use of accommodation strategies. The use of adaptive devices (e.g., calculator, communication board, tape recorder, or memory log) or environmental cues or prompts (e.g., color-coded cue cards to prompt for sequential job tasks) are examples of accommodations that may be applied to overcome identified limitations associated with TBI. Modifying work schedules (e.g., working 3/4 days), altering performance demands of particular work tasks (allowing the employee to dictate reports into a tape recorder for transcription rather than preparing a written report), and changing the physical environment in which the client must function (e.g., screening the client from visual or auditory distractions) may also be effective. Finally, by using client strengths (e.g., visual memory), individuals may compensate for areas in which their performance is deficient. Listings of sample accommodations, modifications, and compensatory strategies can be found in Parente (1989) and in Ylvisaker, Szekeres, Henry, Sullivan, and Wheeler (1987).

## Career Counseling and Vocational Exploration

Career guidance including vocational interest and aptitude should be available to clients who are either seeking alternative employment options or who are resuming career development following head injury. An appreciation for the disruption of learning and development associated with head injury and the resulting need for modifications and flexibility in the traditional career counseling approach is required. Detailed knowledge of the client's previous work history and competencies are also critical elements of the counseling process.

As a component of vocational development, clients should have an opportunity to develop an awareness of a wide variety of vocational alternatives. Options and resources including a career library, videotapes, talking with people employed in various types of jobs, and job site visits are suggested. Clients should be encouraged and supported in coordinating and developing exploration options.

## Job Development and Placement

When exploring competitive placements for persons who have sustained TBI, one must determine whether the opportunity to return to a previous job or employer exists. This determination is based upon:

1. The availability of the position;
2. the capacity of the individual to meet the demands of the position;
3. the potential to modify the position to allow the client to return despite limitations in the ability to perform at previous levels.

Modifications might take the form of a reduction or change in duties or responsibilities or allowances for specific accommodations or supports on-site.

Despite the preference to return, in some capacity, to previous employment, most persons who have sustained severe TBI do not return to old jobs. Placements must, therefore, be developed within the local community. Effective job development utilizes an individual client approach in which a specific job is developed for a particular client. Strategies used for job development include emphasizing client assets, assuring or guaranteeing productivity (through job coaching), and highlighting incentives (financial) for hiring the worker with a disability. A great deal of effort goes into preparing the client for interviewing, including didactic training, modeling, and rehearsal. Videotaping equipment is useful for providing direct feedback to clients on their job-seeking skills.

Utilizing the *involvement* of support systems around the individual (e.g., family) may facilitate job development and job maintenance. Each person within the support system of a person who has sustained a TBI is part of a network of individuals. Each of these social networks may provide valuable job leads or opportunities. Using naturally occurring social networks is how most persons without disabilities obtain jobs and should be encouraged as a very normalized strategy for placement of persons with disabilities. Careful attention to, and planning of, job site modifications and accommodations may also enhance the likelihood of developing stable positions.

## EMPLOYMENT OPTIONS

In a job-oriented rehabilitation approach, the emphasis is placed upon a relatively brief treatment period, which is designed to be carried over and implemented in a real work setting. This emphasis allows for "in vivo" treatment of cognitive and behavioral deficits in the client's natural community, through the implementation of programs which have been initially designed and implemented in a treatment environment. This design allows for maximum generalization of treatment approaches to the client's real life problems.

The following "employment options" identify settings in which treatments can be implemented. These range from noncompetitive to competitive placements. In each of these options, implementation of the assessment and treatment strategies described above is recommended. Preemployment and employment options for use in job-oriented rehabilitation of TBI include: job simulations, volunteer placements, specialty evaluations or work trials, transitional employment, and supported work.

The use of *work simulations* is a relatively informal approach to job-oriented rehabilitation. In this approach, aspects of a particular job or work setting are re-created in the rehabilitation environment. The best simulations are those which most closely approximate the real environment. Simulations may be done for brief periods of time and are flexible with respect to varying the demands on the client. Simulations may be designed to evaluate or train specific job skills (e.g., word processing) or to address suspected behavioral or cognitive problem areas (e.g., impulsivity, attentional difficulties). Simulations can be very elaborate with multiple and complex demands placed on the individual, or it can be quite simple, focusing upon one discrete performance area. In using simulations, productivity is not necessarily the objective. Therefore, it can be seen as more of a training or teaching option.

Unpaid, *volunteer placements* may be used both as an assessment and adjustment resource prior to competitive placement. Volunteer options also serve as an excellent resource for vocational exploration, in which clients can experience different vocational environments without having to make a commitment or risk job failure.

A third preemployment option is a *specialty evaluation* or *work trial*. These approaches are designed to evaluate a specific ability or competency, or to provide intervention in a particular area. For example, data entry jobs are frequently considered for persons who may have mobility problems. Because many of the more severely impaired clients who have sustained TBI have motor problems, their ability to utilize a computer keyboard is often questioned. In these cases, a special evaluation of this capability may be requested, along with recommendations for rehabilitation engineering which may enhance performance. Work trials are also used to develop and test intervention strategies, such as the efficacy of an accommodative cuing procedure (e.g., beeping watch) to maintain on-task behavior in a worklike setting.

*Transitional employment* (TE) utilizes positions within the competitive arena which are filled by persons with disabilities for limited periods of time. The positions may be staffed by trainers or coaches and may be used to evaluate employability or to fine tune work behavior and skills. After a period of time in such a position, the worker makes a transition into a competitive job. Some degree of job training or support may be required after TE in the next placement, but it is likely to be reduced as a result of the transitional work experience. When a worker is transitioned, a new person fills the vacated position. Transitional placements may be in an enclave-type setting, which is advantageous because it offers a wide range of work activities and is less staff intensive. In this setting, one or two staff can usually train or supervise several clients. TE is also particularly beneficial for work with TBI clients because of the inherent flexibility to modify conditions and to implement, train, and test out accommodation and compensation strategies.

The options described above all occur prior to competitive placement. *Supported work* (SW) is a relatively novel approach which is designed to enable persons who have sustained TBI to function competitively on a job, despite severe disability. SW has been demonstrated to be an effective rehabilitation technique with the severely retarded, the only population in which this strategy has been thoroughly tested (Brickey, Browning, & Campbell, 1982; Brickey & Campbell, 1981; Kraus & MacEachron, 1982; Revell, Arnold, Taylor, & Saitz-Blotner, 1982; Sowers, Thompson, & Connis, 1979; Wehman, Hill, Goodall, Cleveland, Brooke, & Pentecost, 1982). Because individuals with traumatic head injuries may have multiple disabling conditions, the type of support and/or preparation provided must take into account the cognitive and behavioral manifestations of TBI, as well as the physical limitations which may also result.

In general, SW is characterized by community-based employment in integrated job settings with nonhandicapped co-workers. It is competitive work for competitive pay, in a real work environment. Supported employment is designed for those individuals who, without some type of ongoing support, would not be able to maintain a job. Support is varied with respect to both nature and extent. The degree and type of support are contingent upon the individual's degree and pattern of disability. For example, supported employment programs designed to serve persons who have sustained TBI should involve basic cognitive and behavioral preparation and ongoing supports in areas known to be problematic for these clients (e.g., attention, memory, and impulse control). In addition, programs should be flexible enough to meet individual client needs as determined by prework assessments and on-site (job) evaluations. SW presents an ideal situation in which treatment and accommodation/compensation strategies, that have been previously developed and tested in the clinic setting, can be implemented "in vivo," through the clinical support of the job coach.

Although the efficacy of supported employment with individuals who have sustained TBI has not been fully tested, preliminary information from various programs has indicated that the approach is effective with this severely disabled population (McCue, 1989; Stapleton, Parente, & Bennett, 1989; Wehman, Kreutzer, Stonnington, Wood, Sherron, Diambra, Fry, & Groah, 1988).

An area of major concern in the provision of supported employment services to the chronically brain-damaged client is the level of support required to maintain employment: (1) must be broad based and address not only the client's work needs, but also pre- and postwork issues which may have a detrimental effect upon job maintenance; and (2) must be, in many cases, a long-term or perhaps indefinite commitment. These requirements pose significant cost considerations which limit the applicability of the model to the general population. Typically, the vocational rehabilitation system can only provide a limited amount of support. For example, in Pennsylvania, the amount of financial support which may be provided to vocational rehabilitation clients is typically limited to 100 hours, far less than what is anticipated in persons with severe disability as a result of TBI.

In order to address the cost considerations and limited availability of SW programming for TBI, creative and innovative strategies are required. Once the client has been established in a competitive job and, with initial supports from rehabilitation staff, has acclimated to the demands of the job, exploration of options for continuation of the required level of support should be undertaken. Support may come from resources in the client's natural community. Those which can be provided at little or no cost to the client or to the vocational rehabilitation system should be explored. While each individual's situation may present unique demands and resource possibilities, a number of innovative approaches may be available for continuation of support. These include the following:

*Family Support*: As suggested above, family support is critical to the overall success of supported vocational placement of clients with TBI. Traditionally, support has been required in the earlier phases of the rehabilitation effort. Support in the job development and placement phase is also a necessity. Many issues which have traditionally served as obstacles to successful rehabilitation are addressed through involvement of the family in the placement process. These include dependency/ independence issues, family role issues, and preworkday briefing and postworkday debriefing issues. Supports may be extended into the actual workplace in some instances. For example, an employee might bring written weekly assignments home for assistance in anticipating, planning, and structuring the week's activities. While the possibility of fostering dependency by having family members involved in work supports may occur, the nature of supports need not infringe on the client's sense of independence, given that the client is productive in other aspects of the job.

*Enclave Placements*: In an enclave placement, several employees with disabilities work in close proximity to one another, within a competitive employment setting. Because even the most severely disabled workers typically only require intermittent support from a job coach, several employees can share one job coach, thus resulting in a much more economical application of ongoing work support. The enclave setting also tends to be more conducive to establishing modifications in the work environment, whether they relate to structure (e.g., designing space accessible to wheelchairs) or changes in schedule and/or routine.

*Job Share*: The opportunity to split job responsibilities between two individuals, in order to allow a disabled worker to achieve maximum productivity on a job with minimal supports, may be an effective strategy with TBI survivors. Two basic options may be explored, neither of which requires ongoing external coaching. The first is pairing a disabled client with an able-bodied co-worker. The job requirements of the client's and the co-worker's jobs are analyzed in detail. Aspects of the two positions, which can be performed by the client, are restructured to become the client's job duties. Aspects of both jobs, which may be outside of the client's capabilities, are performed by the co-worker. In this fashion, there is a formal "share" of job responsibilities. The second option is pairing two disabled workers in a similar fashion by identifying two individuals with distinctly different but complementary patterns of strengths and weaknesses. Job development is then conducted to identify two positions in which the clients can share responsibilities. Both options require some initial coaching support, the latter requiring a greater degree of support. However, both options have the potential to provide a natural system of support on an ongoing, no-cost basis. A variant of this approach is using two individuals at 50% effort to meet the demands of a full-time position.

*Co-Worker Support*: After an initial period of job training and support, it is possible to draw upon co-workers and supervisors in the workplace to provide ongoing support to clients. This additional support allows for the withdrawal of professional job coaching. As with other innovative alternatives, this option may only be appropriate under specific conditions. Employers and co-workers in selected instances are often very receptive to using this strategy, which works best when the support required by the co-worker or supervisor is clearly defined and is not demonstrably different from their daily routine. In many instances, employers prefer this option to having nonemployees (job coaches) in the work environment.

*Volunteer Support*: The use of volunteers has been widespread in the helping and rehabilitation professions. The nature of the supported employment needs of persons who have sustained TBI is particularly conducive to the use of volunteers. Specifically, supports are required in the natural environment, not in the clinical setting. Volunteers can work with clients in the work environment which is familiar to them. The use of retired workers is an avenue that can be utilized. These individuals may possess specific areas of vocational expertise (which in many cases may be hard to acquire for a job trainer) which can be used in a support role. Often, retired workers want to maintain some contact with their field and may do so by coaching a client in that area. Another source of volunteers is through advocacy groups where knowledge of the specific type of presentations of disability is present. After an initial period of support by a professional job trainer or coach enables the client to stabilize in the job and identifies ongoing support needs, volunteers with particular areas of expertise may then be paired with disabled workers to provide ongoing supports.

*Client-Funded Support*: Borrowing from the model in which physically disabled individuals independently pay for personal care aids to assist them with some aspects of daily living, it is also possible that clients who require support on the job may pay for that support. This is particularly applicable in higher-level positions where supports may be primarily of a physical nature. It may also be applied in situations where a group of workers may pool financial resources to fund a job coach in a job share or "enclave"-type situation. Again, this option could be explored after an initial period of stability and success has been demonstrated through more traditional rehabilitation supports.

*Previous Employer Support Options*: For some individuals, while a full return to previous work duties is unlikely, it is possible that persons may be able to perform effectively at several aspects of their previous job. In these cases, particularly if an individual has a good history with a previous employer, the employer may be willing to provide modifications and ongoing support. If a return to work is structured and supported initially by professional staff, employers are often willing to take over support responsibilities, particularly if these are well defined.

*Other Third-Party Sources of Funding Support*: Some individuals may be eligible for long-term financial support which relieves the burden of cost for job support services from the vocational rehabilitation agency and the individual. Insurance carriers are often receptive to funding ongoing, indefinite support of clients on jobs, if it can be determined to be an effective rehabilitation intervention. This is particularly the case when the provision of ongoing job supports is less costly than comprehensive or residential placements. While it is obvious that this is not an option for persons who do not have third-party funding resources, for those who do, the possibility should be explored and tested.

## SUMMARY

Job-oriented rehabilitation of persons with TBI requires functionally oriented assessment to identify the obstacles to meeting the everyday and work demands which face the individual. A number of rehabilitation strategies targeted to the amelioration of identified functional limitations must be applied outside of the traditional treatment setting, in the work and living environments. These include direct treatment approaches (such as cognitive rehabilitation and behavior management procedures), accommodations and compensatory strategies, and, in some cases, strategies for circumventing problem areas. Such strategies can be implemented in the natural environment through the intervention of job trainers or coaches who support the client in the community.

Support to the client and employer must be provided for whatever length of time necessary for successful acclimation to work demands. Often, after an initial period of job training or coaching, the degree of support can be faded to periodic technical assistance or troubleshooting. However, some very severely disabled persons may require extensive degrees of support to maintain competitive, integrated employment. While acknowledging the cost of such services, this option is preferable to sheltered placements for persons who have survived TBI. Creative and innovative strategies for the provision of ongoing support to persons in the workplace may need to be explored as part of the job-oriented rehabilitation process.

## REFERENCES

Ben-Yishay, Y., Diller, L., & Rattok, J. (1978). A modular approach to optimizing orientation, psychomotor alertness, and purposive behavior in severe head trauma patients. *Working approaches to cognitive deficits in brain damage* (Rehabilitation Monograph No. 59). New York: New York University Medical Center, Institute of Rehabilitation Medicine.

Ben-Yishay, Y., Silver, S. M., Piasetsky, E., & Rattok, J. (1987). Relationship between employability and vocational outcome after intensive holistic cognitive rehabilitation. *The Journal of Head Trauma Rehabilitation, 2*, 35–48.

Brickey, M., & Campbell, K. (1981). Fast food employment for moderately and mildly retarded adults: The McDonald's project. *Mental Retardation, 19*, 113–116.

Brickey, M., Browning, L., & Campbell, K. (1982). Vocational histories of sheltered workshop employees placed in Projects with Industry and competitive jobs. *Mental Retardation, 20*, 52–57.

Brinkley, S. B. (1989, February). *Selected findings of an informal survey of state agency activities involving TBI.* Paper presented at the National Conference on Traumatic Brain Injury and Community-based Employment, Clearwater Beach, FL.

Brooks, N., McKinlay, W., Symington, C., Beattie, A., & Campsie, L. (1987). Return to work within the first seven years of severe head injury. *Brain Injury, 1*, 5–19.

Cicerone, K. D., & Tupper, D. E. (1990). Neuropsychological rehabilitation: Treatment of errors in everyday functioning. In D. E. Tupper & K. D. Cicerone (Eds.), *The neuropsychology of everyday life: Issues in development and rehabilitation.* Boston: Kluwer.

Crewe, N. M., & Athelstan, G. T. (1984). *Functional Assessment Inventory manual.* Menomonie: University of Wisconsin–Stout.

Dennerll, R. D., Rodin, E. A., Gonzalez, S., Schwartz, M. S., & Lin, Y. (1966). Neuropsychological and psychological factors related to employability of persons with epilepsy. *Epilepsia, 7*, 318–329.

DeTurk, J. (1975). Neuropsychological measures in predicting rehabilitation outcome. *Dissertation Abstracts International, 36*, No. 1, p. 437-B. Ann Arbor, MI: University Microfilms International.

Dikmen, S., & Morgan, S. F. (1980). Neuropsychological factors related to employability and occupational status in persons with epilepsy. *Journal of Nervous & Mental Disease, 168*, 236–240.

Diller, L., Fordyce, W., Jacobs, D., Brown, M., Gordon, W., Simmens, S., Orazem, J., & Barrett, L. (1983). *Final Report: Rehabilitation indicators project* (R&D Project No. G008003039). Washington, DC: National Institute of Handicapped Research.

Field, J. H. (1976). *Epidemiology of head injury in England and Wales: With particular application to rehabilitation.* Leicester: Printed for H.M. Stationery Office by Willsons.

Fraser, R., Dikmen, S., McLean, A., Miller, B., & Temkin, N. (1988). Employability of head injury survivors: First year post-injury. *Rehabilitation Counseling Bulletin, 31*, 276–288.

Haffey, W. J., & Johnston, M. V. (1990). A functional assessment system for real-world rehabilitation outcomes. In D. E. Tupper & K. D. Cicerone (Eds.), *The neuropsychology of everyday life: Issues in development and rehabilitation.* Boston: Kluwer.

Halpern, A. S., & Fuhrer, M. J. (1984). *Functional assessment in rehabilitation.* Baltimore: Paul H. Brooks Publishing.

Heaton, S., Chelune, G., & Lehman, R. (1978). Using neuropsychological and personality tests to assess the likelihood of patient employment. *Journal of Nervous & Mental Disease, 166*, 408–416.

Indices, Inc. (1979). *Functional limitations: A state of the art review* (RSA Grant No. 13 P 59220/3 01). Falls Church, VA: Author.

Kay, T., Ezrachi, O., & Cavallo, M. (1988). *Annotated bibliography of research on vocational outcome.* New York: New York University Medical Center, Research and Training Center on Head Trauma and Stroke, Publication No. 185-1.

Killiam, S., Diambra, J. F., & Fry, R. L. (1990). Supported employment phase II: Job-site training and compensatory strategies. In P. Wehman & J. Kreutzer (Eds.), *Vocational rehabilitation for persons with traumatic brain injury.* Rockville, MD: Aspen Publishers.

Kraus, A., & MacEachron, A. (1982). The supported work model. *American Journal of Mental Deficiency, 86*, 650–653.

Kreutzer, J. S., Wehman, P., Morton, M. V., & Stonnington, H. H. (1988). Supported employment and compensatory strategies for enhancing vocational outcome following traumatic brain injury. *Brain Injury, 2*, 205–223.

McCue, M. (1989, September). *"In vivo" treatment of cognitive and behavioral deficits in the workplace.* Paper presented at the Third Annual Conference on Cognitive Rehabilitation: Community Reintegration Through Scientifically Based Practice, Clearwater Beach, FL.

Mackworth, N., Mackworth, J., & Cope, N. (1982). Cognitive-visual assessment of head injury recovery to predict social outcome by measuring verbal speeds and sequencing skills. *Head injury project final report.*

San Jose, CA: Santa Clara Valley Medical Center.

Morris, J., Ryan, J., & Peterson, R. (1982, August). *Neuropsychological predictors of vocational behavior*. Presented at the meetings of the American Psychological Association, Washington, DC.

Naugle, R. I., & Chelune, G. J. (1990). Integrating neuropsychological and "real-life" data: A neuropsychological model for assessing everyday functioning. In D. E. Tupper & K. D. Cicerone (Eds.), *The neuropsychology of everyday life: Issues in development and rehabilitation*. Boston: Kluwer.

Newnan, O. S., Heaton, R. K., & Lehman, R. A. (1978). Neuropsychological and MMPI correlates of patients' future employment characteristics. *Perceptual & Motor Skills, 46*, 635–642.

Oddy, M., Coughlan, T., Tyerman, A., & Jenkins, D. (1985). Social adjustment after closed head injury: A further follow-up seven years after injury. *Journal of Neurology, Neurosurgery, & Psychiatry, 48*, 564–568.

Parente, R. (1989, September). *Compensatory strategies: Design and implementation*. Paper presented at the Third Annual Conference on Cognitive Rehabilitation: Community Reintegration Through Scientifically Based Practice, Clearwater Beach, FL.

Prigatano, G. P. (1989, February). *Maintaining work after traumatic brain injury: Experiences from two neuropsychological rehabilitation programs*. Paper presented at the National Conference on Traumatic Brain Injury and Community-based Employment, Clearwater Beach, FL.

Revell, G., Arnold, S., Taylor, B., & Saitz-Blotner, S. (1982). Project transition: Competitive employment services for the severely handicapped mentally retarded. *Journal of Rehabilitation, 48*, 31–35.

Schwartz, M., Dennerll, R., & Lin, Y. (1968). Neuropsychological and psychological predictors of employability in epilepsy. *Journal of Clinical Psychology, 24*, 174–177.

Silver, S. M., Ezrachi, O., Kay, T., Rattok, J., Piasetsky, E., & Ben-Yishay, Y. (1988). *Administration manual for the N.Y.U. Prevocational Checklist*. New York: Research and Training Center on Head Trauma and Stroke, Department of Rehabilitation Medicine, New York University Medical Center.

Sowers, J., Thompson, L., & Connis, R. (1979). The food service vocational training program: A model for training and placement of the mentally retarded. In G. T. Bellamy, G. O'Connor, & O. C. Karan (Eds.), *Vocational rehabilitation of severely handicapped persons*. Baltimore: University Park Press.

Stapleton, M. C., Parente, R., & Bennett, P. (1989). Job coaching traumatically brain injured individuals: Lessons learned. *Cognitive Rehabilitation, 7*, 18–21.

Wehman, P., & Goodall, P. (1990). Return to work: Critical issues in employment. In P. Wehman & J. Kreutzer (Eds.), *Vocational rehabilitation for persons with traumatic brain injury*. Rockville, MD: Aspen Publishers.

Wehman, P., Hill, M., Goodall, C., Cleveland, P., Brooke, V., & Pentecost, J. (1982). Job placement and follow-up of moderately and severely handicapped individuals after three years. *Journal of the Association for Severely Handicapped, 7*, 5–16.

Wehman, P., Kreutzer, J. S., Stonnington, H. H., Wood, W., Sherron, P., Diambra, J., Fry, R., & Groah, C. (1988). Supported employment for persons with traumatic brain injury: A preliminary report. *The Journal of Head Trauma Rehabilitation, 3*, 82–94.

Ylvisaker, M., Szekeres, S. F., Henry, K., Sullivan, D. M., & Wheeler, P. (1987). Topics in cognitive rehabilitation therapy. In M. Ylvisaker & E. M. Gobble (Eds.), *Community re-entry for head injured adults*. Boston: College Hill Press.

# 23

# Neurological Impairment and Driving Ability

## DANNY WEDDING

Determining when a patient is unfit to drive an automobile because of a neurological defect or disease is a difficult problem both for physicians and for the neuropsychologists they may consult. Driving has symbolic functions that far surpass the utilitarian value of the act itself; for example, it may represent independence, freedom, or masculinity. In addition, the blanket assertion that a patient should no longer drive, albeit a simple decision rule, may fail to address the varied situational demands of driving: the patient who cannot make the rapid decisions required for freeway driving during heavy traffic periods may well retain the capacity for driving to the grocery using-well known and little-traveled streets. Yet one always has lingering doubts—the situational demands of driving to the grocery increase dramatically when a neighborhood child chases a ball in front of an oncoming car.

Some of the many problems experienced by patients who have sustained brain insults include impulsiveness, aggressiveness, difficulty with memory, limited attention span, poor concentration, and personality change. All of these are problems that can potentially affect driving ability and can be measured. Psychological methods should prove useful and should supplement clinical judgment in arriving at decisions about when, or if, patients with cognitive limitations should return to driving; however, neuropsychologists have

---

DANNY WEDDING • Institute of Medicine, National Academy of Sciences, Washington, DC 20418.

*HANDBOOK OF HEAD TRAUMA: Acute Care to Recovery*, edited by Charles J. Long and Leslie K. Ross. Plenum Press, New York, 1992.

not, heretofore, been especially helpful in resolving these pragmatic issues and little research has addressed these problems.

## MAGNITUDE OF THE PROBLEM

### The Aging Driver

Driving in routine situations is an overlearned activity and many individuals continue to drive despite significant neurological problems that limit their ability to solve problems, make decisions, and respond rapidly to the demands imposed by novel stimulus situations. This may be a particular problem with the aging driver. In 1985, there were 15.5 million American drivers aged 65 or older (approximately 10% of all drivers) (Reuben, Silliman, & Traines, 1988). Some investigators have not found systematic relationships between age and accidents (e.g., Liddell, 1982); however, the more common finding is a "U"-shaped distribution with increased likelihood of accidents occurring at either end of the age spectrum. These findings become more compelling when one adjusts for the fact that many aging individuals voluntarily remove themselves from the driving public and the typical driver over the age of 65 drives almost 4000 miles per year less than the average for all drivers (Garcia, 1986). When the accident rate is expressed in terms of accidents/miles driven, drivers over age 60 are shown to have approximately twice as many accidents per million miles as drivers in the age range of 30 to 47 years (Reuben et al., 1988). This increased accident rate can be attributed to multiple causes, including decreased visual acuity, the increased likelihood of neurologic, cardiovascular, and other disease, and the greater use of prescription medications (especially benzodiazepines) in the elderly. Benzodiazepines have been shown to increase significantly the risk of automobile accidents in those patients for whom they are prescribed (Skegg, Richards, & Doll, 1979). Interestingly, although the elderly perform poorly on tests of simple reaction time, their reaction speed in complex situations approximates that of younger subjects and most elderly individuals can stop a moving car within the 2.5-second limit generally assumed by highway engineers making decisions about speed limits and the placement of road signs (Reuben et al., 1988).

Age is a potent risk factor for both dementing illnesses and cerebrovascular disease. Wilson and Smith (1983) took stroke patients who had been cleared for driving by their attending physicians and subjected the patients to actual road tests. These tests demonstrated multiple difficulties with driving in these individuals including problems entering or exiting from traffic and performing multiple tasks in emergency situations. These findings underscore the limits of clinical judgment and the importance of naturalistic assessment of driving in realistic situations.

Another study at the Dementia Research Clinic of the Johns Hopkins Hospital revealed that 30% of patients had at least one accident since the onset of their symptoms and an additional 11% were reported by caregivers to have caused accidents. Although patients who are experiencing cognitive decline secondary to a progressive neurological disease (e.g., Alzheimer's, Parkinson's) often promise to themselves and to their loved ones that they will stop driving once their disease "gets bad enough," the disease process itself may interfere with the judgment necessary to make sound decisions about when to terminate driving.

## Patients with Acquired Brain Impairment

A surprising number of patients continue to drive after sustaining significant head injuries or other major cerebral insults. van Zomeren, Brouwer, and Minderhoud (1987) reviewed numerous studies on the incidence of driving after acquired brain damage and reached the following conclusions: (1) About half of the patients with acquired brain damage have licenses (although not every licensed driver actually drives) and (2) lower percentages of drivers are found in populations treated at rehabilitation centers than in those outside these facilities. This latter finding may reflect the fact that more severe cases are sent for rehabilitation; it may also be a measure of the effective reality orientation that occurs in these programs.

Hopewell and Price (1985) studied a series of 56 patients who sustained traumatic brain injuries but eventually achieved Glasgow Recovery Scale ratings of "moderate" or "good"; 53% of these patients returned to driving. Those unable to return to driving tended to be characterized by one or more of the following factors: (1) an estimated IQ $< 80$; (2) failure on driver simulation tests; (3) significant impairment on clinical rating scales; or (4) posttraumatic amnesia lasting 11 or more weeks. The mean duration of posttraumatic amnesia was 37 days for the group that returned to driving; it was 95 days for the group that did not resume driving.

Sivak, Olson, Kewman, Won, and Henson (1981) designed a methodologically sophisticated study which empirically evaluated the effects of brain damage on driving. These researchers found comparable levels of driving performance when subjects with spinal cord damage were compared to able-bodied controls; however, subjects with a history of brain damage performed significantly worse than either of the other two groups on perceptual and cognitive tests and on both closed-course and open-road driving. Interestingly, good performance on neuropsychological tests correlated with good driving ability; however, different sets of predictor variables emerged for the brain-impaired and non-brain-impaired subjects. In addition, this study found there was minimal correlation between the performance of impaired subjects on a closed-course driving test and a composite measure of driving skill determined *in vivo* with open-road driving, suggesting that actual samples of driving behavior in naturalistic settings may be necessary to assess driving skill with this population. However, it is essential that these driving skills assessments tap many of the variegated skills involved in operating a motor vehicle; the traditional, somewhat perfunctory, written examination and *in vivo* driving test administered by state police departments have not been shown to be predictive of either future driving behavior or accident risk (Wallace & Crancer, 1971).

## Physical Disabilities

There is convincing evidence that the presence of physical disabilities is not a predictor of high risk driving. Insurance companies, using actuarial data, rate physically handicapped drivers as "good risks." There is no evidence of increased risk for drivers with orthopedic handicaps and the California Department of Motor Vehicles has failed to find evidence of increased risk for drivers with physical impairments. A Swiss study of one-eyed drivers demonstrated that this group did not experience more accidents than drivers with full binocular vision. In short, there is compelling evidence that people can adequately compensate for their physical limitations, provided appropriate adjustments are made (van Zomeren *et al.*, 1987).

## NEUROPSYCHOLOGICAL PREDICTION OF DRIVING RISK

Michon (1979) has provided a useful model for conceptualizing driving skill. This model is hierarchically organized and involves three levels of decision-making: (1) strategic, (2) tactical, and (3) operational. Strategic decisions involve considerable planning (e.g., the decision not to drive during inclement weather) and are made without time pressure. Tactical decisions are made while actually driving and involve moderate time pressure (e.g., the decision to change lanes and pass a slow-moving vehicle). Operational decisions include those involved with the moment-to-moment operation of the car and are made under high time pressure (e.g., braking instantly when a child runs in front of the car).

Brain damage can affect decision making at any of these three levels. The patient with an isolated frontal lobe lesion, for example, may have impaired executive functions and will probably experience considerable difficulty at the strategic level (e.g., planning trips, appreciating the importance of avoiding rush hour traffic). The patient with an early dementia may suffer impaired judgment which will affect decisions at all levels but especially at the tactical level (e.g., inappropriate risk taking). The patient with a left visual field defect and hemineglect will have to cope with problems at the operational level (such as drifting to the left while driving or failing to adequately scan the visual world on the left side).

Many writers have suggested that neuropsychological tests should be helpful in predicting what patients are at risk for the resumption of driving after a neurological insult. For example, Chelune and Moehle (1986) describe driving as a task requiring judgment and flexibility, attention, nonverbal memory, constructional skills, and right–left discrimination. They speculate that these skills should be most accurately assessed by tests such as the Category Test, Trail-Making Tests, Speech Sounds and Rhythm tests, Figure Memory, WAIS Block Design, the drawing of crosses from the Aphasia Screening Exam, and assessment of the visual fields. However, there has been surprisingly little empirical support for the utility of neuropsychological tests in predicting driving risk. For example, van Zomeren, Brouwer, Rothengatter, and Snoek (1988) found that conventional neuropsychological tests (e.g., the Benton Visual Retention Test, WAIS Picture Completion and Picture Arrangement subtests, Trails A and B, the Stroop, visual choice reaction times, and finger tapping) were not effective in predicting driving performance. Sivak *et al.* (1981) had obtained modest predictive power with a brain-damaged sample using the Picture Completion and Picture Arrangement subtests but these results were not replicated by van Zomeren and his colleagues. These difficulties may in part result from the failure of specific tests to sample adequately the three domains of decision making described in the Michon (1979) model: Most neuropsychological tests are designed to assess behavior at the operational level. However, ability patterns are only a part—and perhaps a small part—of the variance in driving.

Hopewell and van Zomeren (1990) have argued that there are five major factors that account for most of the variance in driving ability. Listed in descending order of importance, they are:

1. Previous driving and accident/violation history, adjusted for exposure
2. General personality and attitudinal factors
3. Pattern and severity of alcohol/substance abuse
4. Nature and extent of psychiatric disturbance
5. Basic psychomotor abilities (assuming no disqualifying conditions such as blindness exist)

Note that behavioral history is the most salient predictor, while most neuropsychological tests assess abilities only at the 5th level. This may account for the poor ability of neuropsychological tests in predicting driving ability after brain injury. In contrast, the salience and importance of personality variables and emotional factors in predicting accidents is underscored by the work of Selzer, Rogers, and Kern (1968) who documented that 20% of individuals involved in fatal accidents had experienced emotional upheaval during the six-hour period immediately preceding their accident.

Not all studies have produced results suggesting that neuropsychological tests are poor predictors of driving. For example, Gouvier, Maxfield, Schweitzer, Horton, Shipp, Neilson, and Hale (1989) found psychometric measures to be helpful in predicting driving performance in disabled individuals. The greatest predictive accuracy resulted from use of the oral version of the Symbol Digit Modalities Test, which singly accounted for about 70% of the variance in a composite global driving score. Adding a second variable into a multiple regression formula increased predictive accuracy to almost 80%. However, these impressive results need to be replicated and the derived formulas need to be cross-validated on different samples before one can be truly confident about the utility of the Symbol Digit Modalities Test used in this context.

Gouvier and his colleagues (e.g., Gouvier, Schweitzer, Horton, Maxfield, Shipp, Seaman, & Hale, 1988; Hale, Schweitzer, Shipp, & Gouvier, 1987) have also experimented with the use of Small Scale Vehicles (SSVs) as adjuncts to the assessment of brain-impaired patients who are considering returning to driving. These vehicles are modified electric golf carts: patients find them "user friendly" and nonthreatening, they have excellent visibility, and they simulate the experience of driving in a meaningful way with minimal cost. Kewman, Siegerman, Kintner, Chu, Henson, and Reeder (1985) reported positive results with a similar program. The Louisiana group has incorporated the SSV into "Mobile Assessment Laboratories" which provide systematic assessment of driving ability for those clients in a four-state region who are unable to arrange transportation to Louisiana Tech University.

## TREATMENT ISSUES

Patients with right hemisphere lesions tend to have more difficulties with driving than patients with equivalent lesions in the left hemisphere (Bardach, 1971; Quigley & DeLisa, 1983). This may result from the importance of the right hemisphere in assessing visuospatial information and the far greater likelihood for hemiinattention or neglect found with lesions in the right parietal region. Approximately 40% of all patients with right hemisphere damage will experience left-sided inattention or neglect (Diller & Weinberg, 1977). However, patients who are aphasic as a result of left hemisphere injuries often have significant neuropsychological deficits besides their very salient problems with language and cannot safely be assumed to be fit to drive.

Although there has been little work in the area to date, a provocative body of literature is beginning to emerge suggesting that it is possible to teach patients to compensate for acquired visuoperceptual and hemiattentional disorders. This literature was reviewed by Gouvier, Webster, and Warner (1986); it has obvious implications for rehabilitation psychology. Patients with left-sided hemianopsias can be taught to "anchor left" and can become quite proficient at driving, although they must resign themselves to the need for virtually constant head motion as they continually scan the rearview mirror and the two side mirrors on their car.

A number of training centers in the United States are available to help assess and train disabled drivers and most of these centers are equipped to serve the brain impaired client. The staff of these centers are enthusiastic about the potential for retraining driving skills but they are also realistic about risks and sensitive to safety issues. A list of training centers is available from the National Head Injury Foundation.* An annotated bibliography on driving is available from the National Rehabilitation Information Center.†

## SUMMARY

Most patients with physical handicaps and about half of the patients who experience cognitive impairment secondary to brain insults will return to driving (Hopewell & Price, 1985; Quigley & DeLisa, 1983; Shore, Gurgold, & Robbins, 1980). Neuropsychologists should be able to help those patients with cognitive deficits—and the rehabilitation professionals who work with them—to determine the relative risk of driving after an injury. However, despite the enormous significance of this problem and the frequency with which the question is posed to neuropsychologists, we have done little research in this area and many of the findings in the field are inconsistent. However, there appears to be growing interest in this very pragmatic issue and the coming decade may well provide realistic assessment tools, workable conceptual models, and meaningful treatment programs for patients wondering if the time has come to return to driving.

## REFERENCES

Bardach, J. L. (1971). Psychological factors in the handicapped driver. *Archives of Physical Medicine & Rehabilitation, 52,* 328–332.

Chelune, G. J., & Moehle, K. A. (1986). Neuropsychological assessment and everyday functioning. In D. Wedding, A. M. Horton, & J. Webster (Eds.), *The neuropsychology handbook: Behavioral and clinical perspectives* (pp. 489–525). New York: Springer.

Diller, L., & Weinberg, J. (1977). Hemiinattention in rehabilitation: The evolution of a rational rehabilitation program. In E. Weinstein & R. Friedland (Eds.), *Advances in neurology* (Vol. 18, pp. 63–82). New York: Raven Press.

Garcia, J. L. (1986). Driving and aging. *Clinics in Geriatric Medicine, 2,* 577–589.

*National Head Injury Foundation, 333 Turnpike Road, Southborough, MA 01772.
†National Rehabilitation Information Center, 8455 Coleville Road, Suite 935, Silver Spring, MD 20910.

Gouvier, W. D., Webster, J. S., & Warner, M. S. (1986). Treatment of acquired visuoperceptual and hemiattentional disorders. *Annals of Behavioral Medicine*, *8*, 1–20.

Gouvier, W. D., Schweitzer, J. R., Horton, C., Maxfield, M., Shipp, M., Seaman, R. L., & Hale, P. N. (1988). A systems approach to assessing driving skills among TBI and other severely disabled individuals. *Rehabilitation Education*, *2*, 197–204.

Gouvier, W. D., Maxfield, M. W., Schweitzer, J. R., Horton, C. R., Shipp, M., Neilson, K., & Hale, P. (1989). Psychometric prediction of driving performance among the disabled. *Archives of Physical Medicine & Rehabilitation*, *70*, 745–750.

Hale, P. N., Schweitzer, J. R., Shipp, M., & Gouvier, W. D. (1987). *Archives of Physical Medicine & Rehabilitation*, *68*, 741–742.

Hopewell, C. A., & Price, R. J. (1985). Driving after head injury. *Journal of Clinical & Experimental Neuropsychology*, *7*, 148.

Hopewell, C. A., & van Zomeren, A. H. (1990). Neuropsychological aspects of motor vehicle operation. In D. E. Tupper & K. D. Cicerone (Eds.), *The neuropsychology of everyday life*. New York: Kluwer.

Kewman, D., Siergerman, C., Kinter, H., Chu, S., Henson, D., & Reeder, C. (1985). Simulation training of psychomotor skills: Teaching the brain-injured to drive. *Rehabilitation Psychology*, *30*, 11–27.

Liddell, F. D. K. (1982). Motor vehicle accidents (1973–1976) in a cohort of Montreal drivers. *Journal of Epidemiology & Community Health*, *36*, 140–145.

Michon, J. A. (1979). Dealing with danger. *Summary report of a workshop in the Traffic Research Center,* State University, Groningen, The Netherlands.

National Head Injury Foundation, Inc. (1987). *Nationwide disabled drivers training centers and transportation services.*

National Rehabilitation Information Center. (1987). *Driving: An annotated bibliography.*

Quigley, F. L., & DeLisa, J. A. (1983). Assessing driving potential of cerebral vascular accident patients. *American Journal of Occupational Therapy*, *37*, 474–478.

Reuben, D. B., Silliman, R. A., & Traines, M. (1988). The aging driver: Medicine, policy, and ethics. *Journal of the American Geriatrics Society*, *36*, 1135–1142.

Rimel, R. W., Giodani, B., Barth, J. T., Boll, T. J., & Jane, J. A. (1981). Disability caused by minor head injury. *Neurosurgery*, *9*, 221–228.

Selzer, M. L., Rogers, J. E., & Kern, S. (1968). Fatal accidents: The role of psychopathology, social stress, and acute disturbance. *American Journal of Psychiatry*, *124*, 46–54.

Shore, D., Gurgold, G., & Robbins, S. (1980). Handicapped driving: An overview of assessment and training. *Archives of Physical Medicine & Training*, *61*, 481–486.

Sivak, M., Olson, P. L., Kewman, D. G., Won, H., & Henson, D. L. (1981). Driving and perceptual/cognitive skills: Behavioral consequences of brain damage. *Archives of Physical Medicine & Rehabilitation*, *62*, 476–483.

Skegg, D. C. G., Richards, S. M., & Doll, R. (1979). Minor tranquilizers and road accidents. *British Medical Journal*, *281*, 1309–1312.

van Zomeren, A. H., Brouwer, W. H., & Minderhoud, J. M. (1987). Acquired brain damage and driving: A review. *Archives of Physical Medicine & Rehabilitation*, *68*, 697–705.

van Zomeren, A. H., Brouwer, W. H., Rothengatter, J. A., & Snoek, J. W. (1988). Fitness to drive a car after recovery from severe head injury. *Archives of Physical Medicine and Rehabilitation*, *69*, 90–96.

Wallace, J. E., & Crancer, A. (1971). Licensing exams and their relation to subsequent driving record. *Behavioral Research in Highway Safety*, *2*, 53–65.

Wilson, T., & Smith, T. (1983). Driving after stroke. *International Rehabilitation Medicine*, *5*, 170–177.

# 24

# Forensic Issues in Head Trauma

## Neuropsychological Perspectives of Social Security Disability and Worker's Compensation

### ANTONIO E. PUENTE

Specific concerns have arisen over the past few years in the application of the rapidly developing field of clinical neuropsychology to the legal setting. Due to the intrinsic nature of head trauma, a significant and increasing number of these types of cases eventually have legal implications.

### GENERAL APPROACH TO FORENSIC CASES

Regardless of whether the case involves Social Security or worker's compensation, a general approach is advisable. Throughout this chapter, several themes will be emphasized. All are provided as a means to decrease ambiguity and provide the courts with the best possible neuropsychological data so a proper administrative and/or legal decision may be reached:

1. Understand the referral and the questions that are to be answered.
2. Understand the rules, regulations, and laws of the type of case involved (e.g., Social Security).
3. Rely on objective information.

ANTONIO E. PUENTE • Department of Psychology, University of North Carolina at Wilmington, Wilmington, North Carolina 28403-3297.

*HANDBOOK OF HEAD TRAUMA: Acute Care to Recovery*, edited by Charles J. Long and Leslie K. Ross. Plenum Press, New York, 1992.

4. Avoid inferences, always provide conclusions that closely parallel the data.
5. Be as comprehensive as feasible.
6. Scrutinize your evaluation, otherwise another professional will do so (much to your dismay).
7. Do not take adversarial positions.
8. Neuropsychological data are not absolute.
9. Clarify confounds, focus on premorbid function.
10. Remain ethical, as the courtroom with its high pay and excitement can lead one astray from correct professionalism.

## THE IMPORTANCE OF OBJECTIVE DATA

The issue of measurable deficits is critical in a neuropsychological evaluation due to difficulties in assessing the validity of "psychological" symptoms and, in turn, of subjective symptoms such as those noted with postconcussive syndrome. However, the question of validity according to Larson (1970) is associated with the issue of malingering. Specifically, "the issue comes down to the presence of responsible conscious volition on the part of the patient to invent, protract, misinterpret, or exaggerate his complaint." Considering the subjectivity of most head injury symptoms, it should come as no surprise to note that malingering is perceived to be such a critical issue. As much as feasible, neuropsychological symptoms should be differentiated from faking.

Objective data are based on scientifically derived knowledge. A neuropsychologist must obviously know the appropriate literature both on head injury and on vocational issues. For example, the information contained in this book by Mapou, Long and Schmitter, and McCue is indispensable to those dealing with forensic issues in head injury. In addition, knowledge about how to apply such data to the courtroom is also critical (e.g., Taylor & Elliott, 1989; Gilandas & Touyz, 1983).

## QUESTIONING THE VALIDITY OF
## FORENSIC NEUROPSYCHOLOGICAL INFORMATION

There is little question that a considerable amount of money as well as personal outcomes hinge on the outcome of head injury cases. Thus, the importance and validity of neuropsychological testimony assume a critical role often more so than medical testimony because of the functional aspects of neuropsychological data.

However, acceptance of neuropsychological data has not been automatic, even from the perspective of other psychologists. Recently, Faust and colleagues (e.g., Faust, Guilmette, Hart, Arkes, Fishburne, & Davey, 1988) published a study examining the judgment accuracy of clinical neuropsychologists. Results indicated that "virtually no systematic relations were obtained among a series of training and experience variables and accuracy across a series of diagnostic judgments" (p. 159). The authors further state that it is acceptable to conclude that "about one in three normal individuals are misdiagnosed as abnormal" (p. 160). The conclusion questions the usefulness of neuropsychological judgment by "experts."

In a more recent review of the literature, Wedding and Faust (1989) addressed the question of clinical judgment and statistical factorial prediction in clinical neuropsychology. They conclude that clinical neuropsychological judgment is open to serious question due to judgment errors. The authors indicate that one or more of the following issues may contribute to judgmental errors: hindsight bias, confirmatory bias, overreliance on salient data, underutilization of base rates, and failure to analyze covariation.

Overall, these studies reflect the "mood" of the courtroom. Specifically, the validity of neuropsychological data is open to question. The question of validity may be phrased less eloquently in the courtroom. Indeed, the question is simply posed of how a non-physician can testify about issues involving the physical status of the body. After all, understanding physical dysfunction is not in the domain of training for psychologists. Of course, Faust has rephrased the question of validity in a more scholarly manner. But the question of validity remains critically unanswered and poses serious threat to the admissibility of neuropsychological data for the legal system.

## AVOIDING INHERENT DIFFICULTIES OF FORENSIC CASES

While not providing specific suggestions as to how to combine these two extremes, Wedding and Faust (1989) do suggest that certain corrective procedures should be taken into account to avoid problems in the courtroom. The authors suggest the following: know the literature on human judgment, do not depend on insight alone, avoid premature abandonment of useful decision rules, regress extreme estimates, limit focus on the esoteric, avoid overreliance on highly intercorrelated measures, start with most valid information, consider alternative hypotheses, consider disconfirmatory information, think Bajesian, collect appropriate norms, and obtain feedback.

An alternative to these specific recommendations is to consider the data presented by the clinical neuropsychologist as open to question. Not only will the data be scrutinized but it will be done in such a manner as to place the burden of proof not on the court, or on the attorney, but on the neuropsychologist. A common error, besides the ones outlined by Faust and Wedding, is to equate clinical and forensic cases in terms of procedures and outcomes. Realizing that the evaluation will be attacked, the neuropsychologist's approach should be to anticipate every possible question and concern by completing the best possible evaluation feasible. Even if such an approach is used, possible complications could arise. If they do, consider them as constructive criticism to be incorporated in future professional activity. In short, the forensic evaluation is similar to submission of a manuscript for editorial review. Close scrutiny by colleagues and other professionals will occur before the data are accepted as useful.

## GENERAL ASSESSMENT ISSUES

More preparation and effort are typically involved for the forensic evaluation than in standard clinical evaluation. Moreover, head injury cases have specific issues that distinguish them from other forensic cases. Thus, care must be taken to be aware of both psychological and neuropsychological issues and how they interact.

## Referral

Clients may be referred from one or more sources. Theoretically supporting the position of the client, an evaluation may be requested by an attorney or legal representative of the client. The referral question is typically associated with the question of deficits. In contrast, referrals from insurance companies or their representatives, often rehabilitation nurses or agencies, focus on strengths. An interest in potential confounding factors is rarely encouraged by this type of referral. While these referrals may be initiated by the primary treating or consultative physician, they are generated by the insurance carrier because of question of the validity of the patient's behavior. The physician or other health care professional who is generally interested in the welfare of the client tends to be a less adversarial referral.

Regardless of the referral source, the task of the clinical neuropsychologist should always remain the same. Specifically, the role should be to provide as accurate, scientific data about the patient's neurobehavioral function as allowable within the constraints of the knowledge available at the time of the evaluation. To participate in an adversarial role not only negatively affects the welfare of the client but the discipline as well. Adversarial positions are unethical.

Another issue is that of available information. It is not unusual for an evaluation to be accompanied by little or no prior data. Since neuropsychologists rarely are the first health professional to evaluate a client, prior records are usually available from other sources and should be obtained. These records are critical to the full appreciation of the complexity of the client's functioning. Of particular importance are work histories and related premorbid data. This information can often be obtained from job descriptions, annual evaluations, and co-worker interviews. School transcripts are also a wealth of information. Additional data can be obtained from the armed services as well as school or university records. Grades and standardized scores serve as an excellent picture of premorbid functioning.

A final issue involves third parties. These could include defense attorneys, insurance companies, and other health care professionals. Again, these relationships should be clarified from the beginning. Clear channels of communication, with emphasis on written communication, are essential to avoid conflicts and misunderstanding. Additionally, specific roles for all parties must be clarified. To obtain objectivity, neuropsychologists should consider themselves as consultants in these cases delegating primary care (including psychological) duties to other health care professionals. If therapy is required, another psychologist (not involved with the case) should assume this duty.

## Professional Issues

Most referral sources, and almost all patients, have a misunderstanding of many of the aspects of a neuropsychological evaluation. These include discussing the case with referral sources, obtaining and reviewing premorbid records, testing and scoring time, dictation, discussion with attorneys and referral sources, depositions, affidavits, and/or court appearances. All of these issues must be understood by the neuropsychologist and should be clarified to all parties involved in the evaluation.

A critical issue is that of reimbursement. Forensic cases can have a significant impact on the financial status of both the individual and the employer so much so that this financial concern carries over into the evaluation process. In order to minimize this potential ethical complication, it is advisable to provide initial cost estimates with potential reasons for later changes. Related to reimbursement is the mode of payment. To ensure the likelihood of minimal complications, a contract similar to that noted in Figure 24.1 may be useful. It is of the utmost importance for all concerned that the cost as well as the method of payment and/ or reimbursement be clearly stated and potential conflicts resolved prior to initiating the evaluation. A contract (Figure 24.1) may also be secured before initiation of the evaluation.

## Evaluation

Educating the patient is an often ignored preliminary step in any evaluation, especially in a head injury case where malingering as well as lack of knowledge makes the gathering of useful data a difficult task. Thus, the patient and possibly the family should be provided with a brief introduction to the field of clinical neuropsychology. Specific emphasis should be placed on the evaluation questions and procedures as well as their relationship to the legal questions.

Record keeping should be considered prior to initiating the evaluation. Records can be subpoenaed by the courts, especially if taken to the stand during testimony. While some forensic experts suggest that records should not be reviewed by others, the possibility does exist for all of the records to be reviewed. Thus, careful record keeping is required. While many neuropsychologists consider the use of a technician acceptable (e.g., Seretny, Dean, Gray, & Hartlage, 1986), it is important to record and qualify who performed each portion of the evaluation since this will be questioned during testimony.

By far the greatest error in forensic cases is the tendency to make incorrect inferences based on the obtained information. The legal system encourages the simplification of matters but simplification poses problems of ethics and clinical validity. It is preferable to report data and arrive at tentative conclusions than face the wrath of a knowledgeable attorney, or worse, a competent neuropsychologist (hired by the opposing counsel) to review and critique your report.

---

I hereby authorize Antonio E. Puente, Ph.D. to release to my attorney(s) _____ any and all information which he may request concerning examination of and treatment given to _____ in connection with injuries sustained as a result of an occurrence on or about the _____ day of _____, 19____ .

I also further authorize and direct my attorney(s) to pay Antonio E. Puente, Ph.D., to satisfy his total bill for all professional and testimonial services rendered to me.

I also understand that if favorable legal settlement does not occur, I remain personally liable for payment of the total bill for professional and testimonial services rendered to me by Antonio E. Puente, Ph.D.

Signature _____ Date _____

Accepted and Agreed by _____ , Attorney

---

FIGURE 24.1. Authorization for release of medical information and for payment of medical expenses.

### Court-Related Issues

The key to court appearance is preparation. The first person to prepare for a court or court-related appearance (e.g., deposition) is the neuropsychologist. Careful analyses of histories, clinical, and psychometric data and their presentation precede another review of the inferences and conclusions. Behavioral rehearsal of potential questions from the attorney should help in clarifying rather than confusing the issues. The client should also not be overlooked. They should be advised of potential procedures and complications.

Some attorneys prefer a signed written statement rather than a court appearance in an effort to clarify questions about the evaluations. Legal representatives may prefer to draft the statement or affidavit themselves. If so, caution should be taken not to oversimplify complex issues.

A deposition is a comprehensive interview conducted by both sets of attorneys in the presence of a court reporter. This may be preliminary to later testimony. As with any form of data presentation, extreme care should be taken not to incorrectly present the issues or the intended inferences or conclusions.

While some neuropsychologists prefer not to appear in court, the likelihood of such an appearance in a head injury case is relatively high. This is especially true in mild head injuries where individuals may have no detectable neurological or neuroradiological deficits. When the opportunity for presenting neuropsychological data arises, the neuropsychologist's task is to educate the court, whether it be a judge, a commissioner, or a jury.

The educational process is fourfold. First, educate regarding your qualifications, especially as they pertain to work-related injuries as well as to neuropsychological disorders. Second, provide information about the field of clinical neuropsychology. It is imperative that both strengths and limitations of neuropsychological data be addressed. Anatomical issues should be avoided while behavioral or functional variables should be emphasized. Next, a thorough understanding of the accident, client, and the residuals should be considered. Treatment and rehabilitative potential and approaches should also be presented.

## SOCIAL SECURITY DISABILITY

Social Security Disability serves as an excellent introduction to forensic neuropsychology for several reasons. First, specific guidelines and test procedures are published, thus providing specific direction for assessments. In addition, this type of case is not seen as adversarial. Finally, the emotional and financial risks are not as intense as personal injury or worker's compensation. Mastery of Social Security Disability cases should serve as a strong foundation for other forensic cases.

### Referral

There are two primary, albeit opposing, sources of referral. The Social Security Administration (SSA) may request a consultative psychological examination. This can occur only if the psychologist's credentials have been approved by the SSA and he or she is listed as a service provider for the state office of the SSA. Alternatively, attorneys or legal representatives of a claimant may request neuropsychological services. As a rule, if the SSA requests the evaluation, few records are furnished and a standard intellectual examination is all that is required. Most of these requests occur early in the disability application process. In contrast, attorneys often request neuropsychological consultation after initial rejection for disability has occurred. Most often these referrals require more comprehensive tests and comprehensive records are usually available. Regardless, one of the most difficult cases for SSA evaluation is closed head injury where the postconcussive syndrome or mild head injury cases are considered as faking or malingering.

## Evaluation

The evaluation for SSA cases is dictated by two major issues. First, specific guidelines or listings for impairment have been published and must be met for an individual to be considered disabled. Second, specific tests have been approved by the SSA for meeting these guidelines.

To meet a listing, an applicant must: (1) directly meet or fit a listing, (2) have a combination of impairments, (3) have limited medical improvements related to employment, or (4) not be able to perform a previous or related work.

There are nine separate listings for categorizing mental impairments (Social Security Administration, 1986). These are organic mental disorders, schizophrenia, paranoid or other psychotic disorders, affective disorders, mental retardation and autism, anxiety-related disorders, somatoform disorders, personality, and substance addiction disorders. The most applicable of these for neuropsychologists is the organic mental disorders listing. Table 24.1 provides the definition or listing of organic mental disorder encompassing two separate categories, termed Parts A and B. Part A contains many of the basic symptoms of "organicity" (e.g., memory impairment), while Part B, Activities of Daily Living (ADL), addresses the effects of these symptoms on functional abilities. Both Parts A and B must be met in order to qualify under a listing.

Tests and testing procedures are outlined for the evaluation of mental impairments. In their "Final Report" of August 1985, SSA stated, "Broad-based neuropsychological assessments using for example, the Halstead–Reitan or the Luria–Nebraska batteries may be useful in determining brain function deficiencies, particularly in cases involving subtle findings such as may be seen in traumatic brain injuries" (pp. 36–57). These supplement the WAIS, MMPI, Rorschach, and TAT. However, on May 29, 1986, SSA revised the original list of acceptable psychological tests to include the following 11 tests: Boston Diagnostic Aphasia Examination, McCarthy Scale of Children's Abilities, the Stanford–Binet Intelligence Scale (3rd ed.), Wechsler Intelligence Scale for Children-Revised, Wechsler Adult Intelligence Scale-Revised, the Peabody Picture Vocabulary Test-Revised, the Luria–Nebraska Neuropsychological Battery, the Millon Behavioral Health Inventory and Adolescent Personality Survey as well as the Clinical Multiaxial Inventory, and the Kaufman Assessment Battery for Children. According to the SSA, the Luria–Nebraska is "a better technique because it provides a low cost, portable, relatively brief alternative to the Halstead–Reitan Neuropsychological Battery" (pp. 19417).

Table 24.2 provides specific suggestions as to how the North Carolina Disability

TABLE 24.1.   Organic Mental Disorders Listings[a]

**Organic Mental Disorders:** Psychological or behavioral abnormalities associated with a dysfunction of the brain. History and physical examination or laboratory tests demonstrate the presence of a specific organic factor judged to be etiologically related to the abnormal mental state and loss of previously acquired functional abilities.

The required level of severity for these disorders is met when the requirements in both A and B are satisfied

**A. Demonstration of loss of specific cognitive abilities or affective changes and the medically documented persistence of at least one of the following:**

  1. Disorientation to time and place; or
  2. Memory impairment, either short-term (inability to learn new information), intermediate, or long-term (inability to remember information that was known sometime in the past); or
  3. Perceptual or thinking disturbances (e.g., hallucinations, delusions); or
  4. Change in personality; or
  5. Disturbance in mood; or
  6. Emotional lability (e.g., explosive temper outburst, sudden crying, etc.) and impairment in impulse control; or
  7. Loss of measured intellectual ability of at least 15 IQ points from premorbid levels or overall impairment index clearly within the severely impaired range on neuropsychological testing (e.g., the Luria–Nebraska, Halstead–Reitan, etc.); AND

**B. Resulting in at least two of the following:**

  1. Marked restriction of activities of daily living, or
  2. Marked difficulties in maintaining social functioning, or
  3. Deficiencies of concentration, persistence or pace resulting in frequent failure to complete tasks in a timely manner (in work settings or elsewhere); or
  4. Repeated episodes of deterioration or decompensation on work or worklike settings which cause the individual to withdraw from this situation or to experience exacerbation of signs and symptoms (which may include deterioration of adaptive behaviors).

[a]From *Disability evaluation under Social Security: A handbook for physicians.* Social Security Administration, 1986. Washington, DC: Author.

Determination Section suggests a report be written. The style may not be as much of an issue as the content. Since psychologists may be reviewing these reports, careful presentation of psychometric data is important. More critical, however, is the issue of addressing activities of daily living, especially Part B of the listing. Findings from the evaluation must be equated to functional residual capacity. Not to address ADL will jeopardize the potential impact of the neuropsychological assessment. A final issue with regards to the report involves whether to state if a claimant has met a listing. Unless requested by the referral sources, this type of analysis may be best left to the court.

## Court-Related Issues

Social Security cases rarely involve court testimony. Typically the report is sufficient. If questions arise they will usually be from the claimant's legal representative and, usually, an affidavit or deposition may answer any questions present. If a court appearance is required, the process is administrative rather than adjudicative. An administrative law judge (ALJ) acts more as a fact finder than an arbitrator and the purpose of an appearance by the neuropsychologist would be to provide clarification of report data, to present new information, or possibly to interview the client for the ALJ. There are no juries and the courtroom usually contains an ALJ, the legal representative, and a court reporter.

TABLE 24.2.   North Carolina Disability Determination Services:
Specific Reporting Requirements of Psychological Assessments

**A. History**
1. Source and estimate of reliability.
2. Description of complaints including when they prevented work if appropriate.
3. Family, social environmental and occupational history.
4. Past medical history (hospitalizations, therapy, drugs and dosage, etc.).

**B. Clinical Interview**
We need enough descriptive detail from your clinical interview on the following items to allow us to independently confirm your conclusions.
1. Description of appearance to include physical, dress, grooming, posture, attitude and behavior. Note how the patient came to the examination (alone or accompanied, distance and mode of travel).
2. Detailed description of daily activities (a typical day). Note if applicant is dependent on others and in what areas he/she requires assistance.
3. Note ability to follow simple directions.
4. Cooperation with examiner—note ability to understand the spoken word.
5. Emotional reaction: depressed, elated, anxious, angry, suspicious, friendly, fearful, flat, blunted, inappropriate or appropriate, etc. Include faces, posture, involuntary movements, tears or other observations which lead to your conclusions.
6. Describe speech as to relevancy, coherence, pressure, retardation, neologisms, etc.
7. Describe ability to read, write and perform simple calculations.
8. Judgment: Ability or inability to avoid physical danger such as cars, fire, etc.

**C. Test Results and Protocols**
1. Standardized intelligence *test results*: Report Performance and Verbal subtest scores in addition to the Full Scale I.Q. score on the Wechsler Intelligence scales (WAIS, WISC, WISC-R, and WPPSI). Both the verbal and performance measures are necessary in conjunction with the Wechsler scales.
2. In instances where administration of certain subtests or subscales may not be feasible because of the applicant's condition or circumstances, an explanation for this limitation is required.

**D. Summary**
1. The claimant's problems should be integrated into the test results and the effect on his ability to carry out work-related activities such as:
   a. Understand, retain and follow instructions.
   b. Sustain attention to perform simple repetitive tasks.
   c. Ability to relate to others including fellow workers and supervisor.
   d. Tolerate the stress and pressures associated with day to day work activity.
2. Statement of capability to manage funds is necessary.
3. Comment on any physical or mental impairment that may have affected I.Q. scores and estimate the extent the scores were changed if possible.

We do not require a statement as to whether the patient is or is not disabled because the determination of disability is an administrative decision which also involves consideration of age, education and vocational history.

This report must be reviewed and signed by the psychologist who actually performed the examination.

## WORKER'S COMPENSATION

If a worker is completely disabled, he or she may qualify to receive Social Security benefits. If the worker is injured on the job (whether completely or partially disabled), then he or she is eligible for worker's compensation benefits. Unlike Social Security, worker's compensation may provide support relative to the amount of functional residual or dysfunction. Thus, one may receive a percentage rating reflecting cumulative impairment. Due to the increased financial implications, such cases are more aggressively challenged by both insurance carriers and attorneys which results in greater burden on the neuropsychologist to provide exhaustive, accurate, and relevant information.

## Referral

As with Social Security, referrals may be generated from the two opposing sides. An insurance carrier may request the evaluation, often through a rehabilitation agency or nurse. The focus, as indicated earlier in this chapter, will be on strengths as well as on malingering. In contrast, attorneys (often retained after an undesirable settlement offer) are more interested in deficits. Another potential referral is the treating physician. Whether the physician realizes the potential for a work-related head injury case to result in legal issues or otherwise, the original consult may be perceived as a standard clinical referral. In many respects, physician referrals represent less adversarial, possibly even more balanced, approaches to the head injury symptoms. Another issue of importance and potential complication is that of reimbursement, especially if the worker is not involved with an insurance program. It may be useful to obtain clearance from appropriate reimbursement agencies or insurance carriers in order to avoid this problem.

## Evaluation

Prior to any comprehensive evaluation, thorough premorbid data must be obtained. Specific records should be obtained from schools, trade or vocational training centers, and/ or universities in order to formulate potential premorbid intellectual abilities. Special emphases should be placed on standardized tests and their potential equivalence to the current evaluation. Of greater concern in compensation cases is vocational history. Comprehensive histories with job descriptions and annual evaluations are a must. In addition, interviews with supervisors or co-workers may be of value. Of related importance is the concern for premorbid family and social function which may be accomplished with interviews of family and friends.

As with any evaluation, the initial step should be to complete a comprehensive clinical interview. Additionally, serial evaluations may help in addressing issues of validity. Similarities should be developed and discrepancies should be noted. Effort should be made to develop a comprehensive clinical understanding of the patient.

Industrial commissions do not have a preference (as do the Social Administration) for specific tests, or for flexible or standardized batteries. The worker's ability to return to work is in question and should direct fact-finding. Tailoring the evaluation both to the complaints or the residual effects of the alleged trauma as well as to the work tasks described in the job description will help clarify the necessary vocational question. Related work potential may be similarly considered by using appropriate tests. While this approach implies the merits of a flexible or nonstandardized approach, Industrial Commissioners and Boards appear to prefer known batteries and norm-referenced tests and results.

Care should be taken with the use of a technician. While considered acceptable and common neuropsychological practice, attorneys will question the credibility of test results not directly obtained by the neuropsychologist. Related confounding variables including fatigue, time and day(s) of testing, and medications, take on a more important role in determining the residual neuropsychological capacity of the worker than in many cases.

By far, the greatest error in worker's compensation cases is the tendency to make incorrect inferences. While this approach is often encouraged by the legal system in order to simplify matters, it poses grave clear problems of ethical and clinical validity. It is preferable to report data and limit the conclusions.

Another issue is that of incongruent findings. These may include findings of prior neuropsychological evaluation and medical examinations or tests. Incongruent findings need to be considered and addressed rather than ignored or belittled. Further effort and analysis should reveal potential correlations between data sets.

A report for worker's compensation should differ from a standard clinical report. Beyond the usual, special emphasis should be placed on premorbid functioning and work tasks. Additionally, emphasis should be placed on both residual symptoms as well as abilities, especially as they pertain to work-related activities. If feasible, directly address the potential limitations of performing the previous employment as well as the likelihood of vocational rehabilitation. As a consequence of the additional and detailed information, such reports may be considerably longer than standard reports.

A major aspect of the report, indeed that segment that clearly differentiates this report from other neuropsychological reports, is a rating. This is a percentage of impairment based on published guidelines by the American Medical Association (1984, 1989). As can be seen from Table 24.3, there are several variables that must be taken into account such as intellectual ability. Each variable is assigned a rating from 1 to 5. Then a composite rating is

TABLE 24.3.  American Medical Association Guidelines
for the Evaluation of Psychiatric Impairment

| Mental status | Class and percentage of impairment | | | | |
|---|---|---|---|---|---|
| | 1<br>0–5% | 2<br>10–20% | 3<br>25–50% | 4<br>55–75% | 5<br>Over 75% |
| Intelligence | Normal or better | Mildly retarded | Moderately mildly | Moderately severely | Severely retarded |
| Thinking | No deficit | Slight deficit | Moderate deficit | Moderately severe deficit | Severe deficit |
| Perception | No deficit | Slight deficit | Moderate deficit | Moderately severe deficit | Severe deficit |
| Judgment | No deficit | Slight deficit | Moderate deficit | Moderately severe deficit | Severe deficit |
| Affect | Normal | Slight problem | Moderate problem | Moderately severe | Severe problem |
| Behavior | Normal | Slight problem | Moderate problem | Moderately severe problem | Severe problem |
| **Activities of daily living** | | | | | |
| Ability | Self-sufficient | Needs minor help | Needs regular help | Needs major help | Quite helpless |
| **Rehabilitation or treatment potential** | | | | | |
| Potential | Excellent | Good | Good for partial restoration | Condition static | Condition will worsen |

From American Medical Association, *Guide to the Evaluation of Medical Impairments* (2nd ed.). Washington, D.C.: Author, 1984.

arrived upon presumably using an average rating of all these variables. In addition, prognosis and rehabilitation potential are taken into account. Note that this rating system is derived from the second edition of the AMA guidelines. The third edition does not provide guidelines for a rating, instead the multiaxial system of the DSM-III-R is presented (AMA, 1989). This poses serious problems for the head injury case since the DSM-III-R system is woefully inadequate with regards to organic brain syndrome.

Several factors are worth noting relative to head injury. First, while it may be seen as more appropriate to use the system provided for neurological disorders, it would be inappropriate since the behavior addressed in head injury cases fits better with the mental impairments category. Next, while some of the variables may superficially "fit" (e.g., perception), they are best suited to address functional disorders. Definitions of these variables should be carefully considered. Third, prognosis and rehabilitation potential (often ignored in compensation cases) have special significance with symptoms associated with head injury. Severity of the accident, age, education and a host of other psychobiological variables (see Puente & McCaffrey, 1992) play a role in the rating provided. For example, a 26-year-old graduate student with a closed head injury being evaluated 3 months posttrauma would have a significantly different prognosis than a 66-year-old migrant worker with little formal education, open skull injury, being evaluated 18 months posttrauma. In other words the rating must be placed in the client's psychosocial and biopsychological context.

## Court-Related Issues

As with every forensic case, preparation is a key factor. Behavioral rehearsal of anticipated questions and situations should help decrease situationally driven emotion while increasing the unbiased presentation of important data.

While affidavits can be used in worker's compensation, depositions are preferred by attorneys. Often these depositions are preliminary, or fact finding, to the actual court appearance. As with the court appearance, it should not be unusual to find one side attempting to present the client premorbidly as a highly functioning worker while the other side suggests that, premorbidly, the worker was marginally functioning.

As with Social Security cases, there are no juries in compensation cases even though the court is a more formal proceeding. The two opposing legal representatives present to a commissioner of the case through the use of witnesses, reports, etc. (similar to a criminal or civil court case). The commissioner reviews the evidence at a later date and renders a decision. This decision may be appealed to the full commission, later to the state Court of Appeals, and if necessary the state Supreme Court. As in all forensic cases, the role of the neuropsychologist is to educate the court about clinical neuropsychology, his or her qualifications, the client, and potential relation of current functional status to premorbid functional status from a neuropsychological perspective.

In some cases it may become difficult, if not impossible, to present neuropsychological data. Probably the best known example of this is the Horne versus Goodson case in the state of North Carolina. In 1980, a 2000-lb log fell from several feet in the air striking Edward Horne in the fronto-parietal area of his cranium. The force drove the man several inches into the ground, broke all of his teeth, and fractured several of his vertebrae. Eventually, a cursory neurosurgical evaluation found him "perfectly well" and encouraged him to return to work (with a verbal prescription of taking BC headache powder, PRN).

With significant vocational, personal, and social behavioral changes present, he was eventually referred to the author for a neuropsychological evaluation. A comprehensive evaluation found him to be impaired and suggested he stop driving logging trucks. The case was heard by a single commissioner and the case was rejected because neuropsychological data were not medical and therefore not admissible or creditable. An appeal to the full commission resulted in the same response. Before submitting the case to the North Carolina Court of Appeals, an amicus brief was submitted on behalf of Mr. Horne by the North Carolina Psychological Association and the American Psychological Association (available from the Office of Professional Practice, APA). Based on the comprehensive amicus outlining the history and usefulness of both clinical neuropsychology and the materials presented for evidence, the Court of Appeals reversed the decision. In October of 1989, the original commissioner "retried" the case and despite taking the original and subsequent evaluations into account, came to the same conclusion. This decision was again appealed and eventually reversed. Case law has been made allowing for the presentation of neuropsychological data in the courtroom. It is important to note that the author avoided localization issues and simplified statements about causation. Behavioral data derived from exhaustive neuropsychological tests were the foundation for the reversal of this case.

## SUMMARY

Head injury cases result in litigation. Since many of the cases involve workers, disability and compensation issues are of critical concern. This chapter presented information as to how neuropsychological data may help those in administrative positions make the best judgment about a client's posttrauma functional residual capacity. In this chapter, general forensic guidelines were initially presented followed by suggestions on how to apply them in Social Security and worker's compensation cases. In all situations several principles emerge. Individuals with head injuries are often perceived as psychiatric cases because of their behavioral presentation. Malingering and faking are often provided as explanations by nontrained health personnel for the unusual behavior of individuals with head injury. Further, to many of those involved with Social Security and worker's compensation, neuropsychology is not well understood.

Thus, the purpose of the neuropsychologist is to educate by providing accurate and useful information about the client's residual capacity from a neuropsychological perspective. Emphasis should be placed on understanding premorbid functioning as well as work-related tasks. Care should be taken not to make unwarranted inferences and sweeping generalizations. Above all, the neuropsychological practitioner should emphasize the scientific context of clinical neuropsychology. To do otherwise will endanger the client's welfare, the validity of neuropsychological evaluation, the career of the neuropsychologist, and the current vitality of the field.

## REFERENCES

American Medical Association (1984). *Guides to the evaluation of medical impairments* (2nd ed.). Washington, DC: Author.

American Medical Association (1989). *Guides to the evaluation of medical impairment* (3rd ed.). Washington, DC: Author.

Department of Health and Human Resources (1985). *Evaluation of mental impairments*. *Federal Register*, August 28, 5, 157, 35038-35070, Part V, Department of Health and Human Services, 20 CFR Part 404.

Faust, D., Guilmette, T. J., Hart, K., Arkes, H. R., Fishburne, F. J., & Davey, L. (1988). Neuropsychologists' training, experience, and judgment accuracy. *Archives of Clinical Neuropsychology*, *3*, 145–163.

Gilandas, A. J., & Touyz, S. W. (1983). Forensic neuropsychology: A selective introduction. *Journal of Forensic Sciences*, *28*, 713–723.

Larson, A. (1970). Mental and nervous injury in workmen's compensation. *Vanderbilt Law Review*, *23*, 1243–1263.

Puente, A. E., & McCaffrey, R. J. (1992). *Psychobiological variables in neuropsychological assessment*. New York: Plenum Press.

Seretny, M. L., Dean, R. S., Gray, J. W., & Hartlage, L. C. (1986). The practice of clinical neuropsychology in the United States. *Archives of Clinical Neuropsychology*, *1*, 5–12.

Social Security Administration (1985). *Operational report of the Office of Hearings and Appeals*. Washington, DC: U.S. Government Printing Office.

Social Security Administration (1986). *Disability evaluation under Social Security: A handbook for physicians*. Washington, DC: U.S. Government Printing Office.

Taylor, J. S., & Elliott, I. (1989). *Appellate court review of neuropsychological evidence*. Columbus, GA: Taylor & Hays.

Wedding, D., & Faust, D. (1989). Clinical judgment and decision making in neuropsychology. *Archives of Clinical Neuropsychology*, *4*, 233–265.

# Index